Cerebrovascular Ultrasound in Stroke Prevention and Treatment

EDITED BY

Andrei V. Alexandrov MD, RVT

Professor and Director
Comprehensive Stroke Center
University of Alabama at Birmingham
Director, Neurovascular Ultrasound Laboratory
University of Alabama Hospital
Birmingham, AL 35249, USA

SECOND EDITION

WILEY-BLACKWELL

A John Wiley & Sons, Ltd., Publication

This edition first published 2011, © 2008, 2011 by Blackwell Publishing Ltd

Blackwell Publishing was acquired by John Wiley & Sons in February 2007. Blackwell's publishing program has been merged with Wiley's global Scientific, Technical and Medical business to form Wiley-Blackwell.

Registered office: John Wiley & Sons Ltd, The Atrium, Southern Gate, Chichester, West Sussex, PO19 8SQ, UK

Editorial offices: 9600 Garsington Road, Oxford, OX4 2DQ, UK
111 River Street, Hoboken, NJ 07030-5774, USA
The Atrium, Southern Gate, Chichester, West Sussex, PO19 8SQ, UK

For details of our global editorial offices, for customer services and for information about how to apply for permission to reuse the copyright material in this book please see our website at www.wiley.com/wiley-blackwell

The right of the author to be identified as the author of this work has been asserted in accordance with the Copyright, Designs and Patents Act 1988.

All rights reserved. No part of this publication may be reproduced, stored in a retrieval system, or transmitted, in any form or by any means, electronic, mechanical, photocopying, recording or otherwise, except as permitted by the UK Copyright, Designs and Patents Act 1988, without the prior permission of the publisher.

Wiley also publishes its books in a variety of electronic formats. Some content that appears in print may not be available in electronic books.

Designations used by companies to distinguish their products are often claimed as trademarks. All brand names and product names used in this book are trade names, service marks, trademarks or registered trademarks of their respective owners. The publisher is not associated with any product or vendor mentioned in this book. This publication is designed to provide accurate and authoritative information in regard to the subject matter covered. It is sold on the understanding that the publisher is not engaged in rendering professional services. If professional advice or other expert assistance is required, the services of a competent professional should be sought.

The contents of this work are intended to further general scientific research, understanding, and discussion only and are not intended and should not be relied upon as recommending or promoting a specific method, diagnosis, or treatment by physicians for any particular patient. The publisher and the author make no representations or warranties with respect to the accuracy or completeness of the contents of this work and specifically disclaim all warranties, including without limitation any implied warranties of fitness for a particular purpose. In view of ongoing research, equipment modifications, changes in governmental regulations, and the constant flow of information relating to the use of medicines, equipment, and devices, the reader is urged to review and evaluate the information provided in the package insert or instructions for each medicine, equipment, or device for, among other things, any changes in the instructions or indication of usage and for added warnings and precautions. Readers should consult with a specialist where appropriate. The fact that an organization or Website is referred to in this work as a citation and/or a potential source of further information does not mean that the author or the publisher endorses the information the organization or Website may provide or recommendations it may make. Further, readers should be aware that Internet Websites listed in this work may have changed or disappeared between when this work was written and when it is read. No warranty may be created or extended by any promotional statements for this work. Neither the publisher nor the author shall be liable for any damages arising herefrom.

Library of Congress Cataloging-in-Publication Data
Cerebrovascular Ultrasound in Stroke Prevention and Treatment
Edited by Andrei V. Alexandrov. – 2nd ed.
   p. ; cm.
  Includes bibliographical references and index.
   ISBN 978-1-4051-9576-8 (hardback)
  1. Cerebrovascular disease–Ultrasonic imaging.   I. Alexandrov, Andrei V.
  [DNLM: 1. Stroke–ultrasonography.   2. Stroke–diagnosis.   3. Stroke–therapy.
WL 355 C41427 2010]
  RC388.5.C4345 2004
  616.8'107543–dc22
                                                                         2010024035

A catalogue record for this book is available from the British Library.

Set in 9/12pt Minion by Aptara Inc., New Delhi, India

1 2011

Contents

List of Contributors, iv

Preface, vi

Foreword, viii

Preface to the First Edition, ix

Foreword to the First Edition, x

Acknowledgment (First Edition), xii

Practice of Ultrasound: an Introduction, xiii

Part I How to Perform Ultrasound Tests, 1

1 Principles of Extracranial Ultrasound Examination, 3
   Andrei V. Alexandrov, Alice Robinson-Vaughn, Clotilde Balucani & Marsha M. Neumyer

2 Intracranial Cerebrovascular Ultrasound Examination Techniques, 13
   Andrei V. Alexandrov, Marta Rubiera, Paola Palazzo & Marsha M. Neumyer

3 Anatomy of the Brain's Arterial Supply, 26
   Joel Cure

Part II Hemodynamic Principles, 45

4 Integrated Assessment of Systemic and Intracranial Hemodynamics, 47
   Anne W. Alexandrov

5 Practical Models of Cerebral Hemodynamics and Waveform Recognition, 68
   Andrei V. Alexandrov

Part III Criteria for Interpretation, 85

6 Diagnostic Criteria for Cerebrovascular Ultrasound, 87
   Georgios Tsivgoulis, Marsha M. Neumyer & Andrei V. Alexandrov

Part IV Ultrasound in Stroke Prevention and Treatment, 145

7 Ultrasound in Stroke Prevention: TCD and Sickle Cell Disease, 147
   Fenwick T. Nichols III, Robert J Adams & Anne M. Jones

8 Cardiovascular Risk Factors and Carotid Ultrasound, 158
   Tatjana Rundek & Joseph F. Polak

9 Applications of Functional Transcranial Doppler (fTCD), 177
   Konstantinos Vadikolias & Georgios Tsivgoulis

10 Transcranial Doppler in the Detection and Quantitation of Patent Foramen Ovale and Other Right-to-Left Circulatory Shunts, 187
   Annabelle Lao, Cindy J. Fuller & Jill T. Jesurum

11 Ultrasound in Neurocritical Care, 198
   Andrew D. Barreto & James C. Grotta

12 Cerebral Vasospasm after Subarachnoid Hemorrhage, 207
   Mark R. Harrigan, David W. Newell & Andrei V. Alexandrov

13 Intra-Operative TCD Monitoring, 214
   Zsolt Garami & Alan B. Lumsden

14 Intracranial Stenosis, 228
   Vijay K. Sharma & K.S. Lawrence Wong

15 Ultrasound in Acute Stroke: Diagnosis, Reversed Robin Hood Syndrome and Sonothrombolysis, 240
   Andrei V. Alexandrov, Robert Mikulik & Andrew Demchuk

16 Ultrasound and Gaseous Microspheres, 252
   Flemming Forsberg & Andrei V. Alexandrov

17 Neurosonology Pearls, 262
   Georgios Tsivgoulis, Clotilde Balucani & Vijay K Sharma

Index, 275

List of Contributors

Robert J. Adams MD
Professor of Neurology
Medical University of South Carolina
Charleston, SC, USA

Anne W. Alexandrov PHD, FAAN
Professor and Director
NETSMART Program
Comprehensive Stroke Center
Department of Neurology
University of Alabama at Birmingham
Birmingham, AL, USA

Clotilde Balucani MD
Stroke and Neurosonology Fellow
Comprehensive Stroke Center
University of Alabama Hospital
Birmingham, AL, USA
and
PhD Student
Department of Neurology
University of Perugia
Perugia, Italy

Andrew D. Barreto MD
Assistant Professor, Director Neurosonology Laboratory, Department of Neurology, Stroke Division, University of Texas–Houston Medical School
Houston, TX, USA

Joel Cure MD
Professor and Neuro-Radiologist
Department of Radiology
University of Alabama Hospital
Birmingham, AL, USA

Andrew Demchuk MD, FRCPC
Associate Professor of Neurology
Director, Stroke Program
Department of Clinical Neurosciences
University of Calgary
Calgary, Alberta, Canada

Flemming Forsberg PHD
Professor and Director of Research
Department of Radiology
Thomas Jefferson University
Philadelphia, PA, USA

Cindy J. Fuller PHD
Research Scientist
Swedish Heart and Vascular Institute
Seattle, WA, USA

Zsolt Garami MD
Director, TCD Center
The Methodist Hospital
Houston, TX, USA

James C. Grotta MD
Professor and Chairman, Department of Neurology, Stroke Division, University of Texas–Houston Medical School
Houston, TX, USA

Mark R. Harrigan MD
Assistant Professor of Neurosurgery and Radiology
University of Alabama at Birmingham
Birmingham, AL, USA

Jill T. Jesurum PHD
Scientific Director
Swedish Heart and Vascular Institute
Seattle, WA, USA

Anne M. Jones RN, BSN, RVT, RDMS
Lecturer, Department of Neurology
Wake Forrest University Medical Center
Winston-Salem, NC, USA

Annabelle Lao MD
Attending Neurologist
Santo Thomas University
Manila, Philippines

Alan B. Lumsden MD
Professor and Chairman, Department of Cardiovascular Surgery
Medical Director, Methodist DeBakey Heart and Vascular Center
The Methodist Hospital
Houston, TX, USA

Robert Mikulik MD, PHD
Director, Stroke Program
Department of Neurology
Masaryk University
Brno, Czech Republic

Marsha M. Neumyer BS, RVT, FSVU, FAIUM, FSDMS
International Director
Vascular Diagnostic Educational Services
Harrisburg, PA, USA

David W. Newell MD
Professor of Neurosurgery
Department of Neurological Surgery
Director, Seattle Stroke Center
University of Washington
Seattle, WA, USA

Fenwick T. Nichols III MD
Professor, Department of Neurology
Medical College of Georgia
Augusta, GA, USA

Paola Palazzo MD
Department of Neurology
Campus Bio-Medico University
Rome, Italy

Joseph F. Polak MD, MPH
Professor of Radiology
New England Medical Center
Tufts University
Boston, MA, USA

Alice Robinson-Vaughn
NVT(C)
Chief Technologist
Neurovascular Ultrasound Laboratory
University of Alabama Hospital
Birmingham, AL, USA

List of Contributors

Marta Rubiera, MD
Stroke Unit, Neurology Department,
Hospital Vall d'Hebron
Barcelona, Spain

Tatjana Rundek MD, PHD
Associate Professor of Neurology
Department of Neurology
Miller School of Medicine
University of Miami
Miami, FL, USA

Vijay K. Sharma MD, RVT
Director of Neurosonology
Division of Neurology
National University Hospital
Singapore and Chinese
University of Hong Kong
Prince of Wales Hospital
Hong Kong
China

Georgios Tsivgoulis MD, PHD, RVT
Adjunct Assistant Professor and Director of Stroke
  Research
Comprehensive Stroke Center
University of Alabama Hospital
Birmingham, AL, USA
and
Lecturer in Neurology
Democritus University of Thrace
Alexandroupolis, Greece

Konstantinos Vadikolias MD, PHD
Assistant Professor of Neurology
Democritus University of Thrace
Neurology Department
University Hospital
Alexandroupolis, Greece

K.S. Lawrence Wong MD
Professor of Neurology
Department of Medicine and
Therapeutics, Chinese
University of Hong Kong
Prince of Wales Hospital
Hong Kong
China

Preface

This edition was prepared during challenging times in my career. I took on the leadership position to organize the acute stroke care team at the University of Alabama Hospital, the home of Tinsley Harrison's internal medicine and Champ Lyons' surgery heritage, that is located in the buckle of the Stroke Belt of the United States. A number of accomplished physicians and scientists paid their dues in fighting this disease in Alabama prior to my arrival at UAB. The list (by no means complete) includes James Halsey, J. Garber Galbraith, Leland Clark, James Morawetz, Winfield Fisher, Gary Roubin, Dennis Doblar, Vijay Misra, Georg Deutsch, Camilo Gomez, Rodney Soto, Sean Orr, Joseph Horton, Michelle Robbin, Edward Faught and Robert Slaughter. Dr Ray Watts, Chairman of the Department of Neurology, with the help of Drs Halsey, Rebecca Sugg and Andrew Barreto, recruited me and my wife, Anne Alexandrov, to UAB in 2007.

Our goal was to build a Stroke Team standing up to a meaning of the words – Comprehensive Stroke Center. We started with education at multiple levels of health professionals about a proactive, "reasons to treat" approach to stroke, removing the word "diversion" from stroke patients access to UAB, instituting shared stroke assessment, treatment and prevention protocols across all physicians on service, opening a dedicated universal-bed concept Stroke Unit and engaging multi-disciplinary care providers in this process.

Prior to start of "code stroke" in 2007, only four intravenous tPAs and just one intra-arterial thrombolysis procedure were given at UAB Hospital comprising less than 3% and 0.5%, respectively, of consecutive stroke patients being treated with reperfusion therapies. In 2008, these numbers were 38 (13%) and 20 (7%) and in 2009 we reached 100 (20%) and 40 (9%).

This could not have happened without our Team members who share the same "find reasons to treat" philosophy towards stroke care: stroke attendings Karen Allbright, Damon Patterson, John Brockington, John Rothrock; our interventionalists Damon Patterson, Mark Harrigan, Joseph Horton, Ed Underwood, Vijay Misra; our neurologists who help at multiple levels, Ivan Lopez, Jennifer deWolfe, Harrison Walker; our clinical and research fellows Aaron Anderson (winner of the 2009 Golden Plumber Award for the best Neurology Resident performance on Stroke service), Luis Cava (2010 Golden Plumber), Thang Huy Nguyen (who also contributed photographs to this edition with his remarkable camera skills), Marta Rubiera, Yi Zhang, Clotilde Balucani, Paola Palazzo, Kristian Barlinn; our nurse practitioner and clinical trial coordinator Mary Brethour and April Sisson; our sonographers Alice Robinson-Vaughn, Limin Zhao; and our Stroke Center staff who try to keep up with all of us: Alexis Jernigan and Sarah Bullock.

A special thanks to Georgios Tsivgoulis, a superb stroke neurologist and sonographer who bravely followed me to Alabama, helped us start this process and continues to conduct very productive research with us and our gurus in biostatistics/epidemiology George and Virginia Howard; and to Anne Alexandrov who coordinates multiple clinical and research protocol developments, education of staff and for her pivotal role in creation of the universal-bed Stroke Unit.

Our Team includes *all* nurses: first on M8 under the leadership of Elizabeth Toomey and Beth Clarkson and now on the Stroke Unit under Kathy Langley, Jill Stewart and Velinda Block, who offered tremendous support to innovations in care and research being delivered in this Unit.

Other members of our Stroke Team include *all* of the University Emergency Medicine faculty physicians, residents and nurses among whom I particularly would like to mention Janyce Sanford, Sarah Nafziger, Christopher Rosco, Henry Wang and Andy Thomas for their continuing support and fighting many political battles for us; Neurosurgery Department faculty physicians, residents and the Neuro-Intensive Care Unit staff with particular acknowledgement of vascular neurosurgeons Winfield Fisher and Mark Harrigan; Neuro-Radiologists Glenn Roberson, Joseph Horton, Joseph Sullivan, Robert Chapman and Joel "The Oracle" Cure; the Neuro-Vascular Laboratory staff at the

UAB Heart and Vascular Center; Vascular Surgeons under the leadership of Will Jordan; Neuro-Rehabilitation specialists Eugene Taub, Victor Mark and Bill Baker; Palliative Care Team staff and physicians Heather Herrington and Rodney Tucker; and of course the backbone of Stroke service – *all* our current Neurology Residents and graduates among whom I particularly would like to mention Andrew Barreto (now at UT-Houston, with whom we continue close collaboration), Bijay Pandy (2008 Golden Plumber), Tiffany Pineda (2009 Golden Plumber runner-up, for "No Ear-Plugs Needed" resident performance on stroke service), Victor Sung (2009 Golden Plumber runner-up) and Hayden Countryman Long (2010 Golden Plumber runner-up). Their endless efforts on the most difficult clinical rotation made a huge difference in many patient lives.

Andrei V. Alexandrov, MD, RVT
Birmingham, AL

Foreword

Neurosonology – dead or alive?

Alive and Kicking!

With the advent of modern imaging technologies and non-invasive assessment of extra- and intracranial brain vessels by both CT angiography and MR angiography, some clinical neuroscientists feel that this may initiate the end of the decades of neurosonology. Is this true or a misconception?

Back in the old days, more than 35 years ago, neurologists in Europe applied continuous wave sonography to explore cervical vessels, mostly the common carotid, the carotid bifurcation and the internal and external branches. Few even tried to insonate the vertebrals. With more and more advanced ultrasound technology, despite the major investments in CT imaging and, later on, MRI imaging, both pulse transcranial and B-mode-neurosonology were developed.

Of note, European neurologists, mostly in Scandinavia, Germany, Austria and Switzerland, made neurosonology part of the basic diagnostic techniques that neurologists offer, on the same level as EEG, EMG or evoked potential testing. Certification for physicians and, some time later, also for technicians was introduced. Basically, at the end of their 5-year training period, virtually every neurology resident in Germany will be an experienced neurosonologist, many of them certified by the National Ultrasound in Medicine Society.

In contrast, in North America, neurosonology was largely considered to be a technician's area of expertise, with physicians only interpreting the results and putting them in perspective. Only in a few centers, such as Seattle and Houston, did academic neurosonography create their own school of physicians trained in ultrasound and applying this technique to their patients. This may, in the future, become more popular.

Sonography is not the tool for the *one time* assessment of the brain-supplying arteries and the intracranial vessels. This can be done more reliably with CTA and MRA. Neurosonology is a monitoring instrument which allows repetitive assessments without side effects and exposure to radiation during procedures such as in re-canalization therapies, in patients with dissections or floating thrombi or, with additional ultrasound contrast, in the monitoring of emboligenic conditions. Furthermore, there may be hope for a therapeutic application of ultrasound. First steps in that direction have been made, and more steps will follow. Finally, three- and four-dimensional techniques and evaluations may help with individualizing treatment decisions, when it comes to the description of plaque morphology and differentiating "hot" plaques from "resting" plaques.

In Europe, several textbooks on neurosonology are available, many of them in their 3rd or 4th edition. This 2nd edition of the book by Andrei Alexandrov and co-workers represents a valid and profound counterbalance to European neurosonology, putting the techniques and future applications into perspective and setting the case for a more physician-applied neurosonology. The book is balanced and comprehensive and therefore could become the standard neurosonology volume for North America. Maybe at some point in time, a joint neurosonology textbook with contributors from North America, Europe and also Asia will follow.

Werner Hacke, MD, PHD
Professor and Chairman
Department of Neurology
University of Heidelberg
Germany
February 2010

Preface to the First Edition

This book is about vascular examination of patients suffering from stroke and relevance of this information to treatment decisions. This book is for clinicians who are eager to learn, prepared to observe and would not stop explorations.

Ultrasound sharpens clinician's ear and provides a stethoscope, an observation tool. And, like a microscope, an ultrasound probe needs a scientist to point it in the right direction. However, to paint a global picture, a complex ultrasound system also needs an artist to bring the art and science of medicine together. Ultrasound enables to monitor the cardiovascular system and brain responses to treatment in real time, a blessing on the way to develop stroke therapies and a handy tool to tailor treatment when the current evidence is meager.

I indebted to my friends and colleagues who spent countless time sharing their expertise in this book. Working with a Stroke Treatment Team is a thrill and this book is the result of many observations, often at obscene hours, that made us believe that stroke is treatable.

Andrei V. Alexandrov, MD
2004, Houston, TX

Foreword to the First Edition

Ultrasound: What's in the Waveforms?

The greatest advances in understanding and treating stroke have occurred in the past 30 years. This progress has coincided with and largely resulted from our dramatically improved ability to diagnose stroke and its subtypes, characterize its location and severity and understand its causes rapidly, accurately and in real time. This has taken some of the charm out of clinical stroke care as the senior readers of this book will still remember even the most astute clinicians' conclusions based on a careful history and physical exam proven wrong at the post mortem table. But the positive benefits of technology and improved diagnostic capability far exceed our nostalgia for the "good old days" when we relied mainly on our clinical acumen. What constitutes our improved ability to diagnose stroke? Unlike many other diseases, precise diagnosis of stroke depends almost entirely on imaging.

Our diagnostic capability took its greatest leap forward with the development of brain imaging, first with X-ray computed tomography and more recently with magnetic resonance imaging. Brain imaging has enabled us to quickly and accurately differentiate between infarct and hemorrhage, determine the location and surmise the probable cause and establish the age and severity of most strokes rapidly and painlessly. Brain imaging is now the first step in stroke diagnosis and treatment and has been called the "EKG of stroke." This technology is now available in the vast majority of hospitals in the developed world and, more than any other component of our clinical management, distinguishes 21st century stroke care.

Physiologic imaging developed almost concomitantly with structural brain imaging. Our ability to investigate cerebral blood flow and metabolism using radio-labeled tracers enabled us to see that acute and chronic stroke is a dynamic and potentially reversible process that would eventually yield to timely and precise therapeutic intervention. Pioneering studies using xenon and positron emitting isotopes demonstrated reduced cerebral blood flow distal to chronic extracranial and intracranial occlusion or vasospasm, and, most importantly, revealed the "ischemic penumbra" of reversibly damaged brain tissue in acute stroke patients that has yielded so far to timely reperfusion and, at least experimentally, to so called "neuroprotective" therapies targeting downstream consequences of interrupted blood flow. Furthermore, the linkage of cerebral blood flow and metabolism discovered with physiologic imaging has generated our ability to carry out "functional imaging." This technology is not only helping us understand the functional anatomy of simple and complex behaviors, but has also given visible proof of the plasticity of brain function. This has given a huge boost to research into treatment aimed at amplifying stroke recovery.

Imaging the vascular bed is the third critical aspect of stroke diagnosis. The seductive complexity of the brain draws our attention, but the stroke clinician must never lose sight of the fact that stroke is first and foremost a disease of the blood vessels nourishing that organ. Vascular imaging has been available to clinicians longer than our ability to image the brain parenchyma. Catheter arteriography can reveal the anatomy of extracranial and intracranial occlusive disease, aneurysms and arterio-venous malformations and for decades has been a standard part of the pre-operative evaluation of patients with severe forms of these conditions. However, it was not until the advent of "non-invasive" techniques, using ultrasound and more recently magnetic resonance and CT-angiography, that vascular imaging has become part of the routine evaluation of all stroke patients. Such testing has become critical to answer essential clinical questions that impact management of every stroke patient such as the cause of bleeding in patients with intracranial hemorrhage and the precise location, nature and severity of arterial occlusion or narrowing in patients with transient ischemic attack or ischemic stroke.

The advantages of ultrasound for vascular diagnosis are well known. It is a fast, portable, non-invasive, repeatable and inexpensive technique. The application of ultrasound to clinical stroke care over the past decades has revealed a number of clinical determinations that are best made by this technique and that directly impact on clinical decision-making. Among various clinical situations, the most established ones include:

- the early detection and characterization of extracranial atherosclerosis and occlusive disease especially at the carotid bifurcation,
- the consequences of proximal arterial occlusive disease on the distal cerebral vasculature,
- the natural history and response to treatment of acute arterial occlusion that causes hyperacute stroke,
- the detection of microemboli associated with cardiac and aortic pathology and carotid artery surgical manipulation (and perhaps gauging response to anti-platelet therapy),
- selection of children with sickle cell disease for blood transfusion as an effective tool in primary stroke prevention, and
- the time course and reversibility of cerebral vasospasm after subarachnoid hemorrhage.

Portable ultrasound machines and handy monitoring sets made it possible to bring this technology to bedside and observe remarkable flow changes in stroke patients in real time. However, the field of ultrasonic diagnosis also has it detractors and limitations. For many applications, ultrasound has not been thoroughly tested for its utility, accuracy and validity in multi-center studies. While the benefits of using this methodology for the above indications, as well as for others that undoubtedly will emerge as our exploration of stroke disease continues, may seem self-evident to those of us who live with ultrasound technology and use it every day, this is not so evident to others. Careful outcomes research investigating the accuracy and cost benefit of ultrasound is needed to establish the utility of this technique for any clinical situation where we surmise that it should be routine. Many such studies have been carried out and have established the value of ultrasound particularly for the clinical issues listed above. This book should help identify where such data exist, and more importantly, where more data is still needed.

Finally, early ultrasound technology was indirect, had poor resolution and had high rates of false positive and false negative results. Even now, the technique is "operator dependent" in terms of the accuracy and validity of its results. While, in fact, to some extent these concerns are true of all diagnostic imaging, these limitations have been particularly true of ultrasound. Newer technology has provided significant advances in this regard, but it is necessary for each and every laboratory to maintain strict quality control in order to maximize the information that this powerful technology can provide. This textbook provides a major advance in that regard. Written by experts in the field, it will provide sonographers with the tools needed to enhance the confidence of clinicians in utilizing ultrasound technology and the clinicians with additional information how to implement this technology in their everyday decision-making.

James C. Grotta, MD
2004, Houston, TX

Acknowledgment (First Edition)

I joined the University of Texas Stroke Treatment Team in 1996 and never regret the loss of life style or many sleepless nights. The best experience one can get is to work together with Team members who would race day or night to see and treat acute stroke patients breaking all speed limits and meeting any strict time windows. With countless hours spent together in the emergency department, angio rooms, specialized care units and late night diners we shared thoughts and debated various ways to treat acute cerebral ischemia.

These observations would never have happened without Jim Grotta, a visionary for stroke treatment, who started this Team long before I joined it. He has led us to the highest percentage of consecutive stroke patients being treated with thrombolytics to date. This work would have never been accomplished without those who made it happen in Houston, current and former Team members, many of whom are now heading their own Stroke Teams in the Unites States, Canada and other countries (I apologize for not listing many more Stroke Team members who worked hard in Houston prior to 1996): Fahmi Al-Senani, Scott Burgin, Alex Brunser, Sergio Calleja, Morgan Campbell, Chin-I Chen, Oleg Chernyshev, David Chiu, Ioannis Christou, Andrew Demchuk, Ashraf El-Mitwalli, Robert Felberg, Zsolt Garami, Christiana Hall, Susan Hickenbottom, Yasuki Iguchi, Jennifer Ireland, Scott Kasner, Derk Krieger, Lise Labiche, Marc Malkoff, Robert Mikulik, Lewis Morgenstern, Elizabeth Noser, Nicholas Okon, Paisith Piriyawat, Marc Ribo, Hashim Shaltoni, Ken Uchino, Carlos Villar-Cordova, Teddy Wein and Frank Yatsu.

The words Stroke Treatment Team would remain just words without acknowledging everyday work of nurses, who took care of our patients and who carried out our pivotal as well as negative clinical trials. The Team is blessed with outstanding nurses who keep physicians on their toes: Patti Bratina, Sheila Ford, Dawn Matherne, Robin Saiki, Sandi Shaw, Dora Vital and Anne Wojner.

The Team could never be complete without interventionalists, cardiovascular surgeons, neurosurgeons, critical care, emergency physicians, scientists and proactive hospital nurse administrators who also made an enormous effort to be there on time and to brain-storm creative ways to combat the most resistive clinical and scientific problems: Jaroslaw Aronowski, Eddy Cacayourin, Linda Chi, Guy Clifton, Tony Estrera, Tom Flanigan, Brent King, Dong Kim, Steve Koch, Bill Maggio, Joseph Nates, David Robinson, Hazim Safi, Richard Smalling, Joon Song and Roger Strong.

This work would also have never been possible without Houston Fire Department, City Paramedics and many Emergency Room nurses, physicians and neurology residents.

2004, Houston, TX

Practice of Ultrasound: an Introduction

A variety of ultrasound tests have been introduced for the detection and monitoring of cerebrovascular disease in the past 50 years [1–10]. Advantages of ultrasound testing include its non-invasive nature, portability, real-time information and versatility. Imagine that one can sample tissues and flow behavior in real time at a rate of 5000 times per second. So far, no other imaging modality in wide use for stroke today comes close to this temporal resolution. Furthermore, ultrasound waves contain a mechanical pressure momentum resulting in energy transmission to tissues that in itself can yield a therapeutic effect.

Current and disappointing reality is that when a stroke patient gets an ultrasound evaluation, it is often limited to assessment of the extracranial portion of the carotid arteries, with an even more limited look at the vertebral arteries. Evaluation of brain vessels is reduced to a snapshot offered by a non-invasive angiography, if any. While in training, physicians dealing with stroke are not getting enough exposure to learning cerebral hemodynamics and the vastness of mechanisms of how strokes occur or can be reversed beyond the meager choice of approved therapies. This edition, in addition to the first, is intended to cover the gap for vascular neurologists to learn how ultrasound can enrich their ability to diagnose, evaluate and treat stroke and for sonographers to understand what information clinicians need from their tests. From the clinical applications standpoint, cerebrovascular ultrasound at present can:

1 differentiate normal from diseased vessels and states,
2 uncover plaques and identify the most dangerous ones,
3 grade categories of stenosis in major pre-cerebral and intracranial vessels,
4 localize the disease process including acute occlusions,
5 detect progression of a variety of diseases, including cerebral circulatory arrest,
6 detect, localize and quantify cerebral embolism,
7 detect right-to-left shunts,
8 assess the ability of collateral circulation to maintain cerebral blood flow or succumb to steal and
9 monitor and even augment thrombolysis.

A single test procedure or a single transducer cannot yet accomplish all of these tasks. Sonographers have to learn how to use a combination of extracranial and intracranial tests and keep up with the progress in the field.

Prerequisites to a successful practice of cerebrovascular ultrasound include knowledge of anatomy, physiology of cardiovascular and nervous systems, fluid dynamics and pathological changes in a variety of cerebrovascular disorders [11–21] and also the basics of ultrasound physics and instrumentation [22–24]. No single textbook is sufficient in preparation for proficiency examinations, nor could it serve as a sole source of reference material in day-to-day practice. I use multiple sources and continue to learn from previously written texts (not limited indeed to the classic contributions referenced in this section) as well as continuing medical education conferences, research papers and presentations at numerous ultrasound and stroke-related meetings.

In the 6 years that have passed since the first edition of this book, I received multiple suggestions on how to improve it. Also, the aim of this second edition is to update the description of cerebrovascular ultrasound testing methods and criteria for interpretation and to illustrate how ultrasound provides information helpful in patient management.

The practice of ultrasound (both performance and interpretation) should be a mandatory part of the residency training for physicians of different specialties as well as the Vascular Neurology training pathway. It still remains problematic in the United States to have all neurology trainees learn these skills during residency while the depth of ultrasound education varies greatly worldwide. As a result, there is skepticism towards ultrasonography [25] that is largely based on the lack of knowledge of how to perform, interpret and use the results of ultrasound tests in clinical practice and research.

Indeed, ultrasound testing has shortcomings since it is very operator dependent. But so are most tests in medicine! The accuracy of ultrasound testing varies between practitioners of different skill, knowledge and experience. Even the most experienced of us are not invincible. Constant learning and improvement are keys to reaching the best possible outcomes of ultrasound testing.

Sonographers have to meet the requirements such set by the board examinations of the American Registry of

Diagnostic Medical Sonographers (ARDMS, www.ardms.org) or other national and international boards and societies. Most vascular practitioners pass the Registered Vascular Technologist (RVT) examination that focuses mostly on vascular ultrasound "from jaw to toe" leaving transcranial Doppler (TCD) largely untested. International or regional requirements for technologists' credentials also vary. The American Society of Neuroimaging and the Neurosonology Research Group of the World Federation of Neurology are making progress in providing certification examinations on all continents where there is an interest in verifying the knowledge and skills of physicians and sonographers.

Interpreting physicians have to demonstrate competence through training such as Fellowship or by completing the required number of hours of continuing medical education in ultrasound methods and supervised interpretation of a set number of cases for each imaging modality. These requirements are outlined in the regulatory documents of the Intersocietal Commission of Accreditation of Vascular Laboratories (ICAVL, www.icavl.org) that recognizes two physician credentials outlined below as qualifications to serve as a director of a vascular ultrasound laboratory.

The American Society of Neuroimaging (www.asnweb.org) also offers a peer-reviewed multiple-choice proficiency examination in neurosonology that covers physics, clinical application and interpretation of the carotid/vertebral and transcranial ultrasound methods. This is the only organization to date that assesses knowledge specific to the neurovascular field including TCD. The Registered Physician Vascular Interpreter (RPVI) examination by ARDMS tests peripheral and carotid vascular testing knowledge and does not cover TCD (www.ardms.org).

In addition to credentialing, consistent application, local validation of ultrasound testing and interpretation and continuing quality improvement are the keys to successful practices [26].

Ultrasound offers a wealth of information, including real-time assessment of patho-physiological changes and monitoring of patients with cerebrovascular diseases. Often, this information finds no place in clinical decision-making as skeptics would say, "it has not been tested in randomized clinical trials." Not everything that we do as clinicians can or should be tested in these trials. Ultrasound can be very helpful in clinical decision-making if the results are provided in a timely fashion and the practicing physicians are prepared to use this information to select the best management strategy and often to go beyond "proven" (often meager) standards in the best interests of the patient.

I consider TCD and carotid duplex as an extension of the neurological examination as these tests enable me to confirm the vascular origin of patient symptoms, detect and localize the disease process and monitor the progress of therapies. This approach is outlined in detail in a companion book entitled *Neurovascular Ultrasound Examination and Waveform Interpretation*. That book also contains basics of ultrasound physics and fluid dynamics complementary to this edition and provides more illustrative case examples of diagnostic findings and considerations in differential diagnosis.

I am indebted to my peers, colleagues who challenged my thinking, those who became my mentors through ongoing debates and ultimately friends: Marsha Neumeyer, Joseph Polak, John Pellerito and Charles Tegeler. The numerous courses that we taught together made me in the first place continuously learn ultrasound and re-think what I thought I knew. Likewise on the clinical side, Andrew Demchuk, James Grotta, Carlos Molina, Peter Schellinger and my team at UAB contributed greatly to my continuing explorations of stroke. I also gratefully acknowledge all contributors to this book who donated their time and shared their expertise – their chapters bring you on a continuing journey of learning stroke and ultrasound. I would like to thank Rune Aaslid, PhD, pioneer of TCD, for generously providing his original drawing of the circle of Willis, as well as his input in advising me on cerebral hemodynamics.

In short, ultrasound remains an exciting field that offers new possibilities and challenges. It requires investment of time and effort to learn, yet it is rewarding in practice if you master these skills. You will start to see the disease process from new angles as real-time patho-physiological changes unfold and hopefully become a better practitioner.

Andrei V. Alexandrov, MD, RVT
Birmingham, AL

References

1 Strandness DE, McCutcheon EP, Rushmer RF. Application of a transcutaneous Doppler flowmeter in evaluation of occlusive arterial disease. *Surg Gynecol Obstet* 1966;**122**(5):1039–45.

2 Spencer MP, Reid JM, Davis DL, et al. Cervical carotid imaging with a continuous-wave Doppler flowmeter. *Stroke* 1974;**5**:145–54.

3 Barber FE, Baker DW, Nation AW, et al. Ultrasonic duplex echo-Doppler scanner. *IEEE Trans Biomed Eng* 1974;**21**(2):109–13.

4 Budingen HJ, von Reutern GM, Freund HJ. Diagnosis of cerebro-vascular lesions by ultrasonic methods. *Int J Neurol* 1977;**11**(2–3):206–18.

5 Aaslid R, Markwalder TM, Nornes H. Noninvasive transcranial Doppler ultrasound recording of flow velocity in basal cerebral arteries. *J Neurosurg* 1982;**57**:769–74.

6 Spence JD, Coates RK, Pexman JA. Doppler flow maps of the carotid artery compared with the findings on angiography. *Can J Surg* 1983;**26**:556–8.

7 Bogdahn U, Becker G, Schlief R, et al. Contrast-enhanced transcranial color-coded real-time sonography. *Stroke* 1993;**24**:676–84.

8 Rubin JM, Bude RO, Carson PL, *et al.* Power Doppler US: a potentially useful alternative to mean frequency-based color Doppler US. *Radiology* 1994;**190**(3):853–6.

9 Burns PN. Harmonic imaging with ultrasound contrast agents. *Clin Radiol* 1996;**51**:50–5.

10 O'Leary DH, Polak JF, Kronmal RA, *et al.* Carotid-artery intima and media thickness as a risk factor for myocardial infarction and stroke in older adults. Cardiovascular Health Study Collaborative Research Group. *N Engl J Med* 1999;**340**(1):14–22.

11 Krayenbuehl H, Yasargil MG. *Cerebral Angiography*, 2nd edn. Stuttgart: Georg Thieme, 1982.

12 Bernstein EF. *Vascular Diagnosis*, 4th edn. St. Louis, MO: Mosby-Year Book, 1993.

13 Polak JF. *Peripheral Vascular Sonography: a Practical Guide*. Baltimore, MD: Williams & Wilkins, 1992.

14 Strandness DE. *Duplex Scanning in Vascular Disorders*, 2nd edn. New York: Raven Press, 1993.

15 Zweibel WJ. *Introduction to Vascular Ultrasonography*, 4th edn. St. Louis, MO: Harcourt Health Sciences, 2000.

16 von Reutern GM, Budingen HJ. *Ultrasound Diagnosis in Cerebrovascular Disease*. Stuttgart: Georg Thieme, 1993.

17 Tegeler CH, Babikian VL, Gomez CR. *Neurosonology*. St. Louis: Mosby, 1996.

18 Hennerici M, Neuerburg-Heusler D. *Vascular Diagnosis with Ultrasound. ClinicalReference with Case Studies*. Stuttgart: Georg Thieme, 1998.

19 Hennerici M, Mearis S. *Cerebrovascular Ultrasound: Theory, Practice and Future Developments*. Cambridge: Cambridge University Press, 2001.

20 Bartels E. *Color-Coded Duplex Ultrasonography of the Cerebral Arteries: Atlas and Manual*. Stuttgart: Schattauer, 1999.

21 Babikian VL, Wechsler LR, eds. *Transcranial Doppler Ultrasonography*, 2nd edn. Woburn, MA: Butterworth Heinemann, 1999.

22 Edelman SK. *Understanding Ultrasound Physics*, 2nd edn. The Woodlands, TX: ESP, 1997.

23 Kremkau FW. *Diagnostic Ultrasound: Principles and Instruments*, 5th edn. Philadelphia, PA: Harcourt Health Sciences, 1998.

24 Zagzebski JA. *Essentials of Ultrasound Physics*. St. Louis, MO: Mosby, 1997.

25 Ringelstein EB. Skepticism toward carotid ultrasonography. A virtue, an attitude or fanaticism? *Stroke* 1995;**26**:1743–6.

26 Katanick SL. Accreditation of vascular ultrasound laboratories. In: Tegeler CH, Babikian VL, Gomez CR, eds, *Neurosonology*. St. Louis, MO: Mosby, 1996:484–88.

I How to Perform Ultrasound Tests

1 Principles of Extracranial Ultrasound Examination

Andrei V. Alexandrov[1], Alice Robinson-Vaughn[1], Clotilde Balucani[2] & Marsha M. Neumyer[3]

[1]University of Alabama Hospital, Birmingham, AL, USA
[2]University of Alabama Hospital, Birmingham, AL, USA and University of Perugia, Perugia, Italy
[3]Vascular Diagnostic Educational Services, Harrisburg, PA, USA

Introduction

A simple observation gives origins to clinical examinations, analysis and scientific exploration. Being able to observe Nature at work or in distress often offers clues that clinicians and scientists need to get an idea as to what could be going on and come up with a hypothesis to explain it. Ultrasound, with its unprecedented temporal resolution, is an elegant tool to probe living tissues. This first chapter describes how we evaluate the extracranial vasculature, then subsequent chapters continue the journey into cerebral vessels, hemodynamics and specific disease states.

Anatomy of the cerebrovascular arterial system

The choice of transducer placement and subsequent repositioning determines the success of visualizing the target structures and staying with the spatial course of the pre-cerebral vessels. Therefore, sonographers performing vascular ultrasound examinations must think "in 3-D," or three dimensions, about the vessel being investigated and put together transducer positioning with vessel intercept and further "go with the structure or flow" to complete scanning.

A sonographer should further imagine how this arterial segment would look on an angiogram. We strongly encourage those learning and interpreting ultrasound to be familiar with cerebral angiograms [1] since angiography is the gold standard for the assessment of the accuracy of ultrasound testing, and ultrasound performance is often judged by vessel appearance on invasive or non-invasive angiograms. The following section deals with normal vascular anatomy and describes a standard protocol for carotid and vertebral duplex testing on the neck. More details of anatomy and angiographic images are provided in Chapter 3.

The common carotid artery

Scanning starts with a quick brightness-modulated (B-mode) surveillance in a transverse transducer position of the common carotid artery (CCA) up to its bifurcation. Color flow or power mode can be added to visualize flow in the vessel lumen (Figure 1.1).

On the right, the brachiocephalic trunk or innominate artery, arises from the aortic arch and then bifurcates into the subclavian artery and the CCA. On the left side, both the common carotid artery and the left subclavian artery usually originate directly from the aortic arch. The CCA is easily assessable on the neck where it runs in parallel with the jugular vein and the initial assessment starts right above the clavicle (Figure 1.2). It is further assessed in its mid-portion as the transducer slides cephalad over the sterno-cleido-mastoid muscle (Figure 1.3).

At approximately the level of the fourth vertebra, which is at the level of the upper border of the thyroid cartilage, the CCA bifurcates into the internal and external carotid arteries (Figure 1.4). The carotid bulb represents dilatation at the distal CCA extending into the proximal internal carotid artery. The carotid bulb bears unique flow patterns yielding a boundary separation zone and its wall has numerous baro- and chemo-receptors. The size and location of the carotid bulb are variable.

Most atherosclerotic disease occurs at the level of the bifurcation due to marked changes in vessel geometry resulting in increased shear stress, fluid stagnation and increased particle residence time on the postero-lateral wall of the bulb [2].

The internal carotid artery

Beyond the carotid bulb, the internal carotid artery (ICA) returns to a normal caliber (Figure 1.5) and courses in a relatively straight line up the neck into the skull to supply blood

---

Cerebrovascular Ultrasound in Stroke Prevention and Treatment, 2nd edition. Edited by Andrei V. Alexandrov. © 2011 Blackwell Publishing Ltd.

PART I How to Perform Ultrasound Tests

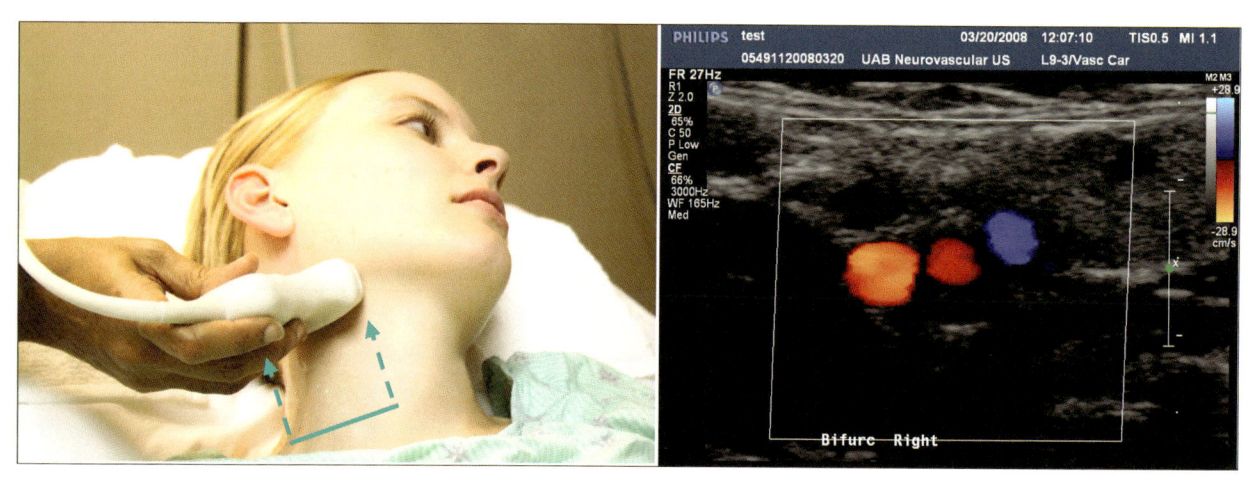

Figure 1.1 Transverse positioning of the duplex transducer depicts carotid bifurcation on the neck. Arrows indicate a proximal initial placement of the probe and its ascent to the bifurcation as the initial step to extracranial vascular examination. The left side of the ultrasound B-mode and color flow image is oriented towards the midline. Red color shows arterial flows, blue indicates the jugular vein.

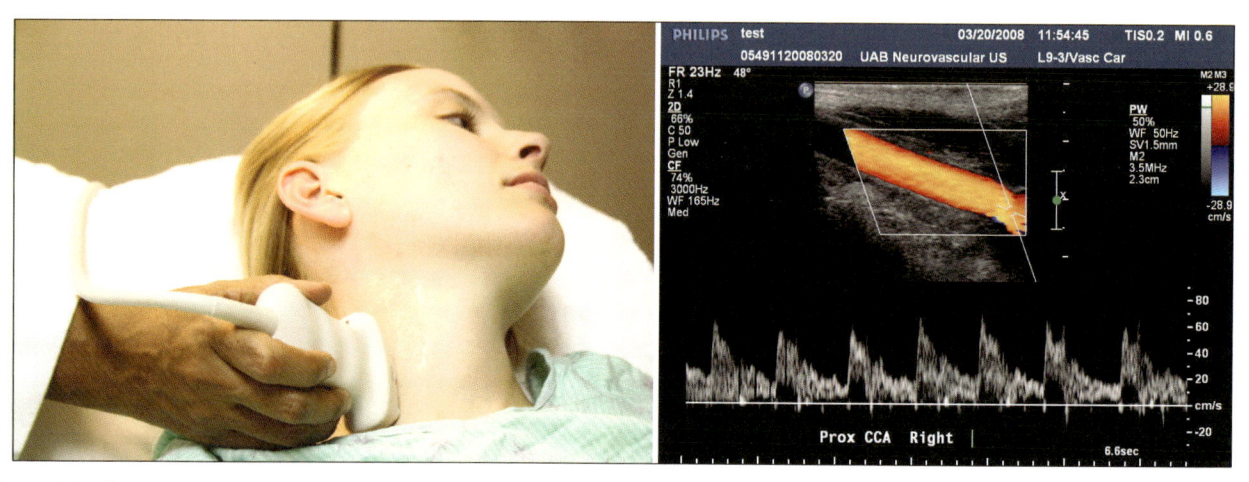

Figure 1.2 After transverse sweeps, a longitudinal position of the probe yields depiction of the proximal common carotid artery close to its origin from the brachio-cephalic trunk on the right side of the neck. Note that ultrasound image is aligned with the middle of the vessel by keeping "the ends of pipe open." The left side of the ultrasound image is oriented cephalad. Doppler sampling shows the velocity spectra at a 60° angle of insonation.

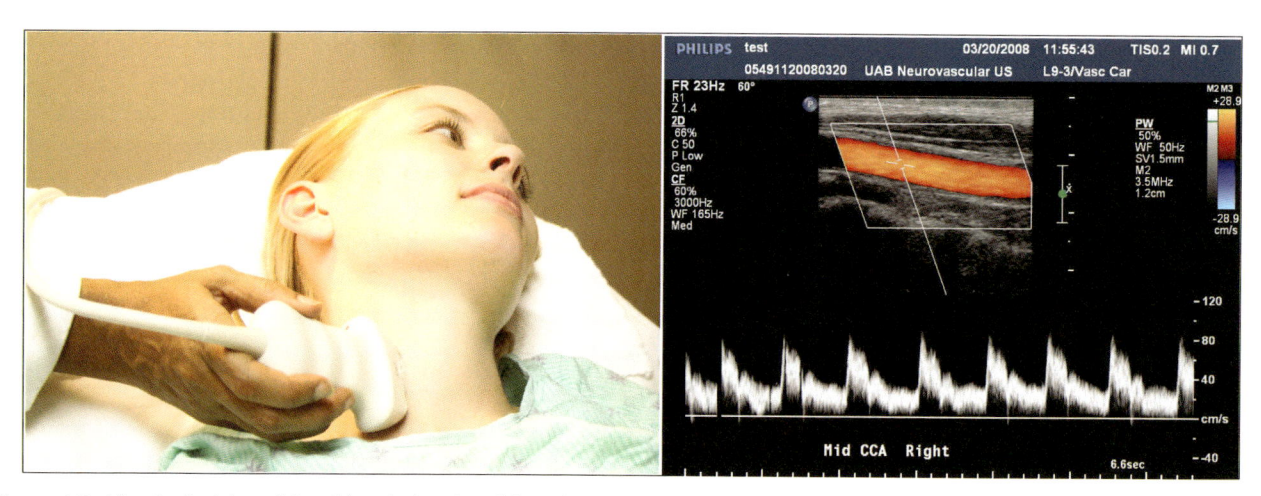

Figure 1.3 A longitudinal view of the mid-cervical portion of the right carotid artery shows B-mode, color flow and Doppler spectra of the artery and flow through it.

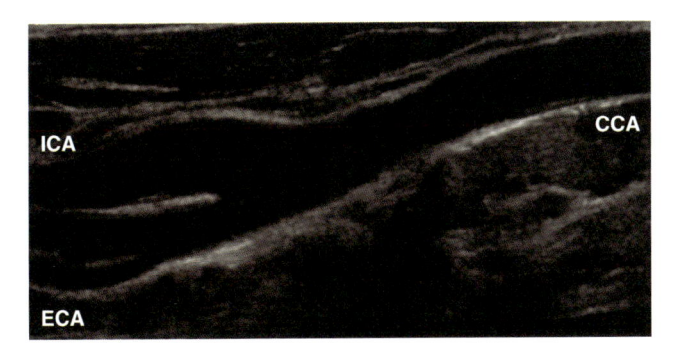

CHAPTER 1 Principles of Extracranial Ultrasound Examination

Figure 1.4 The "tuning fork" of the carotid bifurcation on B-mode.

flow to the eye and brain. As a rule, the ICA has no branches within the neck. After entering the skull, the ICA makes an S-shaped curve in the region of the carotid siphon. The ICA entrance to the skull marks a vulnerable area where arterial wall dissections may occur due to fixed ICA position. The first major branch of the ICA is the ophthalmic artery that supplies the eye. After giving off the ophthalmic artery, the ICA divides into the middle cerebral artery (MCA) and the anterior cerebral artery (ACA), a part of the circle of Willis. This is covered in Chapters 2 and 3.

The external carotid artery

The extracranial carotid artery (ECA) supplies the muscles of the face, forehead and scalp (Figure 1.6). To switch between the ICA and ECA, a sonographer often must reposition the transducer from lateral to more medial angulation since both vessels are seldom visualized together in one plane for sufficient interrogation. The ECA has branches that could be visible while scanning its proximal segment. The ICA divides into eight branches on the neck. Several of these branches, i.e. ascending pharyngeal, facial, internal maxillary and superficial temporal arteries, communicate via anastomoses with the ICA. The occipital artery is the only ECA branch that communicates with the vertebral artery circulation. It is important to recognize these branches because the ECA fairly often becomes a collateral source for blood flow to the brain when the ICA is critically stenosed or occluded.

The vertebral artery

The vertebral arteries (VA) arise from the subclavian arteries and its origin can be found with transducer sliding towards the clavicle and aiming deep and lateral to the CCA (Figure 1.7). The VA passes medially in the neck to enter the bony canal at the C6 vertebrae and it further courses cephalad through the transverse processes of the vertebrae (Figure 1.8). It enters the base of the skull by looping around the atlas and ascending through the foramen magnum. At this point, the right and left vertebral arteries join together to form the basilar artery. The basilar artery terminates in the posterior cerebral arteries, which make up the posterior portion of the circle of Willis.

Components of ultrasound examination

Continuous wave (CW) Doppler

Although this technology is now regarded more of historic interest due to technological advances in imaging, knowledge of CW Doppler is required for board examinations and occasionally the skill of using the so-called "pencil probe" may be useful.

Dr Eugene Strandness and co-workers first reported the use of a transcutaneous flowmeter to evaluate occlusive arterial disease in 1966 [3]. Extracranial carotid and vertebral examinations with CW Doppler were reported by Drs Merrill Spencer and Michael von Reutern and colleagues in the 1970s [4,5].

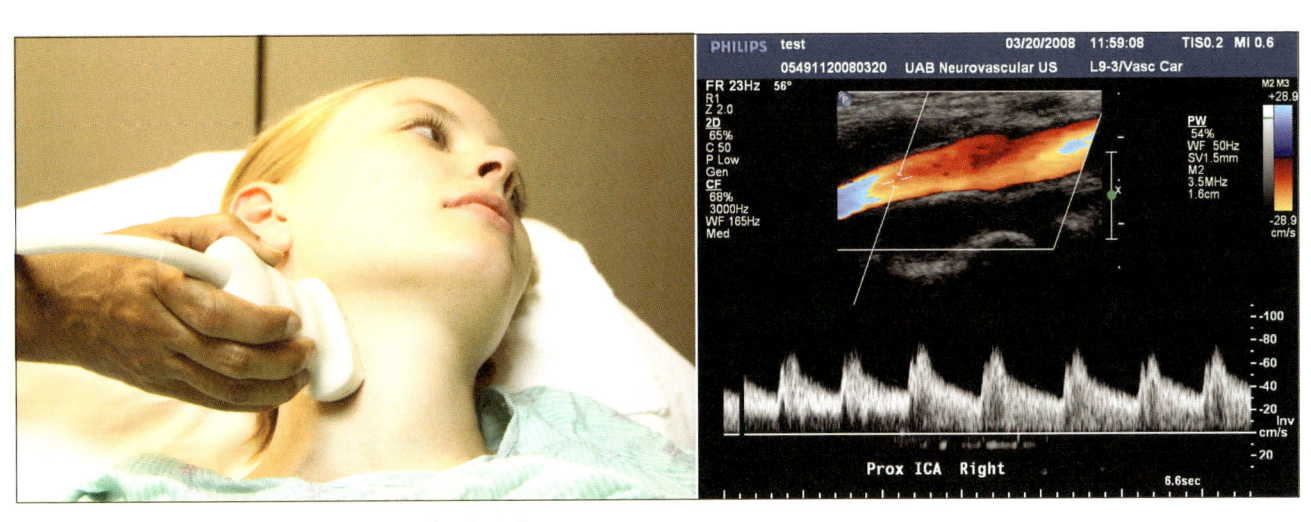

Figure 1.5 Insonation of the proximal ICA just after the bulb.

PART I How to Perform Ultrasound Tests

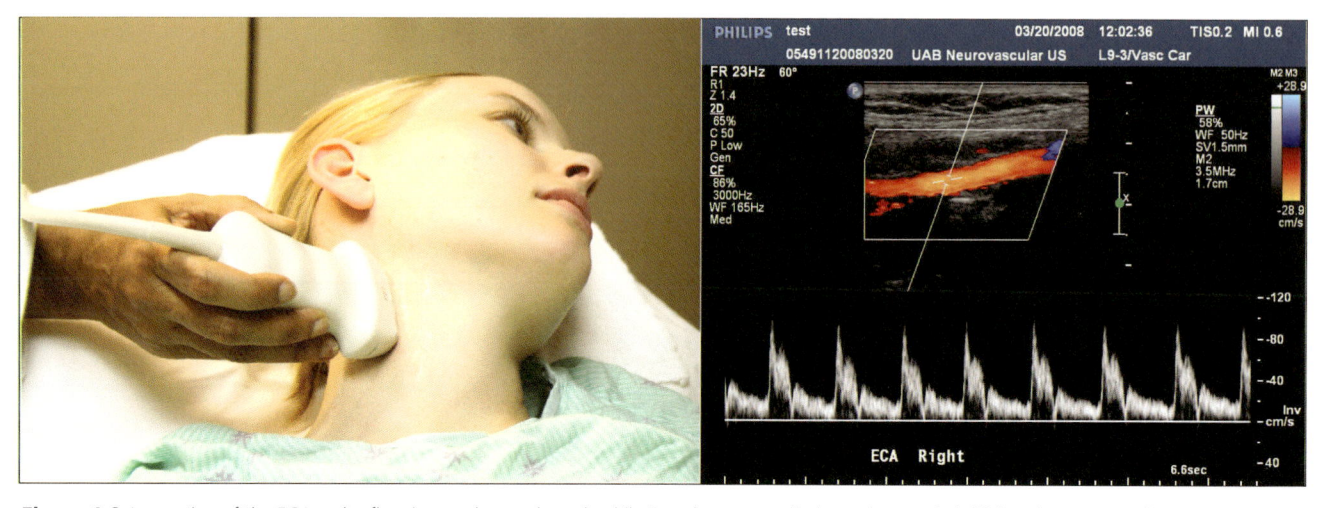

Figure 1.6 Insonation of the ECA: color flow image shows a branch while Doppler spectra display a characteristic high resistance waveform.

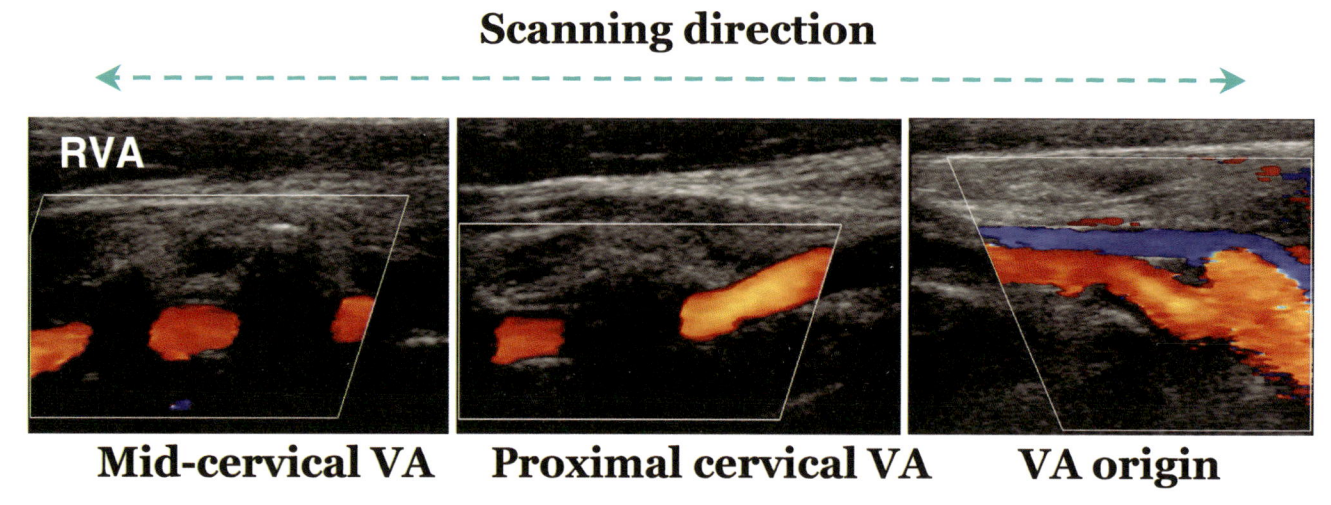

Scanning direction

Mid-cervical VA   Proximal cervical VA   VA origin

Figure 1.7 Insonation of the origin of the vertebral artery. Arrows show the further extent of the vertebral artery examination on the neck.

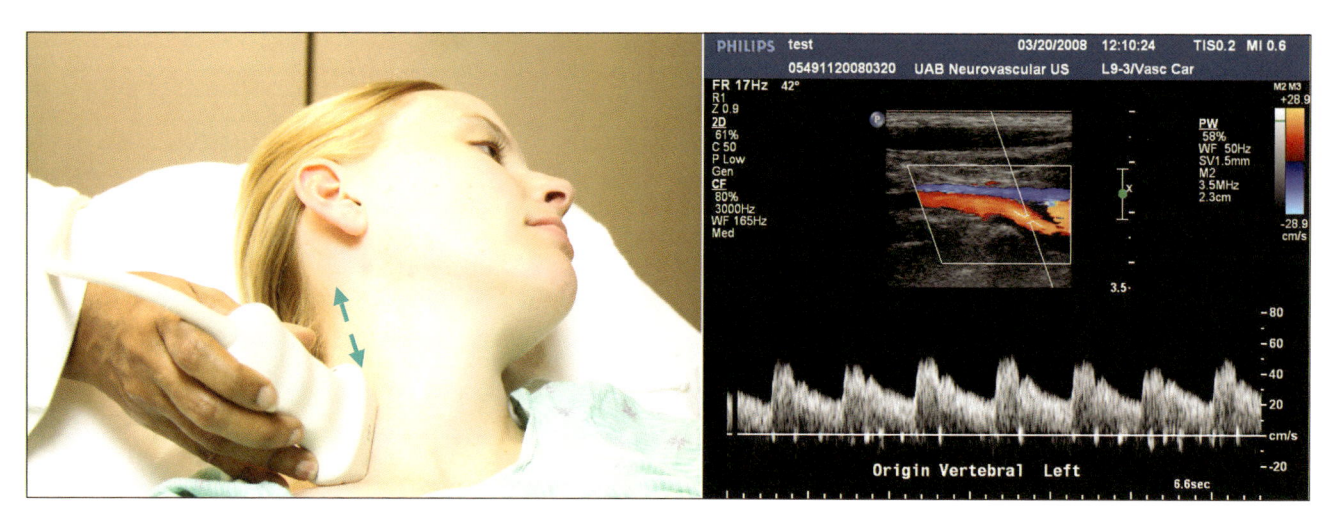

Figure 1.8 Doppler spectra in a proximal cervical segment of the vertebral artery visualized with B-mode and color flow.

Insonation with CW probe

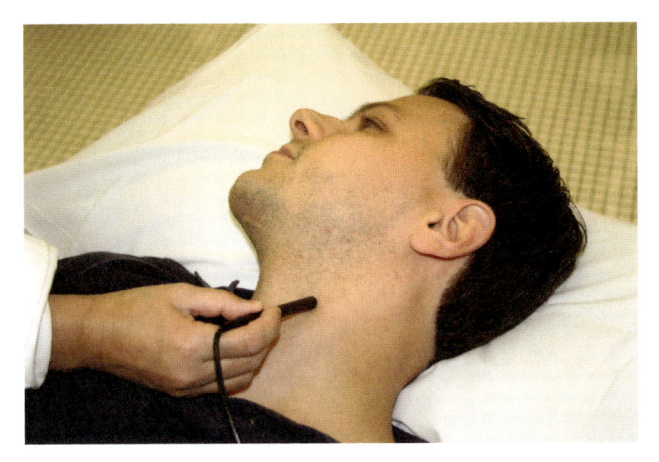

Figure 1.9 Insonation with continuous wave (CW) transducer.

With this technology, one crystal continuously emits the signal and another crystal continuously receives returned echoes, and this "non-imaging" transducer looks like a pencil (Figure 1.9). CW Doppler displays Doppler frequency shifts including maximum frequency trace without an artifact due there being no limitations related to pulse repetition frequency. Current CW systems can differentiate between positive and negative Doppler shifts and create a bi-directional spectral signal that shows flow direction as towards or away from the transducer. However, CW Doppler shows no information regarding the structure, i.e. image, or the depth from which the signals originated.

The advantage of this ultrasound test is its ability to display Doppler frequency shifts from moving objects without an artifact called aliasing. With the recent development of direct imaging and pulsed wave Doppler methods, CW Doppler is rarely performed and is not reimbursed in the United States as a *sole* test used for evaluation of the carotid vessels. Perhaps the only remaining indications for CW Doppler for carotid arteries are extensive (>2 cm) shadowing of the bifurcation, arterial lesions extending above the level of lower jaw or a quick bifurcation screening before or with (not as a substitute for) direct imaging investigation.

The B-mode image

The B-mode image is created from the amplitude of backscattered echo signals that are displayed in gray scale along beam propagation (depth) and the length of transducer/skin interface (Figures 1.1 and 1.2). The gray shade of the signal on-screen displays the strength of the returning echo while its location relates to the depth of tissue reflector. Several crystals are sequentially activated with electronic pulses or the transducer is rotated mechanically (steering) to create multiple scan lines. The scan lines are put together to generate an image (or "frame"). Since the average speed of sound propagation in soft tissues is 1540 m s^{-1} ("a mile per second"), multiple frames are generated in a second, creating an illusion of a real-time picture ("movie making" with ultrasound).

The maximum depth of sound penetration is determined by the emitting frequency of the ultrasound transducer, which is usually 4–12 MHz for extracranial imaging and 2–4 MHz for intracranial imaging. Higher frequencies have smaller pulse lengths and allow better spatial resolution but less penetration due to increased sound scattering. Time-gain compensation (TGC) is applied to improve visualization of structures with increasing depths of insonation. The smallest distinguishable distance between two reflectors along the ultrasound beam axis (axial resolution) is directly proportional to the spatial length of the pulse. Lateral resolution (or resolution perpendicular to the direction of an ultrasound beam) is also dependent on transducer geometry since it is the highest in the focal zone. The focal zone is determined as the narrowest point between converging (near-field) and diverging (far-field) parts of the ultrasound beam. Note that an ultrasound scanner can create multiple focal zones to optimize different parts of the image. Therefore, linear or curved array transducers with larger surface, dynamic electronic focusing and multiple narrow width beams have better lateral resolution.

B-mode imaging artifacts include the following:

1 Shadowing (no image can be generated along ultrasound beam axis behind a bright reflector). Changing the transducer position and planes of insonation may minimize shadow appearance. Shadows can originate from perpendicular insonation of vessel walls, plaque calcification (Figure 1.7) and transverse vertebral processes (Figure 1.3).
2 Reverberation (multiple bright echoes that often have a regular shape and layered position are displayed along the axis of ultrasound beam when echoes bounce many times between two strong reflectors).
3 Mirror image [a false image (also known as phantom image or reflection artifact) is created when obliquely scanning a strongly reflecting boundary]. Vessel visualization in transverse and longitudinal planes often resolves confusion associated with this artifact.
4 Plane-of-section (three-dimensional structure is inadequately displayed on a two-dimensional monitor). Using imagination for three-dimensional spatial relationships, the transducer position should be changed to generate adequate sectional planes.

B-mode imaging is used to identify the carotid and vertebral arteries, carotid intima–media complex, atherosclerotic plaques and anatomic anomalies. B-mode imaging can also be used to perform intracranial studies where it shows contralateral skull line, midline structures including the third ventricle and brain parenchymal structures.

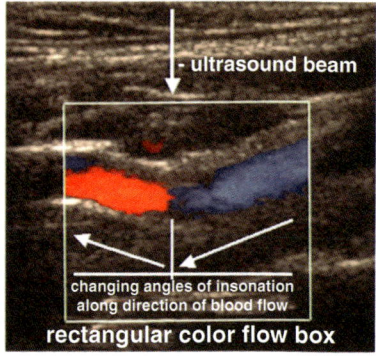

PART I How to Perform Ultrasound Tests

Figure 1.10 Changes in color flow assignment relative to the middle of the transducer within a rectangular color flow box.

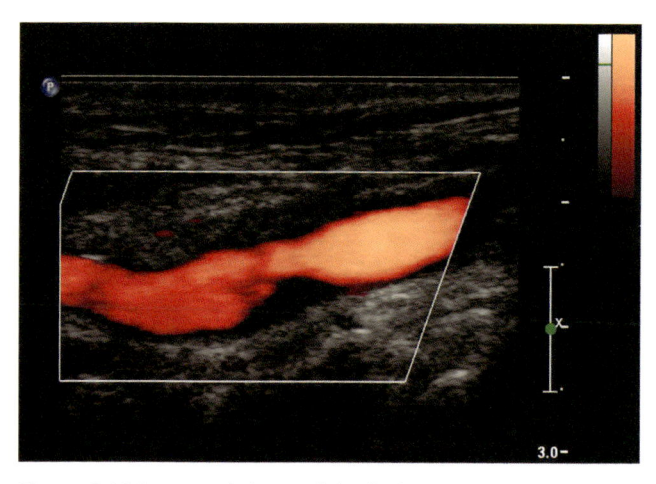

Figure 1.11 Power mode image of the distal CCA, proximal ICA and a small hypoechoic plaque at the ICA bulb.

The color-flow Doppler image

Color-coded Doppler flow image (CDFI) displays the average (or mean) shifts in the frequency of returned echoes backscattered from moving objects, usually red blood cells. The color scale can be selected manually, ranging from two colors (red and blue) to a rainbow palette. At least two distinctly different colors are used to display clearly the direction of flow relative to transducer midline (Figure 1.10). According to the Doppler effect, objects moving towards the transducer will increase the frequency of backscattered echoes relative to emitted frequency and vice versa. However, color assignments are operator dependent.

Therefore, CDFI is used to identify moving blood and display the direction of flow. No Doppler frequency shift occurs at a 90° angle between ultrasound beam and moving blood stream (Figure 1.8). CDFI often contains artifacts:

1 Aliasing (abrupt change from the maximum velocity in one flow direction to the maximum velocity in the opposite direction without crossing the zero line). It can be present in a normal vessel if the scale settings are inadequately low to display flow velocity, i.e. a sonographer uses a low pulse-repetition frequency (Figure 1.9). It can also be present with maximum scale settings in stenosed vessels due to elevated flow velocities. Scale setting control and comparison of vessel course and B-mode findings help to differentiate imaging artifact from pathological finding.

2 "Bleeding" (the presence of moving blood outside the vessel). This artifact can be produced by an oblique strong reflector (mirror image) or by tissue motion adjacent to the vessel. In both circumstances, changing the transducer position and color gain setting helps to optimize the image (Figure 1.10).

Occasionally, CDFI may be unable to depict blood flow since its spatial resolution is lower than the B-mode image. Also, there is a trade-off between B-mode and superimposed CDFI images: larger CDFI boxes require slower frame rates that decrease B-mode resolution and vice versa. CDFI may not be able to display blood flow adequately in tortuous and deep-located vessels and also vessels affected by the low flow states, i.e. near-occlusion. Other forms of flow imaging may be used in these circumstances.

The power Doppler image

Power Doppler imaging displays color-coded intensities of the returned echoes that contain Doppler frequency shifts. Unlike CDFI, power mode Doppler shows direction-independent changes in the energy of signals backscattered by moving objects. Therefore, power mode images are usually created with brightness-adjusted uni-color scales (Figure 1.11). Power mode images show the course of the vessel without color change due to flow direction. Power mode can be used to visualize tortuous and deep-located vessels, branches and slow-moving blood. "Flashing" is the most common artifact that is created by tissue motion and, similarly to "bleeding," displays artifactual flow signals outside the vessel lumen. This can be corrected by changing the gain settings and color box size.

The color velocity image

The color velocity imaging (CVI) display is similar to CDFI; however, the color-encoded velocities are derived from time-domain processing of returned echo signals. For example, the CVI image represents the movement of red blood cell clusters in time along the vessel course. It allows a better trade-off between B-mode and color flow information in terms of image resolution due to better utilization of scan lines. CVI can also display functional flow lumen better. It is also used in some laboratories to calculate flow volume estimates in the carotid arteries.

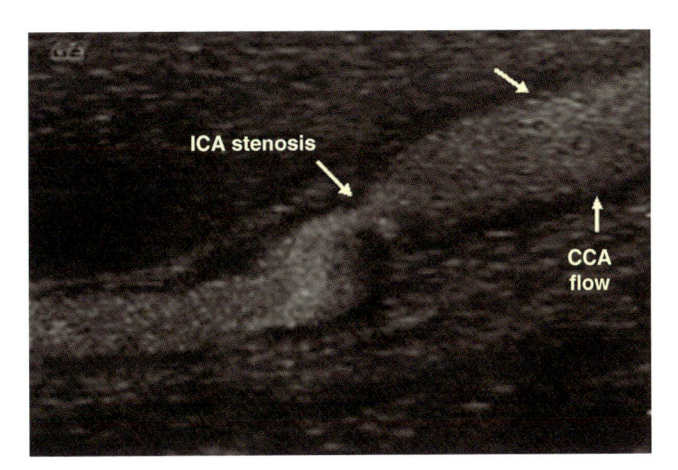

Figure 1.12 B-flow imaging of the carotid stenosis.

B-Flow and compound imaging
Brightness-mode display can also be used to generate flow images since moving blood changes the strength of reflected signals relative to surrounding structures. Combined with electronic focusing and multiple focal zones, such images can provide high-resolution structural scans (Figure 1.2) and superimpose flow signals in gray scale over a B-mode image (Figure 1.12). The B-flow scans avoid aliasing and offer potentially better trade-off between tissue motion and moving blood signals.

Harmonic imaging
An emitted frequency of a diagnostic ultrasound pulse wave passing through tissue can change due to reflection off a moving object (Doppler shift) or during faster sound transmission through fluid compressed at the peak intensity of the ultrasound wave (harmonics). This frequency change occurs mostly during wave propagation (less during reflection). The result is the appearance of the second harmonic frequency that is twice the emitted frequency. This mechanism of non-linear interaction of ultrasound with body tissues allows the use of harmonic frequencies to image tissues with and without contrast substances, and new-generation duplex scanners provide this option. Potential clinical utility of harmonic imaging in cerebrovascular ultrasound includes application of contrast agents for tissue perfusion studies, including brain parenchyma, differentiation of a complete occlusion from subtotal stenosis and better delineation of plaque and vessel wall morphology.

Doppler velocity spectral display
A pulse-wave ultrasound beam can also be used to detect Doppler shift in the returned echoes since moving blood or tissues will change the emitted frequency. This phenomenon is used to measure flow velocity simultaneously with structural and color flow imaging. To obtain velocity values close to real speed of blood, angle correction is applied, which is discussed in the scanning protocol in the next sub-section.

Extracranial duplex ultrasound examination technique and scanning protocol

The extracranial duplex examination should include transverse and longitudinal B-mode scans of the vessels. Examination can start with transverse scanning since it allows fast identification of CCA, jugular vein, the level of bifurcation and the presence of atherosclerotic disease. The transverse examination begins with the most proximal segment of the common carotid artery following its course towards the distal portion, passing through bifurcation and ending at the level of the mandible with visualization of the distal cervical segment of the internal carotid artery (Figure 1.13). The transverse plane permits appreciation of vessel diameter, presence of pathology and anatomic anomalies. The examination is repeated in the longitudinal plane (Figures 1.1 and 1.2), beginning again with the most proximal segment of the CCA and extending the scan throughout the bifurcation, internal and external carotid arteries. The vertebral artery is examined at its origin and also in the mid-cervical segment of the neck (Figure 1.3).

To optimize the gray-scale image, set the dynamic range to 40–50 dB and the time-gain compensation (TGC) as appropriate to the depth of the common carotid and vertebral arteries.

Imaging in the transverse plane
1 With the patient's head turned slightly away from the side being examined, place the ultrasound probe low on the neck, anterior to the sterno-cleido-mastoid muscle, just above the clavicle. The left side of the image should be oriented towards midline structures, i.e. trachea.
2 Locate the proximal segment of the CCA in the transverse plane. Slowly move the probe along the length of the CCA.
3 At the distal end of the CCA, locate the dilatation that identifies the carotid bulb.
4 Slowly move the probe through the region of carotid bulb and note the bifurcation into the internal (ICA) and external (ECA) carotid arteries.
5 Follow the course of the ICA and ECA to the level of mandibule. Document any evidence of pathology, vessel tortuosity and abnormal anatomy.

Imaging in the longitudinal plane
1 Return to the proximal segment of the CCA with the ultrasound probe rotated to image in the longitudinal axis. The left side of the image should be oriented cephalad.
2 Begin with the probe placed anterior to the sterno-cleido-mastoid muscle.

PART I How to Perform Ultrasound Tests

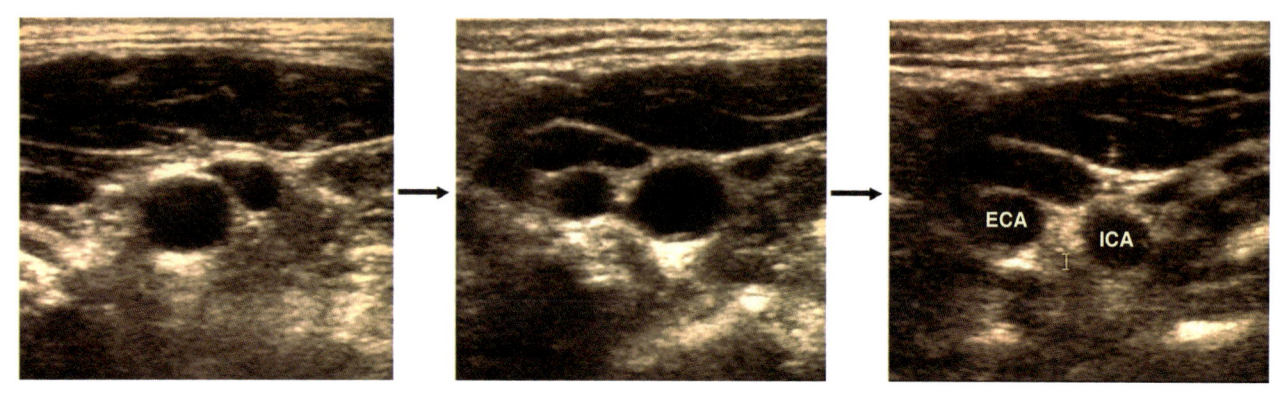

Figure 1.13 Transverse scanning of the proximal CCA, bifurcation, ECA and ICA (from left to right).

3 Image the widest longitudinal axis of the CCA by directing the sound beam perpendicular to the anterior wall of the vessel.
4 Optimize the image so that the normal linear reflectivity of the arterial wall is apparent.
5 Slowly move the probe along the course of the vessel and into the carotid bulb.
6 With the distal CCA and bulb in view, slowly rock the transducer side-to-side to reveal the origins of the internal and external carotid arteries. Care must be taken to angle the probe along the origins to avoid transecting the views of each artery.
7 In turn, follow the courses of the ICA and ECA, optimizing the image for accurate evaluation of anatomy and pathology. Document any evidence of pathology, vessel tortuosity or abnormal anatomy.

Color flow ultrasound evaluation of flow dynamics

1 Return to the longitudinal image of the proximal CCA.
2 Choose the appropriate color pulse repetition frequency (PRF) by setting the color velocity scale for the expected velocities in the vessel. For normal adult arteries, the velocity range is usually around or under 100 cm s^{-1} (or 2.5 kHz Doppler frequency shift). Note that most criteria will use a 125 cm s^{-1} cut-off for velocities elevated due to carotid stenosis. Adjust the scale further to avoid systolic aliasing (low PRF) or diastolic flow gaps (high PRF or filtering) in normal vessels.
3 Optimize the color power and gain so that flow signals are recorded throughout the lumen of the vessel with no "bleeding" of color into the surrounding tissues.
4 Avoid using large or wide color boxes since this will slow frame rates and resolution of the imaging system. Use color boxes that cover entire vessel diameter and 1–2 cm of its length. Align the box, i.e. select appropriate color flow angle correction, according to the vessel geometry and course.

5 Slowly move the probe throughout the course of the CCA, bulb, ICA and ECA.
6 Identify and record regions of flow disturbance, inappropriately high or low velocity signals or the absence of flow signals.
7 To find the vertebral artery, return to the CCA (longitudinal view, transducer position anterior to the sterno-cleido-mastoid muscle). Steer the color beam towards the proximal CCA. Rock the probe slightly to the lateral aspect of the neck to image the vertebral artery as it courses through the transverse processes of the vertebrae ("shadows"). "Heel–toe" the probe above the clavicle to image the origin of the vertebral artery as it arises from the subclavian artery. Confirm that the direction of flow in the VA is the same as the CCA.

Doppler spectral evaluation of flow dynamics

1 Return to the longitudinal image of the CCA.
2 Use the color flow image as a guide for Doppler examination (Figure 1.14).
3 Begin the examination using a Doppler sample volume size of 1.5 mm positioned in the middle of a normal vessel (Figure 1.14).
4 Consistently follow one of the choices for angle correction: parallel to the vessel walls or to the color flow jet.
5 Adjust the Doppler spectral power and gain to optimize the quality of the signal return.
6 Slowly sweep the sample volume throughout the length of the CCA, bulb, ICA and ECA.
7 Perform temporal artery tapping when insonating ECA to differentiate between the ECA and ICA flows. Also note the presence of arterial branches that may be present at the proximal ECA stem.
8 Identify regions of flow disturbance or where flow is absent.
9 Record flow patterns in the proximal and distal CCA, the proximal, mid and distal ICA and the proximal ECA

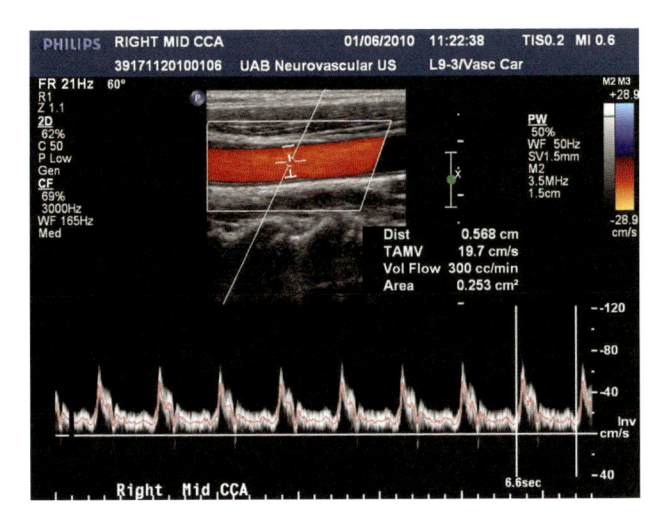

Figure 1.14 Placement of sample volume in the CCA using color flow image as a guide. A small (1.5 mm) gate is used for Doppler spectral measurement and a large (10 mm) gate is used for the flow volume measurements.

at appropriate angles of insonation. Additionally, include Doppler spectral waveforms proximal, within and distal to all areas where flow abnormalities were observed.

10 Locate the origin or proximal segment of the vertebral artery (Figure 1.7). Record flow patterns paying careful attention to flow direction. Follow accessible cervical segments of the vertebral artery (Figure 1.8). Change the angulation of the color box and Doppler sample along with the course of the artery.

Extracranial duplex examination should provide the following data

1 Peak systolic velocity in all vessel segments.
2 End-diastolic velocity in all vessel segments.
3 Ratios of the ICA to CCA peak systolic velocities.
4 Documentation of the Doppler spectral waveform morphology from the CCA, ICA and ECA.
5 Flow direction and peak systolic velocity of the vertebral arteries.
6 Views demonstrating the presence and location of pathology.
7 Images of plaque morphology and surface features.

Tips to improve accuracy

1 Consistently follow a standardized scanning protocol.
2 Perform a complete examination of the carotid and vertebral arteries.
3 Sample velocity signals throughout all arterial segments accessible.
4 Use multiple scan planes.
5 Take time to optimize the B-mode, color and spectral Doppler information.
6 Videotape or create a digital file of the entire study including sound recordings.
7 Always use the highest imaging frequencies to achieve higher resolution.
8 Account for any clinical conditions or medications that might affect velocity.
9 Integrate data from the right and left carotid and vertebral arteries.
10 Do not hesitate to admit uncertainty and list all causes for limited examinations.
11 Expand Doppler examination to intracranial vessels when indicated.

Tips for optimizing color flow set-up

1 According to standardized protocols, the carotid bifurcation should be to the left of the image. This orientation should then clearly indicate the appropriate direction of flow in the common carotid artery and jugular vein. The arterial and venous flow directions are then given color assignments with respect to flow towards or away from the transducer. Traditionally, flow towards the transducer is assigned red (common carotid) and flow away from the probe is assigned blue (jugular vein). The direction of flow relative to the probe will change if the probe is rotated 180° or if the color box is steered in the opposite direction, i.e. the vein will appear red whereas the artery will appear blue. When this occurs, the color should be changed back to the original assignment to avoid confusion. It must also be noted that the color will change along the course of an artery if the flow direction varies throughout the cardiac cycle (triphasic, to-and-fro) or if the vessel changes direction relative to the orientation of the sound beam.

2 The zero baseline of the color bar (PRF) is set at approximately two-thirds of the range with the majority of frequencies allowed in the red direction (for flow towards the brain). This setting allows you to display higher arterial mean frequency shifts (velocities) without aliasing artifacts. You should make allowance for some flow in the reverse (blue) direction to allow for changes in flow direction (i.e. ICA bulb, post-stenotic dilatation). When the transducer is rotated 180°, the color will change (note point 1 above) and the zero baseline will shift with the color changes to accommodate flow in the forward direction. You will need to adjust both the color assignment and the zero baseline to the initial set-up for consistency.

3 The color PRF and zero baseline may need to be readjusted throughout the examination to allow for the changes in velocity that occur with tortuousity and stenosis. It is important to adjust the PRF in the following situations:

Examination of the carotid bulb –
  The color differentiation scale should be set to detect and clearly visualize the slower flow in the boundary separation zone. The range (PRF), however, may need to be set higher to detect increased velocities in the region adjacent to the flow divider.

In the presence of stenosis –
  The color PRF should be increased to display the high velocities and to avoid aliasing.

In the post-stenotic zone –
  The color PRF should be decreased to observe the lower velocities and flow direction changes, if any, found in the region of turbulent flow just distal to the stenosis.

When bruits are encountered –
  The color PRF should be decreased to detect the lower frequencies associated with a bruit. Usually, the frequency of these bruits is less than 1 kHz.

When occlusion is suspected –
  The color PRF should be decreased to detect the pre-occlusive, low velocity, high resistance signal associated with critical stenosis or occlusion and to confirm absence of flow at the site of occlusion.

4 The color wall filter should be set as low as possible. You should note that the color wall filter may automatically increase as you increase the PRF. You may need to decrease the wall filter manually when you decrease the color PRF.

5 The ensemble length (color sensitivity) should be around 12 in systems where this is an adjustable control. You can increase the ensemble length in regions where you want more sensitive color representation. It is important to remember that the frame rate will decrease when the ensemble length is increased (see also point 8 below). There are no circumstances when the ensemble length would be decreased during an extracranial carotid duplex examination.

6 The angle of the color box should be changed to obtain the most acute Doppler angles between the scan lines and the direction of blood flow. This will result in better color display because of more suitable Doppler angles. The angle should always be equal to or less than 60°. Because linear array transducers are steered at angles of 90 and 70° from the center of the array, this may require a "heel–toe" maneuver with the transducer on the surface of the skin to adjust the position of the vessel within the color box. An alternative would be to change physically the orientation of the transducer 180°.

7 The desaturation of color from darker to lighter hues on the color bar indicates increasing Doppler frequency shifts, i.e. increasing velocities. Note that close to the zero baseline, the colors are the darkest. As the velocity increases, the color becomes lighter. You should select colors so that the highest frequency shifts in each direction are of high contrast to each other so that you can readily detect aliasing. For example, you could set the color selections so that low to high velocities are seen as dark blue to light green to aqua in one direction and red to orange to yellow in the opposite flow direction. Aliasing would then appear as aqua adjacent to yellow.

8 The frame rate should be kept as high as possible to capture the very rapid change in flow dynamics that occur with stenosis, especially in the region of the carotid bulb. Remember that frame rate is affected by:

PRF –
  Frame rate decreases with decreasing PRF.
Ensemble length –
  Increasing the color ensemble length will decrease the frame rate.
Width of the color box –
  Increased width will decrease the frame rate.
Depth –
  Deep insonation decreases frame rate.

9 The color box should be kept to a size that is adequate for visualizing the area of interest and yet small enough to keep the frame rate at a reasonable number, approximately 15 or more, to ensure adequate filling of the vessel. The frame rate is usually displayed in hertz on the monitor.

10 The color gain should be adjusted throughout the examination to detect the changing signal strength. If the color gain is not properly adjusted, some color information may be lost or too much color may be displayed. In this case, you will see color in areas where there should be no flow. The gain should initially be adjusted to an "over-gained" level, with color displayed in the tissue and then turned down until the tissue noise just disappears or is minimally present. This is the level at which all color images should be assessed. In situations where there is very low flow or questionable occlusion, an "over-gained" level may be advantageous to show any flow that might be present, e.g. total occlusion versus a near-occlusion or critical stenosis.

References

1 Krayenbuehl H, Yasargil MG. *Cerebral Angiography*, 2nd edn. Stuttgart: GeorgThieme, 1982.
2 Glagov S, Bassiouny HS, Zarnis CK, *et al*. Morphogenesis of the atherosclerotic plaque. In: Hennerici M, Mearis S, eds. *Cerebrovascular Ultrasound: Theory, Practice and Future Developments*. Cambridge: Cambridge University Press, 2001:117–33.
3 Strandness DE, McCutcheon EP, Rushmer RF. Application of a transcutaneous Doppler flowmeter in evaluation of occlusive arterial disease. *Surg Gynecol Obstet* 1966;**122**(5):1039–45.
4 Spencer MP, Reid JM, Davis DL, *et al*. Cervical carotid imaging with a continuous-wave Doppler flowmeter. *Stroke* 1974; **5**(2):145–54.
5 von Reutern GM, Pourcellot L. Cardiac cycle-dependent alternating flow in vertebral arteries with subclavian artery stenoses. *Stroke* 1978;**9**(3):229–36.

2 Intracranial Cerebrovascular Ultrasound Examination Techniques

Andrei V. Alexandrov[1], Marta Rubiera[2], Paola Palazzo[3] & Marsha M. Neumyer[4]

[1]University of Alabama Hospital, Birmingham, AL, USA
[2]Vall d'Hebron Hospital, Barcelona, Spain
[3]Campus Bio-Medico University, Rome, Italy
[4]Vascular Diagnostic Educational Services, Harrisburg, PA, USA

Introduction

The pursuit to understand how the brain works and how it is supplied by blood led Sir Thomas Willis to his landmark 1664 publication, *Cerebri Anatome*. Since then, the network of vessels on the base of the brain has become known as the circle of Willis. Originally, it was depicted in a 1664 drawing by Sir Christopher Wren (Figure 2.1). Three centuries later, the need to detect vasospasm before a delayed ischemic deficit strikes after subarachnoid hemorrhage led Rune Aaslid to perform the first successful ultrasound detection of blood flow signals from the circle of Willis. His artistic take on the circle of Willis and a non-invasive ultrasound approach, now known as transcranial Doppler (TCD), appeared on the cover of the first TCD textbook published in 1986 (Figure 2.1).

In over a quarter or a century since the original paper appeared in 1982 [1], thousands of health professionals have tried to learn TCD. Unlike carotid duplex, skilled sonographers able to perform and understand TCD are still scarce. Many also were disappointed with the non-imaging aspect of TCD and either left the field or switched to transcranial color duplex imaging (TCDI). Despite numerous advances in diagnostic ultrasound, such as harmonic imaging, color flow, power motion Doppler and contrast agents, the skull bone still represents a formidable challenge for signal acquisition and image resolution and the performance of TCD and TCDI remains extremely operator dependent. Regardless of modality, availability of contrast agents or advanced imaging capabilities, education with sufficient supervised hands-on practice and interpretation remains the key to a successful start of practicing intracranial ultrasound. Whether one uses TCD or TCDI, the diagnosis is obtained from waveform interpretation and measurements of flow parameters in the spectral display. Color flow image or power motion screen can provide images highly suggestive of certain pathologies, but the definitive confirmation of flow findings is still derived from the spectral analysis. This chapter describes transducer positioning, the use of anatomic landmarks and appropriate scale settings for the spectral analysis, gray scale and color flow displays.

TCD examination technique

A single-gate spectral TCD was introduced by Rune Aaslid in 1982 to assess cerebral hemodynamics non-ivasively [1]. The four "windows" for insonation (Figure 2.2) are temporal, orbital, foraminal and submandibular [2]. The transtemporal approach allows velocity measurements in the middle (MCA), anterior (ACA), and posterior (PCA) communicating arteries [1–6]. The transorbital approach is used to insonate the ophthalmic artery (OA) and internal carotid artery (ICA) siphon. The transforaminal approach allows insonation of the terminal vertebral (VA) and basilar (BA) arteries through the foramen magnum. The submandibular approach is used to obtain ICA velocities as it enters the skull.

Interestingly, since the 1987 publication by Hennerici *et al.* [5], no major peer-reviewed journal had a dedicated experts' article on how to perform a complete TCD examination that aimed to provide a consensus approach and recommended a set of insonation steps and measurements that should be taken into consideration as test performance standards. As a result, a number of practices perform very limited TCD examinations (often restricted to the proximal MCA and ACA segments) while regulatory agencies require "bilateral" TCD examinations without specifying the extent of transtemporal examination or the use of orbital, foramenal or submandibular windows. Thus, 20 years after the landmark publications on TCD, the American Society of Neuroimaging Clinical Practice Committee assembled an international group of experts to define what represents the test performance standard, i.e. a complete TCD examination.

Cerebrovascular Ultrasound in Stroke Prevention and Treatment, 2nd edition. Edited by Andrei V. Alexandrov. © 2011 Blackwell Publishing Ltd.

PART I How To Perform Ultrasound Tests

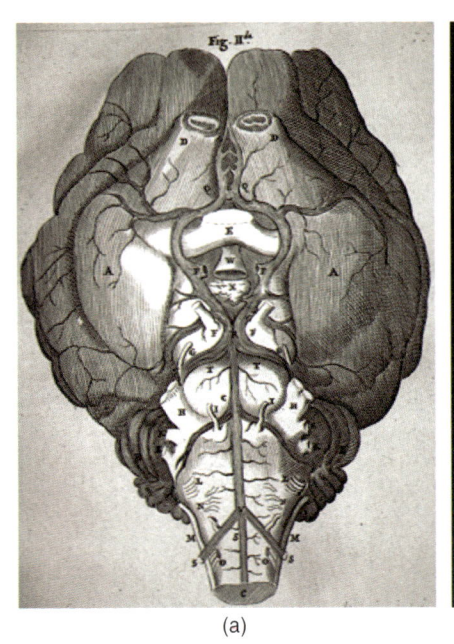

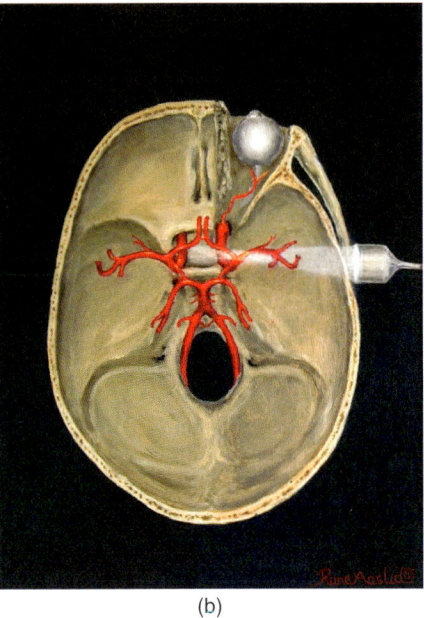

(a) (b)

Figure 2.1 Circle of Willis as depicted by (a) Sir Christopher Wren (1664) and (b) Dr Rune Aaslid (1986). The authors are indebted to Rune Aaslid for providing a high resolution digital copy of his painting of the circle of Willis.

The text below largely represents their paper [6], and also the present authors' personal recommendations on how to improve scanning techniques.

Where to start?

For a typical diagnostic TCD examination, use a fast 3–5 s sweep speed that allows you to see details of the waveform and spectrum (Figure 2.3). If your ultrasound machine provides a large monitor, adjust the sweep speed so that you are not too tired at the end of examination to hold the transducer steady to complete long sweeps without artifacts or displacement of the sample volume. This is particualrly important if you use the envelope to provide automated cal-culations of the velocity. For the envelope to provide correct calculations, the entire sweep has to be completed with an even-intensity, optimized waveform. Longer acquisition periods will result in varying intensity and velocities, particularly in restless or uncooperative patients.

To shorten the time necessary to find the window for insonation and to identify different arterial segments with a single-gate spectral TCD, the examination should begin with the maximum power and gate settings (i.e. power 100%, gate 10–15 mm) for the transtemporal and foramenal approaches. Although this recommendation seemingly violates the rule of using ultrasound power "as low as resonably achievable" (ALARA), it allows the time necessary to find windows and to complete the examination to be shortened, thus satisfying the second safety rule of "reducing the overall patient exposure to ultrasound energy." The goals of

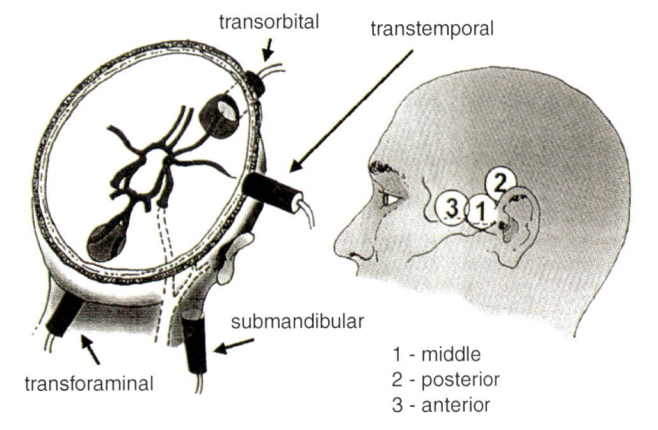

Figure 2.2 Acoustic windows for transcranial Doppler examination.

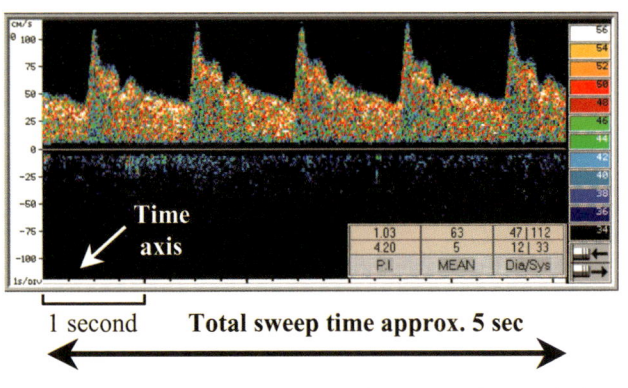

Figure 2.3 Spectral Doppler recording with time as the horizontal axis.

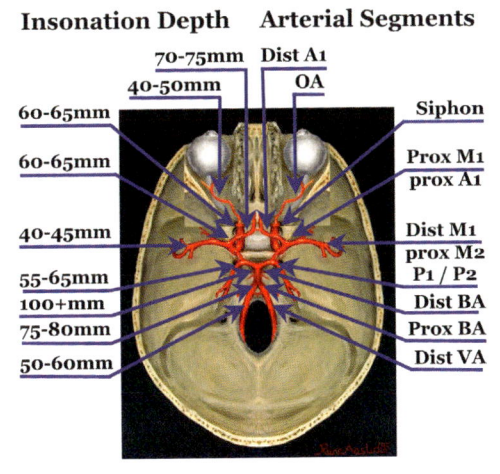

Figure 2.4 Proximal intracranial segments for transcranial Doppler examination.

a "non-image-guided" single-gate spectral TCD examination are as follows:
1 to follow the course of each major branch of the circle of Willis with spectral display;
2 to identify, optimize and store the highest velocity signals;
3 to obtain TCD spectra from at least two key points per artery (Figure 2.4); and
4 to identify, optimize and store any abnormal or unusual waveforms.

Transtemporal insonation steps (Figure 2.5)

Step 1: Set the depth at 50 mm (most TCD units start with this depth since the mid-point of the M1 MCA segment was established at an average of 50 mm depth in cadaver skulls [7]).
Place the probe above the zygomatic arch and aim it slightly upwards and anterior to the contralateral ear/window.
Find any flow signal (window) and avoid too anterior and too posterior angulation.
Find a flow signal directed towards the probe which resembles MCA flow. A normal MCA flow is a low-resistance waveform (Figure 2.2) similar to the ICA flow pattern.
By decreasing the depth, follow the signal to the distal M1 key-point of insonation without losing the signal. Often, a slight adjustment of the probe angulation is needed.
Store the distal M1 MCA signal at 45 mm. If bi-directional signals are found, store the highest velocity signal in each direction (distal M1–proximal M2 branches). Arbitrarily, M2 branches should appear at 40 mm depth or less. However, the anterior temporal branch may arise much deeper.
Step 2: Follow the signals until they disappear at shallow 30–40 mm depths.
Store any abnormal signal.
Return to the distal M1 MCA signal.
Step 3: Follow the M1 MCA stem to its origin at 60–70 mm depthsdepending on the size of the adult patient skull. Pay attention to the sound and velocity changes since insonation of the terminal ICA is also possible at these depths.
Find the ICA bifurcation at approximately 65 mm (range 58–70 mm in adults) and obtain both proximal M1 MCA and proximal A1 ACA signals.
Store a bi-directional signal of the bifurcation (M1/A1).
Step 4: Follow the A1 ACA signal to 70–75 mm depth.
Store the distal A1 ACA signal at 70 mm.
Step 5: Follow the distal A1 ACA signal to the midline depth range (75 – 80 mm). The A1 ACA signal may disappear or a bi-directional signal may appear at the midline depth.
Store any abnormal signals.
Return to bifurcation at 65 mm.
Step 6: Find the terminal ICA signal just inferior and sometimes slightly posterior to the bifurcation at 60–65 mm. If the probe is angled inferior and anterior to the ICA bifurcation at 60–70 mm depths, the distal part of the supraclinoid siphon can be found through the temporal window.
Store any abnormal signal.
Return to the bifurcation at 65 mm.
Step 7: Set the depth at 63 mm and slowly turn the transducer posteriorly by 10–30°. Usually there is a flow gap between the ICA bifurcation and the PCA signals.
Find PCA signals directed towards (P1) and away from (P2) the probe at a depth range of 55 – 75 mm.
Store the PCA signals with the highest velocity.

Transorbital insonation steps (Figure 2.6)

Step 1: Decrease power to the minimum (17 mW) or 10%. Set the depth at 50–52 mm, place the transducer over the eyelid and angle it slightly medially.
Determine flow pulsatility and direction in the distal ophthalmic artery.
Store the distal OA signals at 52 mm.
Step 2: Increase the depth to 60–64 mm and find the ICA siphon flow signals. The siphon signals are usually located medially in the orbital window.
Store bidirectional signals at 62 mm (C3 or the siphon genu). If only unidirectional signals are obtainable, store signals directed towards (C4 or the lower limb of the siphon) and away from (C2 or the upper limb) the probe.

Transforaminal insonation steps (Figure 2.7)

Step 1: Set the system back to full power.
Place the transducer at midline 1 inch (2.5 cm) below the edge of the skull and aim it at the bridge of the nose.
Set the depth at 75 mm (presumed location of both terminal VAs and proximal BA).
Identify a flow signal directed away from the probe, i.e. find the window. This signal can be arbitrarily assigned to the terminal vertebral arteries (slightly lateral probe angulation) or the proximal basilar artery (medial and slightly upward angulation).

PART I How To Perform Ultrasound Tests

Increasing the depth, follow the flow directed away from the probe. This depth increase presumably focuses the beam on the proximal BA in most adults.

Store the proximal BA signal arbitrarilly assigned to the depth of 80 mm.

Step 2: Follow the basilar artery to 90 mm (mid-BA segment). Bi-directional signals may be found at various depths with a low resistance flow in the cerebellar arteries directed towards the probe.

Store any abnormal signals.

Step 3: Follow the distal BA segment to a depth of 100+ mm until it disappears or is replaced by the anterior circulation signals.

Store the highest velocity signal obtained at the most distal depth of the basilar artery insonation.

Step 4: Follow the stem of the basilar artery backwards while decreasing the depth of insonation to 80 mm and confirm previous findings.

Step 5: Place the probe about 1 inch (2.5 cm) laterally to the midline and aim towards the bridge of the nose or slightly towards the contralateral eye.

Find the vertebral artery (VA) flow signal directed away from the probe.

Follow the course of the terminal VA segment intracranially from 80 to 40 mm.

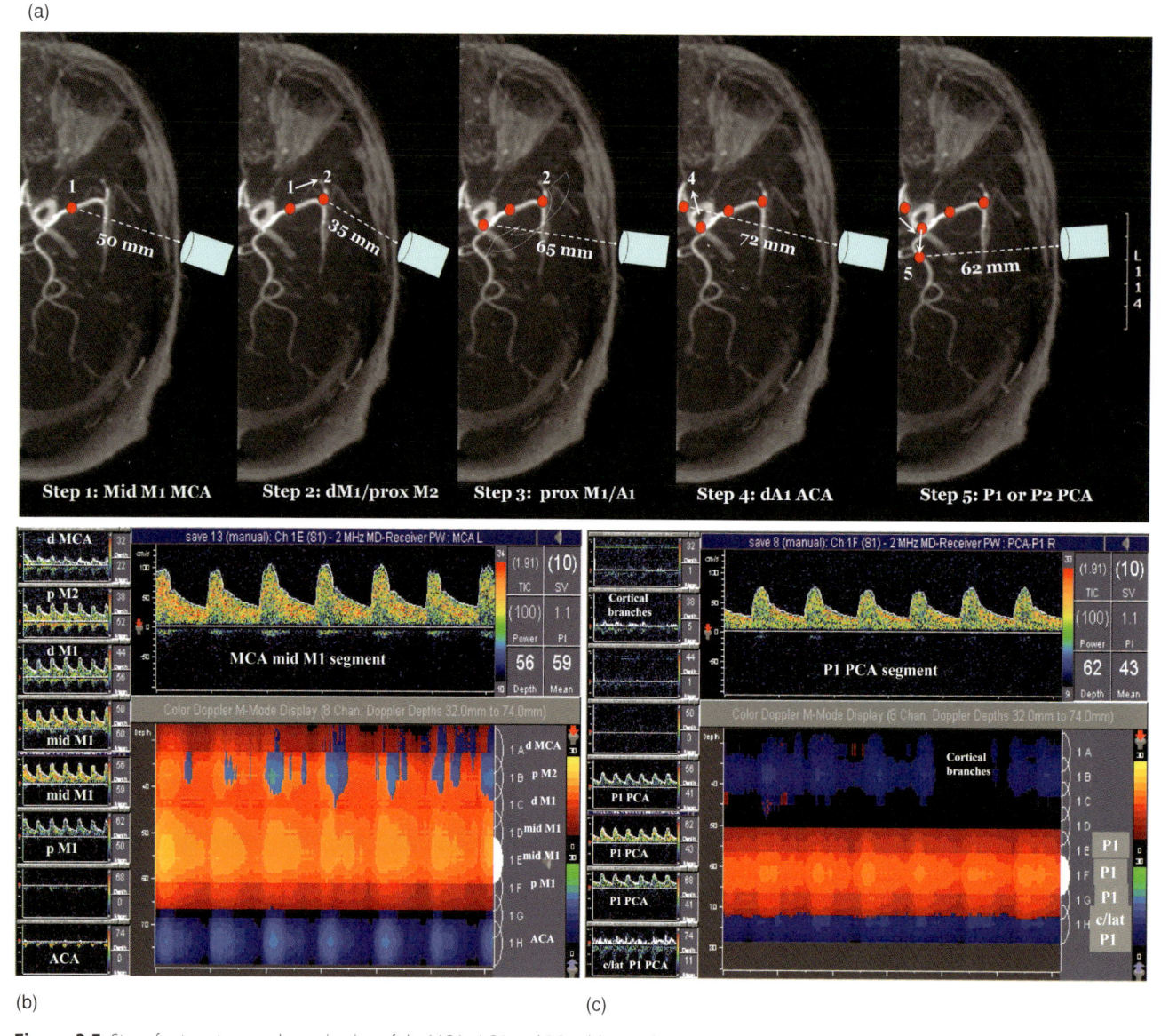

Figure 2.5 Steps for transtemporal examination of the MCA, ACA and PCA. (a) Transducer positioning and angulation relative to anatomic structures as shown by MRI. Lower images represent M-mode and spectra detected from the upward-and-anterior (b) and straight-in/slightly-posterior (c) transducer angulations.

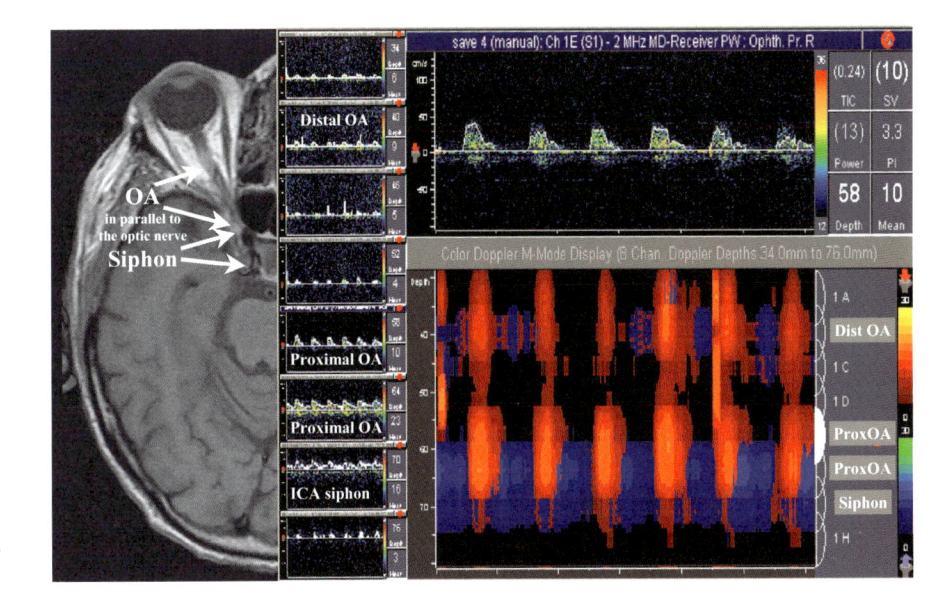

CHAPTER 2 Intracranial Cerebrovascular Ultrasound Examination Techniques

Figure 2.6 Transorbital insonation (spectra and M-mode) relative to anatomic structures as shown by MRI.

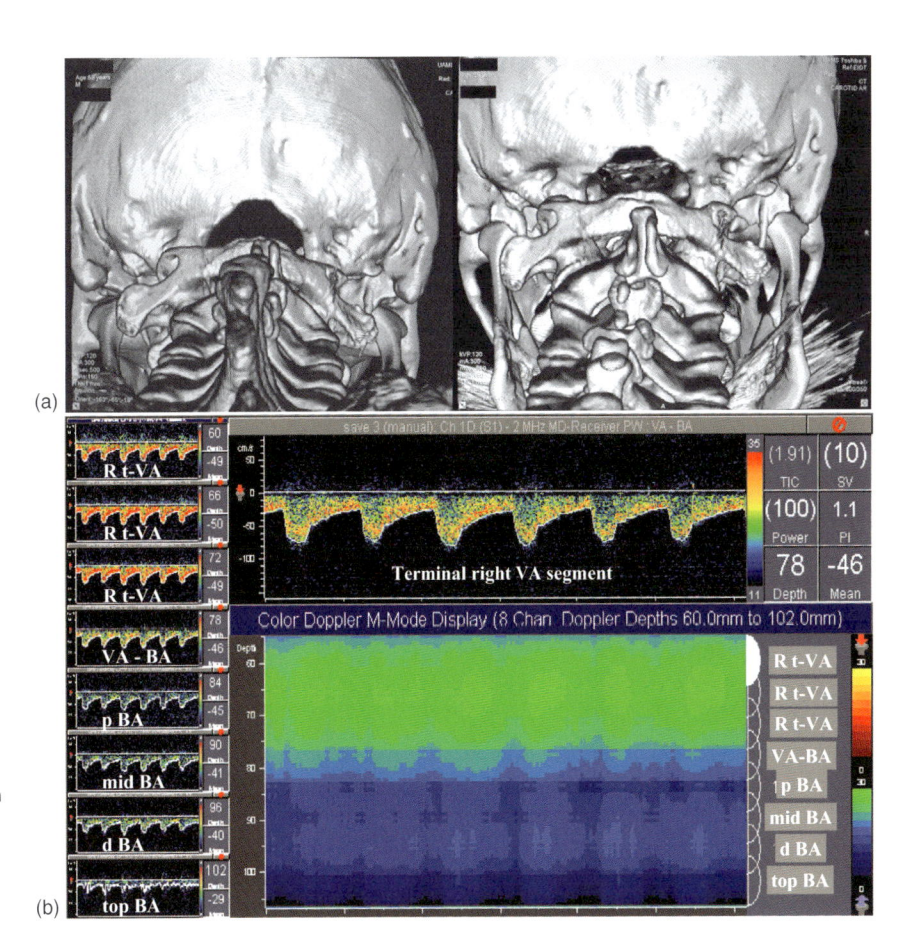

Figure 2.7 Transforaminal examination through foramen magnum (image (a) reconstructed from CT, courtesy of Dr William Culp) (b) Spectra and M-mode findings of the terminal VA and basilar artery stem.

PART I How To Perform Ultrasound Tests

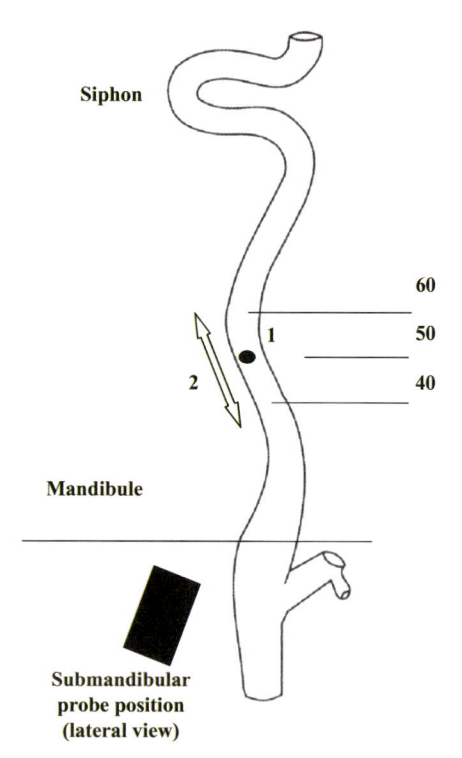

Figure 2.8 Schematic representation of sub-mandibular insonation of the distal ICA prior to its entrance to the skull.

Store the VA signals at 60 mm or at the depth of the highest velocity signal.
Step 6: Place the probe on the contralateral side 1 inch (2.5 cm) off the midline position.
Repeat the VA examination steps for the contralateral vessel from 80 to 40 mm.
Store the VA signals at 60 mm or at the depth of the highest velocity signal.

Submandibular insonation steps (Figure 2.8)
Step 1: Place the probe laterally under the jaw anterior and medial to the sterno-cleido-mastoid muscle. Aim the transducer upwards and slightly medially.
Set the depth at 50 mm.
Find a low-resistance flow directed away from the probe.
Step 2: Increase the depth from 50 to 60 mm and decrease to 40 mm.
Store the distal ICA signal at the depth that shows the highest velocity signal.
At a shallow depth, perform the temporal artery tap to differentiate from the external carotid artery flow signals.

Practical advice
1 Avoid too anterior or too posterior angulation of the probe at the begining of the transtemporal examination.
2 Do not settle on the first signal obtained. Always keep searching for higher velocity signals.
3 Once the highest signal has been found, avoid losing signals when switching the depth of insonation: follow the course of the arteries with slight angulation of the probe over the same window whenever possible. Remember the normal depth ranges (Figure 2.4) and flow direction (Figures 2.6–2.9) for the circle of Willis and supplying vessels for adults.
4 Try not to take the probe off the skull until investigation of all segments through that window is completed.
5 Try not to lose arterial flow signals while switching between the segments of the same artery.
6 Memorize the transducer position and angulation if the patient is restless or insonation is being interrrupted.
7 Use insonation across the midline to locate contralateral MCA/ACA signals if one temporal window is suboptimal, absent or not accessible. [Insonation across the midline can be difficult without imaging. You can measure the

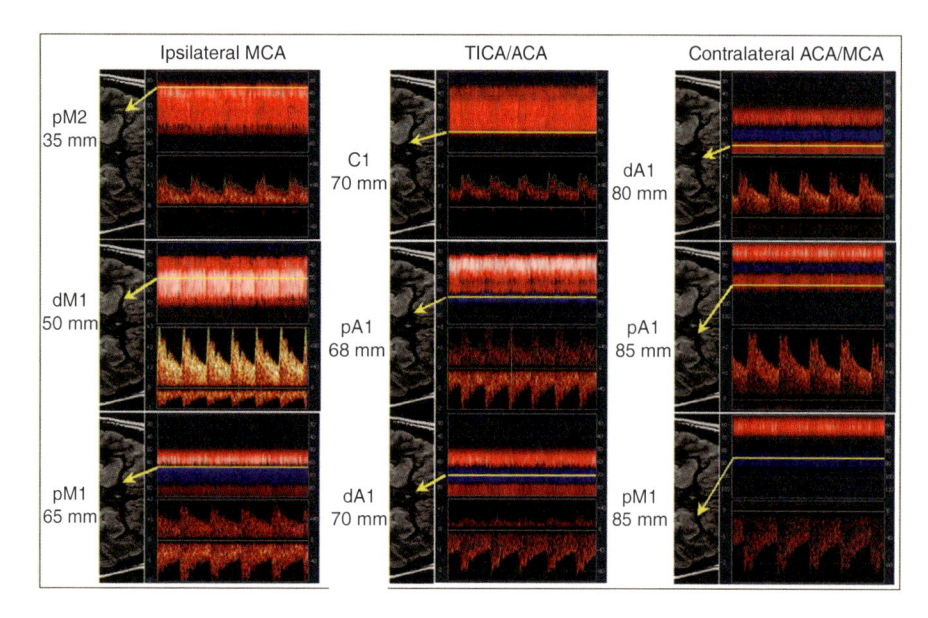

Figure 2.9 Uni-lateral and across-midline insonation (power motion Doppler and spectra) of the anterior circulation vessels with corresponding anatomic segments depicted by MRI scan inserts.

18

CHAPTER 2 Intracranial Cerebrovascular Ultrasound Examination Techniques

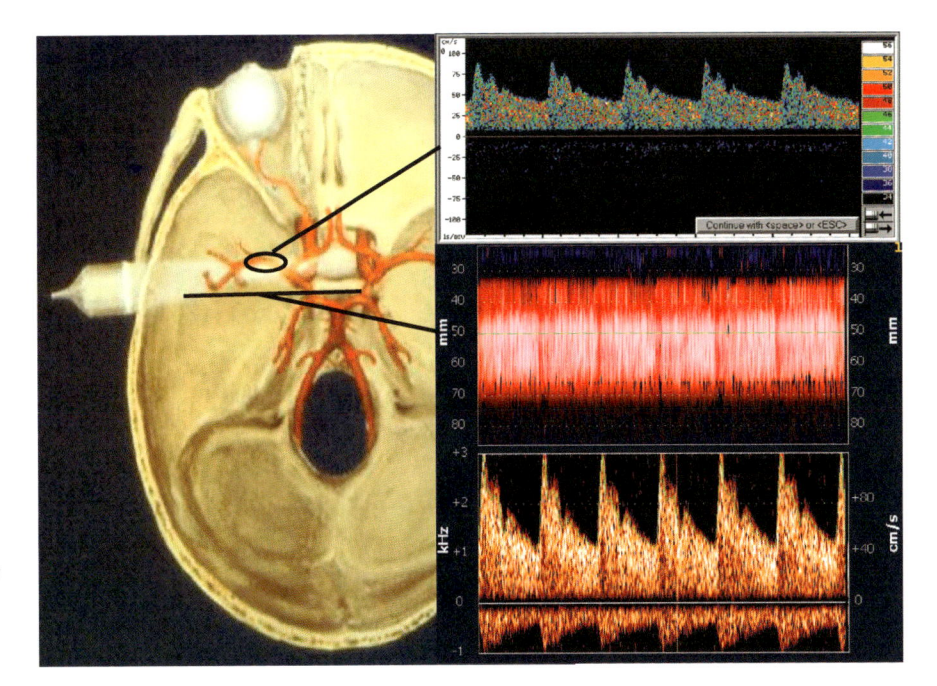

Figure 2.10 Relative extent of insonation by a traditional single-gate TCD and a newer generation single-transducer power motion Doppler system.

diameter of the patient's skull to determine the midline depth. In most adults, midline is located between 70 and 80 mm. Once you cross the midline, the vessel identification becomes reversed: contra-lateral A1 ACA is directed towards the probe (range 75–85 mm), while others are directed away from the probe: M1 MCA (range 85–105+ mm), TICA (80–85 mm) and P1/P2 PCA (75–83 mm). The top of the basilar segment at midline depths and the very proximal contra-lateral P1 PCA can be directed towards the probe from the transtemporal window.]

8 Do not overgain the signals (the background should not contain any noise signals).

9 In case of weak signals, boost the signal and/or gain settings and apply manual measurements.

10 Perform a complete examination, document the mean flow velocities, pulsatility indices and flow direction in all major arteries (Figure 2.10) and double-check missing arterial segments.

11 Remember that vessel identification is operator dependent. Gain experience from studying normal individuals and patients with angiographically documented arterial pathology.

12 Consistently apply insonation protocol for TCD examinations. Use notes to document information pertinent to interpretation.

M-mode or PMD/TCD examination technique

Transcranial power motion mode Doppler (PMD) was recently invented by Mark Moehring [3]. PMD, or M-mode, simultaneously displays flow intensity and direction over 6 cm of intracranial space (Figure 2.10). An advantage offered by this mode of insonation is to display all flow signals obtainable at a given position and direction of the transducer. The promise of PMD is to make TCD examination easy even for an inexperienced person since it takes a long time to acquire the skills to find windows of insonation with a single-channel spectral TCD.

PMD is combined with a single-channel spectral analysis (Figure 2.10). Using a single transducer, a clinician can search for a window of insonation without "blindly" choosing a depth for spectral analysis and without relying on sound recognition/arm coordination. PMD shows flow signals on a color-coded, real time display that may serve as a guide for proper spectral analysis (Figures 2.6–2.10). A standard PMD/TCD insonation protocol is provided below:

A standard PMD/spectral TCD insonation protocol for an average-sized adult patient

Transtemporal insonation

1 Set the PMD display at 30–80 mm depth range.

2 Apply the transducer to the middle aspect of the temporal window above the zygomatic arch and close to the ear lobe.

3 Maintain slightly upward and anterior angulation of the probe.

4 Set noise levels to allow minimal background signal on the PMD display.

5 If no flow signals appear, advance the transducer in slow, circular movements towards the anterior temporal window.

PART I How To Perform Ultrasound Tests

6 While advancing the transducer, keep changing the probe angulation from the anterior to perpendicular direction relative to the temporal bone.

7 Find a window with maximum spatial presence of the middle cerebral artery (MCA) flow signature between 30 and 70 mm depths. In other words, attempt to fill the PMD screen with color flow signals over the MCA depth range.

8 Readjust the probe angulation to detect flow signals in the M2 MCA segments (depths 30–45 mm), terminal ICA (depths 60–70 mm) and anterior cerebral artery (ACA) (depths 60–75 mm).

9 Return to the view of the MCA origin and slightly rotate the transducer 10–30° posteriorly and downwards to detect flow in the posterior cerebral artery (PCA depth range is 60–70 mm).

10 At all transducer positions, note if the contra-lateral flow signals can be displayed (depth ≥75 mm in most adults).

11 Sequentially advance the TCD sample volume in 1 mm steps over all arterial segments detected by PMD to display spectral information.

Transorbital insonation

1 Decrease the power output of the unit to 10%.

2 Set the PMD depth at 30–80 mm range.

3 Place the transducer over the closed eyelid and angle it slightly medially.

4 Align the transducer position to display flow signatures at depths of 40–70 mm.

5 Determine pulsatility and direction of flow in the ophthalmic artery.

6 Sample spectral information from the distal ophthalmic artery (depths 40–55 mm) and ICA siphon (depths 55–70).

Transforaminal insonation

1 Set the PMD depth at 60–110 mm range.

2 Place the transducer suboccipitally at the midline and aim towards the bridge of the nose and detect any flow signal moving away from the probe.

3 Align the transducer position to display maximum flow signatures between 75 and 100 mm.

4 Sample spectral information from the proximal (80 mm), middle (90 mm) and distal (100+ mm) portions of the basilar artery.

5 To find the terminal vertebral arteries, set the PMD depth at 30–80 mm range.

6 Place the transducer laterally 0.5–1 inch (1.25–2.5 cm) off the midline and aim towards the orbits. Avoid angulation to the contra-lateral side.

7 Sample spectral flow signals from all segments of the terminal vertebral artery and repeat the examination on the other side. Note that a small sample volume for spectral TCD delivers higher intensities with a PMD/spectral TCD unit. The trade-off between sensitivity and spatial resolution may remain optimal even with a small 3 mm spectral gate.

Useful rules to remember

1 TCD velocities do not measure cerebral blood flow volume. However, changes in the mean flow vlocity or disapearance/reappearance of the end diastolic flow may correlate with changes in the cerebral blood flow.

2 Cerebral blood flow and mean flow velocities decrease with age.

3 An increase in blood pressure may increase flow velocities while chronic hypertension often increases pulsatility of flow by affecting the end diastolic velocity.

4 Hyperventilation decreases the mean flow velocity and increases pulsatility of flow through vasoconstriction.

5 Hypercapnia increases the mean flow velocity and decreases pulsatility of flow through vasodilation.

6 A waveform pattern is determined by various factors, including cardiac output and blood pressure, and also the brain autoregulatory or vasomotor responces and focal or diffuse arterial lesions.

7 A waveform pattern can also be determined by the downstream circulatory conditions such as compensatory vasodilation, loss of autoregulation or increased resistance due to elevated intracranial pressure (ICP).

8 Cerebral blood flow and mean flow velocity are inversely proportionate to vessel radius and length and blood viscosity.

9 When homologous arterial segments are compared, normal variations of up to 30% in flow velocities and pulsatility indexes can be expected.

10 Variations in the angle of insonation can account for up to 15% and the resistance of downstream vasculature during breathing cycles for another 15% of a normal velocity/pulsatility difference.

11 Normal variations of up to 100% in flow velocities between homologous segments such as PCA or VA can be attibuted to the tortuous vessel course, angle of insonation changes, anatomic variants of the circle of Willis and hypoplasia/atresia.

12 Anatomic variations of the circle of Willis are common: it is normal (symmetric, with all proximal segments and communicating arteries properly developed) in only about 20% of patients.

13 If an intracranial artery is not found, this impression itself does not mean that this artery is occluded.

Tips to improve accuracy

1 Perform a complete and thorough examination and store actual sound recordings when possible.

2 Try not to lose flow signals when changing the depth of insonation ("go with the flow").

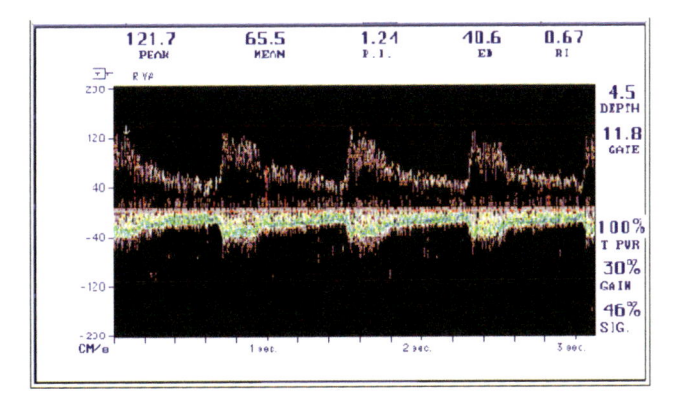

Figure 2.11 Mirror image (spectra above the baseline) artifact with a bright reflector (terminal VA) during transforamenal TCD examination.

3 Target clinically involved arterial segment(s) or suspected level of occlusion(s).

4 Use headphones and the maximum pulse repetition frequency possible, particularly when searching for weak, high-pitch jets, i.e. stenoses.

5 To focus on a specific segment, decrease the gate or sample volume, and increase gain, if necessary.

6 Avoid mirror artifacts (do not overgain with older generation TCD units, decrease power or sample volume) (Figure 2.11).

7 Account for medications and clinical conditions which change the flow volume/velocity.

8 Do not hesitate to admit uncertainty and list all probable causes.

Previous studies have established normal values and variations for depth of insonation [1,2,4–6] and a multicenter study was performed to validate TCD findings [7]. Some variation between the depths of insonation can be expected due to the differences in patient skull diameters and sample volumes used for insonation. Regardless of which scanning protocol or depth ranges are adopted, a local validation of TCD findings must be performed at each laboratory.

Transcranial color duplex imaging

Transcranial color duplex imaging (TCDI) is performed with a phased array transducer. Most often the Doppler carrier frequency is in the range 2–3.5 MHz with an imaging frequency up to 4 MHz. It is important to optimize not only the B-mode image, but also the color and spectral Doppler information for accurate evaluations [8–15]. Although TCDI provides a convenient flow imaging map, a single-channel spectral Doppler interrogation remains the mainstay of diagnosis, even with newer transcranial ultrasound techniques.

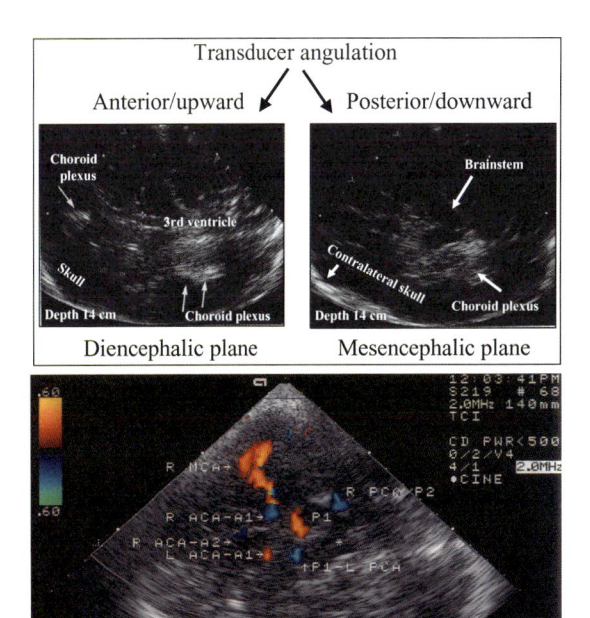

Figure 2.12 Transducer angulation, resulting B-mode images and color flow depiction during transtemporal transcranial color duplex examination (images courtesy of Dr Eva Bartels).

The B-mode image

The anatomic landmarks vary with the acoustic window chosen and transducer angulation (Figure 2.12). It is important to:

1 pay careful attention to the width and depth of the sector image;

2 optimize signal return throughout the depth of the image using time gain compensation (TGC);

3 place the focal zone at the level of the area of interest or immediately inferior to this region;

4 achieve appropriate gray-scale contrast by adjusting the dynamic range so that the echo intensity clearly defines intracranial bony and soft tissue anatomy.

The color Doppler image

The color Doppler image represents Doppler-shifted frequencies within a designated area of interest, the color box. Fairly often, the entire circle of Willis can be displayed within the color box. If this is not the case, the anterior (Figure 2.13) and posterior circulation can be studied separately. It is important to:

1 optimize the color display by proper choice of colors to represent forward and reverse flow: choose contrasting colors to represent forward and reverse high-velocity signals;

2 use a high frame rate because you are expecting arterial signals with moderate antegrade velocity;

PART I How To Perform Ultrasound Tests

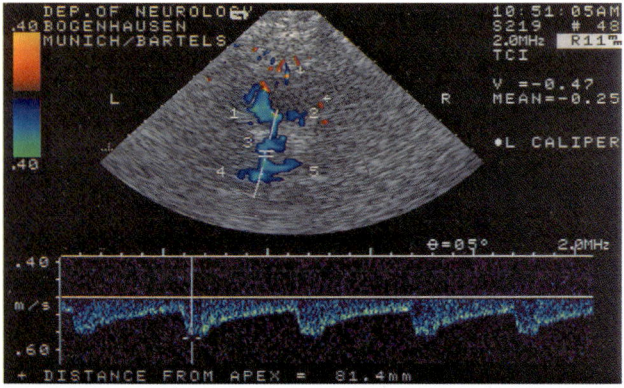

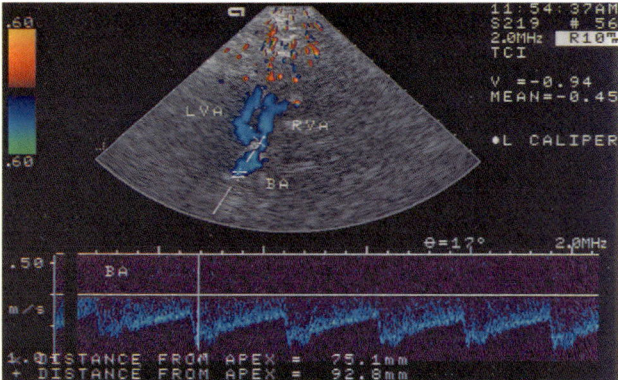

Figure 2.13 Transforamenal transcranial color duplex examination and spectra (courtesy of Dr Eva Bartels).

3 adjust the color gain so that the lumen of the vessels is filled without evidence of "bleeding" of color into the surrounding tissues;
4 change the color velocity scale (PRF) often throughout the course of the examination to detect variations in velocity that occur with vessel tortuosity, stenosis and occlusion;
5 keep the wall filter as low as possible so that detection of low-velocity, low-amplitude signals will not be overlooked;
6 remember that "seeing is believing": do not assume that what you see on the image is all detectable vasculature – open up out-of-plane segments by using your knowledge of anatomy and "go with the flow" principle.

Doppler spectral analysis

The Doppler spectral display contains diagnostic information similar to "non-image-guided" TCD. However, TCDI allows angle correction and the velocity values will be different from those for a non-image-guided TCD that assumes a zero angle of insonation [16,17]. The TCDI display should document the peak systolic, mean and end-diastolic velocities, the resistance index (RI) or the pulsatility index (PI). The following are important:
1 Use adequate Doppler power to allow penetration but to limit the duration of high power use.
2 Employ a low wall filter so that low-velocity, low-amplitude signals can be detected.

3 Vary the sample volume size, velocity scale and Doppler gain to obtain characteristic and accurate spectral information from the intracranial arteries.
4 Whenever possible, achieve displays of color jet as long as feasible, particularly if angle correction is sought [17,18].
5 As a rule, we do not require angle correction and sample all segments during routine examinations at a 0° angle.
6 If you use *TCD* criteria, change the angle of insonation to *0° for all vessels*.
7 Correlate audible Doppler signal with the spectral display for *all* accessible arterial segments and make sure that you agree with measurements provided by automated envelope placement.
8 When in doubt, use manual cursor placement to measure velocities.

TCDI examination technique

Unlike transcranial Doppler, the TCDI examination allows the visualization of anatomic landmarks and spatial course of the arteries that are helpful for vessel identification (Figures 2.12 and 2.13). By complementing the duplex examination with color flow or power Doppler and, when available, 3-dimensional imaging, the course of the arteries can be traced and arterial segments can be identified with more certainty.

The acoustic windows that are employed for TCD are also useful for TCDI, i.e. transtemporal, orbital and foramenal. An additional frontal window has recently been described to insonate the origins of A2 ACA segments [19].

Using the transtemporal approach, the examiner should look for the petrous ridge of the temporal bone, cerebral falx, the supracellar cistern, third ventricle and the cerebral peduncles as anatomic landmarks [20]. From the suboccipital (or foramenal) window, the examiner should find the foramen magnum and the occipital bone. B-mode imaging through the orbit should reveal the globe and optic nerve. These are useful anatomic landmarks that allow you to select the transducer position over the best achievable window, optimize image quality and direct interrogation towards structures that surround arteries intracranially.

Using the transtemporal window

1 The study is initiated with the patient lying in the supine position with the head straight.
2 It is best for the examiner to sit or stand behind the patient, with their arm or elbow resting on the pillow beside the patient's ear.
3 Place the ultrasound transducer on the temporal bone in the pre-auricular area anterior to the ear and cephalad to the zygomatic arch. The left side of the image should display the frontal portion of the intracranial structures.
4 Angle the transducer slightly superiorly to visualize the anterior cerebral circulation. You should note that the

ipsilateral anterior circulation is at the top of the image and that you can fairly often see through the midline of the brain to visualize the contralateral anterior circulation. Although infrequent in the majority of patients, you may occasionally visualize the posterior circulation also. When this is possible, the posterior circulation will appear to the right of the monitor while the anterior circulation lies to the left.

5 Begin the examination with the maximum image depth set at up to 16 cm. This will allow visualization of the contralateral skull and interrogation of the entire intracranial field in most adults.

6 Using B-mode imaging, you should be able to identify the lesser wing of the sphenoid bone extending anteriorly and the petrous ridge of the temporal bone extending posteriorly.

7 From this point, angle the transducer slightly superiorly to image the third ventricle. Also pay attention if the image captures falx and peduncles. This will establish the midline structures and relative position of the anterior and posterior circulation vessels.

8 Reduce the imaging depth to 8–10 cm to study the ipsilateral anterior circulation. Set the color controls to allow for equal forward and reverse flow velocities and steer the color box straight down from center.

9 Use as narrow a width of the color box as possible to interrogate the middle cerebral artery to the level of the bifurcation. This will increase the frame rate and prevent aliasing of signals in normal arteries. Although angle correction may be possible over short segments of arteries, it is best to maintain a 0° angle of insonation to prevent velocity overestimation and make measurements comparable with application of TCD diagnostic criteria.

10 Using color flow imaging, follow the course of the middle cerebral artery to its bifurcation. You may need to angle the probe slightly anteriorly and superiorly to image M2 branches, return back to the M1 segment position and then search for the anterior cerebral artery (ACA). The normal ACA will be displayed in blue as it courses away from the transducer towards the midline of the brain. The A2 segment can occasionally be visualized extending anteriorly and upwards after a characteristic turn at the level of ACommA or merging with contra-lateral A1 ACA displayed in red under normal circulatory conditions at midline depths. The ACommA usually cannot be differentiated from the neighboring ACAs because of its small size.

11 When sampling in the region of the bifurcation, the terminal segment of the internal carotid artery (ICA) can be visualized by tilting the transducer slightly inferiorly. Although blood flow is most commonly towards the transducer, the flow direction relative to the ultrasound beam can vary in this often tortuous segment.

12 Angle the ultrasound beam slightly posteriorly and inferiorly to image posterior cerebral artery and posterior communicating artery, if present. This can be achieved by steering the box so that it is positioned over the peduncles. You should note that the posterior cerebral artery wraps around the peduncle. Flow towards the transducer is commonly assigned to the P1 PCA segment and flow away from the transducer is considered to represent the P2 PCA segment distal to the origin of the posterior communicating artery (PCOA). Given the depth of the posterior cerebral artery and the relatively low velocity, the color scale (PRF) may need to be reduced in order to optimize the return signal. If you are able to visualize the top of the basilar artery, you may be able to image both the ipsilateral (red) and contra-lateral (blue) P1 segments.

13 Keeping in mind the anatomy and the appropriate angulation of the sound beam relevant to the axis of the vessels, you should be able to image the functioning posterior communicating artery (PCommA), which is of longer length, as it connects the anterior and posterior segments of the circle.

Using the foramenal window

1 Have the patient sit up on a chair or lie on their side with the head tilted forward ("bring your chin to your chest") to image the vertebral and basilar arteries. This creates an easily accessible acoustic window between the cranium and the atlas of the vertebral column (Figures 2.7, 2.12 and 2.13). The transducer could be placed about 1 inch (2.5 cm) below the skull line at midline or slightly to the right or left with the beam angled towards the bridge of the nose. The first structure that you will encounter is the large anechoic foramen magnum. Surrounding this you will see the brightly echogenic rim of the occipital bone. Blood flow will normally be away from the transducer in the vertebral arteries and a Y-shaped color flow image of the vertebro-basilar junction can be visualized at 6–8 cm depth (Figure 2.13).

2 Examine the Doppler spectra of the vertebral arteries along their course to the confluence forming the basilar artery. You may see the posterior inferior cerebellar arteries (PICAs) branching from the vertebral arteries. Because these small branches course towards the transducer, they should appear in red. It is important to standardize your imaging protocol so that, if you can not image both vertebral arteries together, the right and left vertebral arteries always appear in the same location on the color flow image. It is our custom to orient the transducer so that the right vertebral artery appears to the right of the image and the left vertebral artery to the left of the image.

3 From the level of the junction of the vertebral arteries, press the transducer slightly inferiorly while aiming it superiorly to visualize the course of the mid and distal portions of the basilar artery. Remember that visualization of the "Y" sign does not mean interception of the distal basilar artery. The basilar artery is most commonly imaged at a depth range of 7–11 cm [20]. Since color flow depth range may be less than in the B-mode, a single-gate spectral Doppler interrogation of the distal BA depth may be performed without a color box. Note that the top-of-the-basilar segment can be visualized using the transtemporal approach or with the help of ultrasound contrast substances.

4 If cerebellar branches are detectable along the course of the basilar artery, use them to identify basilar artery segments, i.e. the anterior inferior cerebellar arteries (AICAs) can be found at the proximal basilar artery while the next pair of branches [superior cerebellar arteries (SCAs)] originate from the distal basilar artery. Finally, PCAs originate at the top of the basilar artery.

Using the orbital window

To access the ophthalmic artery (OA) and the carotid siphon, the transorbital window should be chosen (Figures 2.12 and 2.13). Because the sound beam is passing through a fluid-filled chamber at relatively high acoustic output levels, there is legitimate concern for ocular/retinal damage due to possible heat absorption and cavitation. It is very important to know the FDA-approved guidelines for choice of transducer and power settings for the ultrasound systems that you are using for transorbital studies and to adhere to these guidelines. The current FDA derated maximum acoustic output levels for ophthalmic imaging set the limits of spatial peak temporal average (SPTA) intensity at 17 mW cm^{-2} and the mechanical index (MI) at 0.28. Transorbital insonation steps are as follows:

1 The ultrasound probe is placed over the closed eyelid, which is covered with acoustic gel. The patient is asked to look inferiorly and towards the contralateral side. It is important to standardize your scanning protocol so that the nasal aspect of the eye corresponds to the orientation marker on the probe (i.e. the left side of the image towards the midline). This is kept constant for both the right and left eyes.

2 The globe appears as a dark anechoic structure in the center of the image. The optic nerve appears as an anechoic tube extending from the globe into the far field of the image (Figure 2.12). The distal portion of the ophthalmic artery will appear slightly medially at a depth of 3–5 cm. Blood flow is normally directed towards the transducer with relatively high resistance compared with intracranial vessels. You will note sharpened peak systolic and often low diastolic flow components.

3 The carotid siphon can be imaged at a depth of 6–7 cm. The direction of blood flow will vary with the segments interrogated (lower limb, genu, upper limb). Flow signals are bi-directional at the genu, towards the sound beam in the lower limb and away from the sound beam in the upper limb.

4 Of note, turning transducer upwards above the siphon may result in interception of the intracranial vessels such as ACA or terminal ICA, particularly if good acoustic windows are present. We generally do not use this approach nor the frontal windows [19] unless the trans-temporal insonation was unsuccessful.

Using the submandibular window

During a routine extracranial cerebrovascular examination, the cervical portion of the internal carotid artery can be imaged to the level of the ramus of the mandible. To access the segment of the ICA distal to this level, place the transducer at the angle of the mandible, in front of the sterno-cleido-mastoid muscle, and angle it towards the head and slightly medially. The distal ICA can be imaged at a depth of 3–6 cm with flow away from the transducer. To calculate the Lindegaard ratio [21], a measurement of the ICA flow velocity should be taken at a 0° angle of insonation.

Advantages of TCDI over non-imaging techniques

With transcranial imaging, the examiner is able to visualize anatomic landmarks and the spatial relationship of the vessels that can be used for identification of the arteries in the circle of Willis. This leads to increased confidence in vessel identification and this in turn can improve the accuracy of the examination. The course of tortuous arteries can be followed, arterial branching can be identified and the terminal vertebral arteries can be differentiated (left and right), leading to positive evaluation of the basilar artery. Using color flow imaging, the examiner is able to detect regions of disturbed flow, immediately suspect focal stenosis or occlusion and occasionally visualize arterio-venous malformations or large aneurysms. The study can be complemented with power Doppler and three-dimensional reconstruction to assure complete evaluation of all segments of the circle of Willis. Additionally, when performed in combination with extracranial duplex evaluation, this technology has enhanced our clinical approach to patients presenting with acute stroke and has a potential to increase our ability to differentiate between ischemic and hemorrhagic stroke [22].

Limitations of TCDI

To ensure a complete and accurate examination, sonographers must use their knowledge of intracranial anatomy and complete a single-gate spectral analysis even if the color visualization of the circle of Willis is incomplete or suboptimal. In other words, *spectral analysis must be performed at depths that may contain arterial flow signals even if these segments are not or poorly visualized with color flow imaging*. It is particularly applicable to tortuous vessels when an out-of-plane position may result in no color flow signal, yet an attempt must be made to re-angulate the transducer to detect flow in this area. It must be kept in mind that several ultrasound techniques are being used to create the gray-scale image of the intracranial anatomy, the color flow image of the cerebral vasculature and the spectral display of flow patterns in the intracranial arteries and veins. This places high demands on the frame rate and processing capacity of the duplex scanner. TCDI should not be used as a screening test for cerebral aneurysms [23,24]. Furthermore, fewer diagnostic criteria are available for the detection and grading of intracranial disease with TCDI [25,26] Although TCDI allows the assessment of intracranial veins, thrombosis and arterio-venous malformations [27–29], the reliability and clinical utility of TCDI in this setting are still unknown.

Although the advantages of transcranial color flow imaging compared with the non-imaging studies are recognized, there is still a need to develop smaller or adaptable imaging transducers that can be fixed for monitoring on a headframe. Furthermore, software packages of the duplex scanners should allow the performance, measurement and reporting of a variety of specialized TCD tasks such as emboli detection and vasomotor reactivity assessment.

References

1. Aaslid R, Markwalder TM, Nornes H. Noninvasive transcranial Doppler ultrasound recording of flow velocity in basal cerebral arteries. *J Neurosurg* 1982;**57**:769–74.
2. Otis SM, Ringelstein EB. The transcranial Doppler examination: principles and applications of transcranial Doppler sonography. In: Tegeler CH, Babikian VL, Gomez CR, eds. *Neurosonology*. St. Louis, MO: Mosby, 1996: 140–55.
3. Moehring MA, Spencer MP. Power M-mode transcranial Doppler ultrasound and simultaneous single gate spectrogram. *Ultrasound Med Biol* 2002;**28**:49–57.
4. Aaslid R. *Transcranial Doppler Sonography*. Vienna: Springer, 1986: 39–59.
5. Hennerici M, Rautenberg W, Sitzer G, et al. Transcranial Doppler ultrasound for the assessment of intracranial arterial flow velocity - Part 1. Examination technique and normal values. *Surg Neurol* 1987;**27**(5): 439–48.
6. Alexandrov AV, Sloan MA, Wong LKS, et al. Practice standards for transcranial Doppler (TCD) ultrasound. Part I. Test performance. *J Neuroimaging* 2007;**17**:11–8.
7. Monsein LH, Razumovsky AY, Ackerman SJ, et al. Validation of transcranial Doppler ultrasound with a stereotactic neurosurgical technique. *J Neurosurg* 1995;**82**(6): 972–5.
8. Babikian V, Sloan MA, Tegeler CH, et al. Transcranial Doppler validation pilot study. *J Neuroimaging* 1993;**3**:242–9.
9. Bogdahn U, Becker G, Schlief R, et al. Contrast-enhanced transcranial color-coded real-time sonography. *Stroke* 1993;**24**:676–84.
10. Schoning M, Buchholz R, Walter J. Comparative study of transcranial color duplex sonography and transcranial Doppler sonography in adults. *J Neurosurg* 1993;**78**:776–84.
11. Schoning M, Walter J. Evaluation of the vertebrobasilar-posterior system by transcranial color duplex sonography in adults. *Stroke* 1992;**23**:1577–82.
12. Giovagnorio F, Quaranta L, Bucci MG. Color Doppler assessment of normal ocular blood flow. *J Ultrasound Med* 1993;**12**:473–7.
13. Fujioka KA, Gates DT, Spencer MP. A comparison of transcranial Doppler imaging and standard static pulse wave Doppler in the assessment of intracranial hemodynamics. *J Vasc Technol* 1994;**18**:29–35.
14. Bartels E, Fuchs HH, Flugel KA. Color Doppler imaging of basal cerebral arteries: normal reference values and clinical applications. *Angiology* 1995;**46**(10): 877–84.
15. Baumgartner RW, Schmid C. Comparative study of power-based versus mean frequency-based transcranial color-coded duplex sonography in normal adults. *Stroke* 1996;**27**:101–4.
16. Kenton AR, Martin PJ, Evans DH. Power Doppler: an advance over color Doppler for transcranial imaging? *Ultrasound Med Biol* 1996;**22**:313–7.
17. Bartels E, Flugel KA. Quantitative measurements of blood flow velocity in basal cerebral arteries with transcranial duplex color-flow imaging. A comparative study with conventional transcranial Doppler sonography. *J Neuroimaging* 1994;**4**(2): 77–81.
18. Giller GA. Is angle correction correct? *J Neuroimaging* 1994;**4**:51–2.
19. Stolz E, Kaps M, Kern A, et al. Frontal bone windows for transcranial color-coded duplex sonography. *Stroke* 1999;**30**(4): 814–20.
20. Bartels E. *Color-Coded Duplex Ultrasonography of the Cerebral Arteries: Atlas and Manual*. Stuttgart: Schattauer, 1999.
21. Lindegaard KF, Nornes H, Bakke SJ, et al. Cerebral vasospasm diagnosis by means of angiography and blood velocity measurements. *Acta Neurochir (Wien)* 1989;**100**(1-2): 12–24.
22. Becker GM, Winkler J. Differentiation between ischemic and hemorrhagic stroke by transcranial color-coded real-time sonography. *J Neuroimaging* 1993;**3**:41–7.
23. Baumgartner RW, Mattle HP. Transcranial color-coded duplex sonography in cerebral aneurysms. *Stroke* 1994;**25**:2429–34.
24. White PM, Wardlaw JM, Teasdale E, et al. Power transcranial Doppler ultrasound in the detection of intracranial aneurysms. *Stroke* 200;**32**(6): 1291–7.
25. Baumgartner RW, Mattle HP, Schroth G. Assessment of >50% and <50% intracranial stenosis by transcranial color-coded duplex sonography. *Stroke* 1999;**30**:87–92.
26. Lien LM, Chen WH, Chen JR, et al. Comparison of transcranial color-coded sonography and magnetic resonance angiography in acute ischemic stroke. *J Neuroimaging* 2001;**11**(4): 363–8.
27. Stolz E, Kaps M, Domdorf W. Assessment of intracranial venous hemodynamics in normal individuals and patients with cerebral venous thrombosis. *Stroke* 1999;**30**:70–5.
28. Becker G, Bogdahn U. Transcranial color-coded real-time sonography in intracranial veins. Normal values of blood flow velocities and findings in superior sagittal sinus thrombosis. *J Neuroimaging* 1995;**2**:1196–9.
29. Becker GM, Winkler J. Imaging of cerebral arterio-venous malformations by transcranial colour-coded real-time sonography. *Neuroradiology* 1990;**32**:280–8.

3 Anatomy of the Brain's Arterial Supply

Joel Cure
University of Alabama Hospital, Birmingham, AL, USA

Introduction

This chapter reviews the normal and variant anatomy of the craniocervical arterial tree from the aortic arch to the brain. The focus is on anatomy relevant to brain perfusion and stroke pathophysiology. The anatomy is illustrated using a variety of modalities, including conventional, CT and MR angiography.

The aortic arch

After emerging from the left ventricle, the aorta arches in the superior mediastinum before beginning its thoracic descent. The blood supply to the head, neck and upper extremities arises from the top of the aortic arch via the great vessels. In most individuals (approximately 70%) three great vessels arise in proximal to distal order: the innominate artery (also known as the brachiocephalic artery or trunk), the left common carotid artery and the left subclavian artery (Figure 3.1a). The innominate artery represents the common origin of the right subclavian and right common carotid arteries. The course of the proximal subclavian and common carotid arteries is relatively straight in childhood, but may become more redundant and tortuous with age.

Variant great vessel origins and aortic arch anomalies

In the most common anatomic variation of great vessel origins, seen in approximately 13% of individuals [1], the left common carotid artery either shares an origin with the innominate artery or arises more distally from the innominate artery, configurations that have been traditionally known as a "bovine" aortic arch (Figure 3.1b–d). Noting that neither of these configurations mimics the anatomy actually observed in cattle, Layton *et al.* [1] suggested replacing the term "bovine arch" with "common origin of the innominate artery and left common carotid artery" or "origin of the left common carotid artery from the innominate artery." Both of these two variants are more common in black than white individuals. Rarely, one may encounter a "true" bovine arch configuration, in which all of the great vessels arise from a single trunk (Figure 3.1d). In up to 5% of individuals, the left vertebral artery arises directly from the aortic arch, typically immediately proximal to the left subclavian artery origin [2] (Figure 3.1e).

Aortic arch anomalies fall into four categories: (1) double aortic arch (DAA), (2) right aortic arch (RAA), (3) left aortic arch with abnormal branching and (4) interrupted aortic arch (IAA) [3]. With DAA, persistence of the embryonic right dorsal aorta leads to bilateral aortic arches that surround the trachea and esophagus before uniting in the dorsal midline as the descending aorta. One common carotid artery (CCA) and one subclavian artery (SCA) arise from each arch. The right arch is larger in most cases. This arch anomaly is the one most frequently associated with other congenital defects, particularly cardiac anomalies. The vascular ring formed by the duplicated arches may produce stridor and/or dysphagia. RAA is due to persistence of the embryonic right dorsal aorta and involution of the left. The descending aorta in RAA may pass down on either side. Great vessel origins with RAA may have a "mirror image" configuration with respect to the normal configuration (i.e. left brachiocephalic artery, right CCA, right SCA). Patients with this particular variant of RAA anatomy have a high incidence of associated cardiac defects. Alternatively, the left SCA may be aberrant, arising as the last great vessel origin from the proximal descending RAA and passing posterior to the esophagus (Figure 3.2a). The aberrant SCA origin may be focally dilated as a "Kommerell's diverticulum" (Figure 3.2b). Stridor or dysphagia may again complicate the vascular ring created by the RAA and ligamentum arteriosum that passes to the left of the trachea and esophagus between the proximal descending RAA and left pulmonary artery. LAA with an aberrant right subclavian artery is the most common aortic arch anomaly (incidence up to 2.3%) [4] (Figure 3.2c and d). The right vertebral artery usually arises from the right subclavian artery even when the right SCA is aberrant. IAA is fairly rare and most patients die within the first week of life. An arch anomaly associated with protrusion of the

Cerebrovascular Ultrasound in Stroke Prevention and Treatment, 2nd edition.
Edited by Andrei V. Alexandrov. © 2011 Blackwell Publishing Ltd.

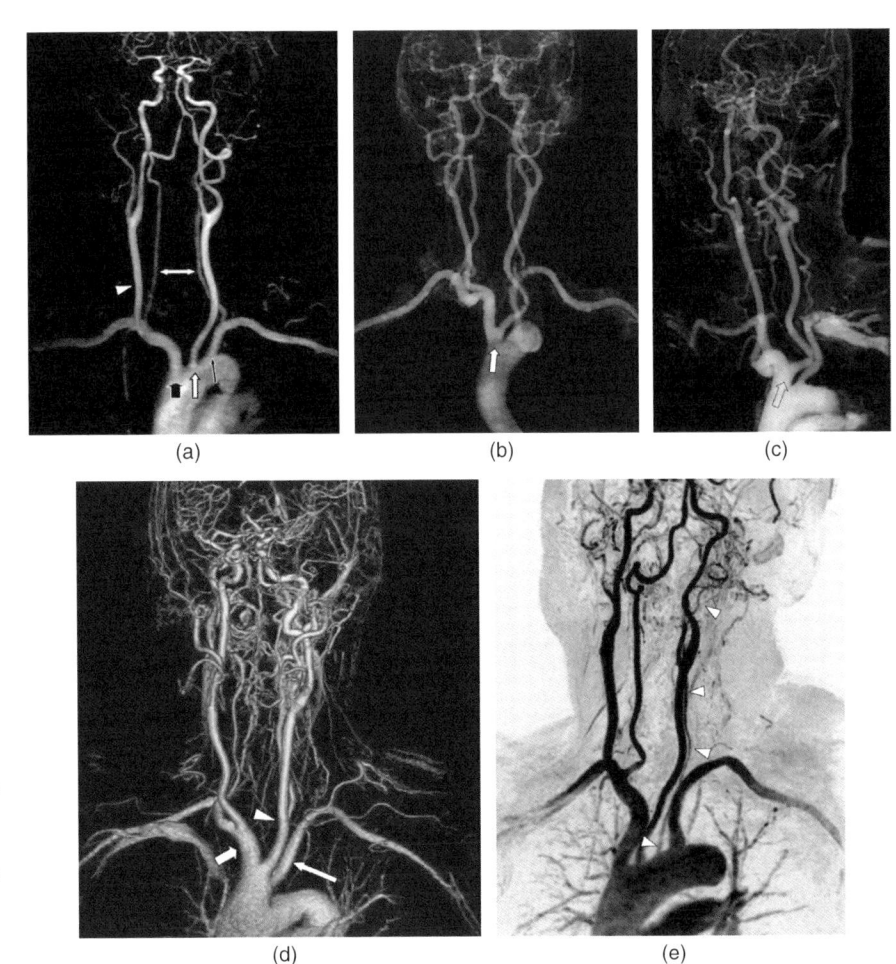

CHAPTER 3 Anatomy of the Brain's Arterial Supply

Figure 3.1 Variants of great vessel origins (contrast-enhanced 3D MR angiograms). (a) The normal configuration of the aortic arch is illustrated. The innominate artery (wide black arrow) originates first, followed by the left common carotid artery (white arrow) and left subclavian artery (thin black arrow). The right common carotid artery (CCA, white arrowhead) arises from the innominate artery. The right subclavian artery continues distal to the right CCA origin. The double-headed arrow indicates the vertebral arteries. (b) The arrow indicates a common origin of the innominate artery and left common carotid artery. (c) The arrow indicates a left common carotid artery origin from the innominate artery. (d) A true bovine arch (in a human). The innominate artery (thick arrow), left common carotid artery (arrowhead) and left subclavian artery all originate from a large common trunk arising from the aortic arch. (e) The arrowheads indicate a direct left vertebral artery origin from the aortic arch.

arch into the base of the neck is known as a "cervical aortic arch" (Figure 3.2e).

The anterior circulation

The anterior circulation consists of the internal carotid arteries and their vascular territories. These territories include the orbits, the superior, medial and lateral aspects of the anterior temporal lobes, the frontal lobes and the anterior parietal lobes. The right CCA normally arises from the innominate artery, with the right subclavian artery beginning distal to the right CCA origin. The left common carotid artery usually arises directly from the aortic arch (see Figure 3.1a). The CCAs ascend to a variable degree before bifurcating into the internal and external carotid arteries (ICA and ECA, respectively) (Figure 3.3a). In most patients this occurs at about the level of the thyroid cartilage (usually between C3 and C5), but the location of the carotid bifurcation is variable, from as low as the T3 level to as high as C1 (Figure 3.3a and b). The internal carotid arteries are normally larger than the external carotid arteries and typically ascend just posterolateral to them, but this relationship is also variable and the vessel size or position should not be used as reliable criteria for differentiation between the external and internal carotid arteries.

The carotid ascends in the "carotid space," a fascia-enveloped compartment that encloses the internal jugular vein and cranial nerves IX–XII above the hyoid level (but only cranial nerve X below the hyoid level). The sympathetic trunk is located immediately medial to the carotid space. The ICA lies along the anterolateral aspect of the cervical spine, anterior to the prevertebral musculature and lateral to the retropharyngeal space. The common and/or internal carotid arteries may course medially, however, and protrude deeply into the retropharyngeal space (Figure 3.3c), where they may be at risk during pharyngeal surgery. Rarely, the ICA and ECA have separate origins from the aortic arch.

The ECA ascends from the carotid bifurcation, giving off the superior thyroid artery, lingual, facial, occipital and postauricular arteries before passing medial to or through the parotid gland. Here it divides into the superficial temporal artery (STA) and internal maxillary artery (IMA) (Figure 3.4a). The ascending pharyngeal artery arises from the most

PART I How To Perform Ultrasound Tests

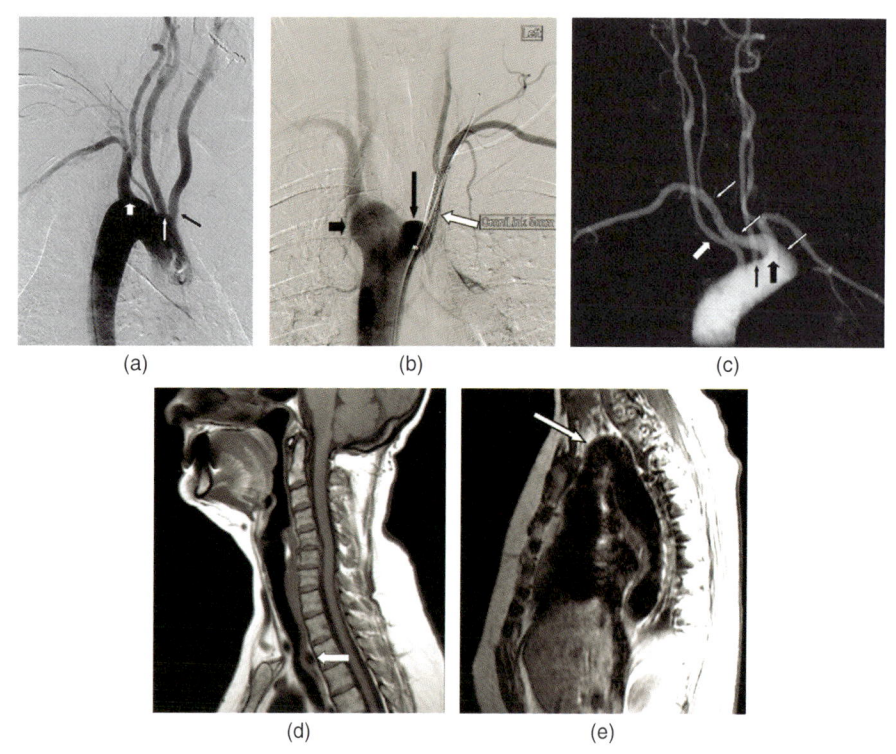

Figure 3.2 Aortic arch anomalies. (a) Right aortic arch with aberrant left subclavian artery, right anterior oblique projection of conventional arteriogram. Wide white arrow indicates right subclavian artery. Narrow white arrow indicates right common carotid artery. Black arrow indicates left common carotid artery. The left subclavian artery is not yet visualized on this injection due to a proximal stenosis. The patient presented with left subclavian steal. The aorta arches toward and descends on the patient's right. (b) Right aortic arch with aberrant left subclavian artery, AP projection, conventional arteriogram [same patient as in (a)]. The wide black arrow indicates the right aortic arch at the level of the right subclavian artery origin. The narrow black arrow indicates a Kommerell's diverticulum associated with the origin of the aberrant left subclavian artery. The stenotic left SCA origin has been stented (white arrow) and the left SCA and vertebral arteries are now well-visualized. (c) Left aortic arch with aberrant right SCA, MRA, left anterior oblique projection. Thick white arrow indicates right common carotid artery. There is no innominate artery. Thin black arrow indicates left common carotid artery. Thick black arrow indicates left SCA. Thin white arrows indicate the aberrant right SCA, originating as the last great vessel origin and passing to the right. (d) Sagittal T1 weighted MR image demonstrates aberrant SCA (arrow) passing posterior to esophagus and trachea. Note mild tracheal narrowing anterior to this. (e) Sagittal T1 weighted MR image demonstrates a cervical aortic arch (arrow) protruding into the base of the neck above the level of the manubrium.

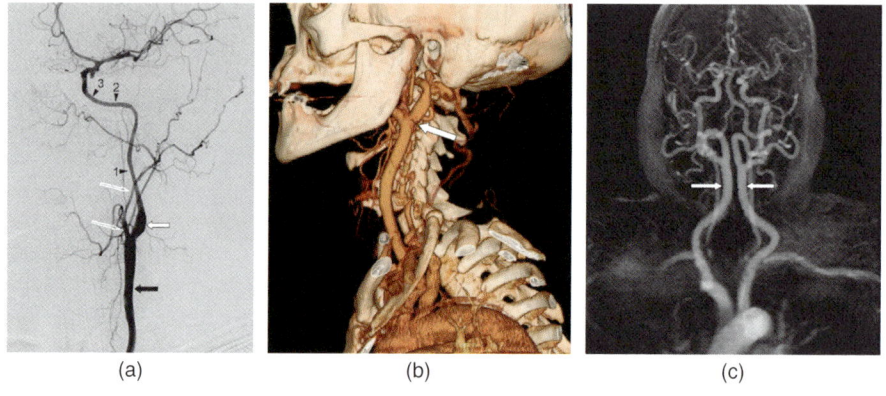

Figure 3.3 Cervical carotid arteries. (a) Normal left carotid bifurcation, left CCA injection, conventional angiogram. Black arrow indicates left common carotid artery. White solid arrow indicates left internal carotid artery bulb. Outlined white arrows indicate left external carotid artery. 1, 2 and 3 designate the corresponding numerically defined segments of the left internal carotid artery (see text). (b) High left carotid bifurcation, left lateral projection of CT angiogram. Arrow indicates high carotid bifurcation at the C2 level. This anatomic situation is often problematic in patients being considered for endarterectomy, where the diseased segment may lie deep to the mandible. (c) AP projection, MR angiogram. Arrows indicate bilateral "retropharyngeal carotids," indenting the retropharyngeal compartment and coursing quite medially towards the midline.

28

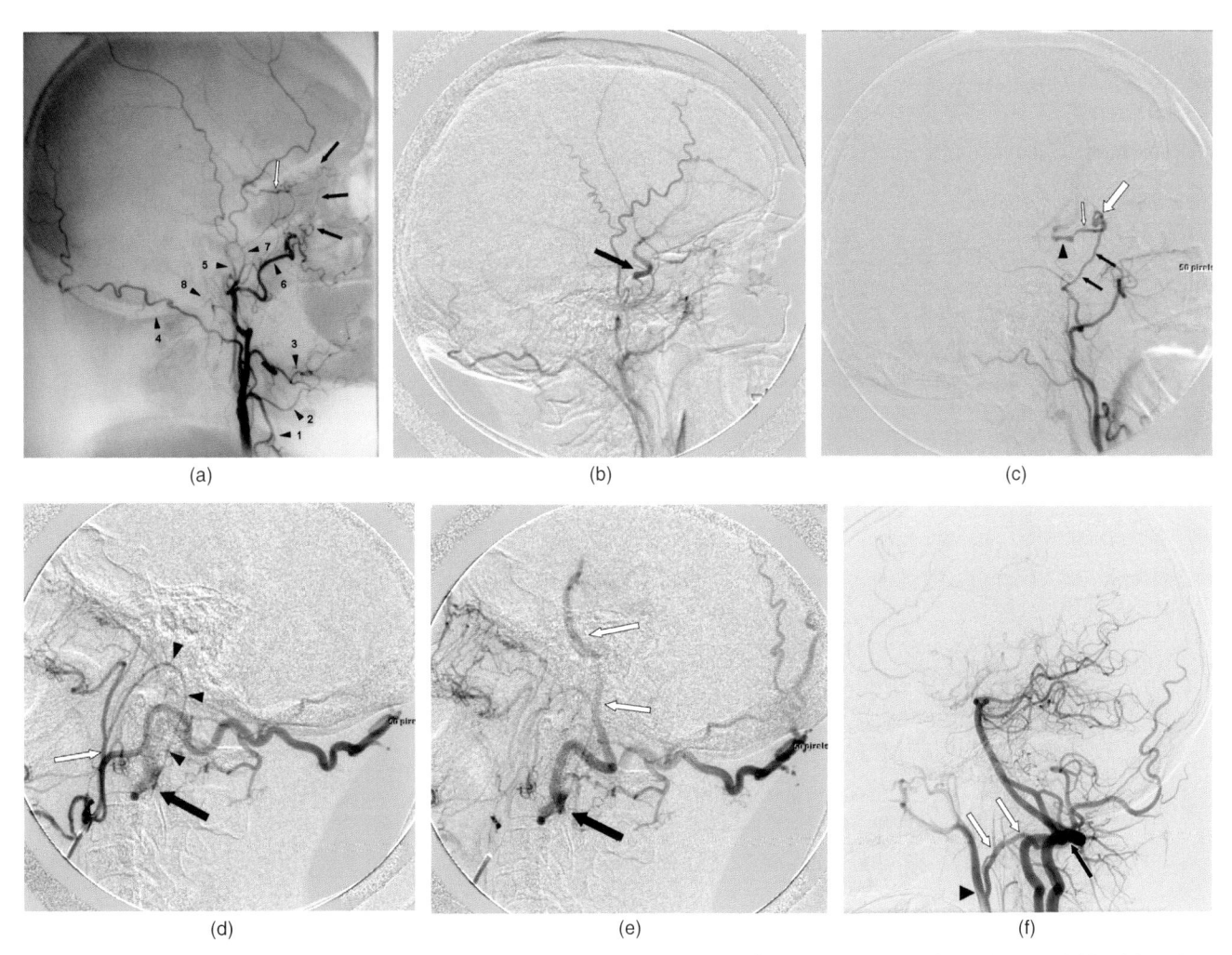

CHAPTER 3 Anatomy of the Brain's Arterial Supply

Figure 3.4 External carotid artery anatomy, collateral pathways. (a) Normal ECA anatomy, right lateral projection, ECA injection, conventional arteriogram. 1, Superior thyroidal artery; 2, lingual artery; 3, facial artery; 4, occipital artery; 5, superficial temporal artery; 6, internal maxillary artery; 7, middle meningeal artery; 8, postauricular artery. Long black arrows trace anastomotic loop from terminal internal maxillary artery to branches of the ipsilateral ophthalmic artery which is filling in a retrograde fashion (indicated by white arrow). (b) Right lateral projection, ECA injection, conventional arteriogram. The C4 segment of ICA (black arrow) filled via collateral flow from external carotid artery branches. The ophthalmic artery filled in a normal antegrade direction. (c) Right lateral projection, ECA injection, conventional angiogram. The anterior division of the middle meningeal artery (black arrows) reconstitutes flow in the supraclinoid ICA (arrowhead) via collateral flow in the recurrent meningeal branch (thick white arrow) of the ophthalmic artery (thin white arrow). (d) Left lateral projection, ECA injection, conventional arteriogram, early phase. Patient had left vertebral artery occlusion. Black arrow indicates early opacification of left vertebral artery via an ascending pharyngeal to vertebral artery anastomosis. Arrowheads indicate an anastomotic branch of posterior division of the ascending pharyngeal artery. The proximal ascending pharyngeal artery is indicated by the white arrow. (e) Left lateral projection, ECA injection, conventional arteriogram, late phase. Black arrow indicates site of anastomosis producing early opacification of left vertebral artery. White arrows indicate vertebral artery. (f) Left lateral projection, left vertebral artery injection, conventional arteriogram. Patient had occlusion of left common carotid artery. Vertebral (black arrow) artery fills occipital artery (white arrows) in a retrograde fashion with collateral flow to left ECA (arrowhead).

proximal aspect of the ECA or from the carotid bifurcation. The superficial temporal artery supplies the scalp. Branches of the IMA supply the cranial dura mater (middle meningeal artery), extracranial musculature (deep temporal arteries), sinonasal region and maxillary alveolus and palate and portions of the face. In addition to their primary role supplying the soft tissues and viscera of the extracranial head and neck and the dura, branches of the ECA are important sources of collateral blood flow in cases of CCA, ICA or vertebral artery (VA) stenosis or occlusion. These collateral pathways take various forms including ECA to ECA, ECA to ICA and ECA to VA (Figure 3.4b–d). Flow may pass in either direction through these pathways depending on the pattern of vascular stenosis or occlusion.

Proximal ECA branches including the superior thyroid, lingual, facial and ascending pharyngeal arteries may

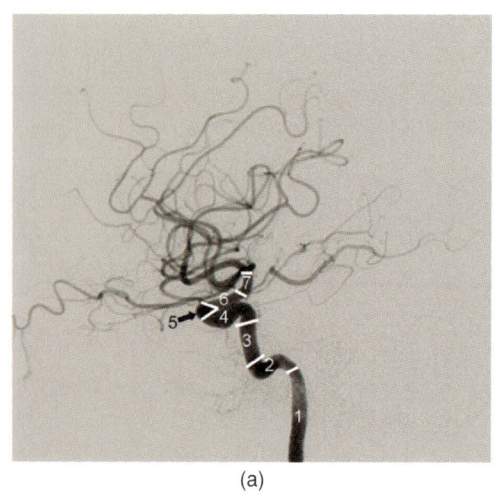

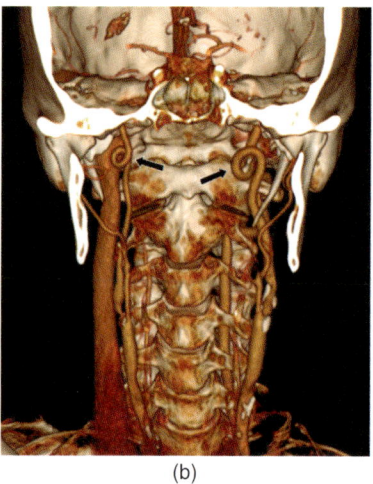

Figure 3.5 Internal carotid artery segments. Left lateral projection, ICA injection, conventional angiogram. 1, Cervical segment; 2, petrous segment; 3, lacerum segment; 4, cavernous segment; 5, clinoid segment; 6, ophthalmic segment; 7, communicating segment.

provide side-to-side collateral flow in cases of contralateral proximal CCA occlusion via end-to-end anastomosis with their contralateral counterpart or other contralateral ECA branches (ECA to ECA). The ascending pharyngeal artery anastomoses with cavernous branches of the ICA and the caroticotympanic branch of the ICA and may be a source of ECA to ICA collateral flow in cases of ICA occlusion. The IMA may similarly provide ECA to ICA collateral flow between distal IMA branches and cavernous branches of the ICA via the foramen rotundum and vidian canal. Several ECA branches anastomose distally with ethmoidal branches of the ophthalmic artery and may provide collateral ECA to ICA flow in cases of ICA or CCA occlusion. These collateral routes share as a final common pathway retrograde flow in the ophthalmic artery to the ICA. This pattern of collateral flow may involve distal branches of the facial artery, STA, IMA and middle meningeal artery. The middle meningeal artery may anastomose with the anterior falx artery (which arises from the ethmoidal branches of the ophthalmic artery) or fill the ophthalmic artery more directly via the recurrent meningeal branch of the ophthalmic artery (Figure 3.4e). Branches of both the ascending pharyngeal and occipital arteries anastomose with branches of the vertebral artery and may reconstitute flow in either direction when the VA or CCA are occluded (ECA to VA). All of these anastomoses are important avenues of collateral flow in cases of vascular occlusion. However, they are also potentially dangerous conduits that must be anticipated during endovascular procedures when emboli may pass through them into cerebral territories with dire consequences [5–7].

Internal carotid artery segments

The internal carotid artery has been anatomically mapped into segments that have been defined and numbered in various ways, from a four-segment system [8] to a system of seven segments [9]. The following anatomic stroll up the ICA refers to the seven-segment system (Figure 3.5a). The cervical internal carotid artery (C1) begins at the carotid bifurcation and continues to the skull base. Some patients have partial or complete loops in the C1 segment just below the skull base (Figure 3.5b) that may complicate endovascular procedures. Upon entering the skull base, the ICA turns anteromedially just anterior and medial to the cochlea and medial to the middle ear cavity. The C2 segment begins at the entrance into the carotid canal and continues its anteromedial course in the petrous temporal bone before turning and exiting anteriorly above the foramen lacerum and underneath Meckel's cave as the C3 segment. The C4 segment commences at the petrolingual ligament (a dural reflection spanning the petrous apex and sphenoid lingula). C4 has a horizontal segment surrounded by the venous sinusoids of the cavernous sinus that is both preceded and followed by long and short vertical segments, respectively. The C4 segment may be tortuous in some patients and "knuckles" of this tortuous segment may be mistaken for aneurysms on axial MR or CT images. Actual aneurysms arising in this segment may produce sixth cranial nerve palsies or, if they rupture, may be associated with direct carotid cavernous fistulas. This segment is commonly affected by atherosclerosis and may also be narrowed by cavernous sinus meningiomas or the inflammatory cellular infiltrate of Tolosa–Hunt syndrome. Upon exiting the cavernous sinus through an anterior ("proximal") dural ring inferomedial to the anterior clinoid process, the ICA turns cephalad as the clinoid (C5) segment before emerging into the intradural compartment at the level of a second, distal dural ring, adjacent to the anterior clinoid process. C5 represents the upper half of the anterior genu of the ICA. Aneurysms in the C5 segment may be associated with coincident third cranial nerve palsy and optic neuropathy as they grow to obstruct the superior orbital fissure and protrude upwards against the anterior clinoid process and falciform ligament. This rigid ligament extends from

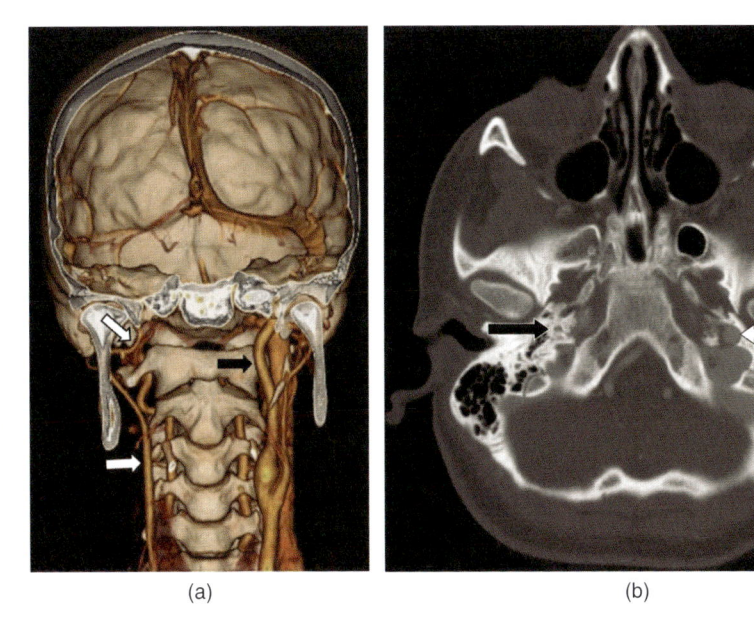

CHAPTER 3 Anatomy of the Brain's Arterial Supply

Figure 3.6 Right ICA aplasia, CT angiography. (a) CT angiogram AP view with cutaway of anterior osseous structures. The left ICA is indicated by a black arrow. No ICA is evident on the right. The smaller right CCA terminates as the ECA (white arrows). (b) Axial source image from the CTA. Black arrow indicates tiny right carotid canal. Normal left carotid canal is indicated by white arrow.

the anterior clinoid process to the tuberculum sella at the entrance to the optic canal and lies above the optic nerve and ophthalmic artery. C6 continues from the distal dural ring/anterior clinoid process to just proximal to the posterior communicating artery (PComA) origin. The S-shaped curve seen on lateral views formed by the C4–C6 segments is referred to as the carotid siphon. At the PComA origin the ICA takes a final, more vertical, turn and continues to its terminal bifurcation as C7, the communicating segment.

In the more simplified four-segment system of ICA nomenclature, C1 represents the cervical ICA, C2 the petrous segment of the ICA, C3 the cavernous segment and C4 the supraclinoid segment, extending from the anterior clinoid process to the terminal ICA bifurcation. Note that the rest of this book uses the four-segment system to reference ultrasound findings since most intra-skull segments are inaccessible to direct ultrasound interrogation. Some authors refer to these segments in reversed order, i.e. C1 = supraclinoid segment; however, despite these differences, the sequence of major anatomic parts remain the same, whether counted up- or downstream.

Internal carotid artery agenesis is rare and when encountered it is usually unilateral [10]. The presence of a small, bony carotid canal on CT images helps to differentiate ICA hypoplasia from acquired carotid narrowing (Figure 3.6). Absence or hypoplasia of the ICA is associated with an increased risk of intracranial aneurysms [11–13].

Intracranial ICA branches

The cervical ICA (C1) has no branches. Intracranial ICA branches are shown in Figure 3.7a and b. Branches of the C2 segment include the caroticotympanic artery and occasionally the vidian artery. The caroticotympanic artery (the first branch of the ICA) passes into and supplies the middle ear. It anastomoses with the inferior tympanic artery (a branch of the ascending pharyngeal artery). The vidian artery passes through the vidian canal (pterygoid canal) and connects the ICA with branches of the distal IMA in the pterygopalatine fossa. These branches represent anastomotic bridges to the ECA that may be important in cases of acquired ICA occlusion (see above). A persistent stapedial artery (PSA) may also arise from the C2 segment. The PSA represents an anomalous origin of the middle meningeal artery in which the embryonic stapedial artery persists as a C2 branch, passing into the anteromedial middle ear cavity and traversing the stapes footplate and cochlear promontory and then continuing into the middle cranial fossa via the tympanic facial nerve canal. Patients with a PSA may present with pulsatile tinnitus. CT scans of these patients demonstrate absence of the foramen spinosum and enlargement of the tympanic facial nerve canal [14].

Patients with an *aberrant* ICA also typically present with pulsatile tinnitus and a red retrotympanic mass (Figure 3.8). The aberrant ICA follows the course of the inferior tympanic branch of the ascending pharyngeal artery into the middle ear and exits the anteromedial middle ear cavity along the course of the caroticotympanic artery to resume its normal petrous course. This anomaly may actually represent an anastomotic loop formed by the inferior tympanic artery with the caroticotympanic artery that bypasses an aplastic segment of the cervical and proximal petrous internal carotid artery [14]. Correct identification of this anomaly is crucial to avoid disastrous biopsy of the ICA in the middle ear. Cases of coexisting persistent stapedial artery and aberrant ICA have also been reported both unilaterally and bilaterally [15]. The C1–C4 segments are surrounded by branches

PART I How To Perform Ultrasound Tests

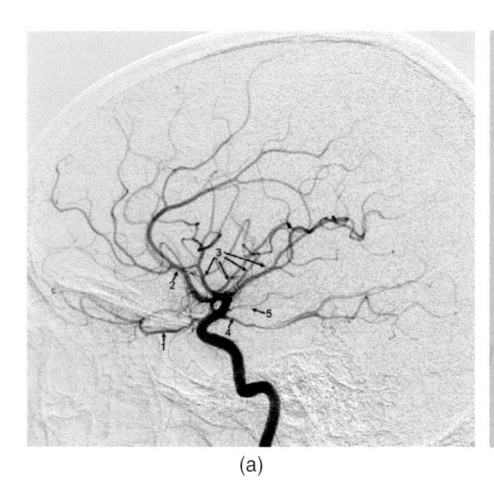

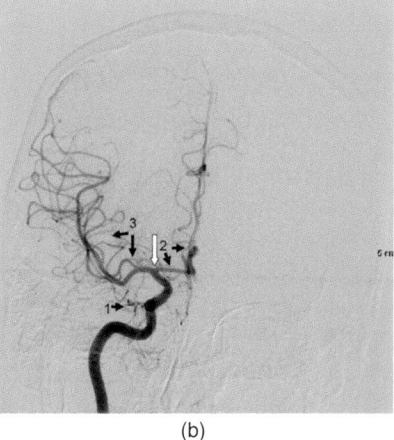

Figure 3.7 Intracranial ICA branches, (a) Left lateral projection, left ICA injection. 1, Ophthalmic artery; 2, anterior cerebral artery; 3, middle cerebral artery (arrows indicate sylvian branches); 4, posterior communicating artery; 5, anterior choroidal artery. (b) AP projection, right ICA injection. 1, Ophthalmic artery; 2, anterior cerebral artery; 3, middle cerebral artery. White arrow indicates terminal right ICA bifurcation.

of the carotid autonomic plexus (derived from the superior cervical ganglion), an anatomic arrangement that explains the association of Horner syndrome with carotid pathology, particularly arterial dissections [16,17].

C3 has no branches. C4 yields the meningohypophyseal artery (that supplies the tentorium, clivus and pituitary gland) and the inferolateral trunk (which supplies cranial nerves III–VI in the cavernous sinus, the gasserian ganglion and the dural walls of the cavernous sinus). These branches have significant roles in the external to internal anastomotic flow in cases of ICA occlusion, with anastomoses to the distal IMA via the artery of the foramen rotundum, directly with dural branches of the MMA and with the more proximal IMA via the artery of the foramen ovale [18] (see Figure 3.4b). The C3–C4 junction or C4 segment are the usual sites of origin of the persistent trigeminal artery, the most common of the primitive carotid–basilar anastomoses. C5 usually has no important branches, although the opthalmic artery occasionally arises from this segment.

C6 gives rise to the ophthalmic artery (OA) and also multiple perforating arteries, including the superior hypophyseal arteries that supply the pituitary gland and infundibulum and perforators that supply the optic chiasm. The OA typically arises above the anterior clinoid process, below the optic nerve, although in a minority of arteries the vessel arises more proximally, even from within the cavernous sinus [19]. Rare cases of OA originating from the middle meningeal artery have also been described and it is important to recognize this anomaly in cases where surgery involving the middle meningeal artery or trans-arterial embolotherapy are planned (e.g. preoperative embolization of meningiomas) [20]. The OA continues into the orbit inferolateral to the optic nerve before rising and crossing just over the top of the nerve to reach the medial orbital wall. This crossover can be seen on lateral arteriographic projections of the artery in the mid-orbit. The recurrent meningeal branch of the ophthalmic artery is a potentially important collateral pathway passing through the superior orbital fissure to connect the middle meningeal artery with the ophthalmic artery (see Figure 3.4c). In addition to supplying the globe, the ophthalmic artery sends branches to the lacrimal gland, extraocular muscles and orbital periosteum (periorbita). Extraorbital branches of the ophthalmic artery (e.g. the ethmoidal arteries) form important anastomoses with ECA branches (see above). The C6 segment enters the subarachnoid space (an important anatomic feature that makes it prone to vasospasm secondary to subarachnoid hemorrhage).

The C7 (communicating) segment commences at the posterior communicating artery (PComA) origin and gives rise to the PComA and anterior choroidal arteries. The C7 segment ends at the terminal ICA bifurcation. The PComA connects the ICA to the junction of the P1 and P2 segments of

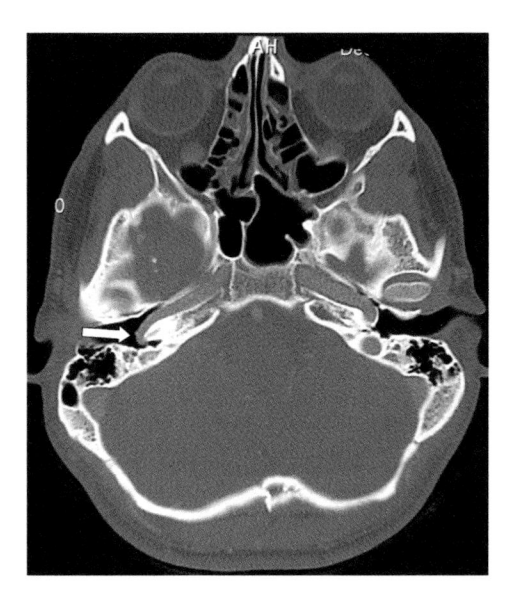

Figure 3.8 Aberrant internal carotid artery. Patient presented with pulsatile tinnits. Axial non-contrast CT image in a bone window. White arrow indicates the aberrant ICA projecting into the right middle ear cavity. Note the appearance and position of its normal contralateral counterpart.

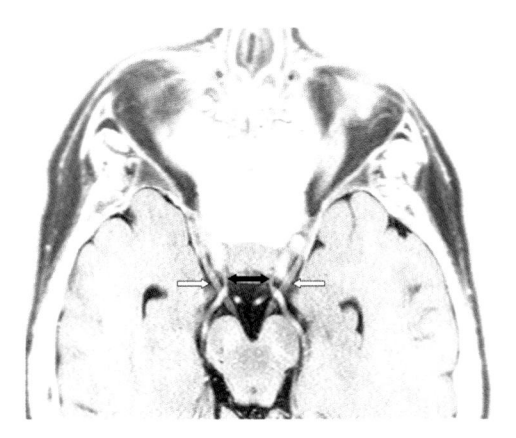

Figure 3.9 Anatomic proximity of posterior communicating arteries (double-headed arrow) and third cranial nerves (white arrows). This intimate proximity explains the common association of third cranial nerve palsies with posterior communicating artery aneurysms.

the posterior cerebral artery and is a key component in the circle of Willis (see below). The PComA courses medial to and slightly above the oculomotor nerve in the suprasellar and interpeduncular cisterns (Figure 3.9). Their proximity explains the common association of oculomotor palsy with PComA origin aneurysms. (Since the oculomotor nerve exits the midbrain and passes anteriorly between the PCA and SCA, SCA aneurysms may also be responsible for oculomotor palsies.) Its long spatial course and exposure to several vessels make it a target for compression by aneurysms. A funnel- or coned-shaped enlargement (infundibulum) of the PComA origin may be seen in up to 6% of hemispheres [8]. The risk of hemorrhage from an infundibular vascular origin is very low, but cases have been reported [21]. Furthermore, cases have been reported of progression of an infundibulum into a true aneurysm [22]. Angiographic differentiation of an infundibulum from an aneurysm may be difficult, but clear demonstration that the PComA arises from the *apex* of the cone is strong evidence for an infundibulum rather than an aneurysm. The situation in which the PComA is the dominant source of flow to the ipsilateral PCA, coexisting with ipsilateral P1 hypoplasia, is known as a fetal configuration of the PCA, as it represents the anatomic configuration that exists in early gestation. Perforating arteries arising from the PComA supply the optic tract, thalamus (thalamoperforating arteries), hypothalamus, subthalamic region and internal capsule.

The anterior choroidal artery (AChA) usually arises just above the PComA. It passes posteriorly within the cistern between the medial surface of the uncus and cerebral peduncle to enter the choroidal fissure above the temporal horn of the lateral ventricle. Branches of the AChA supply the optic tract, middle third of the cerebral peduncle, lateral geniculate body and origin of the optic radiation, posterior two-thirds of the posterior limb of the internal capsule, globus pallidus, hippocampus, fornix and the lateral ventricular choroid plexus (within the temporal horn and body of the lateral ventricle as far forward as the foramen of Monro). A reciprocal relationship exists between the PComA and AChA territories. For example, in patients with a small PComA, the AChA may take over the supply to the genu and anterior third of the posterior limb of the internal capsule. Anastomoses between the AChA and lateral choroidal branches of the PCA on the surface of the choroid plexus are common and may also be encountered along the lateral surface of the lateral geniculate body and on the medial temporal lobe near the uncus. These anastomoses may mitigate the clinical and imaging effects of AChA occlusion.

Anterior cerebral artery

The terminal ICA bifurcation produces the medially directed A1 segment of the anterior cerebral artery (ACA) and the laterally directed M1 segment of the middle cerebral artery (MCA). The A1 segment of the anterior cerebral artery arises at the medial end of the sylvian fissure and courses anteromedially, above the optic nerve and chiasm, into the interhemispheric fissure where it is joined to its contralateral counterpart by the anterior communicating artery (AComA) (Figure 3.10a). Beyond the anterior communicating artery, the vessel continues upwards as the A2 segment (Figure 3.10b), coursing upwards anterior to the lamina terminalis and callosal rostrum. The ACA segment passing in front of the callosal genu is designated the A3 or precallosal segment. The artery then swings around to course above the top of the corpus callosum (A4, supracallosal segment). The A5 segment begins about half way back the horizontal segment of the ACA and ultimately rounds the splenium of the corpus callosum (postcallosal segment). The division between the A4 and A5 is described as occurring just behind the coronal suture on lateral angiographic projections [8]. This anatomic localizer is impossible to apply on CT or MR angiograms. The ACA distal to the AComA is also known as the pericallosal artery. A more simplified numbering system divides the ACA into only three segments: A1 (proximal to the AComA), A2 (AComA to top of genu of corpus callosum) and A3 (the distal segment arching over the corpus callosum).

The A1 segment is the most commonly hypoplastic segment of the circle of Willis (see below). A hypoplastic A1 segment is frequently accompanied by a large AComA. In this situation, a greater than normal volume of blood from the opposite A1 must pass through the AComA to perfuse both ACAs adequately, including the contralateral part distal to the hypoplastic A1 segment. Likely reflecting this flow perturbation or associated embryologic defects in formation of the arterial media, anterior communicating

PART I How To Perform Ultrasound Tests

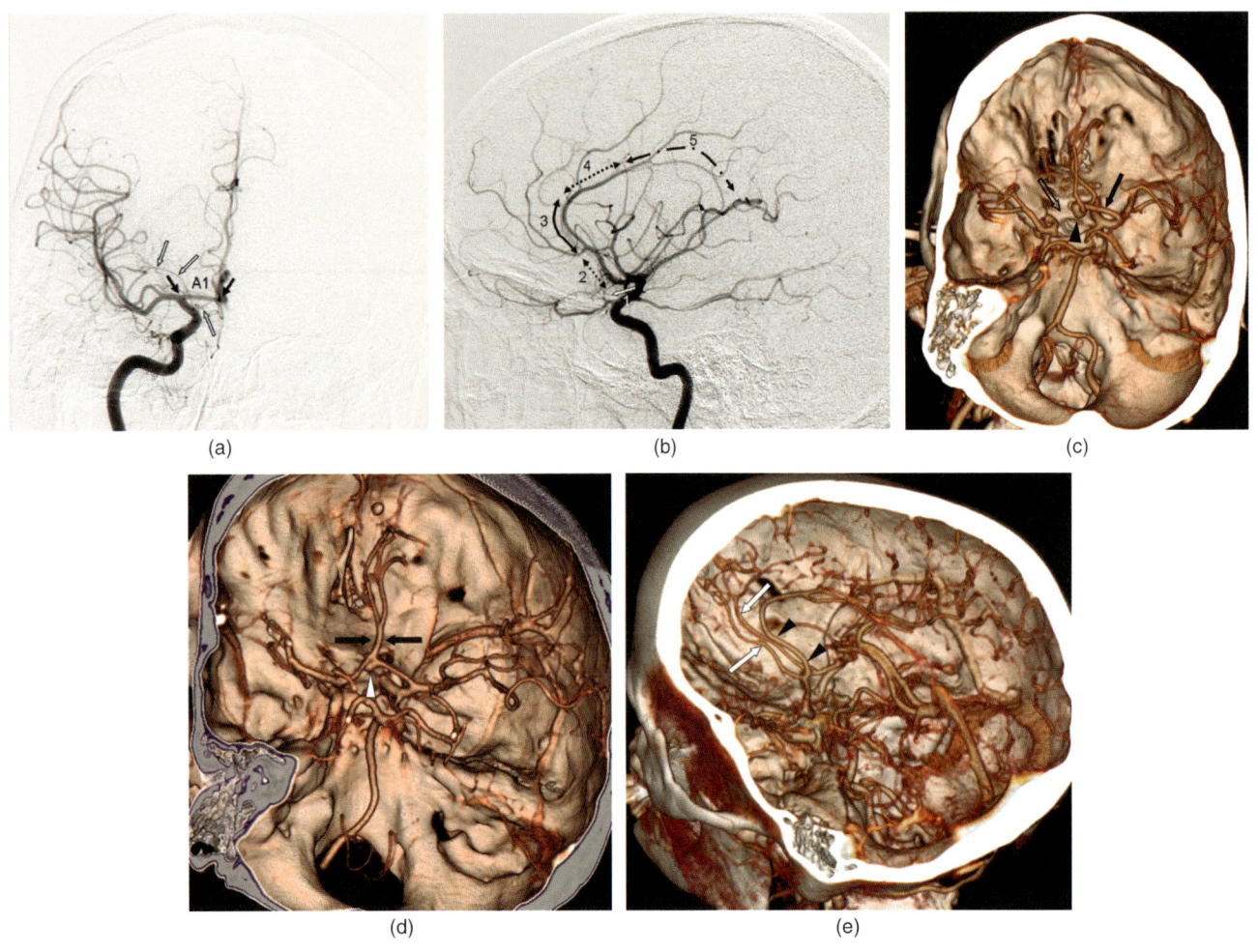

Figure 3.10 Anterior cerebral artery. (a) AP projection, RICA injection. Extent of A1 segment is indicated by black arrows. Outlined arrows indicate recurrent artery of Huebner. (b) Left lateral projection, left ICA injection, conventional angiogram. Single- and double-headed arrows indicate the numbered segments of the ACA. (c) Superior oblique view, CT angiogram. Right A1 segment is indicated by solid black arrow. Aplastic left A1 segment would normally be located at tip of "outlined" black arrow. Note anterior communicating artery origin aneurysm (arrowhead). (d) Superior oblique view, CT angiogram. Black arrows indicate azygous A2 segment. Note associated aneurysm (arrowhead). (e) Superior oblique view, CT angiogram. Arrowheads indicate "median artery of the corpus callosum." The "normal" adjacent bilateral ACAs are indicated by white arrows.

artery aneurysms often coexist with A1 hypoplasia (Figure 3.10c). The AComA is frequently fairly oblique in orientation (rather than directly transverse) and may be difficult to profile on catheter angiograms. Studying AComA anatomy is less problematic with CT or MR angiograms, which, once acquired, can be viewed from any desired angle. Infundibular (funnel-shaped dilatations) origins of one or both ends of the anterior communicating artery are common. The anterior communicating artery may be duplicated or fenestrated in some patients, but absence of the AComA is rare. The azygos (undivided) ACA has an estimated incidence of 0.3–2% [23]. This anomaly consists of a single A2 segment arising from the confluence of the A1 segments, with absence of the AComA. The azygos ACA gives rise to the pericallosal and callosomarginal arteries at a variable distance from its origin. There is an association between forms of holoprosencephaly and the azygous ACA. Another AComA variant is the presence of an artery arising from the center of the AComA and passing upwards around the callosal genu where, after dividing, it may supply branches to both paracentral lobules. This variant has been given various names, most commonly the accessory anterior cerebral artery or median artery of the corpus callosum. The angiographic appearance suggests "three" pericallosal arteries (Figure 3.10e).

The recurrent artery of Huebner (Figure 3.10a) usually arises from either the proximal A2 or distal A1 segment in the immediate vicinity of the AComA. It then passes laterally in front of the A1 and M1 segments to pierce the anterior perforated substance and supply the anterior caudate nucleus, antero-inferior aspect of the anterior limb of the internal capsule, the uncinate fasciculus, anterolateral globus pallidus, the anterior third of the putamen and

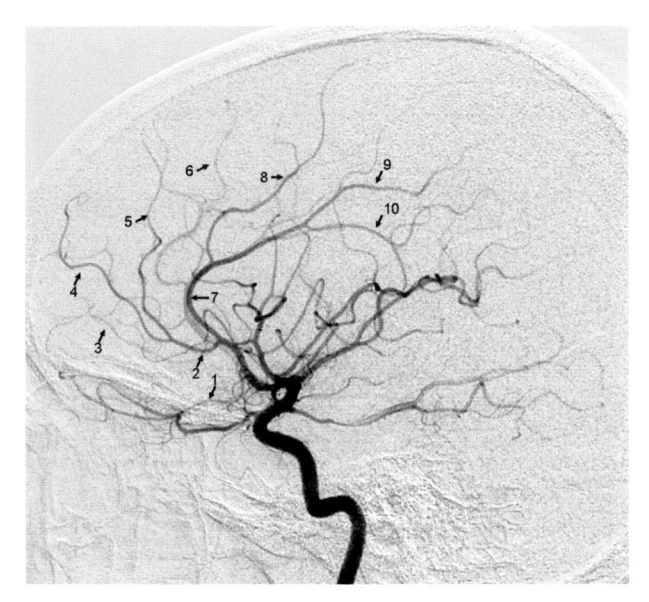

CHAPTER 3 Anatomy of the Brain's Arterial Supply

Figure 3.11 Anterior cerebral artery branches. Left lateral projection, left ICA injection, conventional angiogram. 1, Orbitofrontal; 2, callosomarginal; 3, frontopolar; 4, anterior internal frontal; 5, middle internal frontal; 6, posterior internal frontal; 7, pericallosal; 8, paracentral; 9, superior parietal; 10, inferior parietal.

occasionally the anterior hypothalamus. Small perforating arteries arise from the A1 and A2 segments to supply the anterior perforated substance, medial-most aspect of the Sylvian fissure, inferior surface of the frontal lobe, dorsal surface of the optic nerve and optic chiasm, suprachiasmatic hypothalamus and optic tract. Perforators arising from the AComA supply the upper surface of the optic chiasm and anterior hypothalamus, the fornix, rostral corpus callosum, septal region and anterior cingulate gyrus.

The callosomarginal artery (Figure 3.11), the largest branch of the pericallosal artery, usually arises from the A3 (precallosal) segment, but may arise anywhere from just distal to the AComA to the A4 segment. It courses in or adjacent to the cingulate sulcus parallel to the pericallosal artery and gives rise to branches that supply the medial cerebral hemispheres and paramedian zones of cortex along the cerebral convexities, including portions of the premotor, motor and sensory cortex. The position of the callosomarginal artery, just above and lateral to the inferior margin of the falx, places it in harm's way in cases of subfalcial herniation. Here, the vessel may be sufficiently compressed along the margin of the falx to produce ACA territory infarction.

The anatomy and arterial distribution of branches from the callosomarginal and pericallosal arteries is variable and complementary (Figure 3.11). Cortical branches of the ACA include the orbitofrontal, frontopolar, anterior, middle and posterior internal frontal, paracentral and superior and inferior internal parietal arteries. The orbitofrontal and frontopolar arteries usually arise from the A2 segment. The anterior and middle internal frontal and callosomarginal arteries usually arise from A3. The posterior internal frontal artery may arise from A3, A4 or the callosomarginal artery (in descending order of frequency). The pericallosal artery is the source of the cortical branches of the ACA more frequently than is the callosomarginal artery. However, the cortical branches most likely to arise from the callosomarginal artery are one of the internal frontal arteries (most commonly the middle internal frontal artery) or a paracentral artery. The paracentral artery usually arises from the A4 segment. The superior parietal artery may arise from A4 or A5 or the callosomarginal artery. The inferior parietal artery usually arises from A5 just anterior to the splenium of the corpus callosum.

The orbitofrontal artery descends from its origin to the floor of the anterior fossa to supply the gyrus rectus, olfactory apparatus and medial orbital surface of the frontal lobe. The frontopolar artery passes along the medial surface of the frontal lobe to supply the medial and lateral surfaces of the frontal pole. These vessels may be enveloped or displaced by anterior fossa floor meningiomas. The internal frontal arteries ascend to supply the anterior, middle and posterior aspects of the medial and lateral surfaces of the superior frontal gyrus as far posteriorly as the precentral sulcus and anterior-most paracentral lobule. The paracentral artery courses into the superior aspect of the paracentral lobule and supplies portions of the premotor, motor and sensory cortex. The internal parietal arteries supply the medial hemispheres and paramedian convexity posterior to the paracentral lobule. The superior parietal artery supplies the superior precuneus. The inferior parietal artery supplies the posteroinferior cuneus and adjacent cuneus.

The ACA also supplies the corpus callosum via straight perforating vessels (short callosal arteries). These are usually branches of the pericallosal and posterior pericallosal arteries [24]. These vessels continue through the corpus callosum to supply the subjacent fornix and portions of the anterior commissure. In a majority of patients, the AComA gives rise to either a subcallosal or median callosal artery which contributes to blood supply to the corpus callosum. The uncommon precallosal artery may arise from the A2 or AComA and pass upwards between the pericallosal artery and lamina terminalis to supply the anterior diencephalon and the rostrum and inferior aspect of the genu of the corpus callosum.

The vascular territory of the ACA usually conforms to a parafalcial zone of the medial superior cerebral convexity and the medial cerebral cortex. The proximally occluded ACA yields a characteristic infarct pattern (Figure 3.12a–c).

Middle cerebral artery

The middle cerebral artery (MCA) is the larger of the two branches arising from the terminal ICA bifurcation,

PART I How To Perform Ultrasound Tests

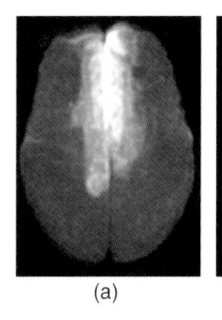

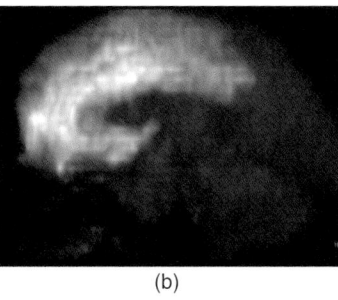

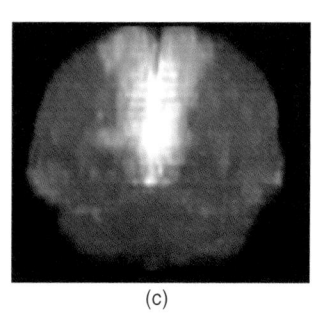

Figure 3.12 ACA vascular territory. 3D maximum intensity projections of diffusion-weighted MRI images in patient with bilateral ACA territory infarctions. (a) Craniocaudal projection; (b) lateral projection; (c) AP projection. Infarct zones occupy medial cerebral hemispheres.

averaging 3.9 mm in diameter at its origin [8] (Figures 3.7a and 3.13). It arises in the medial-most end of the sylvian fissure and continues laterally beneath the anterior perforated substance, where the perforating lenticulostriate arteries arise from its superior surface. Further laterally it bifurcates into upper and lower divisions that supply the insular, suprasylvian and infrasylvian (frontal, parietal and temporal) opercular cortex, most of the lateral cerebral convexity and portions of the base of the cerebral hemisphere. Rhoton [8] divided the MCA cortical territory into 12 areas: the orbitofrontal, prefrontal, precentral, central, anterior parietal, posterior parietal, angular, temporo-occipital, posterior temporal, middle temporal, anterior temporal and temporo-polar areas.

Although the MCA bifurcates in most individuals (anterior and posterior divisions), in some patients there is an MCA *trifurcation* (with superior, middle and inferior divisions) and, more rarely, even more elaborate branching into more than three trunks. The trunks distal to the MCA bifurcation may be of similar size or the superior or inferior trunk may be dominant. The cortical territories that are perfused by the trunks differ in pattern with each of these variants. By convention, the MCA is divided into four segments (Figure 3.7a), M1 (sphenoidal segment) extending from the MCA origin to the vertical turn into the medial Sylvian fissure and including the MCA bifurcation, M2 (insular segment), the vertical portion located in the medial sylvian fissure and ascending beside the insula, M3 (opercular segment), the portion in the lateral sylvian fissure commencing at the circular sulcus and extending obliquely laterally between superior temporal lobe and frontal and parietal opercula, and M4 (cortical segments), coursing up or down along the lateral and superior cerebral convexity. Most MCA branching occurs in the M2 segment. The orientation of the anterior M4 branches is more vertical, whereas posterior M4 branches have a more horizontal course, paralleling the axis of the Sylvian fissure. The highest M3–M4 turn on routine AP angiographic projections and the most posterior MCA branch visualized on lateral angiographic views is the angular artery.

The perforating branches of the MCA (the lenticulostriate arteries) are best depicted on catheter angiograms and are poorly depicted on CT and MR angiograms (Figure 3.13b). Most arise proximal to the MCA bifurcation. They are divided into medial, intermediate and lateral groups. The intermediate and lateral vessels penetrate the anterior perforated substance to supply most of the upper internal capsule and the body and head of the caudate nucleus. The medial group perfuses the area inferomedial to this, including the lateral globus pallidus, the superior aspect of the anterior limb of the internal capsule and the anteriosuperior aspect of the head of the caudate nucleus [8].

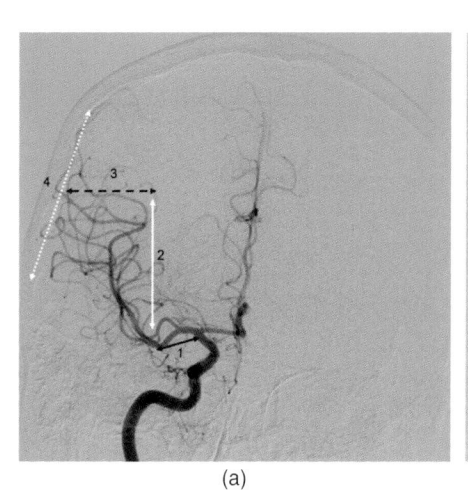

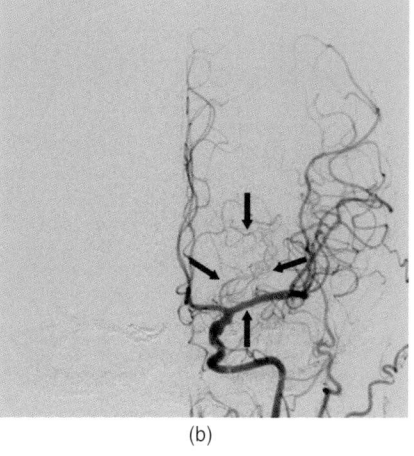

Figure 3.13 Middle cerebral artery anatomy. (a) AP projection, right internal carotid artery injection, conventional angiogram. Double-headed arrows demarcate the segments of the right middle cerebral artery. (b) AP projection, left internal carotid artery injection, conventional angiogram. Arrows indicate perforating arteries of MCA (lenticulostriate arteries).

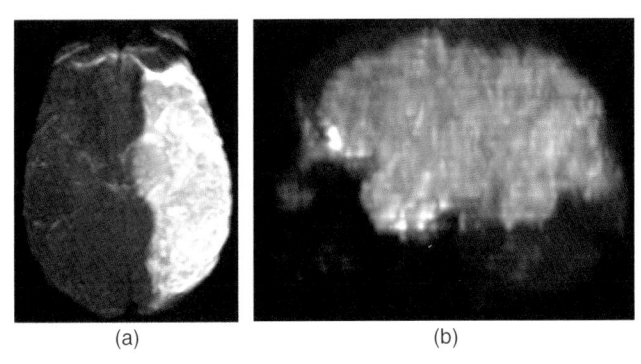

Figure 3.14 Middle cerebral artery vascular territory. 3D maximum intensity projection of diffusion-weighted MRI images in patient with left MCA territory infarction. (a) Craniocaudal projection; (b) lateral projection; (c) AP projection.

The vascular territory of the MCA includes most of the cerebral cortex exclusive of the paramedian ACA territory, the medial and lateral cortical territories of PCA branches and most of the "basal ganglia region" exclusive of the thalami. Even with total MCA occlusion, the size and shape of MCA infarcts are variable, reflecting this territory but influenced by the adequacy and pattern of collateral blood flow (Figure 3.14).

The posterior circulation

The posterior circulation consists of the "vertebrobasilar arterial system" and supplies the cerebellum, brainstem, thalami, posterior parietal lobes (posteriorly and medially), posterior inferior temporal lobes and occipital lobes.

The vertebral arteries (VAs) arise from the top of the subclavian arteries at the apex of the lateralward curve that each makes as it turns from the superior mediastinum towards the subclavicular fossa (Figure 3.15). Each vertebral artery (V1, extraosseous segment) travels briefly medially, then upwards from its origin to enter the transverse foramina of the cervical spine, usually at the C5 or C6 level, but as high as C3. The V2 (foraminal) segment continues from the lowest (usually C6) traversed transverse foramen cranially to the C1 level. V3 (the extraspinal segment) extends from the C1 transverse foramen to the foramen magnum. V4 represents the final intracranial (intradural) segment.

The cervical vertebral arteries give off muscular and spinal branches. The muscular branches supply the adjacent deep cervical muscles. The spinal branches supply the spinal cord, cervical spinal meninges and cervical vertebra. These branches also anastomose with branches of the ascending pharyngeal, ascending cervical and costocervical arteries. Intracranially, each of the two V4 segments gives off a posterior meningeal artery, posterior and anterior spinal arteries, multiple perforating arteries and a posterior inferior cerebellar artery before uniting to form the basilar artery. The perforating arteries supply the olive and inferior cerebellar peduncle. The posterior meningeal arteries supply the posterior fossa dura and may supply dural-based lesions such as meningiomas and posterior fossa dural arteriovenous malformations. The anterior and posterior spinal arteries supply the cervical spinal cord.

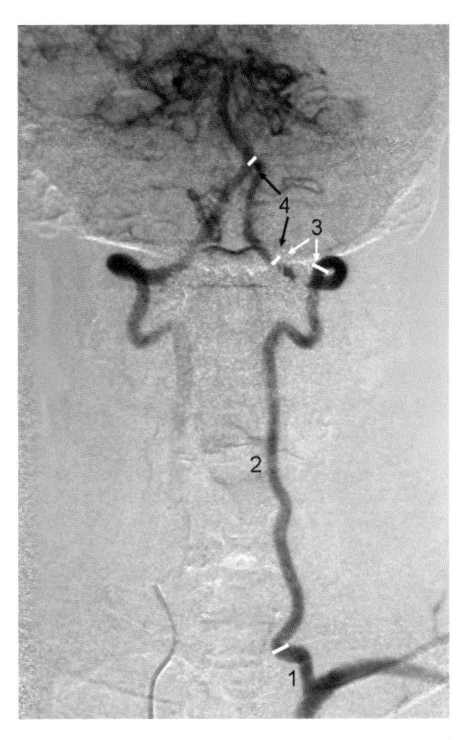

Figure 3.15 Segments of the vertebral artery. AP projection of right vertebral artery injection in a patient with "subclavian steal." Retrograde flow in the left vertebral artery opacifies the entire vessel. Numbers correspond to the numbered segments of the vertebral artery (see text).

Asymmetry of the vertebral arteries is fairly common, with the smaller one often functionally terminating as the posterior inferior cerebellar artery (and having only a hypoplastic or atretic segment between the posterior inferior cerebellar artery origin and the V4 confluence). The left vertebral artery is "dominant" (larger than the right) in 50–60% of individuals [2]. Fenestrations of the VA (duplicate endothelially lined parallel lumens) are common. Most fenestrations occur at the C1–C2 level, but they may be seen intracranially and may be associated with aneurysms (Figure 3.16a and b). The vertebral arteries are rarely duplicated. The basilar artery is of variable length and diameter. It is normally straight, but may become fairly tortuous in some patients. Multiple tiny perforating arteries arise from the basilar artery trunk to supply the ventral brainstem.

Posterior circulation branches

These branches are shown in Figure 3.17. The posterior inferior cerebellar artery (PICA) arises near the inferior olive and

PART I How To Perform Ultrasound Tests

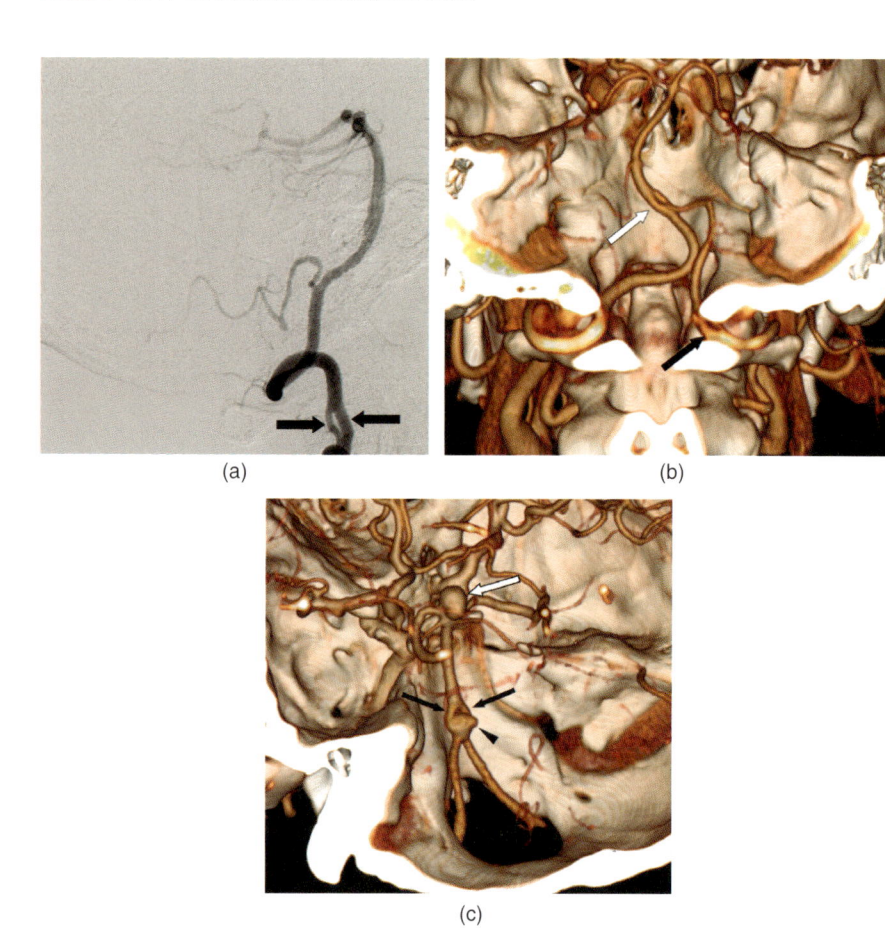

Figure 3.16 Posterior circulation fenestrations. (a) Lateral projection, right vertebral artery injection, conventional angiogram. Arrows indicate right vertebral artery fenestration at C1–C2 level. (b) Posterior projection, CT angiogram. White arrow indicates basilar artery fenestration. Black arrow indicates right vertebral artery fenestration. (c) Posterior oblique projection, CT angiogram. Black arrows indicate basilar artery fenestration. Note aneurysm (arrowhead) within the fenestration. There is also a basilar tip aneurysm (white arrow).

passes posteriorly around the medulla. Proximally, the PICA gives rise to perforating arteries that supply the medulla [25]. The vessel passes just above hypoglossal nerve anteriorly and just inferior to cranial nerves IX, X and XII along the posterolateral medullary surface. Just distal to this the artery loops downwards around the cerebellar peduncle then up in the cerebellomedullary fissure to pass the caudal fourth ventricular roof (where it gives rise to branches that supply the fourth ventricular choroid plexus) before exiting the cerebellomedullary fissure. Here it bifurcates into medial and lateral trunks that descend to provide cortical branches to the inferior vermis, cerebellar tonsils and inferior cerebellar hemispheres. Infarcts in the PICA territory typically affect the posterior, inferior aspect of the cerebellar hemisphere (Figure 3.18).

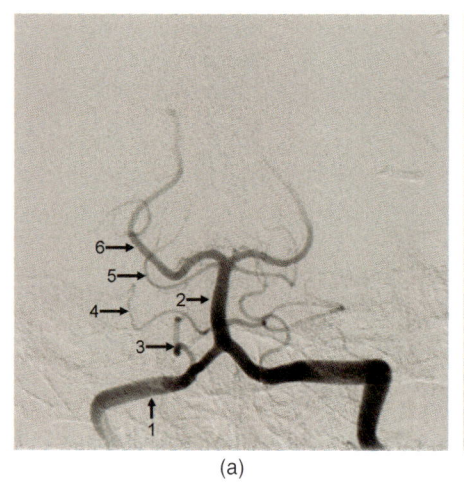

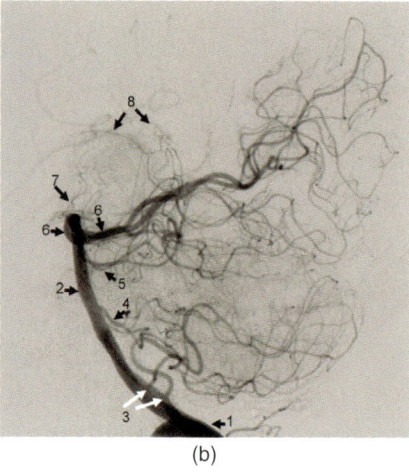

Figure 3.17 Posterior circulation branches. (a) AP projection, left vertebral artery injection, conventional angiogram. 1, Vertebral artery (V4 segment); 2, basilar artery; 3, posterior inferior cerebellar artery; 4, anterior inferior cerebellar artery; 5, superior cerebellar artery; 6, posterior cerebral artery; 7, thalamoperforating arteries; 8, posterior choroidal arteries (medial and lateral). (b) Lateral projection, left vertebral artery injection, conventional angiogram. Branches are numbered as in (a).

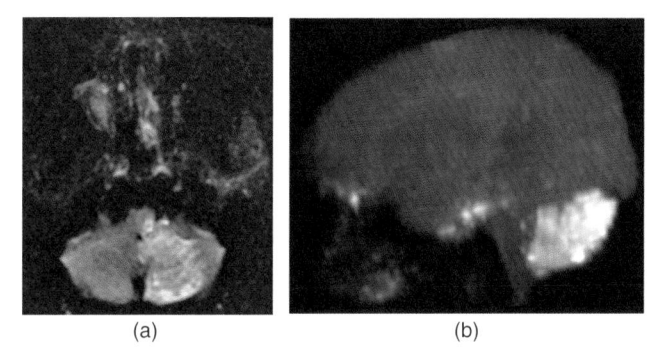

Figure 3.18 3D maximum intensity projection of diffusion-weighted MRI images in a patient with left PICA territory infarction. (a) Craniocaudal projection; (b) lateral projection.

The anterior inferior cerebellar arteries (AICAs) arise from the mid-basilar artery and are usually the smallest of the major cerebellar arteries. The origins of the AICAs on the two sides are frequently craniocaudally asymmetric. The AICA travels laterally from its origin through the central portion of the cerebellopontine angle adjacent to cranial nerves VII and VIII. Proximal AICA perforating arteries supply the brainstem. The artery supplies branches to nerves within and may commonly loop into, the internal auditory canal. The AICA also supplies the labyrinth. The AICA commonly bifurcates to form rostral and caudal trunks. The rostral trunk supplies the superior lip of the cerebellopontine fissure and the adjacent petrosal surface of the cerebellum. The inferior trunk supplies the more inferior aspect of the petrosal surface of the cerebellum, the flocculus and fourth ventricular choroid plexus. Distal branches of the rostral trunk often anastomose with distal branches of the SCA, whereas distal branches of the caudal trunk anastomose with distal PICA branches. There is frequently a reciprocal relationship in PICA/AICA anatomy, with one vessel perfusing a larger than normal portion of the other's territory and an inverse relationship between the sizes of the two. A common finding is a large PICA with a small or absent ipsilateral AICA and contralateral PICA. This has been called the "PICA–AICA" variant. Alternatively, patients may have a dominant AICA and small or absent ipsilateral PICA ("AICA–PICA"

variant). Infarcts in the AICA territory typically affect the anterior, inferior aspect of the cerebellar hemisphere (Figure 3.19).

Distally, the basilar artery gives rise to the superior cerebellar arteries (SCAs) just below the tentorium and just in front of the midbrain. The SCA is occasionally duplicated. The SCA passes below cranial nerves III and IV and above cranial nerve V and travels around the midbrain near the pontomesencephalic junction. Its course may indent the root entry zone of the trigeminal nerve, the most commonly identified cause for neurovascular compression-induced trigeminal neuralgia. In rare cases in which the SCA arises from the PCA, the SCA passes above the oculomotor nerve. SCA branches include perforating arteries that supply the brainstem and cerebellar peduncles and precerebellar branches that supply the deep cerebellar white matter and dentate nuclei. The precerebellar arteries are small vessels that arise from the SCA trunks and cortical branches of the SCA within the cerebellomesencephalic fissure. The SCA divides into the rostral trunk that supplies the vermis and adjacent paramedian upper cerebellar hemispheres and a caudal trunk that supplies the remaining superior cerebellar hemispheres, both superiorly (tentorial surface) and anteriorly (petrosal surface). Infarcts in the SCA territory involve the superior cerebellar hemisphere and vermis and deep cerebellar white matter (Figure 3.20).

Posterior cerebral artery

In most patients, the posterior cerebral arteries (PCAs) arise from the terminal basilar artery immediately above the tentorium, although the basilar artery tip and PCA origins may be a high as the mammillary bodies/third ventricular floor (Figure 3.21). The PCA origins may lie very close to the SCA origins, in which case their proximal course often passes both superiorly and laterally. More commonly, there is a short basilar artery segment between the SCA and PCA origins and the orientation of the proximal PCA is more horizontal. The P1 or precommunicating segment of the PCA begins a course around the ventral midbrain, receiving the posterior communicating arteries at the lateral margin of the

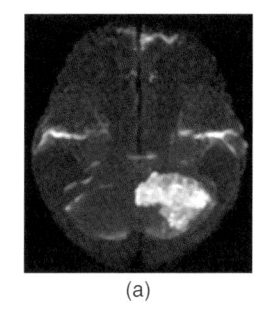

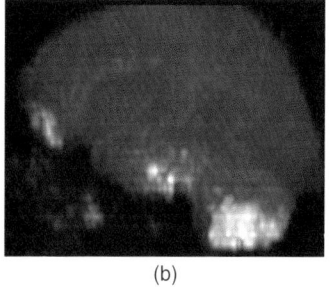

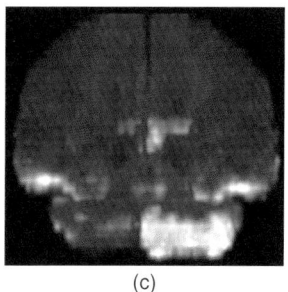

Figure 3.19 3D maximum intensity projection of diffusion weighted MRI images in patient with left AICA territory infarction. a: craniocaudal projection, b: lateral projection, c: PA projection. In this patient, there was some involvement of the usual territory of the PICA. It is common for there to be significant overlap between cerebellar arterial territories.

PART I How To Perform Ultrasound Tests

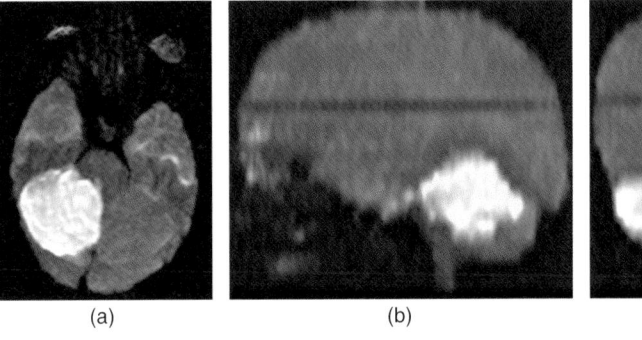

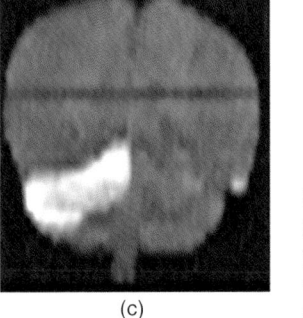

Figure 3.20 3D maximum intensity projection of diffusion weighted MRI images in patient with right SCA territory infarction. a: craniocaudal projection, b: lateral projection, c: PA projection.

interpeduncular cistern. The P1 segment gives rise to the thalamoperforating arteries, the medial posterior choroidal artery, the branch to the quadrigeminal plate and branches to the cerebral peduncle and midbrain tegmentum. The PComA–P1 confluence marks the beginning of the P2 segment. This segment extends laterally and posteriorly, curving around the cerebral peduncle in the crural and ambient cisterns, ending at the level of the posterior margin of the midbrain. The P3 segment continues from the posterior margin of the lateral midbrain surface and terminates at the anterior edge of the calcarine fissure. The P3 segment bifurcates to yield the calcarine and parieto-occipital arteries.

The PCA has central perforating branches (including the thalamoperforating, thalamogeniculate and peduncular perforating arteries) that supply the diencephalon and midbrain, ventricular branches (medial and lateral posterior choroidal arteries) supplying the choroid plexus and walls of the lateral and third ventricles and cerebral branches (inferior temporal group, parieto-occipital, calcarine and splenial arteries) to the cerebral cortex and callosal splenium. The perforating arteries arise primarily from the P1 segment. The hippocampal, anterior temporal, peduncular perforating and medial posterior choroidal arteries arise from proximal P2 segment. The middle, posterior and common temporal and lateral posterior choroidal arteries arise from the distal P2 segment. The thalamogeniculate perforating arteries arise from the proximal or distal P2 segment. The calcarine and parieto-occipital arteries arise from the P3 segment. The inferior temporal artery group (recall that the superior temporal arteries arise from the MCA) supplies the inferior temporal lobe and portions of its medial and lateral aspects. Arteries in this group are variable in size and have a reciprocal/complementary relationship in terms of diameter/area of supply. The hippocampal artery (first cortical branch of the PCA) supplies the uncus, anterior parahippocampal gyrus, hippocampal formation and dentate gyrus. The anterior temporal artery is usually the next cortical PCA branch. It supplies the anteroinferior temporal lobe and may supply the temporal pole and lateral temporal in the region of the middle temporal gyrus. The middle temporal artery supplies the inferior surface of the temporal lobe and is the smallest and least constant branch of the inferior temporal group. The posterior temporal artery is the largest and most branched of the inferior temporal group. It courses posterolaterally to supply the inferior temporal and occipital surfaces of the brain including the occipital pole and lingual gyrus. It is also the most common source of PCA supply to the lateral convexity (the parieto-occipital artery being the next most important source of this). The common temporal artery is seen in less than 20% of hemispheres and when present it supplies most of the inferior surfaces of the temporal and occipital lobes. The parieto-occipital artery courses posteriorly in the parieto-occipital sulcus to supply the posterior parasagittal cortex including the cuneus and precuneus, as well as the lateral occipital gyrus and rarely the precentral and superior parietal lobules. When its origin is more proximal, it may contribute to the territories of more proximal PCA branches, including the thalamus, midbrain, lateral geniculate bodies, lateral and third ventricular choroid

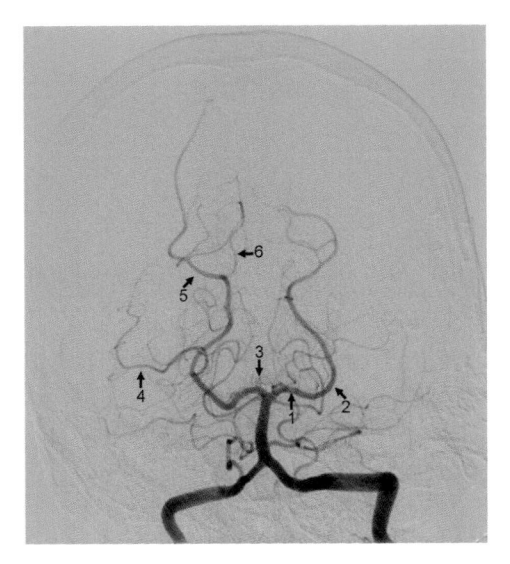

Figure 3.21 PCA branches. AP projection LVA injection, conventional angiogram. 1, P1 segment of PCA; 2, P2 segment of PCA; 3, thalamoperforating vessels; 4, posterior temporal artery; 5, parieto-occipital artery; 6, calcarine artery

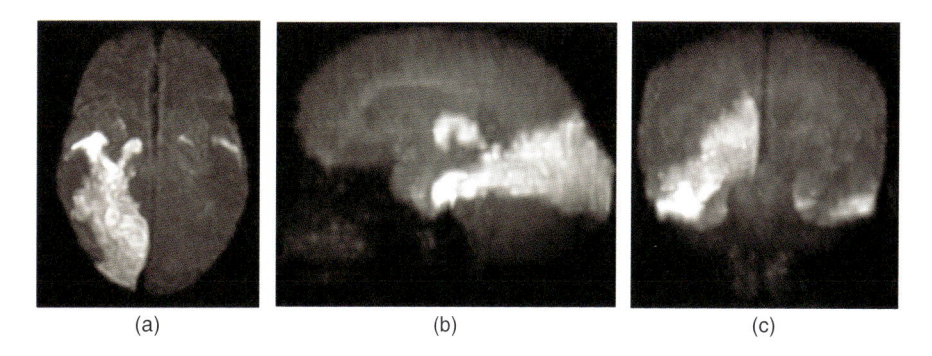

Figure 3.22 3D maximum intensity projection of diffusion-weighted MRI images in patient with right PCA territory infarction. (a) Craniocaudal projection; (b) lateral projection; (c) PA projection.

plexus and splenium. The calcarine artery travels through the calcarine sulcus to supply the visual cortex, occipital pole, lingual gyrus and inferior cuneus. The splenial artery may arise directly from the PCA or one of its branches. The splenial arteries anastomose with branches of the pericallosal artery and may provide collateral flow in cases of ACA or proximal PCA occlusion or stenosis. PCA territory infarcts rarely involve the entire territory, but large PCA infarcts often involve the posterior inferior temporal lobe, occipital lobe, posterior inferior parietal lobe, thalamus and hippocampus (Figure 3.22).

Posterior circulation vessels can recruit multiple collaterals the most important being reversed basilar artery in the dominant VA is obstructed [26]. In this case, basilar flow descends from the top of the basilar towards cerebellar branches and it is supplied via PComAs. Antegrade reconstitution of VA flow distal to VA occlusion may occur via the ascending cervical and/or the costocervical arteries, in addition to occurring across occlusions via bridging muscular branches of the same vertebral artery or opposite vertebral artery. ECA to VA anastomoses may also reconstitute flow in proximally occluded vertebral arteries (see Figure 3.4d and e)

The circle of Willis

The circle of Willis is the central collateral circuit at the base of the brain that helps to preserve blood flow in cases of proximal cerebral vascular occlusion. It consists of "supply" and "bridging" components (Figure 3.23). The "supply" components to the circle of Willis are the internal carotid arteries and basilar arteries. The "bridging" components of the circle of Willis interconnect the supply components and consist of the midline anterior communicating artery and the A1 segments of the anterior cerebral arteries, which connect the right anterior circulation to the left and the parasagittal posterior communicating arteries, and P1 segments of the posterior cerebral arteries, which connect each side of the anterior circulation to the posterior circulation. Hypoplasia or absence of various bridging components is very common [27–29].

Pial to pial anastomotic flow

End-to-end collateral flow at margins (borderzones) of vascular territories or across ischemic zones in a single vascular territory may occur in response to proximal vascular occlusions (Figure 3.24). Dural collaterals may also arise from meningeal or other branches of the ECA.

Primitive anastomoses

A craniocaudal series of primitive vessels connects the anterior to the posterior circulation during embryogenesis like

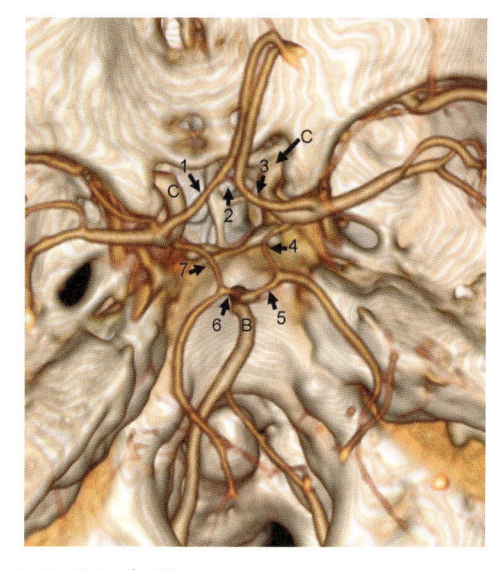

Figure 3.23 Circle of Willis. C, Internal carotid artery; B, basilar artery. 1, Left A1 segment; 2, anterior communicating artery; 3, right A1; 4, right posterior communicating artery; 5, right P1 segment; 6, left P1 segment; 7, left posterior communicating artery.

PART I How To Perform Ultrasound Tests

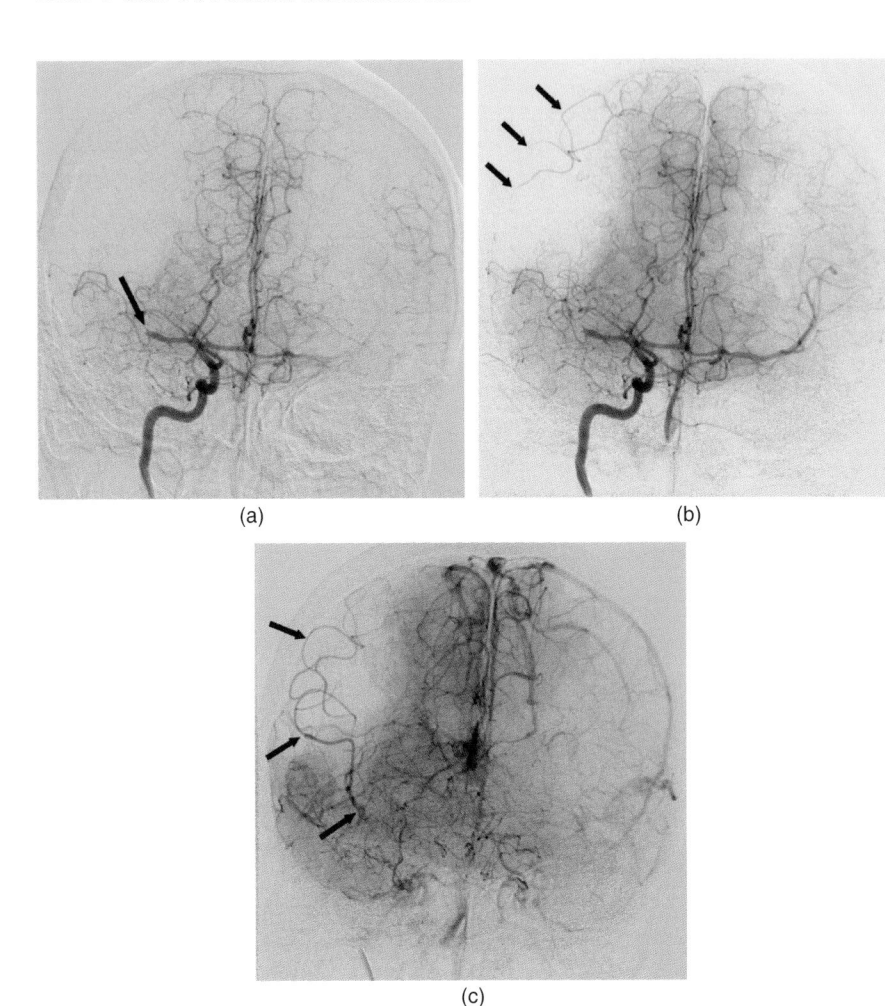

Figure 3.24 Pial to pial anatomotic flow. Right internal carotid artery injection, conventional angiogram. (a) Arrow indicates occlusion of right middle cerebral artery just distal to the anterior temporal artery origin. (b) Arrows demonstrate retrograde filling of distal right MCA branches via pial to pial anatomotic flow from terminal ACA branches. (c) Retrograde flow in right MCA branches continues nearly to the point of proximal occlusion (arrows).

rungs on a ladder. These primitive anastomoses may explain acute simultaneous infarcts in both anterior and posterior vascular territories. Ordinarily, the most superior of these connections persists as the PComA and the others regress. In approximately 20% of patients, the embryonic fetal condition (with the PCA being derived primarily from the ipsilateral ICA via a prominent PComA and a small ipsilateral P1 segment) persists on one side. This is known as a "fetal configuration" or "fetal origin" of the PCA (Figure 3.25a). In some patients there is persistence of one of the other primitive connections as a "carotid–basilar anastomosis." In many patients with these primitive connections, the vertebral and basilar arteries are small proximal to the anastomosis. Three of the primitive connections are named by the cranial nerves that they parallel. Below the PComA the next and the most common of the primitive anastomoses is the primitive trigeminal artery. The persistent trigeminal artery arises near the junction of the C3 and C4 segments of the ICA and passes posteriorly, either lateral to or through the dorsum sella, to connect to the basilar artery (Figure 3.25b).

Numerous variants of persistent trigeminal artery anatomy may be encountered. There is an increased incidence of vascular abnormalities, especially aneurysms, in association with persistent trigeminal arteries [30]. The persistent otic artery is the next lower of the primitive connections, but is rarely visualized angiographically. This passes from the petrous (C2) segment of the ICA to the basilar artery. The next more caudal primitive connection, second in frequency to the persistent trigeminal artery, is the persistent hypoglossal artery, which arises from the cervical ICA and traverses the osseous hypoglossal canal to join the basilar artery. The last of the primitive anastomoses is the proatlantal intersegmental artery [31], which originates from the upper cervical ICA and (type 1, most common variant) passes superolaterally, then medially, over the arch of C1, to pass through the foramen magnum and give rise to the ipsilateral vertebral artery. A second, less frequent variant (type 2), arises from the external carotid artery and connects with the vertebral artery below C1. The vertebral artery then continues upward in the normal fashion, through the C1 transverse foramen.

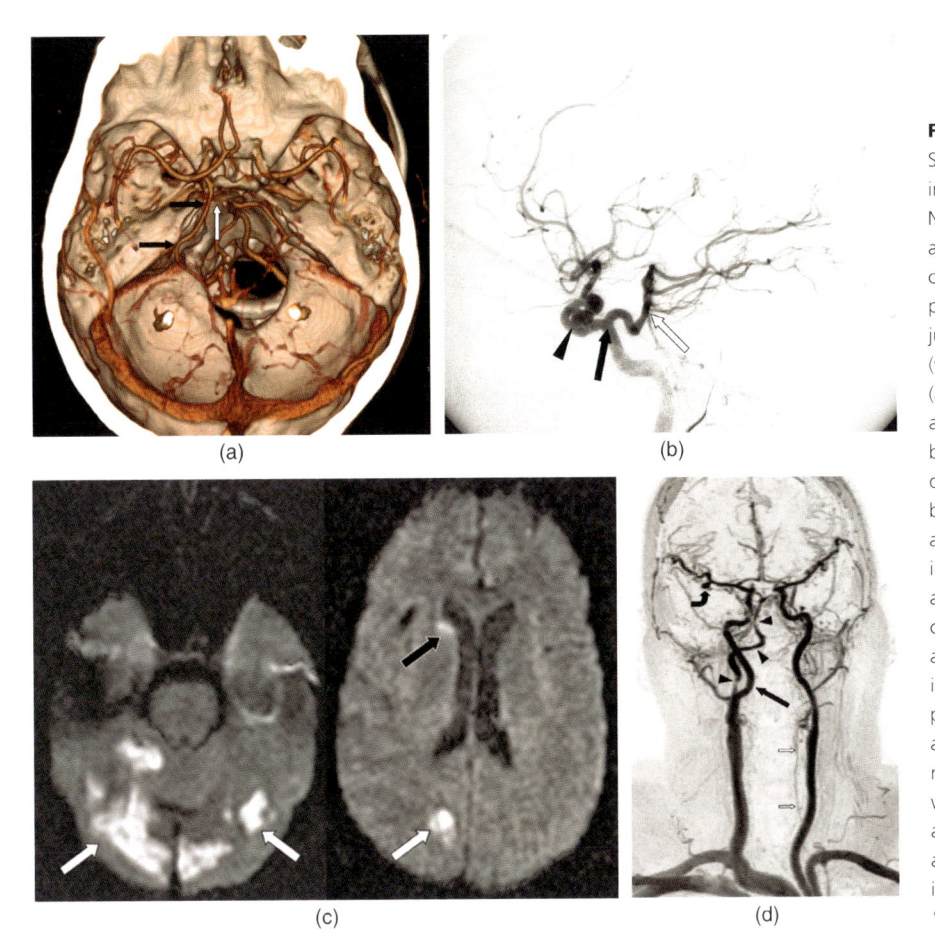

CHAPTER 3 Anatomy of the Brain's Arterial Supply

Figure 3.25 Primitive anatomoses. (a) Superior view, CT angiogram. Black arrows indicate fetal configuration of the left PCA. Note that left P1 segment is hypoplastic (white arrow). (b) Lateral projection, left ICA injection, conventional angiogram. Black arrow indicates persistent trigeminal artery arising at C3–C4 junction and filling the distal basilar artery (white arrow). Note associated aneurysms (arrowhead). Note that the basilar artery appears small proximal to the anastomoses (i.e. below the white arrow). (c) A pair of diffusion-weighted MR images demonstrates bilateral PCA territory infarcts (white arrows) and a synchronous right caudate nucleus infarct in the "anterior circulation" (black arrow). (d) Contrast-enhanced 3D MRA of cervical arteries; same patient as in (c). Black arrow indicates right ICA. Black arrowheads indicate primitive hypoglossal artery (note proximal stenosis adjacent to lowest arrowhead). Curved arrow indicates incidental right MCA bifurcation aneurysm. The cervical vertebral arteries are hypoplastic (outlined arrows). This patient's anomalous vascular anatomy helps explain the pattern of brain infarction with simultaneous involvement of "anterior" and "posterior" vascular territories.

References

1 Layton KF, Kallmes DF, Cloft HJ, et al. Bovine arch variation in humans: classification of a misnomer. *AJNR Am J Neuroradiol* 2006;**27**:1541–42.

2 Tay KW, U-King-Im JM, Trivedi RA, et al. Imaging the vertebral artery. *Eur Radiol* 2005;**15**:1329–43.

3 Atkin GK, Grieve VR, Vattipally KH, et al. The surgical management of aortic root vessel anomalies presenting in adults. *Ann Vasc Surg* 2007;**21**:525–34.

4 Hara M, Satake M, Itoh M, et al. Radiographic findings of aberrant right subclavian artery initially depicted on CT. *Radiat Med* 2003;**21**:161–5.

5 Kagetsu NJ, Berenstein A, Choi IS. Interventional radiology of the extracranial head and neck. *Cardiovasc Intervent Radiol* 1991;**14**:325–33.

6 Oguzkurt L, Kizilkilic O, Tercan F, et al. Vertebrocarotid collateral in extracranial carotid artery occlusions: digital subtraction angiography findings. *Eur J Radiol* 2005;**53**:168–74.

7 Smith T. Embolization in the external carotid artery. *J Vasc Intervent Radiol* 2006;**17**:1897–913.

8 Rhoton AL Jr. The supratentorial arteries. *Neurosurgery* 2002;**51**(4 Suppl):S53–120.

9 Bouthillier A, van Loveren HR, Keller JT. Segments of the internal carotid artery: a new classification. *Neurosurgery* 1996;**38**(3):425–32.

10 Okahara M, Kiyosue H, Mori H, et al. Anatomic variations of the cerebral arteries and their embryology: a pictorial review. *Eur Radiol* 2002;**12**:2548–61.

11 Dinc H, Alioglu Z, Erdol H, et al. Agenesis of the internal carotid artery associated with aortic arch anomaly in a patient with congenital Horner's syndrome. *AJNR Am J Neuroradiol* 2002;**23**:929–31.

12 Orakdöğen M, Berkman Z, Erşahin M, et al. Agenesis of the left internal carotid artery associated with anterior communicating artery aneurysm: case report. *Turk Neurosurg* 2007;**17**(4):273–6.

13 Demirgil B, Tuğcu B, Günaldi O, et al. Agenesis of the left internal carotid artery associated with right anterior cerebral artery A1 segment bifurcation aneurysm: a case report. *Minim Invasive Neurosurg* 2007;**50**(5):300–3.

14 Branstetter IV BF, Weissman JL. The radiologic evaluation of tinnitus. *Eur Radiol* 2006;**16**:2792–802.

15 Silbergleit R, Quint DJ, Mehta FA, et al. The persistent stapedial artery. *AJNR Am J Neuroradiol* 2000;**21**:572–7.

16 Walton KA, Buono LM. Horner syndrome. *Curr Opin Opthalmol* 2003;**14**:357–63.

17 Lee JH, Lee HK, Lee DH, et al. Neuroimaging strategies for three types of Horner syndrome with emphasis on anatomic location. *AJR Am J Roentgenol* 2005;**188**:W74–81.

18. Tubbs RS, Hansasuta A, Louka M, *et al*. Branches of the petrous and cavernous segments of the internal carotid artery. *Clin Anat* 2007;**20**:596–601.
19. Matsumura Y, Nagashima M. Anatomical variations in the origin of the human ophthalmic artery with special reference to the cavernous sinus and surrounding meninges. *Cells Tissues Organs* 1999;**164**:112–21.
20. Liu Q, Rhoton AL Jr. Middle meningeal artery origin of the ophthalmic artery. *Neurosurgery* 2001;**49**:401–6.
21. Coupe NJ, Athwal RK, Marshman LA, *et al*. Subarachnoid hemorrhage emanating from a ruptured infundibulum: case report and literature review. *Surg Neurol* 2007;**67**:204–6.
22. Marshman LA, Ward PJ, Walter PH, *et al*. The progression of an infundibulum to aneurysm formation and rupture: case report and literature review. *Neurosurgery* 1998;**43**:1445–8.
23. Auguste KI, Ware ML, Lawton MT. Nonsaccular aneurysms of the azygos anterior cerebral artery. *Neurosurg Focus* 2004;**17**:E12.
24. Türe U, Yaşargil MG, Krisht AF. The arteries of the corpus callosum: a microsurgical anatomic study. *Neurosurgery* 1996;**39**(6):1075–84.
25. Rhoton AL. The cerebellar arteries. *Neurosurgery* 2000;**47**:S29–68.
26. Ribo M, Garami Z, Uchino K, *et al*. Detection of reversed basilar flow with power-motion Doppler after acute occlusion predicts favorable outcome. *Stroke* 2004;**35**:79–82.
27. Krabbe-Hartkamp MJ, van der Grond F-E, de Groot J-C, *et al*. Circle of Willis: morphologic variation on three-dimensional time-of-flight MR angiograms. *Radiology* 1998;**207**:103–11.
28. Waaijer A, van Leeuwen MS, van der Worp HB, *et al*. Anatomic variations of the Circle of Willis in patients with symptomatic carotid artery stenosis assessed with multidetector row CT angiography. *Cerebrovasc Dis* 2007;**23**:267–74.
29. AbuRhama AF, Robinsin PA, Short Y, *et al*. Cross-filling of the circle of Willis and carotid stenosis by angiography, duplex ultrasound and oculoplethmysography. *Am J Surg* 1995;**169**:308–12.
30. Cloft HJ, Razack N, Kallmes DF. Prevalence of cerebral aneurysms in patients witih persistent primitive trigeminal artery. *J Neurosurg* 1999;**90**:865–7.
31. Gumus T, ONal B, Ilgit ET. Bilateral persistence of type I proatlantal arteries: report of a case and review of the literature. *AJNR Am J Neuroradiol* 2004;**25**; 1622–4.

II Hemodynamic Principles

4 Integrated Assessment of Systemic and Intracranial Hemodynamics

Anne W. Alexandrov
University of Alabama at Birmingham, Birmingham, AL, USA

Introduction

Hemodynamics is a term used to describe the flow of blood through the vascular system. The measurement and augmentation of hemodynamics require an understanding of complex physiologic mechanisms that foster systemic autoregulation, the body's ability to adjust blood flow despite marked changes in arterial blood pressure. Learning these principles is a must for every vascular medicine discipline, and stroke is no exception.

Neurological sub-specialization should include exposure to learning general principles of critical and cardiovascular care to ensure sound understanding of systemic hemodynamic principles and how to utilize this information in clinical practice.

Neurovascular ultrasound is an exquisite tool that helps one to understand and integrate systemic and cerebral hemodynamic findings into clinical decision making. All stroke neurologists and critical care specialists who work with neurovascular patients should be trained in neurovascular ultrasound to understand how real-time flow measurement may benefit assessment, treatment planning, and ongoing evaluation of patient management strategies in relation to both local vascular lesions and systemic hemodynamics.

One concept explored in this chapter is autoregulation, which guards brain perfusion and ultimately cellular energy.

Autoregulation is dependent upon complex mechanisms that allow rapid detection of flow alterations coupled with multi-system responses that aim to maintain optimal perfusion, especially to critical organ systems. Chief among these mechanisms is augmentation of myocardial performance through intrinsic and extrinsic means.

Management of many neurovascular conditions often hinges on augmentation of systemic hemodynamic parameters to enhance intracranial blood flow, perfusion and brain tissue oxygenation. The coexistence of cardiac conditions

Cerebrovascular Ultrasound in Stroke Prevention and Treatment, 2nd edition. Edited by Andrei V. Alexandrov. © 2011 Blackwell Publishing Ltd.

such as acute myocardial ischemia or infarction, coronary artery disease, cardiac valvular anomalies and dysrhythmias frequently challenge safe augmentation of systemic flow parameters in neurological patients, yet the heart and systemic vasculature may be enslaved to drive intracranial perfusion when the clinician safely and accurately uses technology and clinical skills to monitor continuously the effects of patient care.

This chapter examines principles associated with systemic and intracranial hemodynamics and the methods commonly used in a critical care setting to assess hemodynamic function. Integrated assessment is illustrated with case studies and management of neurological patients. It builds the foundation for a specific discussion of cerebral hemodynamics and waveform recognition in the following chapter. Most of the following content in this chapter remains unchanged from the first edition, as remain the basic laws and principles of systemic hemodynamics.

Principles of blood flow

The circulatory system is viewed as a closed circuit for simplicity, made up of two major components, the systemic and pulmonary circulation. In reality, if endothelium is considered an organ it would be the largest in the body with a complex function and magnitude of fluid volume and variety of molecules shifted back and forth through it. Integration of hemodynamic principles discussed below with knowledge about vaso-active drugs, blood–brain barrier function and therapeutic agent delivery defines the ever-evolving field of vascular and critical care medicine.

Blood *flow* propagation through these circuits is first driven by the inter-relationship of *pressure* and *resistance* and also the physical characteristics of blood, a complex non-Newtonian fluid. The latter implies that blood would respond to changing circulatory conditions in a way that would differ from water. Manipulation of pressure and resistance variables within the cardiovascular system directly affects blood flow parameters and serves as the basis for clinical hemodynamic augmentation.

PART II Hemodynamic Principles

Blood *viscosity* is primarily determined by hematocrit, the percentage of blood that is made up of cells. Hence red blood cells can change their shape and they can adjust to conditions such as a stenosis, while platelets can be activated by plaque contents not covered by endothelium. These and other complex mechanisms contribute to blood behavior that could not be predicted by simple equations derived for Newtonian fluids. Nevertheless, some basic principles could still be applicable to some extent. An increase in hematocrit results in an increase in friction between successive layers of blood, slowing its propagation velocities and amplifying the pressure necessary to drive blood through the systemic circulation. When combined with reduced internal vessel diameter, an increase in blood viscosity may significantly impair blood flow.

Flow of blood through vessels is primarily determined by two factors:
1 Differences in pressure ($P_1 - P_2$) between the two ends of a vessel; and
2 Vascular resistance to flow.

Ohm's law is often used to describe flow through the vascular system [1,2]. Simply put, it states that blood flow is directly proportional to the pressure difference, but inversely proportional to the resistance:

Blood flow = Δ *pressure/resistance*

The amount of muscle tension within the vascular bed necessary to maintain specific flow pressures varies significantly. The *law of Laplace* describes this, stating that the muscle tension (T) needed to maintain a specific pressure (P) is reduced as the radius (R) is decreased [1]:

$P = T/R.$

The smaller the blood vessel diameter, the less tension is required to maintain a given pressure within the vessel. Applied to human anatomy, the degree of wall tension necessary to maintain perfusion pressure in the aorta would be approximately 10 000 times that necessary to maintain pressure within a capillary bed [2].

Resistance, or impediment to flow, cannot be measured directly and is derived by measurements of blood flow and pressure difference within a vessel [1,2]. Varying degrees of resistance occur in vessels throughout the body. Resistance is a product of changing vessel diameters coupled with proportional increases in blood viscosity, and also the cross-sectional area of vascular beds. The resistance associated with changes in vessel diameter affects the movement of blood flow through a phenomenon known as streamlining or laminar flow [1].

Laminar flow describes the parabolic movement of blood in layers within a blood vessel; the layer closest to the vessel wall moves at the slowest velocity, whereas larger vessels with multiple layers exhibit increased rates of flow at the core of the vessel [2].

Turbulent flow occurs when blood moves at the same time in a crosswise and streamlined fashion. Turbulence is typically the product of obstructions to flow, passage of blood over a rough surface or a sharp change in the direction of flow; it results in an eddy current, with an increase in friction and resistance [2].

Poiseuille's law is often used to describe the impact of resistance on blood flow. Note that this law introduces other variables that influence the resulting flow volume through a given "pipe" or an artery in our case. It states that the flow (Q) of a fluid through a tube is directly proportional to the pressure difference that exists between two ends of a tube ($P_1 - P_2$) to the fourth power of the radius of the tube (r^4) and is inversely proportional to length of the tube (L) and the viscosity of the fluid (n):

$Q = \pi(P_1 - P_2)r_4/8Ln$

where $\pi/8$ serves as a proportional geometric value [1]. Poiseuille's law illustrates how resistance increases in direct proportion to viscosity and vessel length, but decreases in direct proportion to vessel diameter and pressure gradient; in other words, the diameter of a blood vessel is the most significant contributor of all to the rate of blood flow through a vessel. It provides an insight that if blood has to go through a long and narrow channel, distal resistance (i.e. P_2) has to decrease in order to create an "incentive" for the flow to go the longer distance [2].

The inter-relatedness of these concepts in the production of varying rates of blood flow can be illustrated by changes in arterial pressure. An increase in arterial pressure increases the force propelling blood and also distends vessel walls, thereby reducing vascular resistance; the result is an increase in blood flow. Similarly, a drop in arterial pressure results in reduced forward flow secondary to a decrease in vessel diameter from reduced arterial stretch, accompanied by an increase in resistance to flow; blood viscosity further contributes to a decline in flow during low-pressure states as sluggish movement fosters clumping of cells and additional flow resistance. Arterial stretch becomes an important mechanism how nature preserves energy and helps the heart to work.

The cardiac cycle

The cardiac cycle represents the sequential electrical and mechanical events that occur within a single heart beat, namely systole and diastole. At normal heart rates approximately two-thirds of the cardiac cycle consists of diastolic events, allowing for muscle relaxation and filling of the ventricles. Figure 4.1 illustrates the events of the cardiac cycle

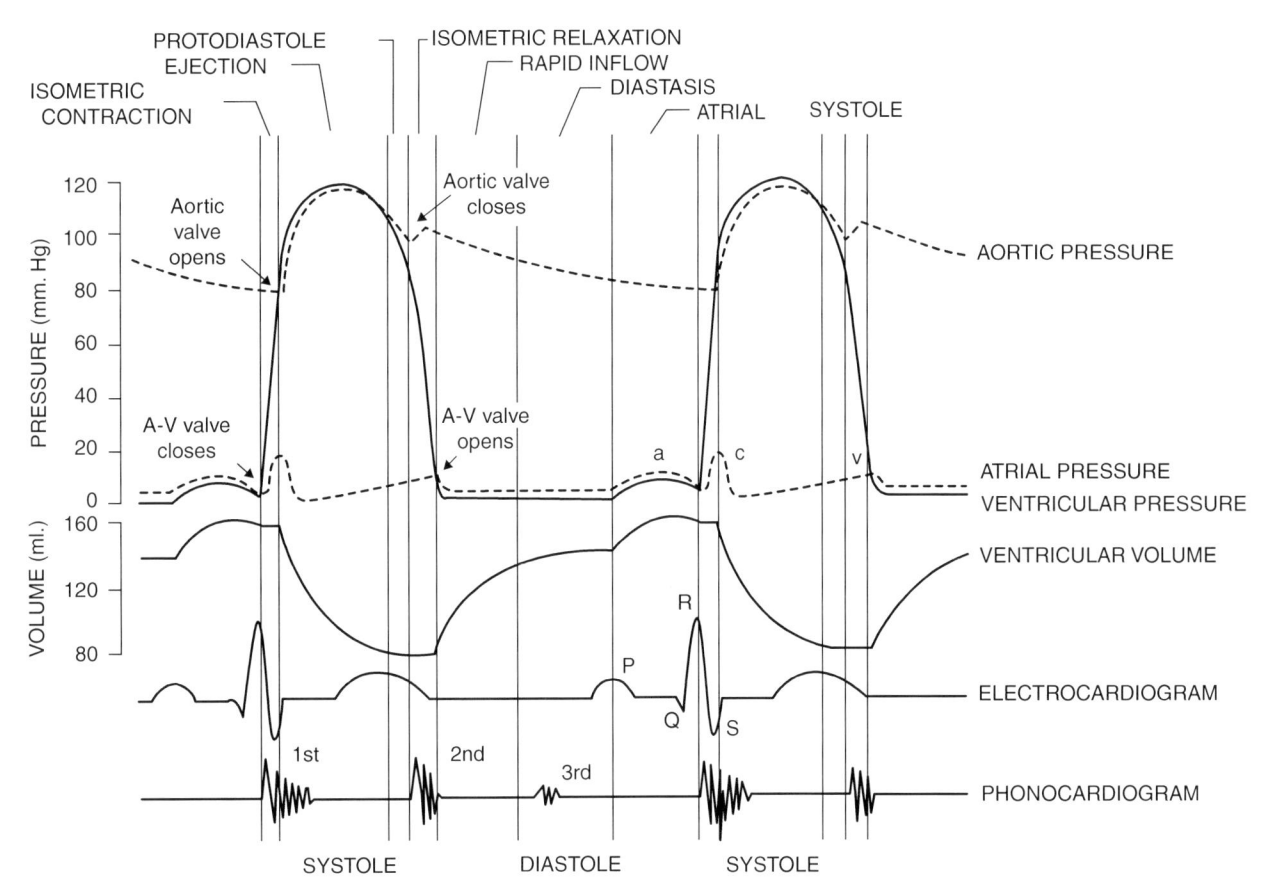

CHAPTER 4 Integrated Assessment of Systemic and Intracranial Hemodynamics

Figure 4.1 Electrical and mechanical events of the cardiac cycle. Note: The interrelationship of the electrical and mechanical events in the cardiac cycle including heart sounds recorded by phonocardiogram and intraventricular volumes. Reproduced with permission from Guyton AC. *Textbook of Medical Physiology*, 9th edn. Philadelphia: W.B. Saunders, 1996.

and corresponding pressure changes associated with blood flow through the heart.

Ventricular systole consists of three phases:

1 In phase 1, also known as *isovolumetric contraction*, the ventricles begin the process of contraction, building wall tension against closed semilunar (aortic and pulmonic) valves. The increase in pressure inside the ventricles causes the atrioventricular (mitral and tricuspid) valves to snap closed.

2 In phase 2, also known as *rapid ventricular ejection*, ventricular pressures exceed those within the aorta and pulmonary arteries, causing the semilunar valves to open as well as ejection of blood under intense pressure.

3 During phase 3, the *reduced ejection phase*, blood ejection slows considerably and intraventricular pressures drop sharply as contraction ends, causing the semilunar valves to close when aortic and pulmonary artery pressures again exceed those within the ventricle.

Under normal resting conditions, each ventricular systole results in a stroke volume of approximately 70–80 ml, constituting about 60% of left ventricular end-diastolic volume [1,2].

Right ventricular (RV) and left ventricular (LV) performances differ significantly during systole due to the physical structure of these very different pumps. The RV exhibits a large surface area capable of moving like a bellows to promote swift ejection of blood to the low-resistance pulmonary system. Because muscle lengthening and shortening are less important contributors to RV contraction, changes within the pulmonary bed that increase resistance are likely to stifle ventricular performance, producing reduced RV output and a backup in intracardiac right heart preload to the systemic venous circulation. The LV has a relatively small surface area and is capable of reducing and increasing its internal chamber circumference through muscle shortening and lengthening [1,2].

Application of the law of Laplace to LV performance demonstrates that wall tension is minimized as chamber size (radius) decreases; in patients exhibiting LV dilation and hypertrophy, significant wall tension is required, amounting to intense myocardial oxygen consumption. A similar clinical picture is illustrated through examination of the process of volume loading; when intraventricular preload

PART II Hemodynamic Principles

exceeds an optimal level, the resulting ventricular dilation requires significant wall tension to maintain optimal chamber pressures and forward flow into the high-resistance aorta. The result of significant ventricular dilation, whether due to excessive fluid hydration, pathologic dilation or hypertrophy, is often the same: congestive failure with backflow to the pulmonary bed and pulmonary edema [2].

Ventricular diastole consists of four phases:

1 In phase 1, also called *isovolumetric relaxation*, ventricular pressure drops dramatically without a change in volume. When ventricular pressure decreases below that within the atria, the atrioventricular valves open initiating the next phase.

2 In phase 2, also called the *rapid filling stage* or the early diastolic filling phase of the ventricles, the low intraventricular pressures present in phase 2 produce a phenomenon known as diastolic suction or recoil, which contributes to rapid blood flow and ventricular filling. When tachycardia is present, diastolic suction/recoil plays a significant role in maintaining ventricular filling despite a shortened filling time.

3 In phase 3, the *period of diastasis* is initiated when blood flow ceases and is marked by an equalization of ventricular and atrial pressures. When the diastolic phase is shortened due to an increase in heart rate, phase 3 may not be present as the process continues on to phase 4.

4 In phase 4, also called the *period of atrial contraction* or late ventricular diastole, heart rate, PR interval length and atrial preload determine the amount of blood that fill the ventricles during atrial kick. Under normal resting circumstances, preload contributed through atrial kick will not greatly affect overall ventricular volumes; however, in periods of stress, loss of atrial kick through processes such as atrial fibrillation may result in a decrease in ventricular preload by as much as 18% or more [1,2].

The arterial system should be viewed as a pressure reservoir that is capable of converting intermittent systolic and diastolic pressures into relatively constant flow through the *Windkessel effect* [1,2]. This effect describes the arterial system's ability to receive pulsatile energy transmission from the heart during systolic ejection and convert this to continuous pulsating waves that foster movement of blood through the systemic circulation. *Distensibility* is the primary factor responsible for maintaining the Windkessel effect's pulsatile transmission: the greater the distensibility or elasticity of the arterial system, the better is the blood flow throughout the circuit. Distensibility and the subsequent elastic recoil of arterial vessels provide for constant forward flow during the diastolic phase of the cardiac cycle, thereby reducing *systemic vascular resistance* (SVR) and the workload of the heart during systole. As elasticity is reduced through processes such as atherosclerosis or chronic hypertension, the resistance to flow from the left heart during systole increases, prompting the need for greater wall tension and an increase in LV workload. Patients with chronic hypertension are often found to have left ventricular hypertrophy on echocardiography and increased flow pulsatility on transcranial Doppler.

Figure 4.2 represents an arterial waveform with the phases of the cardiac cycle identified. As noted previously, the arterial system is capable of maintaining a constant pressure within the vascular system, despite the dynamic events of the cardiac cycle. Because this constant pressure is a more accurate portrayal of physiologic systemic arterial pressure, calculation and assessment of *mean arterial pressure* (MAP) serves as a more reliable marker of systemic arterial pressure [1,2]. MAP was first calculated by recording the area under the arterial pressure curve and dividing the area by the concurrent time period. A more simplistic calculation of MAP is

$$MAP = (\text{systolic pressure} - \text{diastolic pressure})/3 + \text{diastolic pressure}$$

It is important to note that as the pulsatile wave is transmitted across the arterial bed, systolic peak pressures may rise by as much as 20–40 mmHg from baseline aortic root pressure, due to an increase in resistance and arterial pulse pressure.

Pulse pressure, or the difference between systolic and diastolic pressures, may be used to assess arterial capacitance [2]. Normal pulse pressure is approximately 50 mmHg. In the

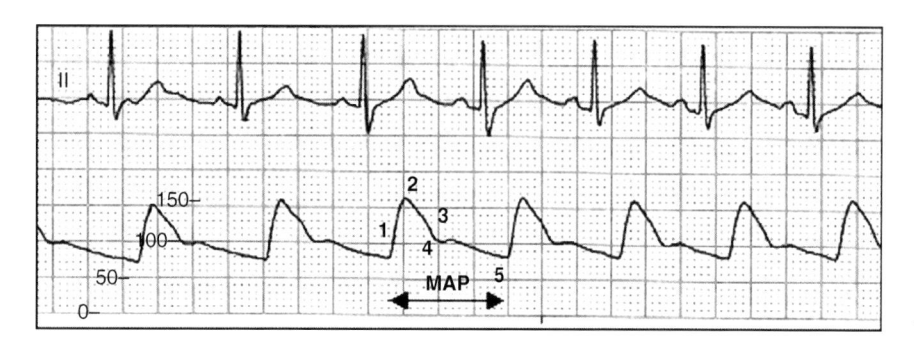

Figure 4.2 Phases of the cardiac cycle arterial waveform. Key to arterial waveform: 1 = isovolumetric contraction; 2 = peak systolic pressure (PSP); 3 = reduced systolic ejection; 4 = dicrotic notch; 5 = end-diastolic pressure (EDP). Note: measurement of arterial pressure is performed by taking PSP over EDP; arterial pressure = 160/80 mmHg; mean arterial pressure (MAP) measured by area under the waveform (107 mmHg).

absence of sepsis accompanied by low diastolic pressures, significant elevations of pulse pressure above this point signify a reduction in arterial compliance, due to processes such as atherosclerosis and/or chronic hypertension, and are associated with increased LV workload due to high resistance to flow. Because arterial compliance directly affects LV workload and the amount of resistance to blood flow during LV systole, pulse pressure also may be used to reflect stroke volume, the amount of blood ejected with each ventricular contraction. Used in this manner, the clinician must critically examine not only systolic and diastolic arterial pressures, but also changes in other accompanying parameters to determine the underlying cause.

For example, a narrowed/decreased pulse pressure occurs in both hypovolemic and cardiogenic shock, signifying decreased cardiac output in the face of elevated SVR; this finding is typically accompanied by low systolic pressures, a normal or often elevated diastolic pressure, an increase in heart rate and delayed capillary refill. Distinct changes in pulse pressure may also be detected in septic shock; pulse pressure may widen/elevate, signifying high cardiac output and low SVR, and is accompanied by low diastolic pressures reflective of vasodilation. All these factors play a role in shaping up spectral Doppler waveforms that can be detected in the carotid, vertebral and intracranial vessels.

Arterial perfusion and venous return

Within the microcirculation, much of the arterial pressure head dissipates, allowing for sufficient pressure gradients to promote forward flow. Dilation and constriction of precapillary sphincters, thoroughfare channels and arterioles promote precise control of blood flowing through capillary networks to match cellular metabolic needs. Diffusion is primarily promoted by solute concentration and pressure gradients. According to the *Starling equilibrium*, filtration and reabsorption across capillary walls depend on the interrelation of four forces:
1 capillary pressure of approximately 30 mmHg which exerts a force to promote filtration through capillary walls;
2 interstitial fluid pressure of approximately 3 mmHg which, through maintenance of a slightly negative pressure, pulls fluid into the interstitial space;
3 interstitial fluid colloid osmotic pressure of approximately 8 mmHg, which promotes osmotic fluid shifts into the interstitium; and
4 plasma colloid pressure (oncotic pressure) of approximately 28 mmHg, which promotes capillary reabsorption [1].

Other factors affecting the exchange of substances across the capillary wall include viscosity of the filtrate and the integrity of the capillary wall. Further considerations about factors that influence flow across Starling's resistors and the "choice" by blood to follow "the path of least resistance" into veins can be found elsewhere [2–4].

The *venous system* serves as a volume reservoir of variable capacity as well as a conduit system for blood flow. Right atrial pressure or *central venous pressure* (CVP) is regulated by the following three contributing factors:
1 total blood volume;
2 the heart's ability to optimally pump blood; and
3 the capacitance of the venous system.

Under normal circumstances, atmospheric pressure approximates CVP (CVP = 0). An increase in total blood volume, reduced left and/or right ventricular pump performance or maximized venous capacitance will result in an elevated CVP.

Intrinsic cardiac determinants of blood flow

Cardiac output (CO) is defined as the amount of blood that is pumped by the left ventricle into the aorta each minute. Normally in adults, the volume of blood pumped by the left ventricle each minute is 4–8 l, with an average cardiac output of approximately 5 l min^{-1}. Cardiac output varies according to body size; because of this *cardiac index* (CI) is a measure that is used to estimate the proportion of blood flow to body surface area (BSA):

$$CI = CO/BSA$$

Normal values for CI are 2.8–4.2 l min^{-1} m^{-2}; an average CI for a healthy 70 kg male is approximately 3 l min^{-1} m^{-2}.

Cardiac output is calculated as

$$CO = \text{heart rate} \times \text{stroke volume}$$

Stroke volume (SV) is the amount of blood ejected from the left ventricle with each contraction. Stroke volume is calculated as

$$SV = \text{left ventricular end-diastolic volume–residual left ventricular blood volume}$$

The residual left ventricular blood volume is determined immediately following systole. The average adult exhibits a stroke volume of 60–100 ml per ventricular contraction [1–3].

The CO equation (heart rate × SV) highlights the dependence of CO on heart rate and factors that influence stroke volume, namely preload, contractility and afterload. To maintain CO within an adequate range, heart rate and/or stroke volume must respond through adjustment of contractile rate or the amount of blood filling the left ventricle for ejection. Spontaneous electrical pacemaker activity,

PART II Hemodynamic Principles

termed automaticity, normally controls adult heart rate in the sino-atrial (SA) node at a rate between 60 to 100 beats per minute. A decrease in CO produces a rapid, dynamic response in heart rate in an attempt to maintain adequate systemic blood flow.

Heart rate augmentation produces distinct processes that may enhance or exacerbate a decline in myocardial performance. Increased heart rates produce an increased cellular influx of calcium into the sarcoplasmic reticulum resulting in an improved myocardial contractile function. This process is called the *Treppe phenomenon* and is capable of offsetting the reduction of left ventricular diastolic filling time occurring in tachycardia [1,2]. As heart rates increase beyond those typical of SA node mediated responses, the diastolic filling time declines sharply; combined with a rise in metabolic substrate production, contractile function is sharply diminished, producing a decrease in CO.

Preload. The term preload is defined as the volume of blood distending the left ventricle at the end of diastole [end diastolic volume (EDVol)]. Since EDVol exerts a pressure within the ventricular system, the term end diastolic pressure (EDP) is also used to reflect preload [1–3]. Preload is determined by the following three factors:
1 total blood volume/venous return
2 vascular resistance/capacitance and
3 myocardial contractility.

Heart rate influences left ventricular preload as EDVol is dependent on the time devoted to diastolic filling which shortens in proportion to increases in heart rate. For example, at a heart rate of 70 beats per minute, diastole represents about 60% of the cardiac cycle resulting in optimal end-diastolic filling, but at a heart rate of 200 beats per minute, diastole comprises only 35% of the cardiac cycle [2].

Contractility. Left ventricular contractility or pump strength is the terminology used to reflect myocardial muscle shortening and the development of muscle tension. A number of extrinsic factors contribute to myocardial contractility; termed *positive inotropic agents*. These substances include:
1 intrinsic circulating sympathetic amines and other synthetic inotropes
2 thyroid hormone and
3 minerals such as calcium and magnesium.

The *Frank–Starling law* [5–6] (also called the length–tension relationship) describes the relationship between preload and resulting contractile force, relating muscle fiber lengthening to the development of tension. Simply stated, optimal myocardial tension is the product of optimal muscle fiber lengthening; lengthening of left ventricular muscle fibers by EDV is directly proportionate to the amount of tension and subsequent contractile force that is produced during systole. Figure 4.3 illustrates the relationship between preload (muscle lengthening) and myocardial contractility. The normal adult left ventricle responds optimally to EDV between 10 and 12 mmHg, pro-

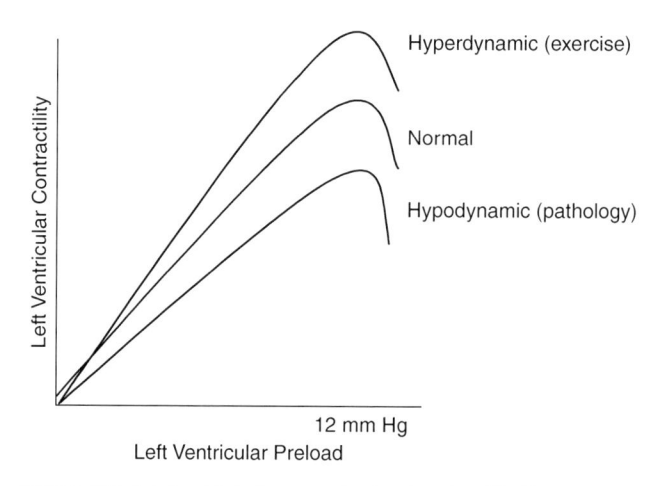

Figure 4.3 Relationship between preload and contractility. Note: myocardial stretch and resulting contractile force in response to preload pressure.

ducing a corresponding myocardial fiber length of 2.2 μm [3]; pressures exceeding this are associated with a decrease in the interdigitation of actin and myosin filaments, with a reduction in contractile site activation (descending limb of the Frank–Starling curve).

Afterload. Left ventricular afterload refers to wall tension and reflects the SVR in the aorta that the ventricle must overcome to eject its volume [2]. An important distinction must be made between left ventricular afterload and SVR. Afterload itself cannot be measured directly in clinical practice, but what is known is that ventricular wall tension must rise to a level that will allow forward flow through the resistance of the systemic arterial bed beyond the aortic valve. During early systole, this is accomplished by building wall tension with the aortic valve in a closed position in phase one of ventricular systole (isovolumetric contraction); this phase represents the point of the cardiac cycle responsible for more than 50% of myocardial oxygen consumption [1,2]. Once wall tension has been optimized and intraventricular pressure rises significantly, the aortic valve opens, enabling forward thrust of blood into the arterial system. Because SVR represents the amount of resistance that the ventricle must build tension against to enable forward flow, SVR serves as a calculated clinical measure that may be used to reflect left ventricular afterload.

Similarly to left ventricular afterload, right ventricular afterload is reflected in the calculated measurement of pulmonary vascular resistance (PVR) [2]. Since the pulmonary vasculature is normally a low-resistance system, the right ventricular afterload is usually an insignificant contributor to overall myocardial oxygen consumption.

Factors capable of influencing left ventricular afterload include a variety of systemic conditions, including body temperature, hypertension, altered aortic distensibility due to atherosclerotic changes, blood viscosity and alterations in vascular resistance due to bacterial endotoxins and severe immune system responses with significant histamine release. Intrinsic cardiac contributors to afterload include structural alterations such as aortic valve stenosis.

Contributors to right ventricular afterload include entities that produce pulmonary hypertension such as chronic obstructive pulmonary disease, pulmonary embolism and use of positive end-expiratory pressure mechanical ventilation settings. Similarly to the left heart, an intrinsic cardiac contributor would be pulmonic valve stenosis.

Arterial blood pressure (ABP) is derived from CO and SVR and intrinsic mechanisms exist to maintain ABP when CO or SVR become altered. Under most circumstances, CO and SVR have an inverse relationship. When cardiac output falls due to reduced contractility or preload values, SVR will increase in an attempt to maintain ABP within normal parameters. Because of this, the use of ABP for rapid detection of clinical changes often provides poor clinical information, as blood pressure may appear normal in the face of early clinical deterioration. When SVR increases due to a primary reduction in contractility, compromised left ventricular function precludes an ability to overcome the increased resistance, stifling forward flow even further. In this scenario, use of medications or devices that reduce SVR may be beneficial, such as dihydropyridine class calcium channel blockers such as nicardipine or clevidipine in combination with a positive inotropic agent, and/or intra-aortic balloon counterpulsation [7]. Similarly, when CO falls due to significant blood loss (alterations in preload), SVR will again increase to maintain ABP; once circulating blood volume is replaced, SVR returns to normal. In sepsis or meningitis, SVR is often significantly reduced, resulting in low vascular resistance to left ventricular outflow. The ventricle compensates with increases in CO often above normal values and transcranial Doppler often shows a general velocity increase above normal values with low-resistance waveforms. When preload is adequately maintained in this scenario, the use of pressors to maintain ABP can often be entirely avoided.

Calculation of SVR requires measurement of the variables mean arterial pressure (MAP), right atrial pressure (RAP or CVP) and CO [2]. The equation for SVR is

$$SVR = [(MAP - RAP) \times 80]/CO.$$

Calculation of PVR requires measurement of pulmonary artery mean pressure (PAM), pulmonary artery wedge pressure (PAWP) and CO [2]. The equation for PVR is

$$PVR = [(PAM - PAWP) \times 80]/CO.$$

Neuro-endocrine mediation of cardiac output

The autonomic nervous system plays an important role in augmenting heart contractility, preload and afterload. Vagus nerve fibers innervate the SA node and atrio-ventricular (AV) conduction tissue. When stimulated, parasympathetic fibers result in reduced SA node automaticity, prolongation of impulse conduction time through the AV node and decreased ventricular contractile force [1,2].

Sympathetic nerve fibers are prevalent throughout the myocardium and the arterial vascular system. Sympathetic β_1 *receptors* within the myocardium increase the rate of firing of the SA node, conduction velocity and myocardial contractility when stimulated by intrinsic sympathetic amines such as norepinephrine, epinephrine and dopamine [1,2]. Stimulation of β_1 receptors may produce an increase in CO up to 20–30% from baseline, primarily as a result of inotropic augmentation [2]. Sympathetic β_2 receptors within vascular smooth muscle produce vasodilation when stimulated by selective adrenergic agents, reducing LV afterload to enhance forward flow. Stimulation of α_1 receptors also located in vascular smooth muscle results in vasoconstriction [1,2].

Within the central nervous system, the pons and the ventrolateral medulla both play a role in cardiac and vasomotor function. Stimulation of pressor regions within the brainstem produces an increase in heart rate, contractility and blood pressure. When the depressor regions are stimulated, profound bradycardia associated with a reduction in myocardial contractility and blood pressure may result. Cortical, limbic and hypothalamic-mediated responses to environmental stimuli may also have a profound influence on myocardial performance [1,2]. Table 4.1 identifies a number of *reflexes that influence vasomotor response*. Cardiac and respiratory reflexes are very closely related; a decrease in pH associated with an increase in $PaCO_2$ results in vasodilation, whereas an increase in pH with a decrease in $PaCO_2$ typically produces some degree of vasoconstriction. *Vasodilation* leads to

1 decrease in peripheral resistance
2 decrease in flow pulsatility and
3 increase in blood flow velocity

and *vasoconstriction* leads to

1 increase in peripheral resistance
2 increase in flow pulsatility and
3 decrease in blood flow velocity.

Hormones may also contribute to alterations in myocardial performance and circulatory mechanisms. Antidiuretic hormone (ADH or vasopressin) may be released from the posterior pituitary in response to decreases in CO associated with a presumed need for volume. In addition to promoting water reabsorption, ADH also possesses potent vasoconstrictive properties. Atrial natriuretic factor (ANF), which possesses both salt- and water-excreting properties, may also be released in response to significant atrial muscle fiber stretch associated with hypervolemia [1,2]. Despite its salt- and water-wasting properties, clinical studies have demonstrated the main benefit of ANF release to be associated with

PART II Hemodynamic Principles

Table 4.1 Reflexes influencing vasomotor response

Reflex	Anatomical location	Cardiac/vasomotor response
Bainbridge reflex	Right atrium of the heart; accelerator receptors	Tachycardia initiated by increased right atrial pressure with receptor distention
Baroreceptor reflex (Marey's law of the heart)	Aortic arch and carotid sinus	Increased arterial pressure stimulates vagal fibers which produces bradycardia and reduced ventricular contractility
Chemoreceptors	Aortic arch and carotid bodies	Hypoxia, hypercapnia, and/or acidosis stimulate receptors to produce tachycardia

arterial and venous vasodilation, which foster reduction of preload and afterload. Aldosterone release is also stimulated by a decrease in CO promoting increased renal tubule reabsorption of sodium and water [1,2].

Microcirculatory flow mechanisms are also mediated by neural control systems. Local blood flow is regulated through arteriole resistance vessels and mechanisms that augment changes in venous capacitance and return. Vasodilating and vasoconstricting prostaglandins also play a role in the augmentation of peripheral circulation, as do endothelial factors such as nitric oxide (NO) which may enhance vasodilation in response to a number of triggers [1,2].

Bedside assessment of systemic hemodynamics

Assessment of systemic hemodynamic parameters necessitates the measurement and interpretation of both non-invasive data from the clinical examination and, when possible, invasive data collected from monitoring technology. For the purposes of this chapter, data specific to those effecting stroke volume and systemic tissue oxygenation will be reviewed; combining these data with those obtained from ECG monitoring and the general physical examination provides an overall picture of systemic hemodynamic status which may be used to direct hemodynamic augmentation.

A common, but inappropriate, practice of accepting values from the numeric display of a bedside monitor, instead of those determined by reading a static graph paper tracing, often places the clinician at risk of misinterpretation of hemodynamic data [2,3,8,9]. All bedside monitor values must be verified against those produced on a graphic strip, as bedside monitors do not always provide accurate waveform values, despite their use of respiratory algorithms. This is especially true when respiratory artifact and/or abnormal waveform morphology related to intrinsic pathology are present. If the clinician is able simultaneously to freeze the ECG and hemodynamic waveform on the bedside monitor, use of a cursor to accurately determine waveform values may be substituted for a paper strip [2,8,9].

As mentioned earlier, stroke volume is derived from three primary contributors, preload, contractility and afterload. Measures of preload consist of both non-invasive data and those obtained through central monitoring systems. Perhaps one of the most undervalued measures of preload, and one that is generally simplistic, is the determination of *jugular venous pressure* (JVP). Because of the proximal location of the right internal jugular vein, measurement of pressures there directly reflect right atrial pressure [2]. To measure JVP, follow these steps:

- Position the patient at a 45° angle with the head and neck in a neutral aligned position.
- Compress the jugular vein at the point just above the clavicle; release the pressure and observe filling of the venous column – if it fills from the top, measurement of JVP will not reliably estimate cardiac preload.
- Identify the following reference points: the top of the fluid column (the meniscus) – reference point; and the angle of Louis (sternal angle) – zero point.
- Measure the vertical distance between the angle of Louis and the meniscus; because the sternal angle lies 5 cm above the right atrium, add the number of centimeters of JVP elevation above the angle of Louis to 5 cm to calculate an estimation of CVP.

Additional assessments related to JVP inspection include noting the presence of the *Kussmaul's sign* and assessment of hepato-jugular reflex. To assess presence of the Kussmaul's sign add the following steps to the procedure listed above:

- Have the patient take a deep breath.
- Observe movement of the meniscus (or the top filling point of the jugular vein) on inspiration.
- Determine a decrease or increase in the filling level.

Normally on inspiration, the intrathoracic pressure decreases, resulting in a decrease in the meniscus level. Kussmaul's sign reflects a pathological increase in meniscus level on inspiration related to decreased cardiac compliance from processes such as congestive failure or cardiac tamponade [2]. Assessment of *hepato-jugular reflex*

involves the addition of the following steps to the above procedure:
- Ask the patient to breathe normally.
- Apply pressure to the right upper quadrant of the abdomen for 10 s; note a rise in JVP filling level and assess whether the rise is sustained throughout the application of pressure or is transient despite pressure application with a return to pre-pressure levels.

Normal findings should include a transient rise of JVP with a return to normal level while pressure continues to be applied. A sustained elevation of JVP throughout the pressure application process signifies a significant increase in LV preload, except in the presence of RV infarction [2]. Lastly, while JVP reflects preload, the clinician assessing JVP data must consider the dynamic interplay between preload, contractility and afterload to determine correctly the meaning of preload elevations.

Invasive hemodynamic monitoring modalities are often useful in the assessment of preload and other variables associated with stroke volume. Normal values and formulas for *invasive cardiac indices* are listed in Table 4.2. Insertion of a CVP line or pulmonary artery (PA) catheter provides the clinician with an improved ability to measure preload parameters directly in an accurate manner. Because invasive catheters require the use of transducers to convert mechanical pressures to numeric data, it is important to make note of *principles associated with transducer maintenance and monitoring*:

1 A fluid interface between catheter and transducer coupled with non-distensible, stiff tubing must be maintained to promote accurate transmission of pressure waves; clinicians must ensure that systems are bubble-free and supported by pressure that prevents a backup of blood into the line. Second, the phlebostatic axis, measured at the level of the tricuspid valve, provides the only known place in the body where central pressures are not influenced by hydrostatic pressure. Because of this, transducer systems used to measure pressures within the heart and arterial system must be leveled and zeroed to atmospheric pressure at the phlebostatic axis to ensure accuracy in measurement. The phlebostatic axis is located at the fourth intercostal space or at the point of half the anterior/posterior diameter of the chest, when the patient is placed in a supine position between 0 and 60° head of bed elevation [2].

2 An important point must be emphasized here due to a practice often observed in neuroscience units of moving the arterial pressure transducer to the level of the foramen of Monro. This practice originated as a method that aimed to approximate MAP within the brain for use in the calculation of cerebral perfusion pressure (CPP); it is not based on

Table 4.2 Invasive cardiac parameters: formulas and normal values

Parameter	Formula[a]	Normal values
Cardiac output (CO)	SV × HR	4–8 l min^{-1}
Cardiac index (CI)	$\frac{CO}{BSA}$	2.8–4.2 l min^{-1} m^{-2}
Stroke volume (SV)	$\frac{CO \times 1000}{HR}$	60–100 ml per contraction
SV index	$\frac{SV}{BSA}$	35–75 ml m^{-2} per contraction
Mean arterial pressure (MAP)	(Pulse pressure/3) + diastolic BP	70–105 mmHg
Central venous pressure (CVP)	Direct measurement; no formula	2–6 mmHg
Pulmonary artery pressure (PAP)	Direct measurement; no formula	PA systole: 15–30 mmHg *over* PA diastole: 5–15 mmHg
Pulmonary artery wedge pressure (PAWP)	Direct measurement; no formula	4–12 mmHg
Systemic vascular resistance (SVR)	$\frac{(MAP) - CVP) \times 80}{CO}$	900–1600 dyne s^{-1} cm^{-5}
SVR index (SVRI)	$\frac{(MAP) - CVP) \times 80}{CI}$	1970–2390 dyne s^{-1} cm^{-5}
Pulmonary vascular resistance (PVR)	$\frac{(PAM) - PAWP) \times 80}{CO}$	155–255 dyne s^{-1} cm^{-5}
PVR index (PVRI)	$\frac{(PAM) - PAWP) \times 80}{CI}$	255–285 dyne s^{-1} cm^{-5}
Venous oxygen saturation (SVO$_2$)	Direct measurement; no formula	60–80%

[a]BSA = body surface area; PAM = pulmonary artery mean; PAWP = pulmonary artery wedge pressure.
Adapted from Whalen DA, Kelleher RM. Cardiovascular patient assessment. In: Kinney MR, Dunbar SB, Brooks-Brunn JA, *et al.*, eds. *AACN Clinical Reference for Critical Care Nursing*. St. Louis, MO: Mosby, 1998; 277–318.

PART II Hemodynamic Principles

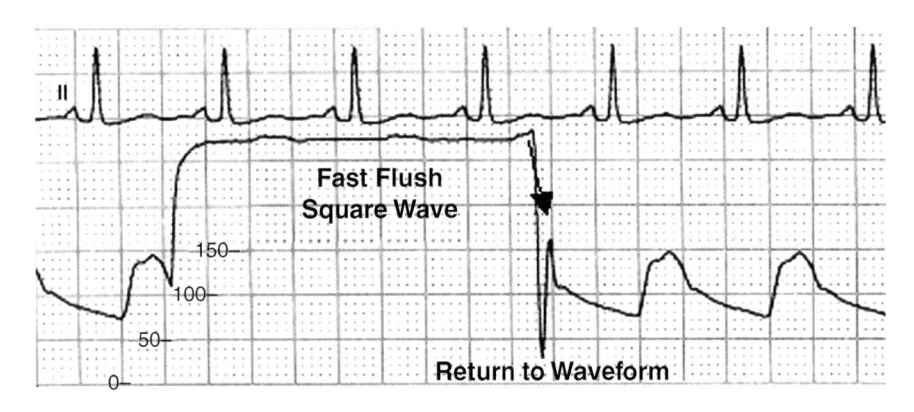

Figure 4.4 Square-wave test with optimal response. Steps to assess square wave: 1, fast flush system and release; 2, count number of small boxes occurring before return of waveform; 3, divide number of small boxes into paper speed (25 mm s^{-1}). Note: one small box before return of waveform; 25/1 = 25 Hz. Ideal frequency response = >25 Hz.

physiologically sound principles of hemodynamic monitoring given the actual location of the catheter in the peripheral arterial bed, coupled with the complex hemodynamics of the intracranial arterial system which can in no way be measured by a simple adjustment of transducer height. Placement of the transducer zero point at any level other than the phlebostatic axis will result in only one finding, distorted pressure values that are not accurate and meaningful in the course of clinical management.

3 To ensure accuracy in invasive hemodynamic measurements, the transducer/monitoring system's dynamic response should be tested. Dynamic response is the ability of the system to reproduce accurately variations in pressure occurring within the vasculature. It is tested through performance of a fast-flush and assessed by the square wave produced. Figure 4.4 provides an example of the correct response to fast-flushing of the catheter. Testing of dynamic response prevents misinterpretation of data obtained from invasive catheters in that overdamped waveforms will underestimate systolic pressures and overestimate diastolic pressures, whereas spiked, underdamped waveforms typically overestimate systolic pressures [8,9].

4 Interpretation of invasive hemodynamic data should be performed with caution. Measurements of pressures within the thoracic cavity are subject to the influence of respiration and pressure changes occurring with the respiratory cycle. The point of end-expiration provides the only time during the respiratory cycle that is minimally influenced by changes in intrathoracic pressure [2,8,9], making measurement at this point critical to the determination of accurate data. In patients breathing without mechanical ventilation, end-expiration is generally the high point on a waveform just before the inspiratory dip, as illustrated in Figure 4.5. However, in patients receiving positive pressure mechanical ventilation, end-expiration may be measured at different points on a waveform depending on the ventilator settings and the presence or absence of spontaneous respiratory effort (Figure 4.6). Use of simultaneous end-tidal CO$_2$ monitoring (capnography or PETCO$_2$) assists with rapid and accurate detection of end-expiration in patients receiving mechanical ventilation [9].

Direct measurement of CVP can be performed through placement of a catheter into the right atrium or by insertion of a pulmonary artery (PA) catheter with measurement of central pressures from the proximal port. Normal CVP varies from 2 to 6 mmHg; Figure 4.7 illustrates a right atrial waveform obtained by CVP catheter. Note the distinct waveforms that reflect specific events in the cardiac cycle. The A-wave reflects right atrial contraction, while the C-wave occurs with closure of the tricuspid valve and the V-wave reflects atrial filling and bulging of the tricuspid valve during right ventricular contraction. Normally the A-wave is the most prominent wave present, while the C-wave may be absent entirely [8,9]. A very large V-wave is often suggestive

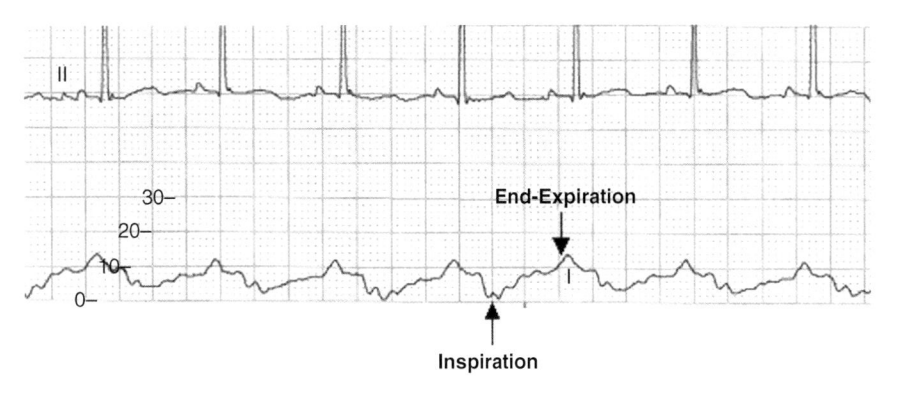

Figure 4.5 End-expiratory measurement in a patient spontaneously breathing without mechanical ventilation [central venous pressure (CVP) waveform]. Key for CVP waveform: 1 = a wave at end-expiration. Note: measurement of CVP is performed by taking the mean of the A wave; CVP = 10 mmHg; measurement taken at incorrect point on waveform would have under estimated CVP at 5–7 mmHg.

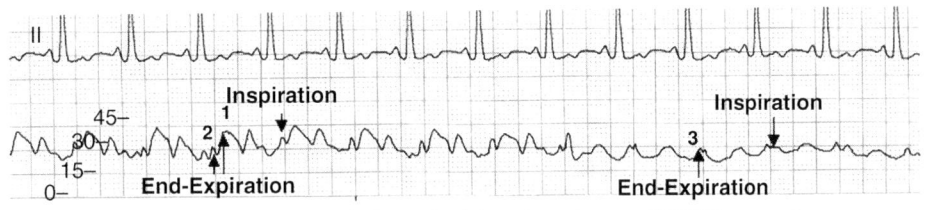

CHAPTER 4 Integrated Assessment of Systemic and Intracranial Hemodynamics

PAP waveform; balloon inflated with migration to PAWP waveform

Figure 4.6 End-expiratory measurement in a patient on positive pressure mechanical ventilation [pulmonary artery pressure (PAP) and pulmonary artery wedge pressure (PAWP) waveforms]. Key for PA waveform (left): 1 = peak systolic pressure (PSP); 2 = end-diastolic pressure (EDP). Note: measurement of PAP is performed by taking PSP over EDP at end-expiration; PAP = 42/28 mmHg; measurement during inspiration would have over-estimated pressures at 45/32 mmHg. Key for PAWP waveform (right): 3 = A wave. Note: measurement of PAWP is performed by taking the mean of the A wave; PAWP = 22 mmHg; measurement during inspiration would have over-estimated pressure at 28 mmHg.

of tricuspid valve regurgitation and can be further assessed by auscultation of a systolic ejection murmur at the fourth intercostal space left sternal border.

Pulmonary artery wedge pressure (PAWP) is another measurement of preload and provides a more accurate picture of LV end-diastolic volume than measures taken within the right atrium (Figure 4.8). The waves present in the PAWP waveform are of similar morphology to those in the CVP waveform, but reflect left heart processes; the A-wave represents left atrial contraction, the C-wave occurs with mitral valve closure and the V-wave reflects atrial filling and bulging of the mitral valve during left ventricular systole [8,9]. Similarly, a giant V-wave is often associated with mitral valve regurgitation and is typically accompanied by a systolic ejection murmur at the cardiac apex. Normal PAWP pressure is between 4 and 12 mmHg [2]. The presence of giant V-waves often causes clinicians to misinterpret left atrial waveforms as pulmonary artery waveforms, but can be easily identified with ECG correlates as a pathological waveform.

Figure 4.7 identifies the correct technique for *measurement of right atrial pressures*, which consists of averaging the peak and lower values of the A-wave. Using the ECG for correlation, the A-wave is found after the P-wave, while the V-wave occurs after the T-wave, but before the P-wave on the ECG; to find the V-wave on a right atrial waveform easily, limit assessment to the components of the waveform occurring within the T–P interval on the ECG. A similar process is used to measure left atrial waveforms obtained by PA catheter in the wedge position. Because of an increase in electrical–mechanical delay, the A-wave on a PAWP waveform is usually found at or just after the QRS complex, whereas the V-wave occurs in close proximity to the P-wave on the ECG (Figure 4.8). When pathological conditions are present that distort or eliminate entirely the production of an A-wave (e.g. tricuspid or mitral stenosis; dysrhythmias producing loss of atrioventricular synchrony, including pacemaker-generated rhythms; atrial fibrillation), right and left atrial pressures may be read at the Z-point, which correlates with the end of the QRS complex on the ECG [8,9].

Pulmonary artery end-diastolic pressure (PAEDP) may also be used as a measure of preload (Figure 4.8). Because the volume of blood at the end of diastole in the pulmonary artery represents the volume that will ultimately fill the left heart, a relationship between PAEDP and PAWP exists. In the absence of pulmonary hypertension, there should be no more than a 6 mmHg difference between PAEDP and PAWP, with the PAEDP running only slightly higher than wedge [2]. Because of this constant relationship, use of the PAEDP as a substitute for PAWP is standard practice in many critical care units, lengthening the life of the catheter's balloon and preventing the need for catheter replacement due to balloon rupture. Normal PAEDP pressures run between 5 and 15 mmHg [2]; the waveform is read just before the systolic upstroke at the end of diastole when ventricular filling is complete.

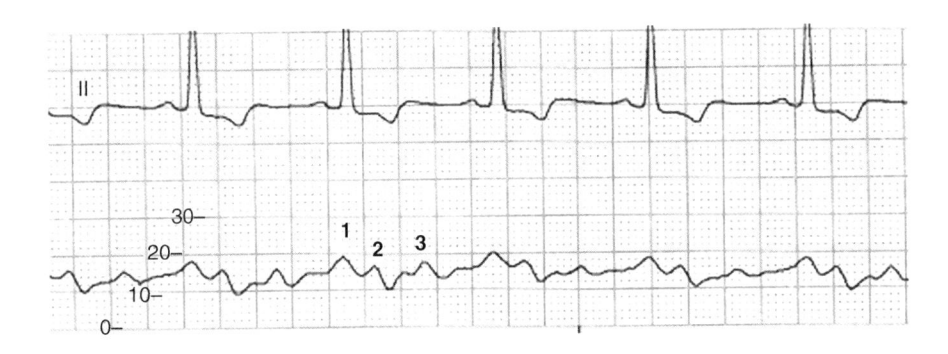

Figure 4.7 Central venous pressure (CVP) waveform. Key for CVP waveform: 1 = A wave; 2 = C wave; 3 = V wave. Note: measurement of CVP is performed by taking the mean of the A wave; CVP = 16 mmHg.

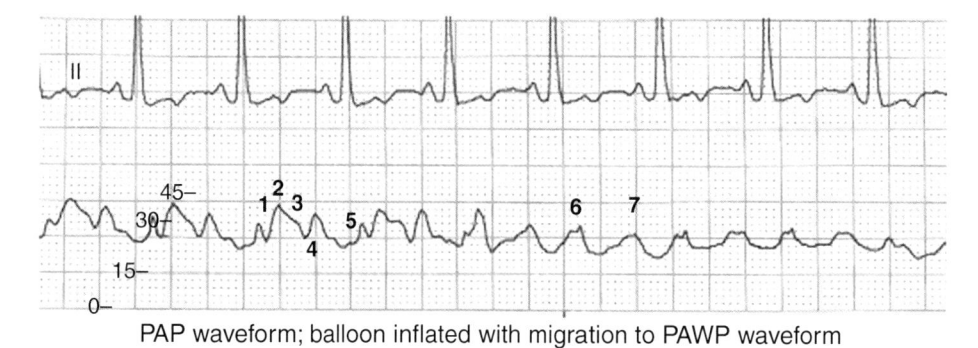

Figure 4.8 Pulmonary artery pressure waveform (PAP) and pulmonary artery wedge (PAWP) pressure waveform. Key for PA waveform (left): 1 = isovolumetric contraction; 2 = peak systolic pressure (PSP); 3 = reduced systolic ejection; 4 = dicrotic notch; 5 = end-diastolic pressure (EDP). Note: measurement of PAP is performed by taking PSP over EDP; PAP = 42/29 mmHg. Key for PAWP waveform (right): 6 = A wave; 7 = V wave. Note: measurement of PAWP is performed by taking the mean of the A wave; PAWP = 27 mmHg.

As stated earlier, preload is affected by not only total blood volume, but also the pumping ability of the heart. Often with significant deterioration in myocardial contractility, preload may become elevated without the addition of fluid to circulatory volume. Hence preload alterations may reflect, indirectly, poor myocardial contractility. Likewise, significant LV or RV afterload may directly alter preload values secondary to an inability of the ventricle to overcome high resistance to forward flow; preload elevates as flow is stifled.

Measurement of contractility as a contributor to stroke volume has been debated by clinicians for many years. Use of calculated variables such as ejection fraction measurements is often considered helpful by clinicians, yet others criticize these values as indirect calculated measures of contractility. Normal values for LVEF and RVEF are 60–75% and 45–50%, respectively. The bottom line is that no measure exists today to determine directly contractile force in real time. Because of this, some practitioners prefer simply to infer contractility from variables that can be measured directly such as CO/CI and preload parameters [2].

Measurement of afterload also relies on use of calculated variables derived from an equation which is an algebraic reformulation of Ohm's law [2]. Because ventricular afterload may not be measured directly, calculated SVR and PVR serve as a reflection of the resistance that the ventricles must overcome to eject their volume. Both SVR and PVR provide the clinician with an estimate of just how hard the ventricle must work to generate wall tension and pressures that will foster forward flow through the semilunar valves.

Increases in SVR have to be examined critically to determine their relationship with other hemodynamic parameters. Because an increase in SVR will occur in response to a decrease in CO/SV, the clinician must analyze critically the precise cause of SVR alterations to determine the necessary clinical action. Similarly, augmentation of SVR with pressor therapy to drive up perfusion pressures must be undertaken cautiously; the effect of significant LV afterload on CO and preload cannot be underestimated, especially in the face of occult or known cardiac dysfunction. Significantly low SVRs are often associated with conditions such as sepsis or systemic immune response syndrome (SIRS) that trigger events that produce widespread vasodilatory processes [2]. Normally SVR values are 900–1600 dyne s^{-1} cm^{-5}.

Alterations in PVR may occur in relation to therapies or pathologic conditions that produce pulmonary hypertension. The normal range for PVR is 155–255 dyne $s^{-1}cm^{-5}$ due to the normally low-pressure pulmonary system [2].

Perhaps the most useful parameter to measure in the patient requiring invasive hemodynamic monitoring is continuous mixed *venous oxygen saturation* or SvO_2. Data relative to body needs in oxygen supply and demand are provided by PA catheters capable of measuring SvO_2. These data are so important that one could argue the logic behind only placing PA catheters capable of providing these data continuously. Oxygen saturation of hemoglobin in the pulmonary artery is presented by digital display; because the pulmonary artery represents the terminal point before the blood can be reoxygenated, measurement of oxygen saturation provides information on tissue uptake or the oxygen extraction demands of the body [2].

Four variables are essential to the assessment of SvO_2:
1 cardiac output (CO)
2 hemoglobin
3 arterial oxygen saturation and
4 tissue oxygen consumption.

Delivery of oxygen, or oxygen supply, is dependent on CO, hemoglobin and arterial oxygen saturation, whereas SvO_2 reflects tissue oxygen consumption. When tissue oxygen needs an increase, the first compensatory measure exerted by the body is an attempt to increase CO. A second compensatory measure is an increase in tissue extraction, which occurs when CO changes are insufficient to meet tissue oxygenation needs [2].

Decreases in SvO$_2$ may be brought about by a number of clinical phenomena that may insult oxygenation and cardiac performance in an occult manner. Chief among these are patient positioning, movement and activities of daily living which may challenge an already compromised cardiopulmonary system [2]. Real-time measurement of SvO$_2$ allows the assessment of the effect of these phenomena on tissue oxygenation supply and demand, promoting improved patient outcomes. Measurement of SvO$_2$ along with other hemodynamic variables enables clinicians to gauge fully the need for specific therapies to augment the oxygen supply and demand equation. Normal SvO$_2$ is 60–80%; significant changes in SvO$_2$ of 5–10% or more for longer than 5 min warrant close clinical investigation to ensure optimal tissue oxygenation [2,9].

The use of *non-invasive CO monitoring* remains controversial. Thoracic electrical bioimpedance is one example of a measure of CO obtained by placement of external electrodes. The electrical impedance change in blood flow through the thoracic aorta is analyzed, producing an estimate of SV; the device multiplies the SV by heart rate to derive CO; EF can also be calculated [2]. Unfortunately, only a "fair" to "satisfactory" relationship has been measured between bioimpedance CO values and those obtained through PA catheter; limitations include the potential for incorrect electrode placement, overestimation of CO during vasopressor therapy, aortic insufficiency and hypovolemia and underestimation of CO during sepsis or hypertensive episodes [2]. Given these limitations, the usefulness of bioimpedance CO measures in neuroscience patient management is doubtful at best.

Relationship between systemic and intracranial hemodynamics

The brain is metabolically dependent on a continuous supply of oxygen and glucose, which are delivered at a rate of approximately 750 ml min^{-1} or 15% of the total CO. Resting *cerebral blood flow* (CBF) is relatively stable despite changes in CO, body position and arterial blood pressure; it amounts to approximately 50 ml per 100 g of brain tissue per minute [1]. Focal changes in CBF correlate with metabolic demands, in that activity in specific brain regions is accompanied by a focal increase in blood flow secondary to autoregulation. When autoregulatory processes are functional, the brain is capable of producing varying levels of arterial perfusion pressures across a wide range of systemic arterial pressures. When autoregulation is dysfunctional, brain perfusion pressures become dependent on systemic hemodynamic flow parameters [2].

The *Monro–Kellie hypothesis*, which was originally postulated in the 1800s [10], describes the relationship of the skull and its contents to pressure dynamics. Intracranial contents (brain tissue, blood and cerebrospinal fluid) interact dynamically and exert a constant pressure within the skull by their volume; the skull itself is incapable of expanding in size, so that changes in the volume of any one of the intracranial contents requires a compensatory change in the volume of another. Under normal circumstances, the dynamic compliant interaction between the intracranial contents ensures constancy of intracranial pressures (ICP) within the normal parameters of 0–15 mmHg [2], making the brain a low-pressure, low-resistance system. When ICP is elevated, the brain's resistance to flow is increased significantly, making critically important the maintenance of optimal systemic hemodynamic performance to ensure brain tissue perfusion.

Direct measurement of *intracranial pressure* (ICP) can be performed using a variety of systems, the most reliable of which is the intraventricular catheter. Because the ventricles are fluid-filled reservoirs, transmission of intraventricular pressure waveforms to bedside monitoring systems provides an ability to view in real time the relationship of systemic hemodynamic flow parameters to intracranial pressure dynamics.

Figure 4.9 represents an intraventricular pressure waveform in a patient with normal intracranial compliance. Note the similarities in waveform morphology to an arterial waveform; this effect is produced by arterial pulsations transmitted through CSF that are subsequently superimposed on the ICP waveform. In particular, note the components reflective of the three phases of ventricular systole, namely isovolumetric contraction, rapid ventricular ejection and reduced ventricular ejection, in addition to ventricular diastole. Discrete *pressure points* (P_1, P_2, P_3) define specific points on the ICP waveform that can be related to the cardiac cycle [2]. P_1 is referred to as the percussion wave and relates to the point of peak systolic pressure. P_2 is called the tidal wave and relates to the reduced systolic ejection phase of the cardiac cycle on an arterial waveform, terminating in the dicrotic notch. P_2 is used to reflect intracranial arterial elastic recoil in that a progressive upward movement of P_2 towards P_1 or complete loss of P_2 indicates reduced arterial compliance. P_3 is initiated immediately following the dicrotic notch on the arterial waveform, which signifies closure of the aortic valve and the onset of ventricular diastole.

Cerebral perfusion pressure (CPP) is a measure that reflects the difference in arterial inflow and venous outflow, typically calculated by subtracting mean venous pressure (MVP) from MAP. Calculation of CPP is performed using a modified equation that substitutes ICP for MVP as the chief resistance factor, producing the following equation:

CPP = MAP − ICP

Optimal CPP is defined as a pressure ≥70 mmHg [2]. Reduction in CPP causes the rate of intracranial arterial

PART II Hemodynamic Principles

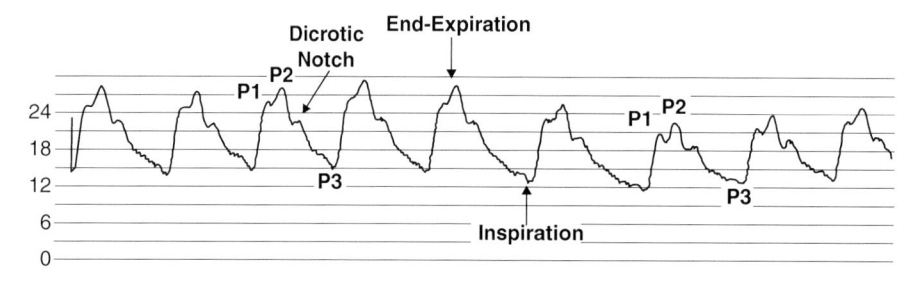

Figure 4.9 Intracranial pressure (ICP) waveform. ICP waveform with respiratory fluctuation; note the drop in pressure due to decreased cardiac output during inspiratory phase. Unlike thoracic pressures, which fluctuate artificially with intrathoracic respiratory pressure changes, measurement at end-expiration is not used in the calculation of ICP, as both inspiratory and expiratory pressures reflect actual pressures generated within the cranial that vary with fluctuations in cardiac output. Key to ICP waveform: P1 = peak systolic pressure; P2= tidal wave; P3 = end-Diastolic pressure. Note: ICP is measured at the point P2; inspiratory and expiratory P2 measurements are averaged; ICP = 26 mmHg.

vasodilation to increase logarithmically. Because autoregulation is an energy-dependent response, sustained periods of oxygen deprivation will devastate the response, making perfusion solely dependent on the balance between MAP and ICP.

Use of the ICP waveform to reflect arterial blood flow through the intracranial circuit requires correlation of the events of the cardiac cycle depicted on the ICP waveform with changes in the waveform morphology. The reduced ventricular ejection phase correlates with the point on the ICP waveform associated with the P_2 waveform; forward flow during this less dynamic phase of the cardiac cycle is normally augmented by changes in arterial compliance secondary to autoregulation. P_2 likely reflects an autoregulatory "bounce" associated with varied perfusion pressures in highly elastic arterial vessels. However, in the case of atherosclerosis, chronic hypertension or increasing ICP, P_2 may be lost or approximate P_1 as the ability for elastic recoil or expansion with varying flow rates may be significantly reduced or lost entirely. As ICP continues to increase, the passive intracranial blood flow occurring during ventricular diastole meets progressively higher degrees of resistance to flow, resulting in loss of a discrete diastolic flow pattern. The overall result of significantly elevated ICP pressures is a flattening of the ICP waveform accompanied by distortion or loss of discrete pressure waves [2].

As mentioned previously, the hemodynamic pressure measurements originating within the thoracic cavity are subject to the influence of inspiratory and expiratory changes and must be measured at end-expiration to ensure accuracy. While inspiratory and expiratory changes often influence the pattern of ICP waveforms, these changes reflect real pressure effects and should be taken into consideration when determining pressure values. Because of its significance as a marker of intracranial arterial compliance, measurement of ICP at the point P_2 has most commonly been advocated, although many practitioners simply calculate a mean pressure using peak systolic and end-diastolic pressure points [2].

Similar to the use of SvO_2 as a marker of systemic tissue oxygenation, neuroscience practitioners use *jugular venous oxygen saturation* ($SjvO_2$) to reflect global brain tissue oxygen consumption and/or *brain tissue oxygen monitoring* ($PbtO_2$) as a direct measure of local tissue bed oxygenation [2,11–17]. Normal $SjvO_2$ is between 55 and 70%. In the absence of a sudden increase in the fraction of inspired oxygen concentration or anemia, $SjvO_2$ levels greater than 75% reflect a state of hyperemia, although discrete areas of ischemia may still be present within the brain. This is a significant limitation of $SjvO_2$ monitoring in that focal ischemic findings tend to be blunted by global oxygenation measures. When $SjvO_2$ levels are less than 55%, a state of oligemia is present. $SjvO_2$ monitoring enables calculation of additional intracranial oxygenation values, including cerebral metabolic rate ($CMRO_2$) and global cerebral oxygen extraction ratio (O_2ER) [2]. Table 4.3 provides the formulas for oxygenation calculations that may be used to fine tune systemic flow parameters to enhance brain tissue oxygenation.[1] Figure 4.10 provides an example of systemic augmentation measures that may be used to enhance brain tissue oxygenation based on $SjvO_2$ and ICP data.

The transcranial Doppler (TCD) waveform should be compared with the ICP values at a closed drainage position and also with the morphology of the ICP waveform. Furthermore, TCD waveforms and velocity data should be

---

[1] $PbtO_2$ monitoring offers the advantage of directly observing changes in tissue oxygenation occurring in real time in relation to other hemodynamic parameters [11–17]. This method uses placement of a catheter directly into a vulnerable tissue bed in the brain, thereby limiting findings to local changes in tissue oxygen. Practitioners can manipulate a number of variables and observe the impact of their interventions on local $PbtO_2$ levels, including $PaCO_2$, PaO_2, temperature and MAP to name a few. Normal $PbtO_2$ values range from 20 to 40 mmHg, with increased time maintained at values ranging less than 15 shown to be associated with death in patients with traumatic brain injury [14]. $SjvO_2$ and $PbtO_2$ values correlate closely, and a number of small studies have tried to discern the value of these tools, as well as device superiority in clinical practice.

Table 4.3 Cerebral oxygenation calculations

Value	Formula[a]
Arterial oxygen content saturation (CaO$_2$)	$1.34 \times$ Hgb $\times$ SaO$_2 + 0.0031 \times$ PaO$_2$
Jugular venous oxygen content saturation (CjvO$_2$)	$1.34 \times$ Hgb $\times$ SjvO$_2 + 0.0031 \times$ PjvO$_2$
Arteriovenous jugular oxygen content difference (AVjDO$_2$) 3.5–8.1 ml dl^{-1}	CaO$_2$ − CjvO$_2$
Cerebral extraction of oxygen (CeO$_2$) 24–42%	SaO$_2$ − SjvO$_2$
Cerebral metabolic rate (CMRO$_2$)	$\dfrac{CBF \times AVjDO_2}{100}$
Global cerebral oxygen extraction ratio (O$_2$ER)	SaO$_2$ − SjvO$_2$/SaO$_2$ *Alternative formula:* $\dfrac{CeO_2}{SaO_2}$

[a]Hgb = hemoglobin; SaO$_2$ = arterial oxygen saturation; PaO$_2$ = partial pressure of arterial oxygen; SjvO$_2$ = jugular venous oxygen saturation; PjvO$_2$ = partial pressure of jugular venous oxygen; CBF = cerebral blood flow.

reviewed in relation to systemic and intracranial hemodynamic parameters. TCD velocities are not the measurement of CBF and therefore TCD can provide only indirect evidence of whether any given therapy is successfully enhancing brain tissue perfusion. Depending on the underlying pathology (e.g. ischemic vessel thrombosis, subarachnoid hemorrhage with vasospasm or increased ICP secondary to traumatic brain injury or intracranial hemorrhage), TCD waveform analysis in combination with assessment of intracranial and systemic hemodynamics can provide important information related to safe augmentation of cardiac performance and arterial pressure.

A number of therapeutic modalities may be used to augment brain tissue perfusion, including α_1 and/or $\beta_{1,2}$ adrenergic agents such as phenylephrine, dopamine and dobutamine, and also volume infusion and in special circumstances intra-aortic balloon pump counterpulsation. Prescribed without complete knowledge of cardiac performance limitations and specific intracranial flow needs, these measures may produce significant harm, instead of therapeutic benefit. The case studies below provide an opportunity to utilize both systemic and intracranial hemodynamic data to direct a plan of care aimed at enhancing brain tissue perfusion.

Insert Ventriculostomy & either SjvO$_2$ or PbtO$_2$ Catheter

Oligemia (ICP > 20 mmHg, SjvO$_2$ < 55%; PbtO$_2$ < 20 mmHg)

1. Treat ICP (ventricular drainage; sedation; neuromuscular blockade; mannitol, etc.).
2. Assess need for transfusion to optimize oxygen carrying capacity.
3. Increase FiO$_2$ to optimize oxygenation; consider increasing PaCO$_2$ to increase intracranial blood flow.
4. Increase mean arterial pressure and cardiac output; assess effect on systemic hemodynamics and titrate volume and pressors cautiously to prevent heart failure.

Hyperemia (ICP < 20 mmHg; SjvO$_2$ > 55%; PbtO$_2$ > 40 mmHg)

1. Assess systemic oxygenation; consider decreasing FiO$_2$ and/or decreasing PaCO$_2$ to achieve intracranial oxygen balance.
2. Assess systemic hemodynamic parameters; titrate medications with hyperdynamic effects to achieve normalization of cardiac output parameters.
3. Balance volume to point of euvolemia determined by systemic hemodynamics (preload/contractility relationship).

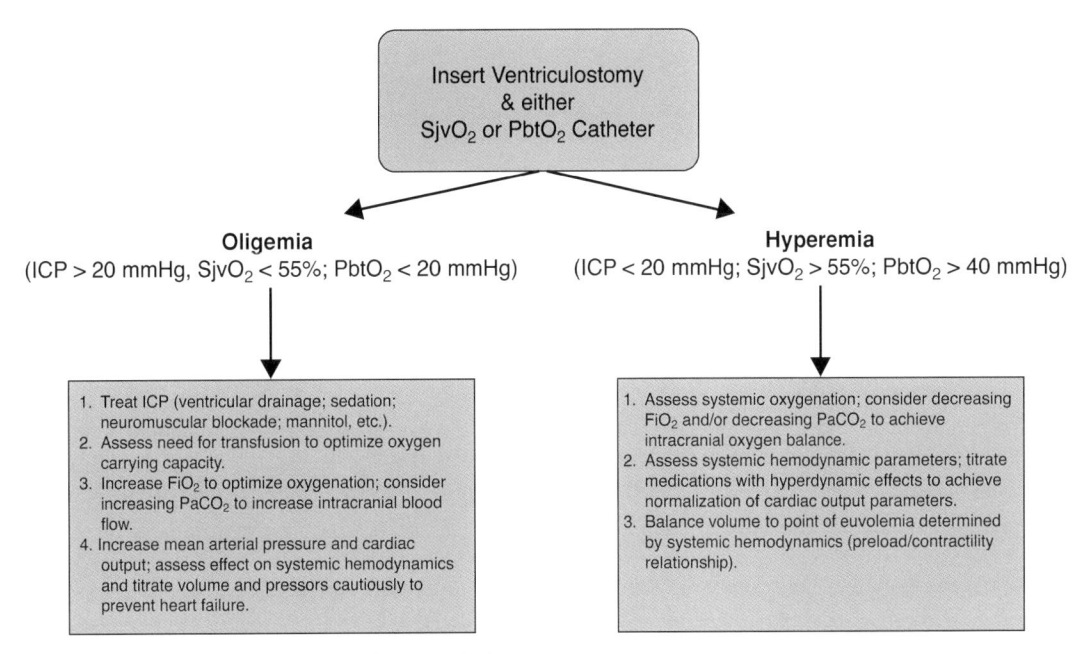

Figure 4.10 Algorithm for oxygenation and intracranial pressure (ICP) management.

PART II Hemodynamic Principles

Case studies in hemodynamic augmentation

Case One

Diagnosis
Traumatic brain injury with diffuse axonal injury (19-year-old male, receiving neuromuscular blockade and sedation on propofol and morphine drips).

TCD waveform analysis
High-resistance waveforms in anterior and posterior circulation, pulsatility index range 1.2–1.6.

Systemic and intracranial hemodynamic parameters and oxygen calculations

Parameter	Data
Core temperature	37.8 °C
Heart rate	78 beats min^{-1}
Arterial pressure (MAP)	118/68 (67) mmHg
Cardiac output	3.8 l min^{-1}
Cardiac index	2.4 l min^{-1} m^{-2}
Stroke volume	48.7 ml per contraction
Stroke volume index	30.4 ml m^{-2} per contraction
CVP	5 mmHg
PAP	$\underline{19}$ / 9
PAWP	7 mmHg
SVR	1305 dyne s^{-1} cm^{-5}
SVRI	2067 dyne s^{-1} cm^{-5}
SvO$_2$	63%
PaO$_2$	97 mmHg
SaO$_2$	98%
CO$_2$	33 mmHg
ICP	35 mmHg
CPP	32 mmHg
SjvO$_2$	45%
AvjDO$_2$	10.8 ml dl^{-1}
CeO$_2$	53%
O$_2$ER	54%
PbtO$_2$	15 mmHg

Interpretation
Elevated ICP with reduced CPP coupled with increased global brain tissue oxygen consumption due to potentially reduced intracranial blood flow. Systemic hemodynamics reflect preload pressures that are within low normal limits in the face of low CO, suggestive of suboptimal left ventricular stretch; systemic tissue oxygen consumption within low normal limits. Current FiO$_2$ on mechanical ventilator of 40%, rate 18 breaths per minute, tidal volume 800 ml. Hemoglobin and hematocrit stable at 12.6 and 36, respectively.

Treatment
- Continue ventricular drainage; administer mannitol.
- Optimize preload: contractility relationship; administer crystalloid and consider addition of colloid (Hespan or 5% albumin) infusion to increase PAWP to 12–14 mmHg and re-evaluate hemodynamic parameters, including effect of volume on MAP.
- If MAP remains below 90 mmHg, add dopamine drip at β_1 range and titrate as needed.
- Decrease ventilator rate to 14 breaths per minute; reassess CO$_2$ in relation to PbtO$_2$.
- Administer antipyretic agent.

Systemic and intracranial hemodynamic parameters and oxygen calculations

Parameter	Data
Core temperature	36.1 °C
Heart rate	95 beats min^{-1}
Arterial pressure (MAP)	155/86 (92) mmHg
Cardiac output	5.2 l min^{-1}ute
Cardiac index	3.3 l min^{-1} m^{-2}
Stroke volume	55 ml per contraction
Stroke volume index	34 ml m^{-2} per contraction
CVP	11 mmHg
PAP	$\underline{36}$
	16
PAWP	14 mmHg
SVR	1246 dyne s^{-1} cm^{-5}
SVRI	1963 dyne s^{-1} cm^{-5}
SvO$_2$	74%
PaO$_2$	99 mmHg
SaO$_2$	100%
CO$_2$	43 mmHg
ICP	24 mmHg
CPP	68 mmHg
SjvO$_2$	57%
AvjDO$_2$	7.9 ml dl^{-1}
CeO$_2$	43%
O$_2$ER	43%
PbtO$_2$	21 mmHg

Interpretation

ICP responded to mannitol and normalization of CO_2. TCD showed an improvement in flow pulsatility (pulsatility index range 0.9–1.2). Systemic hemodynamics improved with volume infusion and administration of β_1 adrenergic agent; SVR decreased in response to improved volume: contractility ratio. Increase in $PaCO_2$ normalizes oxyhemoglobin dissociation and vasorelaxation with improved brain tissue perfusion as reflected in increased $SjvO_2$ and $PbtO_2$.

Treatment

- Maintain PAWP at 14–16 mmHg; monitor urinary volume from mannitol and dopaminergic effects of dopamine infusion and replace intravascular volume as necessary.
- Maintain MAP between 90 and 100 mmHg with volume and dopamine.
- Repeat systemic hemodynamics for significant change in status.

PART II Hemodynamic Principles

Case Two

Diagnosis
Subarachnoid hemorrhage, post-operative day 4 (67-year-old female, spontaneously breathing via nasal cannula at 2 l min^{-1}; vasospasm treated with hypervolemia and phenylephrine vasopressor therapy).

TCD waveform/velocity analysis
Left middle cerebral artery (MCA) vasospasm, maximum mean flow velocity 190 cm s^{-1}, Lindegaard ratio 5.2.

Systemic and intracranial hemodynamic parameters and oxygen calculations

Parameter	Data
Core temperature	36.2 °C
Heart rate	121 beats min^{-1}
Arterial pressure (MAP)	120/93 (102) mmHg
Cardiac output	3.4 l min^{-1}
Cardiac index	2.0 l min^{-1} m^{-2}
Stroke volume	28 ml per contraction
Stroke volume index	16.5 ml m^{-2} per contraction
CVP	17 mmHg
PAP	$\frac{54}{22}$
PAWP	20 mmHg
SVR	2000 dyne s^{-1} cm^{-5}
SVRI	3400 dyne s^{-1} cm^{-5}
SvO$_2$	54%
PaO$_2$	90 mmHg
SaO$_2$	97%
CO$_2$	32 mmHg
ICP	16 mmHg
CPP	96 mmHg
SjvO$_2$	58%
AvjDO$_2$	7.2 ml dl^{-1}
CeO$_2$	39%
O$_2$ER	40%
PbtO$_2$	17 mmHg

Interpretation
ICP/CPP are acceptable; SjvO$_2$ reflects global brain tissue oxygen consumption, but not discrete oxygen deficits which may be occurring in the left MCA territory due to vasospasm. PbtO$_2$ suggests need for improved perfusion in vulnerable left MCA territory. Myocardial performance is suboptimal due to high preload pressures with over-distention of the left ventricle and increased SVR due to both reduction of CO and direct vasoconstriction secondary to α_1 adrenergic therapy. Systemic tissue oxygenation reduced due to poor myocardial performance (increased demand with decreased supply), coupled with pulmonary infiltrates due to volume load.

Treatment
- Diuresis with furosemide to reduce PAWP to 12–14 mmHg and re-evaluate systemic hemodynamic parameters, including cardiac tolerance of MAP values between 95 and 100 mmHg.
- Consider FiO$_2$ 40% by simple face mask until volume overload resolved.

Systemic and intracranial hemodynamic parameters and oxygen calculations

Parameter	Data
Core temperature	36.0 °C
Heart rate	117 beats min^{-1}
Arterial pressure (MAP)	126/98 (107) mmHg
Cardiac output	3.7 l min^{-1}
Cardiac index	2.2 l min^{-1} m^{-2}
Stroke volume	32 ml per contraction
Stroke volume index	18.8 ml m^{-2} per contraction
CVP	10 mmHg
PAP	$\underline{43}$
	17
PAWP	14 mmHg
SVR	2097 dyne s^{-1} cm^{-5}
SVRI	3527 dyne s^{-1} cm^{-5}
SvO$_2$	57%
PaO$_2$	96 mmHg
SaO$_2$	98%
CO$_2$	37 mmHg
ICP	15 mmHg
CPP	92 mmHg
SjvO$_2$	58%
AvjDO$_2$	6.6 ml dl^{-1}
CeO$_2$	40%
O$_2$ER	41%
PbtO$_2$	20 mmHg

Interpretation

ICP/CPP are acceptable; SjvO$_2$ reflects global brain tissue oxygen consumption, but not discrete oxygen deficits which may be occurring in the left MCA territory due to vasospasm. PbtO$_2$ borderline acceptable, but given potential for ischemia due to vasospasm and systemic hemodynamics, further improvement recommended. Repeat TCD examination shows increase in the mean flow velocity (MFV = 205 cm s^{-1}), with a Lindegaard ratio of 5.4. Myocardial performance remains suboptimal despite reduction in preload measures; contractility is unable to overcome high SVR due to a combination of low cardiac output and the vasopressor therapy necessary to optimize perfusion through stenotic arterial segments.

Treatment

- Consider intra-aortic balloon pump counterpulsation to increase cardiac output and reduce left ventricular afterload.
- Titrate vasopressor and volume according to systemic hemodynamic parameters to optimize brain tissue perfusion (target to increase CPP values, decrease the Lindegaard ratio and achieve continuous positive diastolic flow during balloon counter-pulsation).

PART II Hemodynamic Principles

Intra-aortic balloon pump (IABP) waveform; the five points of the IABP are identified as follows (Figure 4.11, bottom waveform):
- ASP assisted systolic pressure (balloon deflation ptoccurs immediately before, reducing left ptventricular workload);
- PAEDP patient aortic end-diastolic pressure;
- PSP peak systolic pressure (unassisted; no balloon ptdeflation occurs before it);
- PDAP peak diastolic augmented pressure (achieved through balloon inflation);
- BAEDP balloon aortic end-diastolic pressure (reduction of afterload achieved by balloon deflation).

Note decreased diastolic perfusion pressures after early balloon deflation resulting in relatively high resistance flow in the middle cerebral artery and likely lower CPP values (Figure 4.11).

Retimed IABP waveform for deflation immediately prior to the next systolic upstroke creates higher positive diastolic flow to the brain in all cycles and low resistance waveforms in the middle cerebral artery (Figure 4.12).

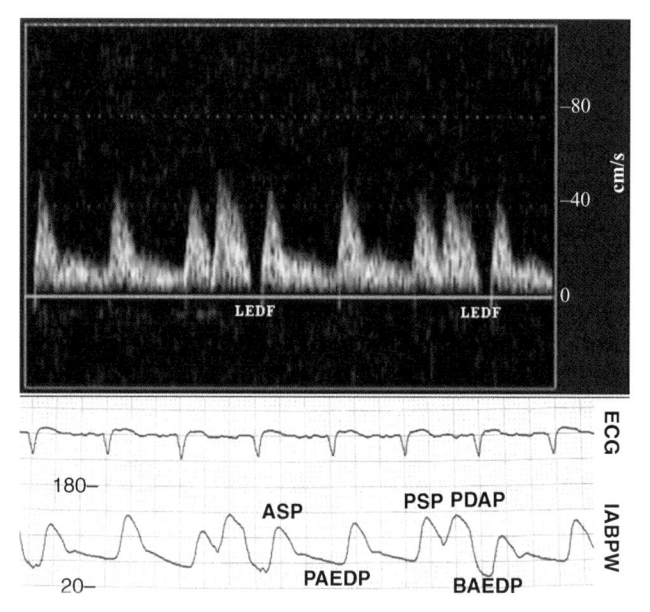

Figure 4.11 Intra-aortic balloon pump waveform (IABPW) and the middle cerebral artery velocity changes with early balloon deflation. Key to IABP waveform: ASP = assisted systolic pressure; PAEDP = patient aortic end-diastolic pressure; PSP = peak systolic pressure (unassisted); PDAP = peak diastolic augmented pressure; BAEDP = balloon aortic end-diastolic pressure; LEDF = loss of end-diastolic flow in the MCA detected by transcranial Doppler (TCD) related to early balloon deflation.

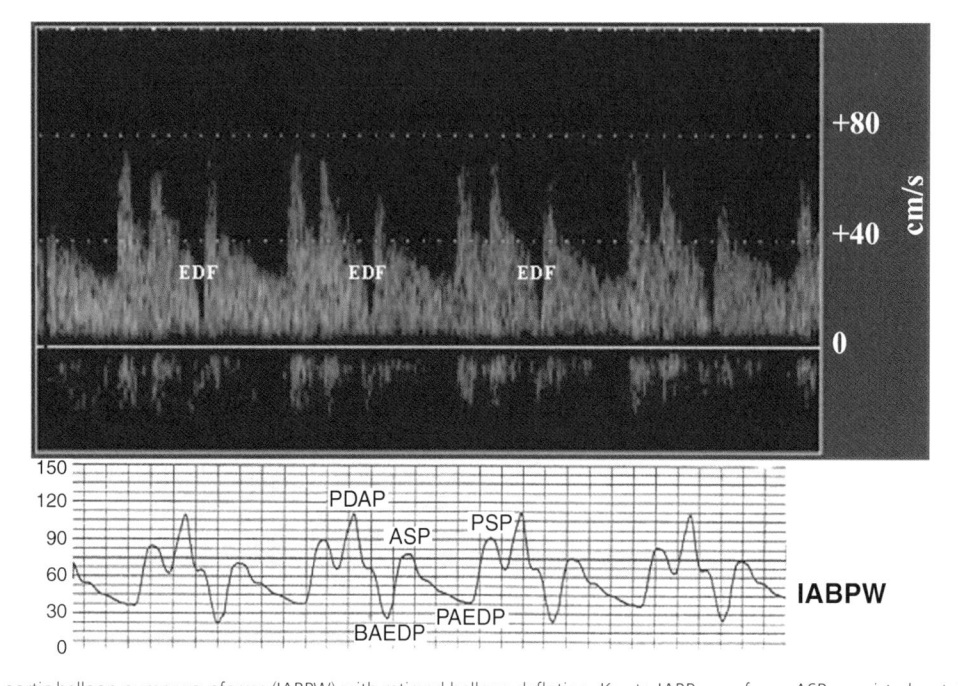

Figure 4.12 Intra-aortic balloon pump waveforms (IABPW) with retimed balloon deflation. Key to IABP waveform: ASP = assisted systolic pressure; PAEDP = patient aortic end-diastolic pressure; PSP = peak systolic pressure (unassisted); PDAP = peak diastolic augmented pressure; BAEDP = balloon aortic end-diastolic pressure; EDF = return of end-diastolic flow and overall low-resistance flow pattern in the MCA on TCD spectral analysis following adjusted balloon deflation.

References

1. Guyton AC. *Textbook of Medical Physiology*, 11th edn. Philadelphia, PA: W.B. Saunders, 2005.
2. Wojner AW. Integrated systemic and intracranial hemodynamics. In Alexandrov AV, ed. *Cerebrovascular Ultrasound in Stroke Prevention and Treatment*, 1st edn. Oxford: Blackwell, 2004.
3. Lim AJ, Goldstein JA, Kern MJ. *Hemodynamic Rounds: Interpretation of Cardiac Pathophysiology from Pressure Waveform Analyses*. Hoboken, NJ: John Wiley & Sons, Inc., 2009.
4. Pranevicius M, Pranevicius O. Cerebral venous steal: blood flow diversion with increased tissue pressure. *Neurosurgery* 2002;**51**:1267–73.
5. Frank O. On the dynamics of cardiac muscle (transl. Chapman CB, Wasserman E). *Am Heart J* 1959;**58**(282):467.
6. Starling EH. *The Linacre Lecture on the Law of the Heart*. London: Longmans, Green & Co., 1918.
7. Wojner AW. Assessing the five points of the intra-aortic balloon pump waveform. *Critical Care Nurse* 1994;**14**(3):48–52.
8. Ahrens TS, Taylor LA. *Hemodynamic Waveform Analysis*. Philadelphia, PA: W.B. Saunders, 1992.
9. Ahrens TS. *Hemodynamic Waveform Recognition*. Philadelphia, PA: W.B. Saunders, 1993.
10. Kelli G. An account of the appearances observed in the dissection of two of the three individuals presumed to have perished in the storm of the 3rd and whose bodies were discovered in the vicinity of Leith on the morning of the 4th November 1821 with some reflections on the pathology of the brain. *Transmissions Med Chir Sci Edinburgh* 1824;**1**:84–169.
11. Dings J, Meixensberger J, Amschler J, Roosen K. Continuous monitoring of brain tissue PO2: A new tool to minimize the risk of ischemia caused by hyperventilation therapy. *Zentralbl Neurochir* 1996;**57**(4):177–183.
12. Dings J, Jager A, Meixensberger J, Roosen K. Brain tissue PO2 and outcome after severe head injury. *Neurological Research* 1998;**20**(Suppl 1):S71–5.
13. van Santbrink H, Maas AI, Avezalat CJ. Continuous monitoring of partial pressure of brain tissue oxygen in patients with severe head injury. *Neurosurgery* 1996;**38**(1):21–31.
14. Valadka AB, Gopinath SP, Contant CF, Uzura M, Robertson CS. Relationship of brain tissue PO2 to outcome after severe head injury. *Critical Care Medicine* 1998;**26**(9):1576–81.
15. Narotam PK, Morrison JF, Nathoo N. Brain tissue oxygen monitoring in traumatic brain injury and major trauma: Outcome analysis of a brain tissue oxygen-directed therapy. *Journal of Neurosurgery* 2009;**111**(4):672–82.
16. Spiotta AM, Stiefel ME, Gracias VH, *et al*. Brain tissue oxygen-directed management and outcome in patients with severe traumatic brain injury. *Journal of Neurosurgery* 2010;**113**(3):571–80.
17. Lang EW, Mulvey JM, Mudaliar Y, Dorsch NW. Direct cerebral oxygenation monitoring – A systematic review of recent publications. *Neurosurgical Reviews* 2007;**30**(2):99–106.

5 Practical Models of Cerebral Hemodynamics and Waveform Recognition

Andrei V. Alexandrov
University of Alabama Hospital, Birmingham, AL, USA

Introduction

The cerebral circulation is exceptional in its requirements. Even when the brain is resting, it has to be provided with a high level of energy. If the flow is interrupted for only a short period, it may have catastrophic consequences for the individual. A broad range of compensatory capacities exist to assure that the supply of nutrients and oxygen is maintained even under adverse circumstances. While the cerebral circulation may seem a complex system, the mechanisms involved are based on basic principles that are easy to formulate and understand. This chapter provides an introduction to basic hemodynamic principles which are the foundation of our interpretation of clinical data.

Ultrasound Doppler provides real-time flow information from arteries and veins. A given level of velocity or a waveform pattern often needs to be seen in relationship to other data to be correctly interpreted and diagnosed. The aim of this chapter is to present practical models of the basic hemodynamic principles that will best explain the findings. Sometimes multiple explanations exist and most often the simplest, yet sufficient, model is the right answer. This chapter describes basic physiological concepts governing cerebral hemodynamics. Several previous publications provide additional considerations about cerebral hemodynamics [1–5]. This chapter further guides the reader through the process of applying spectral Doppler analysis to correct interpretation and differential diagnosis. The illustrations presented contain typical data found during transcranial Doppler (TCD) examinations. Interpretation and discussion of these findings and differential diagnosis are provided.

Cerebrovascular Ultrasound in Stroke Prevention and Treatment, 2nd edition. Edited by Andrei V. Alexandrov. © 2011 Blackwell Publishing Ltd.

The driving force

The brain requires a steady supply of flow and has an unusually low flow resistance even at normal levels of activity. The characteristic waveform pattern of cerebral blood flow, with a high diastolic component, is the result of a low flow resistance. The *pressure gradient* is responsible for providing the energy for driving the flow. In most regions of the circulatory system, the pressure gradient or perfusion pressure is defined as the difference between the inflow arterial blood pressure (ABP) and the outflow vein pressure (VP). In the cerebral circulation, the venous pressure in the outflow sinuses is often lower than that in the veins inside the dura. Therefore, the *cerebral perfusion pressure* (CPP) is defined as the difference between the ABP and the intracranial pressure (ICP), which in turn is equal to the outflow pressure in the so-called bridging veins.

Flow resistance

The driving force, CPP, is counteracted by the flow resistance of the cerebral circulation. This resistance is exceptionally low for a vascular bed (Billy Joel: *"You can't go the distance with too much resistance"*). Most of the resistance is located in the small arterioles and precapillary sphincters where the cerebral blood flow (CBF) is regulated by changes in vessel radius controlled by vascular smooth muscle actuation. The radius is an extremely effective regulator of resistance to flow as expressed by the Hagen-Poiseuille law:

$$\text{Flow rate} = \frac{\pi (P_1 - P_2) r^4}{8 \eta L}$$

where P_1 is the pressure at the beginning and P_2 is the pressure at the end of the flow system, r is the radius of the lumen, π is a constant, η is the fluid viscosity and L is the length or distance that the flow has to travel between the pressure points.

In the pre-TCD days of cerebrovascular studies, it was common to define the cerebrovascular resistance (CVR) as cerebral perfusion pressure divided by cerebral blood flow, which is usually presented as an equation for determining cerebral blood flow:

CBF = CPP/CVR

Although the velocity measured by TCD is *not* flow volume [5,6], Newell *et al.* [7] stated that the flow velocity can reflect CBF in the sense that the velocity *change* can be proportionate to the *change* in CBF if:
1 The angle of insonation remains constant.
2 The perfused territory remains the same.
3 The cross-sectional area of the artery does not change substantially.

Moreover, according to Kontos [6], to calculate the flow volume through an intracranial vessel, its diameter should be precisely measured at the time of velocity assessment, and this cannot be accomplished by current ultrasound methods.

However, the strictly proportional relationship between CBF and CCP expressed by the equation above is not suitable to account for observed changes in waveform pulsatility as encountered in investigational and clinical practice. A more accurate representation of the cerebral pressure–flow velocity relationship is achieved by assuming that flow stops at a so-called critical closing pressure (CPP). This phenomenon was extensively investigated for the myocardial circulation [8] and was later observed in the cerebral circulation [9]. The pressure–flow relationship of the "conventional" CVR model is illustrated in Figure 5.1a and compared with the new model in Figure 5.1(b). In the latter, two parameters are used to describe the model: the slope (*S*) and the cerebral closing pressure (*CCP*, also called the zero-flow pressure).

This concept is indeed important for the understanding of how vascular tone influences the pulsatility of TCD waveforms. Traditionally, two indices have been used to describe the pulsatility of a Doppler velocity waveform: the pulsatility index

$PI = (V_s - V_d)/V_m$

and the so-called resistance index:

$RI = (V_s - V_d)/V_s$

where V_s, V_d and V_m are systolic, diastolic and mean velocities, respectively. As can be seen from the equations, the only difference is the denominator. In theory, the *PI* should be a more linear representation of resistance than the *RI*; however, because the latter is easier to calculate when the waveforms are noisy it may be preferable. We are not aware of any studies that show any clear preference of either index when it comes to accuracy of diagnosis. In any case, both indices are only very approximate indicators of cerebral hemodynamics because they are very much influenced by central arterial hemodynamics via the ABP waveform.

In Figure 5.1, we see that the increasing vascular tone causes an increase in CCP and a decrease in slope (slope is the inverse of resistance). The *PI* and *RI* increase correspondingly. From this we can formulate the first practical *model*:

Vascular tone ↑   arterioles diameter ↓   resistance ↑
  ⇒ MCA velocity ↓   MCA *PI* ↑
Vascular tone ↓   arterioles diameter ↑   resistance ↓
  ⇒ MCA velocity ↑   MCA *PI* ↓

Pressure–flow relationship of stenosis

In stenosis or in vasospasm, pressure energy is lost by the same viscous losses that we described as responsible for

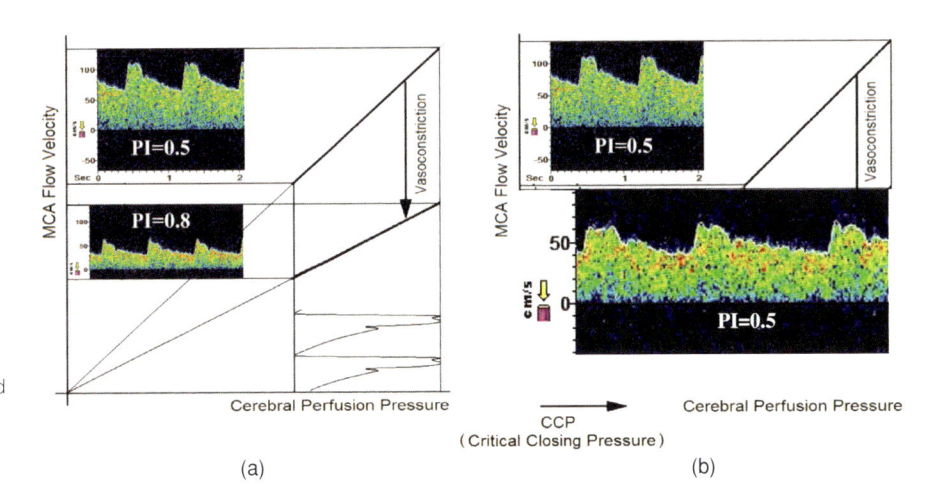

Figure 5.1 Comparison of conventional and new models. Models and spectral waveforms courtesy of Dr Rune Aaslid who generously provided these for this edition.

PART II Hemodynamic Principles

controlling flow in the previous section. The precise calculation of these losses is, however, complicated by the relatively short length of the stenosis (compared with vessel lumen). This means that the flow profile will not be parabolic as is assumed in Poiseuille's law. The viscous pressure loss will typically be 2–4 times higher than predicted by Poiseuille's law above [10].

In addition, pressure is lost by accelerating the flow. This effect begins at the stenosis entrance where the pressure energy driving the flow (i.e. blood pressure) is converted into kinetic energy producing increased velocities. This is described by the *Bernoulli equation of conservation of energy*:

$$P_1 - P_2 = \Delta P = 1 - 2\rho(V_1^2 - V_2^2)$$

where ρ is the density of blood. Theoretically, the kinetic energy could be converted back to pressure again when the flow decelerates after the stenosis. In practice, this is not so, because of irregular stenosis geometry that causes the kinetic energy to be lost in vortex formation and turbulence. In hydrodynamics the Reynolds number is used to predict the occurrence of turbulence. However, in the human circulation, the Reynolds numbers encountered, even in pathological cases, are much lower than those which should cause turbulence in the classical hydrodynamic sense. The observed disturbances in stenotic flow are more a product of the stenosis geometry not being conducive to smooth laminar flow.

Spectral Doppler waveforms provide general evidence for disturbed flow; however, the spectra do not provide quantitative measurements of turbulence. Several flow changes can be found simultaneously in vessels that contain turbulent flow: low-frequency systolic bruits and bi-directional noise, flattening of the waveform and appearance of a "plug-like" flow.

Practical models

Velocity ↑   blood viscosity (=) degree of stenosis ↑
    ⇒ turbulence ↑
Velocity (=) blood viscosity ↑   degree of stenosis (=)
    ⇒ turbulence ↓

Flow velocity in stenosis

In a vessel segment with no bifurcations, the flow velocity and cross-sectional area are linked by the "continuity principle" because the flow volume must be the same throughout the segment [1]:

$$A_1 V_1 = A_2 V_2$$

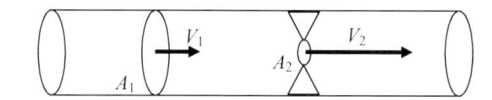

Since fluid is non-compressible and if the average pressure remains the same, the velocity V_2 should increase by an amount inversely proportionate to the reduction in the vessel lumen area:

$$V_2 = V_1(A_1/A_2)$$

Note that the *highest* velocity that theoretically is found within the narrowest cross-section of the stenosis is maintained at the *exit* from a focal stenosis. However, the actual velocity in a stenosis is not simply an inverse function of the stenotic area (A_2) as suggested by this equation. The viscosity, the actual blood pressure, the possible existence of collateral channels and the cerebral autoregulation (see sections below) all influence the observed velocity. The correlation between velocity and stenosis was described by Spencer and Reid [3,4] (see Chapter 6).

Practical models

Degree of stenosis ↑   blood viscosity (=)
    length of stenosis (=)   ⇒ velocity ↑
Degree of stenosis (=) blood viscosity ↓
    length of stenosis (=)   ⇒ velocity ↑
Degree of stenosis (=) blood viscosity (=)
    length of stenosis ↑   ⇒ velocity ↓

Further considerations about hemodynamic changes with an arterial stenosis or spasm are described as follows:

	Practical models		TCD	Condition
Degree of stenosis ↑	length of stenosis (=)	BP (=) ⇒	velocity ↑	focal stenosis progression
Degree of stenosis ↓	length of stenosis (=)	BP (=) ⇒	velocity ↓	focal stenosis regression
Length of spasm ↑	degree of spasm (=)	BP (=) ⇒	velocity (=) or ↓	diffuse vasospasm
Length of spasm ↓	degree of spasm (=)	BP (=) ⇒	velocity (=) or ↑	focal vasospasm

where ↑ means increase, (=) unchanged and ↓ decrease.

Vasomotor reactivity (VMR)

Cerebral blood flow (CBF) rates change with vasodilatory or constricting stimuli that affect the diameter of brain resistance vessels. These changes that occur in the periphery also affect the velocity and waveforms in the proximal branches of the circle of Willis. The middle cerebral artery (MCA) velocity changes by 3–4% per mmHg change in end tidal CO_2 [5]. Determination of vasomotor reactivity requires the recording of end-expiratory pCO_2 and administration of breathing air with increased content of CO_2.

However, a much simpler method to quantify the vasomotor reactivity is very suitable for routine use. Markus and Harrison [11] described a simple measurement of the MCA velocity response to 30 s of breath-holding termed the *breath-holding index (BHI)*:

$$BHI = \frac{MVF_{end} - MVF_{baseline}}{MVF_{baseline}} \times \frac{100}{\text{s of breath} - \text{holding}}$$

Silvestrini *et al.* prospectively evaluated *BHI* in case–control studies and showed that impaired VMR can help to identify patients at higher risk of stroke who have asymptomatic carotid stenosis or previously symptomatic carotid occlusion [12,13].

Practical model

Blood viscosity (=) blood pressure (=) degree of stenosis ↑ ⇒ vasomotor reactivity ↓

Decreased VMR or intracerebral steal [14] may also suggest failure of collateral flow to adapt to the stenosis progression or systemic circulatory changes. Hypercapnia can cause paradoxical reduction in flow velocities distal to a persisting arterial occlusion at the time of normal vasodilation and velocity increase in the unaffected vessels [14]. This velocity reduction indicates that flow was diverted to (or in other words stolen by) normal vessels that have more capacity to vasodilate than vessels already affected by hypoperfusion or ischemia. This has been described as the hemodynamic steal mechanism that can lead to clinical deterioration, i.e. reversed Robin Hood syndrome by analogy with "rob the poor to feed the rich" [14]:

$$\text{Steal magnitude(SM, \%)} = \frac{MFV_{min} - MFV_{baseline}}{MFV_{baseline}} \times 100$$

where MFV_{min} is the minimal velocity detected at the time of vasodilation and velocity increase in the unaffected vessels. Note that this usually occurs 15–25 s from the beginning of voluntary breath-holding. Using currently available technology, the steal is detectable at the level of the circle of Willis in almost one in seven consecutive patients with ischemic strokes or transient ischemic attacks and no other known causes of neurological deterioration [15]. However, a similar mechanism can exist (and possibly be even more prevalent) at arteries beyond the first- and second-level branching.

Cerebral autoregulation

A sudden change in perfusion pressure leads to an immediate change in flow. In the normal circulation, flow is restored after a few seconds. The cerebral circulation has developed an intrinsic mechanism that adjusts the vascular resistance to maintain practically constant CBF in the physiological range of ABP, which is from 50 to 150 mmHg in normo-tensive individuals [16]. Autoregulation guards the brain with a continuous supply of oxygen and glucose necessary for its function. It also prevents hyperperfusion during sudden increases in ABP. Both VMR and autoregulation co-exist and over-ride each other when invoked by various stimuli. As a result, complex dynamic changes in the waveform shape and velocity values can be observed with varying breathing cycles, changes of cardiac output, coughing, sneezing, etc.

Autoregulation also decreases distal resistance to flow when a proximal arterial obstruction develops. When autoregulation has already set the cerebral vessels to maximum dilation to compensate for proximal stenosis or occlusion, no vasomotor response is induced by breath-holding and any significant drop in ABP or blood oxygenation can cause hypoperfusion or ischemia [17].

Cerebral autoregulation can be accomplished through *metabolic* or *myogenic* mechanisms. The metabolic hypothesis postulates that a fast-acting mechanism detects the imbalance between supply and demand of oxygen and adjusts the tone of the resistance vessels to maintain constant flow. The myogenic hypothesis (*Bayliss effect*) postulates that smooth muscles of the resistance vessels respond to changes in the transmural pressure to increase or restrict the incoming flow. Regardless of the priority of each mechanism or the existence of other mechanisms (i.e. neurogenic, etc.), cerebral autoregulation can be disturbed by head trauma or cerebral ischemia and its non-invasive assessment with Doppler ultrasound is still being developed.

Arterial bifurcations and collateral flow distribution

The brain circulation has a wide variety of mechanisms to compensate for arterial lesions by utilizing a complex network of connection between arteries and also regulatory mechanisms that redistribute flow around the obstruction. The pressure gradient distal to a lesion invokes flow around the lesion. This flow is channeled from neighboring vessels through collateral channels. The collateral flow through a well-functioning circle of Willis can maintain an ICA occlusion symptom free in some patients.

As a general rule, flow in a bifurcation involved as a collateral channels is triggered when a lesion is located proximal to its origin and a pressure gradient develops between the donor arteries and the recipient vessels.

Several factors can disturb the regulatory mechanisms and the ability of brain vasculature to maintain adequate perfusion. Systemic blood pressure and cardiac output may decrease, the patient may become dehydrated, platelet function may be activated, an embolus can lodge in the distal vasculature and spreading tissue edema can change overall resistance to flow. The key to interpreting a variety of cerebrovascular ultrasound findings is to interpret flow changes observed at bifurcations in the light of the hemodynamic models and check for flow diversion pathways that compensate for obstructive lesions.

Velocity (branching vessel) ↑   velocity (stem with
   bifurcations) (=)   velocity (proximal to clot) ↓

Reasons: collateral channels "escape hatch" increased resistance.

In case of a distal M1 middle cerebral artery (MCA) occlusion, a practical model of which is illustrated, the anterior cerebral artery (ACA) can serve as flow redistribution channel to deliver blood to the MCA territory via transcortical collaterals. The lenticular-striate arteries or perforators serve as a channel that delivers blood to the internal capsule and more distally via the ascending branches. Applying analogy with a submarine, these branches can act like an "escape hatch" for flow proximal to the occlusion. Thus, sometimes distal M1 MCA occlusion may not cause any significant proximal velocity decrease and angiography in cases like this shows "blush" to perforators.

Practical model of an acute distal M1 MCA occlusion:

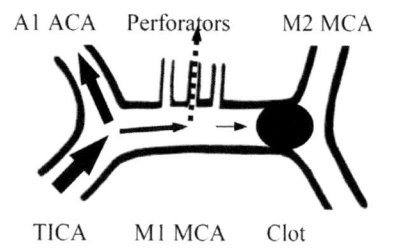

These flow phenomena may further account for variable stroke severity with the distal M1 MCA occlusion and relatively normal or slightly decreased proximal M1 MCA velocity. More information about flow changes at the site of an acute intracranial occlusion are provided by the Thrombolysis in Brain Ischemia (TIBI) residual flow grading system [18] (see Chapters 6 and 15).

These simple models can help in memorizing the effects of the most important factors that determine velocity and pulsatility of flow. Flow models that are invoked to explain actual flow findings should be corrected with respect to cardiac output, blood pressure, heart rate, patient age, vital signs and medications.

How to read waveforms

The flow waveform represents the time dependence of blood flow velocity on cardiac activity [19]. Waveform recognition during Doppler examination starts with hearing the flow signal followed by visual analysis of the signal appearance on screen. Steps to optimize flow signals depend largely on this immediate recognition of the waveform and sonographer skills. Reading any ultrasound findings starts with orientation on screen and identification of machine settings. For Doppler examination, these simple and essential components include:
1 transducer and sample volume (gate) positioning
2 flow direction
3 angle of insonation
4 scale settings and
5 sweep speed.

For the purposes of this chapter, all Doppler recordings were obtained with a large (13 mm) sample volume at an assumed zero angle of insonation. Flow signals towards the probe are displayed above baseline with a constant sweep speed. Scale settings, gain and baseline position were adjusted when necessary. Learn a standard scanning protocol, since consistent practice of ultrasound examination helps not only with vessel identification but also with quality controls and understanding when certain things went missing or how in certain situations one can further improve scanning and interpretation skills [20].

First, using the following five steps, identify the components of a cardiac cycle (Figure 5.2):
1 beginning of systole
2 peak velocities during systole (peak systole)
3 dicrotic notch (closure of the aortic valve signaling the beginning of diastole)
4 end diastolic velocities (end diastole) and
5 the shape and magnitude of flow deceleration during cardiac cycle.

Second, determine if the measurements provided by automated software are representative of the waveforms found. Most instruments provide a spectral outline follower that is shown on screen. If there are spikes of dropouts of this

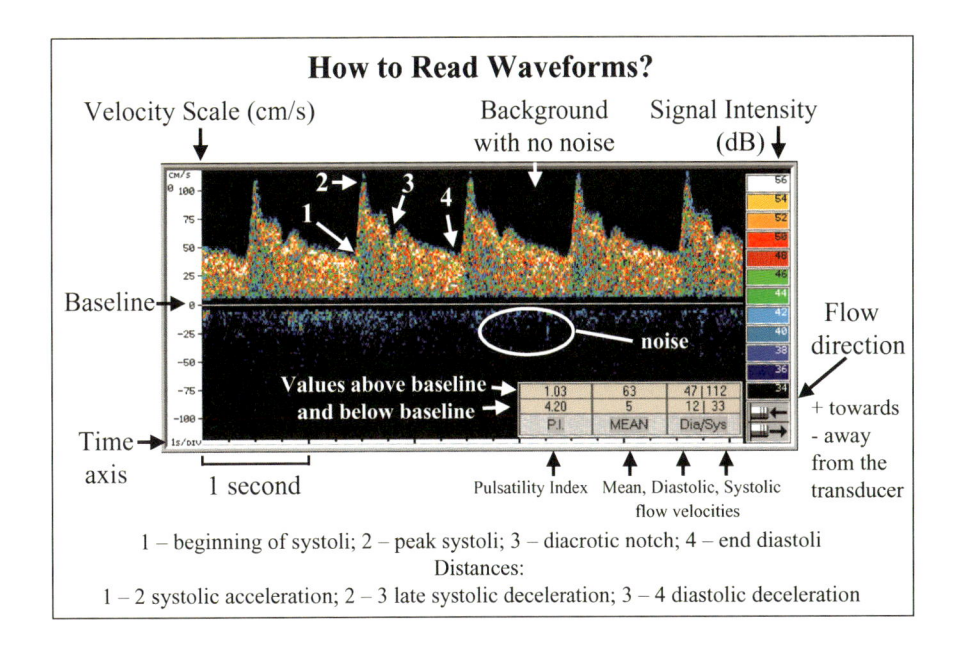

CHAPTER 5 Practical Models of Cerebral Hemodynamics and Waveform Recognition

Figure 5.2 How to read waveforms.

outline, the indicated readings may not be correct and it is advisable to perform manual readings using cursor placement. Doppler flow velocity signal optimization is checked by the following:

1 Signal-to-noise ratio (i.e. the background should contain no or minimal noise).
2 Envelope (or waveform follower) does not over- or underestimate velocities.
3 Scale settings are adequate to display maximum velocities.
4 Baseline (zero line) is positioned to avoid aliasing or sufficiently separate signals.
5 Signal intensity is equal during recording sweep.

Third, the waveform characterization will depend on identification of the following elements of the spectral signal:
1 early systolic upstroke (sharp or slow, delayed)
2 late systolic and diastolic deceleration (continuous, stepwise or flattened)
3 systolic/diastolic velocity difference (flow pulsatility) and
4 other components of the Doppler spectrum (bruit, spectral narrowing, embolic signals, etc.).

Specific waveforms

Normal findings

Case history: An asymptomatic 32-year-old man with arterial blood pressure 130/80.

Interpretation: The waveform (Figure 5.3) shows a sharp systolic flow acceleration and continuous deceleration after the closure of the aortic valve and positive end-diastolic flow. The end-diastolic velocity falls between 20 and 50% of the peak systolic velocity values and this finding indicates normal low resistance to arterial flow.

Case history: An asymptomatic 32-year-old man with arterial blood pressure 130/80.

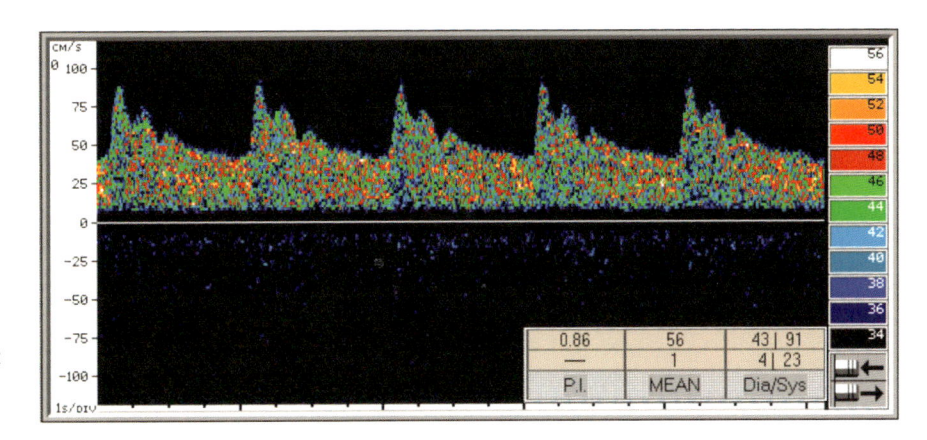

Figure 5.3 A low-resistance unidirectional flow signal. Case history: An asymptomatic 32 years old man with arterial blood pressure 130/80.

73

PART II Hemodynamic Principles

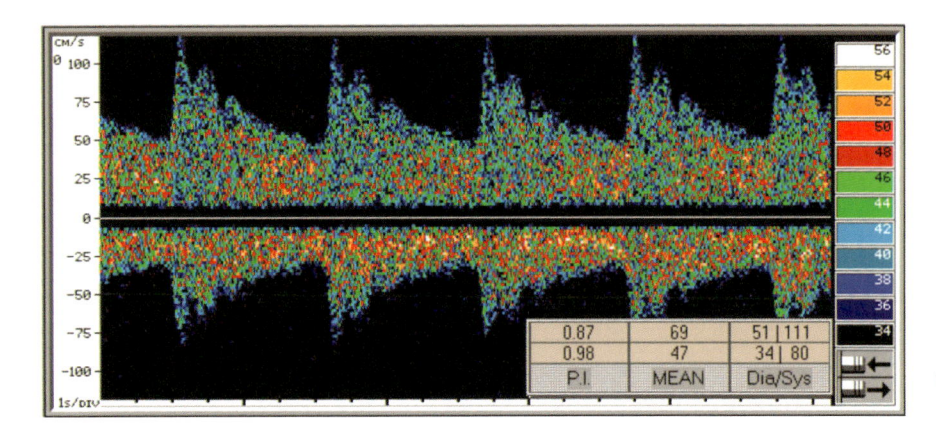

Figure 5.4 Bi-directional flow signals with normal resistance.

Interpretation: The recording (Figure 5.4) shows a bi-directional signal with simultaneous sharp systolic upstrokes and similar continuous deceleration in both flow directions during diastole. Both waveforms show normal low-resistance flow patterns obtained at the ICA bifurcation.

Increased pulsatility of flow

Case history: A 65-year-old man with a new onset aphasia and chronic hypertension.

Interpretation: The waveform (Figure 5.5) above baseline has a rapid systolic upstroke and a rounded peak systolic complex followed by a more abrupt flow deceleration compared with normal waveforms. The end-diastolic velocities below 30% of peak systolic values indicate the relative increase in flow resistance/ABP pulse pressure. If flow pulsatility is relatively similar in branching and contralateral vessels, a pulsatile waveform with normal or elevated mean flow velocity indicates normal vessel patency at the site of insonation and is not suggestive of a distal arterial occlusion. A weak flow signal below baseline in Figure 5.5 is not optimized and measurements are erroneous.

The effects of chronic hypertension on intracranial Doppler recordings usually include an increase in flow pulsatility [21] (pulsatility index values of ≥ 1.2 at our laboratory). Kidwell *et al.* showed that a relative increase in the Gosling pulsatility index above 1.17 correlates with the presence of silent brain damage (T2 hyperintensities) on MRI in patients with chronic hypertension [22].

Case history: A 37-year-old man with closed traumatic brain injury and ICP 52 mmHg. *Interpretation:* The flow signal (Figure 5.6) above baseline shows sharp systolic upstrokes followed by sharp deceleration indicating an overall increased resistance to flow.

Despite elevated pulsatility index in a young individual free of chronic hypertension ($PI = 1.2$), this high-resistance waveform in the middle cerebral artery indicates normal patency of its proximal segment. This patient with traumatic brain injury (TBI) had intracranial pressure of 52 mmHg that produced increased resistance in the distal vascular bed. Elevated pulsatility index values were observed in patients with increased intracranial pressure [23]. The Doppler spectrum shows sharpening of the waveform due to faster flow deceleration. At the same time, the waveform above baseline also has a substantial diastolic flow, indicating that some of this flow may be directed to a low-resistance vascular bed. This can happen in patients with TBI because both edematous (bruised) and normally perfused tissues may be present within the MCA territory. Furthermore, brain areas may be present with disturbed autoregulation or unequal distribution of ICP and mass effect. The waveform above

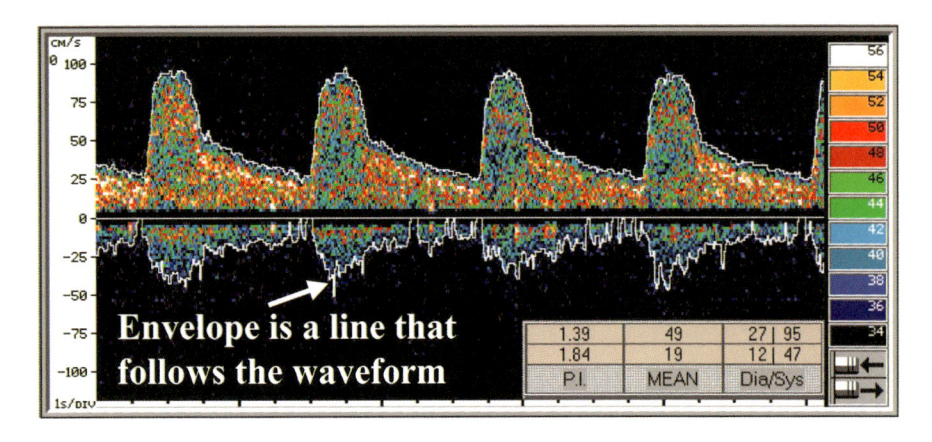

Figure 5.5 Increased resistance to flow with chronic hypertension.

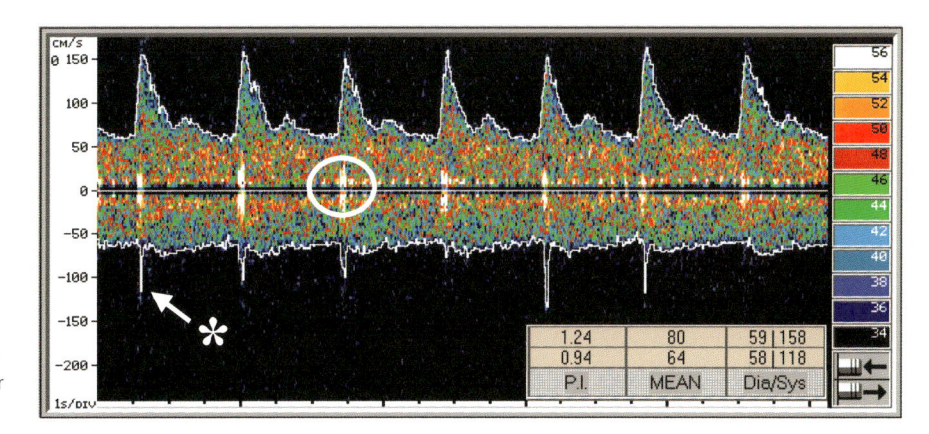

CHAPTER 5 Practical Models of Cerebral Hemodynamics and Waveform Recognition

Figure 5.6 A complex waveform indicating flow to both high- and low-resistance vascular beds.

baseline is reminiscent of a common carotid waveform because CCA supplies both low- and high-resistance vascular beds.

The flow signal below baseline has a low-resistance flow pattern flow seen in a vein. A loud thump-like early systolic sound (circled) is present due to vessel wall motion. This bright reflector disturbs spectral analysis and causes the envelope to spike (marked with *), leading to errors in automated velocity and pulsatility measurements below baseline.

Case history: A 35-year-old man with subarachnoid hemorrhage (grade II, day 2) and liver failure.

Interpretation: Both waveforms above and below the baseline (Figure 5.7) have sharp systolic upstrokes and an abrupt flow deceleration. These pulsatile waveforms with the end-diastolic velocities within 20–25% of peak systolic values indicate high resistance to arterial flow. The difference in automated calculations of *PI* (*PI* below baseline is higher than that above baseline) is attributable to the weakness of the signal directed away from the probe and the underestimation of the diastolic velocity by the envelope (last full cycle on the right).

This patient with subarachnoid hemorrhage has an even more pulsatile waveform (*PI* = 1.7). The differential diagnosis includes increased intracranial pressure, vasospasm and systemic conditions. Although hydrocephalus can be expected to develop by 48 h after the bleeding, this patient has normal ICP values (continuous ventricular drainage and invasive ICP monitor) at the time of TCD examination. A vasospasm that may produce these waveforms at M1 and A1 segment origins should affect both MCA and ACA territories and this will be unlikely event on day 2. Finally, the patient does not hyperventilate since he is alert and breathing room air at a normal pace. In this case, increased *PI* values and a sharp pulsatile waveform are probably a result of spontaneously increased cardiac output (cardiac index = 7) in a young patient with liver failure.

Case history: A 42-year-old woman with closed traumatic brain injury.

Interpretation: The waveforms above baseline (Figure 5.8) show a regular heart rate with variable velocities (sharp systolic upstrokes, stepwise deceleration, normal low resistance). Marked velocity fluctuations can spontaneously occur every four cardiac cycles due to breathing. A cycle with the highest velocities (*) can be used for manual calculations.

Flow velocity and pulsatility fluctuations can also be caused by altered autoregulation (the patient has traumatic brain injury) and changes in the intracranial pressure. Blood

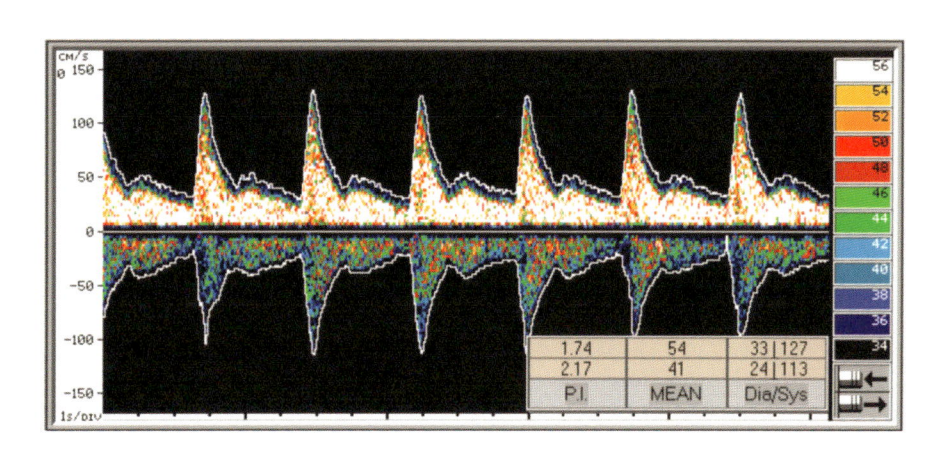

Figure 5.7 Increased pulsatility of flow at a bifurcation.

PART II Hemodynamic Principles

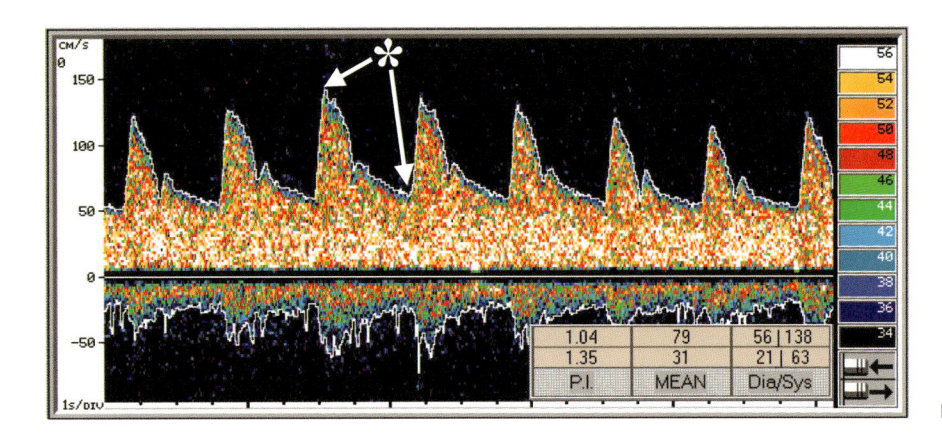

Figure 5.8 Variable velocity and pulsatility.

flow velocity measurements can also be partially affected by changes in the angle of insonation (transducer positioning and, to a lesser extent, vessel pulsation and motion). Changes in flow pulsatility and waveform shape, as seen in this patient, are unlikely affected by the angle of insonation.

Irregular heart rhythm

Case history: A 54-year-old man with an acute small cortical stroke and LVH.

Interpretation: Waveforms above and below the baseline (Figure 5.9) have sharp upstrokes, arrival of maximum systolic velocities towards the end of systole and stepwise flow deceleration. The end-diastolic velocities fall below 30% of peak systole due to irregular heart rate; this also affects estimation of flow resistance (increased values of *PI* calculated with envelope tracings) from only 2–5 cycle-averaged values. A single cycle may be selected for manual measurements.

Measurements that are affected by irregular heart rate include:
1 velocity (underestimation) and
2 pulsatility (overestimation).

A prolonged pause between cardiac contractions (seen in the second cycle, Figure 5.9) leads to lower than usual end-diastolic velocities that artificially decrease the velocity and increase *PI* values. The compensatory pauses after extra-systole should be avoided from being included into measurements or, if extra-systole are too frequent, a higher number of cardiac cycles should be averaged using slower sweep speeds or manual measurements of the highest velocity cycle should be used.

Case history: A 60-year-old woman with recent TIA and atrial fibrillation.

Interpretation: Waveforms towards the probe (Figure 5.10) demonstrate an "irregular–irregular" heart rhythm and sonographers should be familiar with these findings as they could be the only witnesses of paroxysmal atrial fibrillation. The waveforms show irregular arrival of cardiac cycles with sharp upstrokes and variable peak velocities. As a practical rule, a cycle with the highest velocities (marked as *) can be used for manual calculations. However, estimation of flow resistance and representative mean velocity is difficult since the pulse rate and cardiac output are affected.

What is the overall resistance in the MCA as shown in these waveforms? *PI* reading indicates relatively high resistance since the software compares the highest peaks with the lowest minimas in its approximation of where peak systole and end-diastole should be. Despite this artificial *PI* calculation, the resistance in a patent brain vessel during atrial fibrillation is low. Remember that the brain needs a

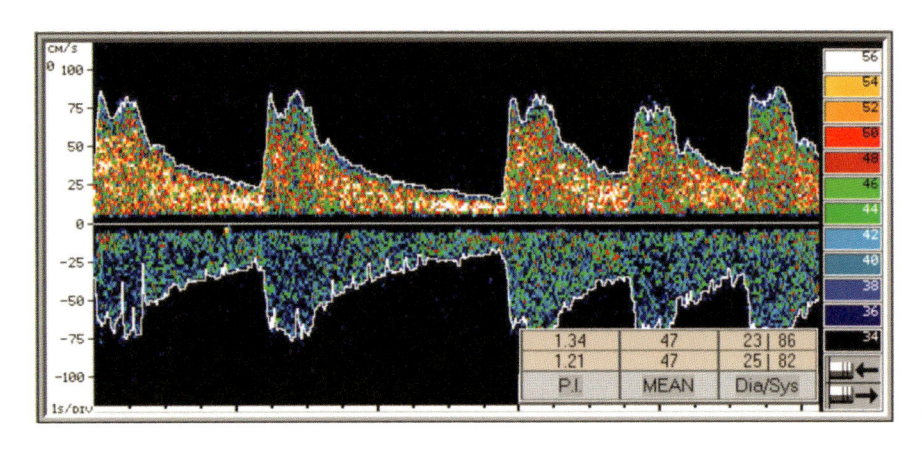

Figure 5.9 Extra-systole.

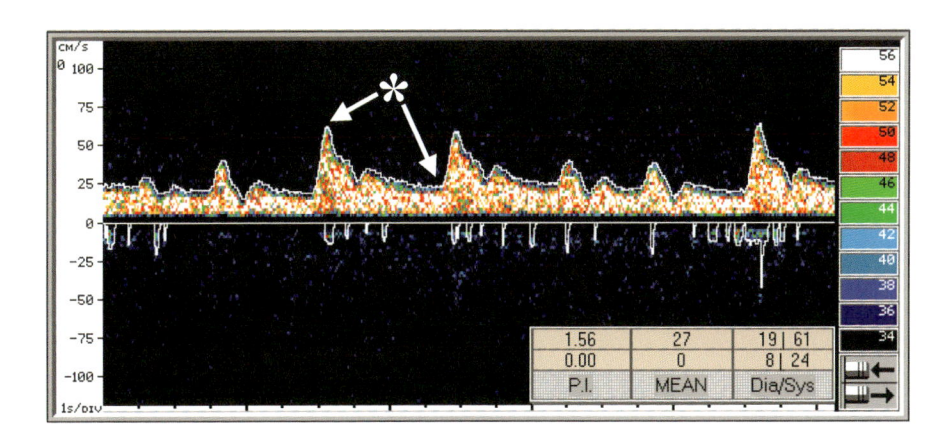

Figure 5.10 Atrial fibrillation.

constant energy supply and it cannot rely on occasional better filling of the left ventricle during atrial fibrillation. Note that despite variable peaks, diastolic velocities remain practically stable after the closure of the aortic valve until the end of diastole. The brain drives diastolic velocities at a steady level despite variations in systolic in-flow. *PI* values are overestimated due to occasionally higher PSV values. Although averaging of 20 cardiac cycles may provide more representative velocity and *PI* values, it is impractical and difficult to accomplish. A less scientific but practical solution is to use manual measurements taken from a cycle with the highest peak and end-diastolic measurements that are often representative of a more synchronized cardiac contraction with better cardiac output. Remember that selection of these cycles would lead to overestimation of *PI*. Nevertheless, this approach also shortens the time of examination and introduces a consistent way of recording velocities for serial studies.

Changes in the systolic flow acceleration

Case history: A 67-year-old man with resolving MCA stroke and carotid occlusion.

Interpretation: The waveform above baseline (Figure 5.11) shows a delayed systolic flow acceleration, flattened systolic complex and slow diastolic deceleration. End-diastolic veloc-

ities above 50% of peak systole indicate very low flow resistance. This waveform is called a "blunted" flow signal.

This waveform shows a delayed systolic flow acceleration that can be found in a patent vessel distal to a high-grade stenosis or occlusion [24]. The MCA usually receives either collateral flow around or residual flow through the ICA lesion and, in order to attract more flow, compensatory vasodilation occurs to reduce overall resistance to flow [low (1.0–0.6) or very low (<0.6) *PI* values]. When these "blunted" waveforms (with MFV generally above 20 cm s^{-1}) are found unilaterally, it is a sign of a proximal (ICA or terminal ICA) hemodynamically significant obstruction. If a delayed systolic flow acceleration is found in both internal carotid branches and the basilar artery, it may be a sign of reduced cardiac output, aortic stenosis or Takayasu's disease. In congestive heart failure, the waveform can look flattened but the initial (although often small) upstroke is preserved.

Case history: A 73-year-old man with MCA stroke and carotid occlusion. *Interpretation:* The waveform above baseline (Figure 5.12) has an upward systolic upstroke. This waveform has to be compared with a non-affected vessel in order to decide if only a *slight* delay in systolic acceleration is present. Regardless, this is *not* a blunted signal since a clear systolic complex is visualized.

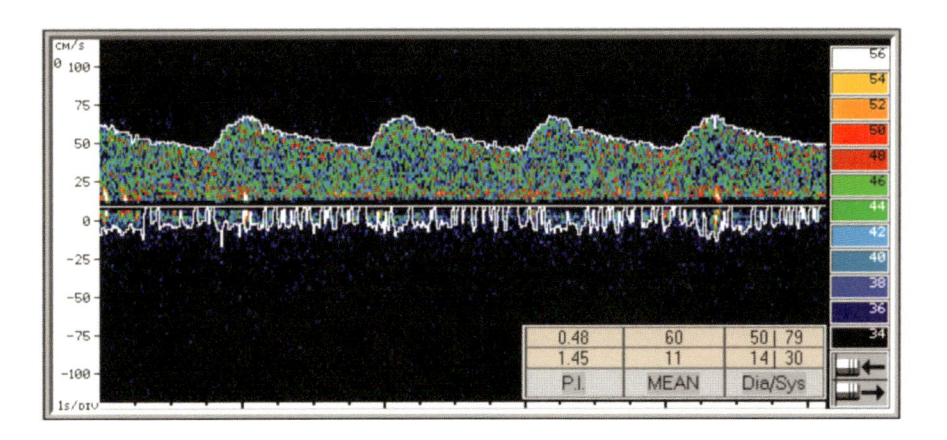

Figure 5.11 A blunted signal.

PART II Hemodynamic Principles

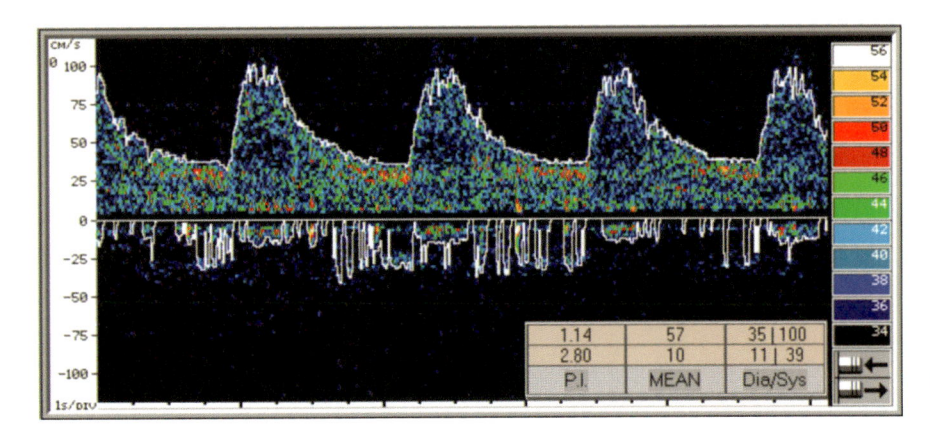

Figure 5.12 Slightly delayed systolic flow acceleration.

This waveform shows only a slight delay in the systolic flow acceleration and a clear systolic complex. This type of flow acceleration can be found in patients with or without hemodynamically significant proximal arterial obstruction. When found at the MCA origin or just posteriorly to a "blunted" MCA signal, this waveform may be attributable to the posterior communicating artery or the posterior cerebral artery with a normal systolic flow acceleration in the presence of an ICA obstruction. In general, remember that the closer one comes to the source of collateral flow, the better the systolic flow acceleration and the higher the velocity are.

Collateralization of flow

Case history: A 70-year-old woman with a recent TIA and carotid occlusion.

Interpretation: The tracing (Figure 5.13) displays a bi-directional signal with normal systolic upstrokes. The waveform below baseline shows higher velocities and lower resistance to flow. This may represent flow diversion to a branch directed away from the probe.

This bi-directional signal represents a typical finding at the MCA–ACA bifurcation with flow diversion to ACA being present. When the ACA becomes the donor vessel for the anterior cross-filling to compensate for a contralateral carotid obstruction, the ACA starts to supply both A2 segments and often the contralateral MCA via contralateral A1 segment reversal. This cross-filling may manifest on the donor site as the mean flow velocity difference ACA > MCA and pulsatility index ACA < MCA due to compensatory flow volume increase and vasodilation. It is important to optimize both MCA and ACA signals to make sure that maximum Doppler shifts are compared at these vessels and not between the terminal ICA and ACA. Simultaneous display of the terminal ICA/ACA signals in a normal individual may yield similar velocity differences (i.e. MFV below greater than above baseline) due to a suboptimal angle of insonation with TICA. If one follows a standard insonation protocol [20], by the time ACA is reached, MCA was surveyed and a velocity decrease due to TICA interception can be suspected.

Aliasing and signal optimization

Case history: A 72-year-old man with a recent TIA and a moderate proximal carotid stenosis.

Interpretation: This recording (Figure 5.14) shows a waveform that exceeds half of the velocity scale (i.e. an artifact called *"aliasing"*). Both envelopes show automated recognition of the velocity values that are erroneous. This waveform

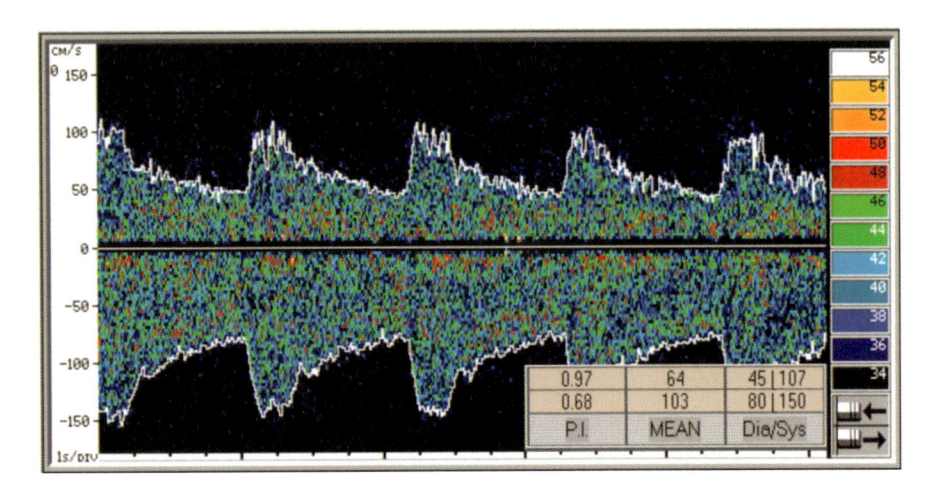

Figure 5.13 Flow diversion.

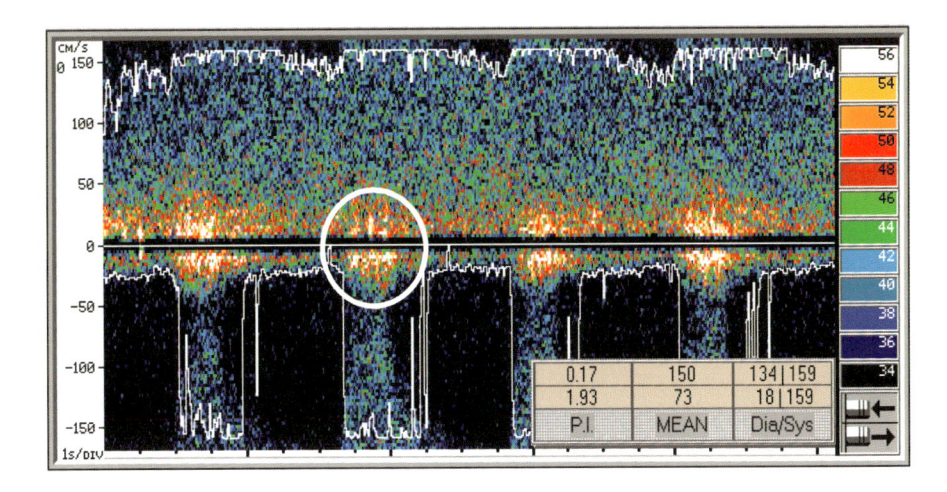

CHAPTER 5 Practical Models of Cerebral Hemodynamics and Waveform Recognition

Figure 5.14 Aliasing.

also contains a low-frequency bi-directional signal heard as a *bruit* (circled).

This waveform is a typical pulse wave Doppler artifact [25]. This artifact inappropriately displays or cuts off the systolic frequencies from the top or the bottom of spectral display. There is often an overlap in maximum velocities between the flow signals towards and away from the probe. This artifact is linked to a pulsed Doppler system handicap in velocity detection posed by half of the pulse repetition frequency (PRF) threshold (or the *Nyquist limit*) [25]. Steps to optimize this signal should include:

1 adjustment of the velocity scale to maximum possible values;
2 moving baseline ("dropping the baseline" or converting the recording into a unidirectional display); and
3 reducing sample volume or gate (this may help to focus the beam at one vessel, thus avoiding or reducing the impact of aliasing on the velocity measurements).

Case history: A 68-year-old man with a recent MCA stroke and MCA stenosis.

Interpretation: The waveform (Figure 5.15) is a signal optimized to reduce aliasing. It has high velocities, bruits, normal systolic acceleration and a normal low-resistance flow pattern. The background contains no noise and the envelope shows a good automated waveform tracing. Other data are needed to confirm if this is a stenotic signal, i.e. focal changes in velocity along the MCA stem and comparison with the contralateral MCA velocity values.

Differential diagnosis includes a compensatory velocity increase if another large vessel lesion is present. From a single depth tracing in the intracranial vessels, it is impossible to tell whether this waveform represents a focal significant velocity increase due to stenosis or hyperemia with collateralization of flow. As shown in Figure 5.15, the MCA flow signal with a mean flow velocity of 117 cm s^{-1} was found at the site of a 50% MCA narrowing unilateral to the hemisphere affected by an ischemic stroke. If found contralateral to a proximal ICA obstruction, similar velocity findings may represent M1 MCA stenosis or flow diversion. A focal MCA stenosis is likely to be found if the distal M1 MCA velocity decelerates by more than 30%. Remember that not all elevated velocities predict the presence of an arterial stenosis. Angiography is insensitive to a mild or even low moderate degree of an intracranial arterial narrowing while

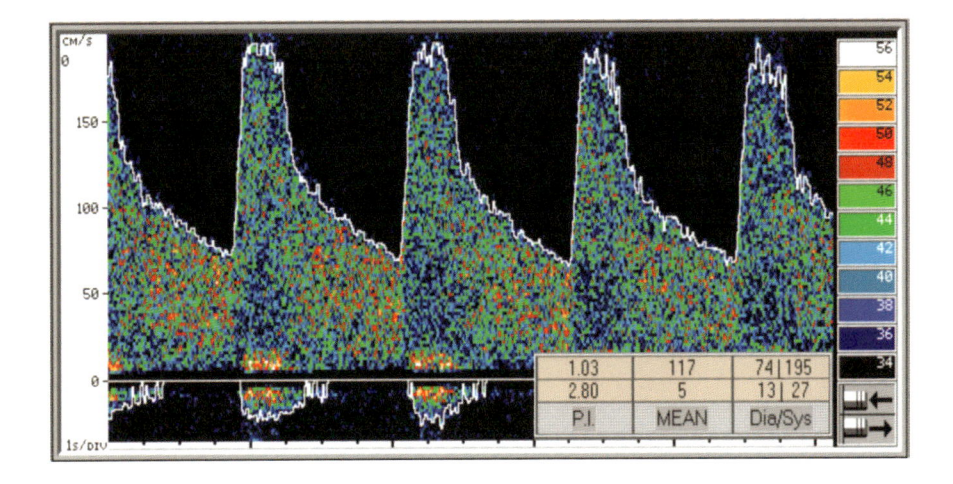

Figure 5.15 A stenotic signal.

PART II Hemodynamic Principles

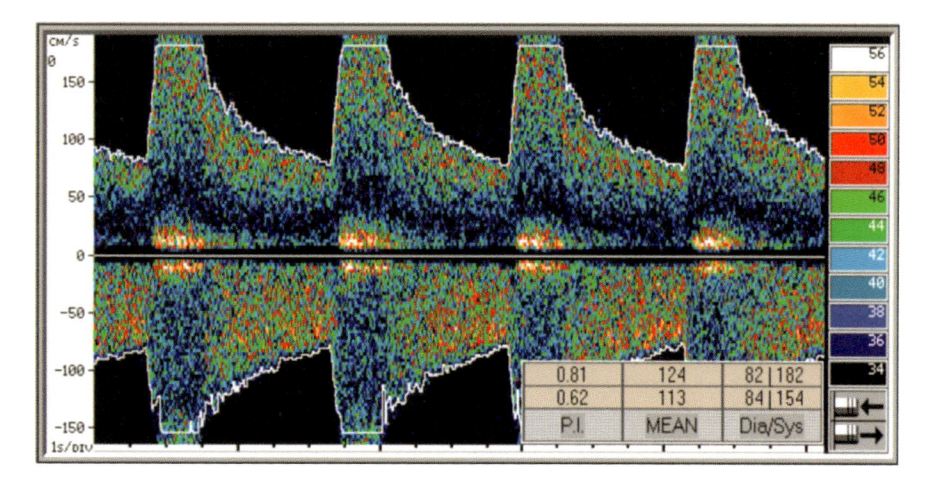

Figure 5.16 Aliasing or optimized signal?

hyperemic flow changes or collaterals can further mimic an arterial stenosis. Apply ratios to non-affected segments that can increase the accuracy of stenosis assessment [26,27] and remember that diffuse or elongated arterial stenoses may not necessarily increase the velocity but rather have normal or decreased values [27].

Case history: A 59-year-old man with an acute stroke and carotid occlusion contralateral to the side of insonation.

Interpretation: The tracing (Figure 5.16) displays a bi-directional signal with abnormally elevated velocities (MFV >100 cm s^{-1}) and minimal aliasing. Both waveforms show normal systolic upstrokes, bruits and low-resistance patterns. Envelopes indicate reasonable signal optimization since automatically measured velocities are indeed abnormal. Further optimization may improve these readings by a small fraction of already obtained velocities. Other data are needed to determine if this is a compensatory or stenotic velocity increase.

The waveforms were found at the ICA bifurcation contralateral to a complete proximal ICA occlusion mostly indicating laminar flow (note an increased intensity spectrum of the MCA waveform towards higher frequencies during the entire cycle) and bruits at bifurcation due to compensatory flow diversion. In acute ischemic stroke, the abrupt development of carotid thrombosis may cause a significant flow diversion and opening of collateral channels. This process may result in acutely elevated velocities in the donor vessels followed by a velocity decrease in the subacute and chronic phases when stroke is completed or vessel dilation was accomplished. Note the spectral broadening in the ACA particularly during diastole when collateral flow has further incentive to move towards dilated contralateral vasculature compared with the unilateral MCA that attempts to auto-regulate the incoming high-velocity laminar flow (PI MCA > ACA).

Case history: A 42-year-old woman with subarachnoid hemorrhage (day 8).

Interpretation: The simultaneous display of four waveforms (Figure 5.17) is due to a large sample volume (or gate) of insonation of 13 mm. Marked as 1, the highest velocities were likely found in a segment with maximal narrowing; 2, elevated velocities in another segment with less narrowing; 3, hyperemic signals likely in a proximal vessel; and 4, branch signals. The differential diagnosis includes the presence of a mirror artifact and hyperemia.

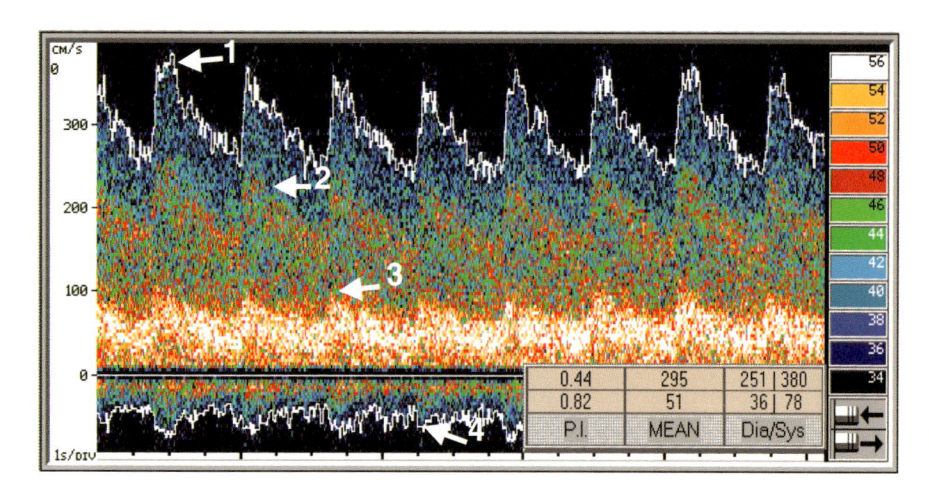

Figure 5.17 Increased velocities, multiple waveforms and severe vasospasm.

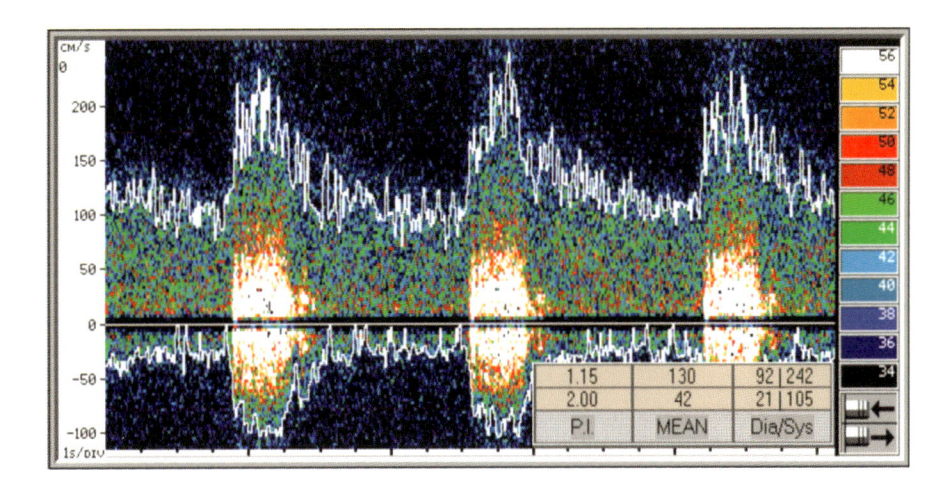

CHAPTER 5 Practical Models of Cerebral Hemodynamics and Waveform Recognition

Figure 5.18 Turbulence, bruits and velocity underestimation.

This is a complex recording obtained in a patient with subarachnoid hemorrhage who developed a severe MCA vasospasm. The use of a large (13 mm) sample volume may produce simultaneous display of waveforms detected at different arterial segments (i.e. terminal ICA, proximal M1, mid M1 MCA or neighboring segments with different patency). Although the highest velocities in the waveform 1 are likely attributable to the site of maximum vasospasm (the mean flow velocity of 295 cm s^{-1}), the presence of mirror artifact [28] and hyperemia (as a potential cause of it being a bright reflector) should be excluded using the Lindegaard ratio [29]. The signal-to-noise ratio appears to be optimized, i.e. no noise in the background. This patient was on hypertension–hemodilution–hypervolemia (triple-H) therapy and hyperemia was mostly ruled out by the Lindegaard ratio of 10 (see also Chapter 6).

Severe stenosis, acute thrombosis and occlusions

Case history: A 65-year-old man with an acute stroke and carotid thrombosis unilateral to the site of insonation.

Interpretation: The tracing (Figure 5.18) displays a loud bi-directional bruit with a turbulent high-velocity signal with a stenotic origin. Minimal aliasing is present. The envelope above baseline indicates weak peak systolic tracings that lead to underestimation of the velocity increase.

Similar waveforms can be found at a severe stenosis with turbulent flow when a sample volume was positioned slightly off the vessel segment that has the highest velocity jet. Remember that the highest velocity jet can usually be found at the maximum narrowing or exit of a focal stenosis. By itself, this waveform is already diagnostic, showing that some flow velocities were lost to turbulence and the peak velocity values may be decreasing as disease progresses towards near occlusion. Velocities taken from such waveforms usually underestimate the highest velocity and this may affect grading of the severity of a lesion.

Case history: A 76-year-old man with a recent TIA.

Interpretation: The tracing (Figure 5.19) displays a turbulent signal of variable intensity with bi-directional bruits. This waveform can be found in a post-stenotic segment. The peak systolic complex is not clearly visualized since a laminar flow profile is not re-established yet.

This waveform, which contains bruits of variable intensity and incomplete spectral velocity tracing, should alert the

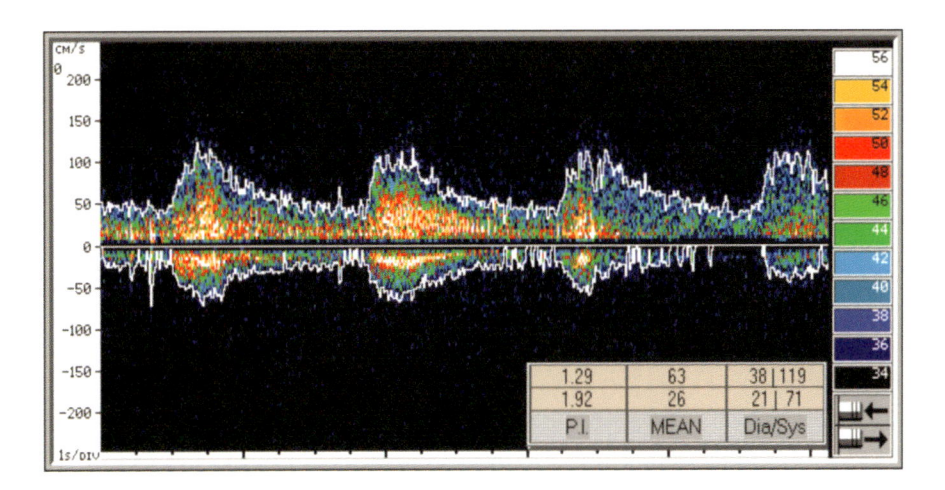

Figure 5.19 Continuous bruit and delayed systolic flow acceleration.

PART II Hemodynamic Principles

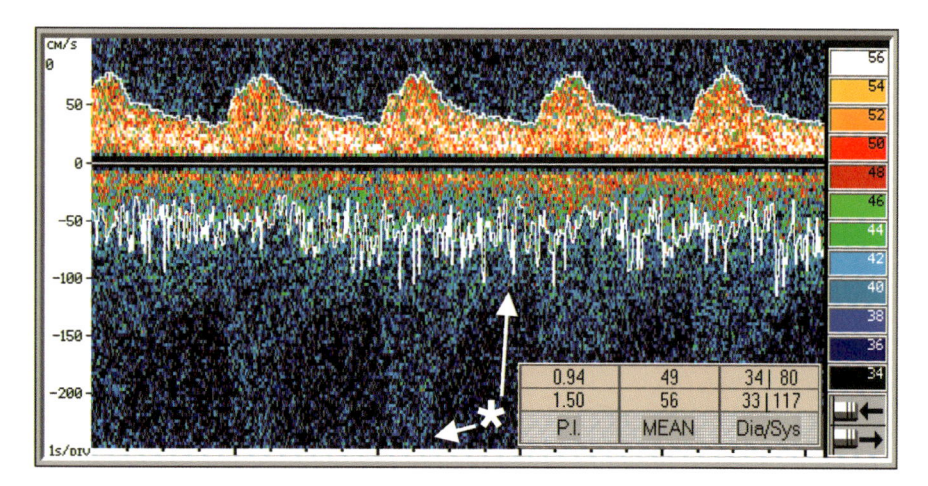

Figure 5.20 A weak signal.

sonographer to expand the search for the highest velocity jet and to suspect a sub-total stenosis with bruits of prolonged duration.

Case history: A 71-year-old woman with an ACA territory stroke and a proximal moderate carotid stenosis.

Interpretation: The tracing (Figure 5.20) shows a bi-directional signal with a low-resistance waveform above baseline that is optimized and has a slightly delayed systolic upstroke. A high velocity weak signal below baseline (marked as *) is not optimized since over-gaining does not change the signal-to-noise ratio and measurements are erroneous.

This recording shows a weak signal suspicious of a focal velocity increase in a branching vessel (below baseline). If a stenosis is located deep in the intracranial vasculature (i.e. depths of insonation 65 mm or more), sound attenuation and limited pulse repetition frequency may preclude its definition and measurement. Increasing gain may help to visualize the waveform but may be insufficient (as in this case) for automated tracings since the signal-to-noise ratio in a weak stenotic signal is low and makes the flow signal indistinguishable. Reducing the sample volume to focus on this specific signal may also reduce the sensitivity of Doppler if burst power is reduced. If waveforms presented in this case are detected, use manual measurements to quantify the velocity increase. The use of power M-mode-guided TCD spectral assessment may lead to the sites of disturbed signals [30] and the use of contrast-enhanced ultrasound agents [31] may help to avoid this technical problem.

Case history: A 75-year-old man with an M2 MCA occlusion and ICA occlusion.

Interpretation: A low-resistance waveform above baseline (Figure 5.21) has a short systolic upstroke and flattened systolic complex. Comparison with a non-affected vessel will help to determine if this is a blunted or damped signal (see TIBI flow grading criteria in Chapters 6 and 15). A high-resistance minimal signal below the baseline has no end-diastolic flow.

This recording shows a complex signal that can be obtained in the intracranial vessels at the site of or just proximal to an arterial occlusion, affecting, for example, the M1 MCA bifurcation. An arterial occlusion can produce a

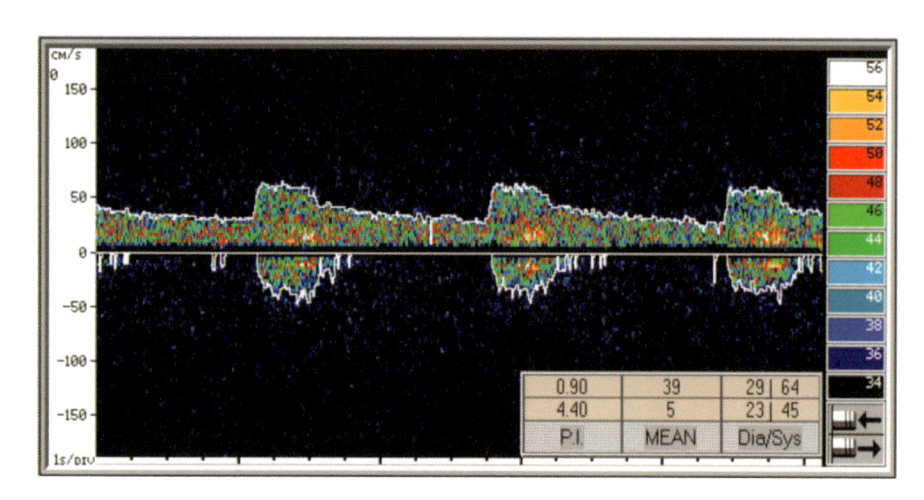

Figure 5.21 A branch occlusion.

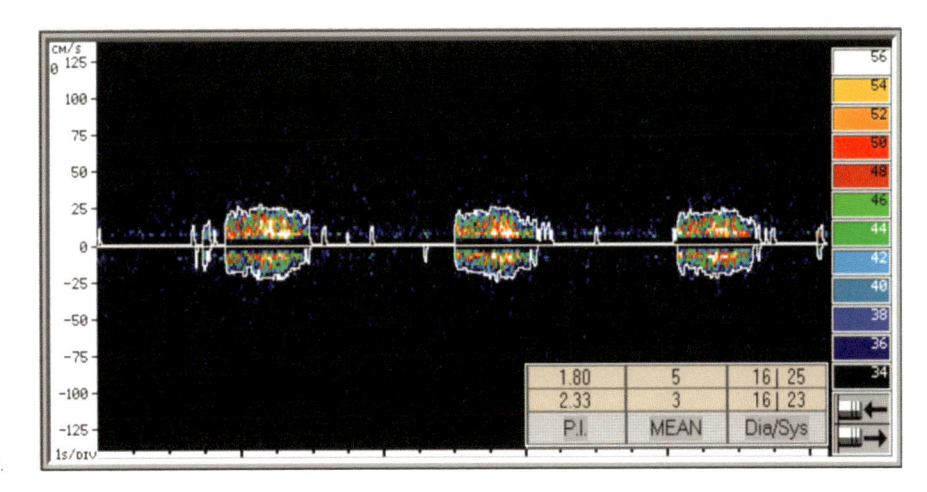

CHAPTER 5 Practical Models of Cerebral Hemodynamics and Waveform Recognition

Figure 5.22 A minimal signal (systolic spike).

variety of residual flow signals [18]. These waveforms can be recognized by abnormal appearances of the systolic complex and end-diastolic flow compared with the unaffected side, including absent end-diastolic flow. Nevertheless, changes in flow pulsatility and velocity are often accompanied by signs of flow diversion or compensatory velocity increase and these findings point to hemodynamic significance of suspected arterial obstruction and potentially the presence of tandem lesions, i.e. MCA and ICA.

Case history: A 62 year old woman with an M1 MCA occlusion.

Interpretation: The tracing (Figure 5.22) shows a minimal bi-directional signal with no end-diastolic flow. This waveform can be representative of a residual flow signal around the MCA thrombus if corroborated by additional findings indicating occlusion at this location. For example, some positive diastolic flow can be found just proximal to this minimal signal and MFV ACA > MCA can be found at 60–65 mm, indicating flow diversion to unilateral ACA. Bruits and vessel intercept at nearly a 90° angle should be considered as a possible "technical error" explanation for the finding of a minimal flow signal by itself.

This recording shows a systolic spike (or a minimal residual flow signal) obtained at the site of an acute MCA occlusion. In this case, systolic spikes with low velocities and bruit-like appearance are seen followed by periods with no diastolic flow, indicating very high resistance to flow and abolishment of brain perfusion at least during diastole. Generally, flow signals obtained at nearly a 90° angle have some recognizable waveform components and the waveforms extending into diastole can be slightly improved by re-angulation of a transducer.

Circulatory arrest

Case history: A 41-year-old woman with TBI and clinical progression to brain death.

Interpretation: The bi-directional waveform (Figure 5.23) represents an extremely high resistance to flow caused by increased ICP. Marked as 1, flow signals above baseline represent sharp spikes with abrupt flow deceleration to zero at the time of closure of the aortic valve and no positive end diastolic flow. Marked as 2, the same blood pool reverses its direction during entire diastole producing the sign of flow reverberation or oscillation.

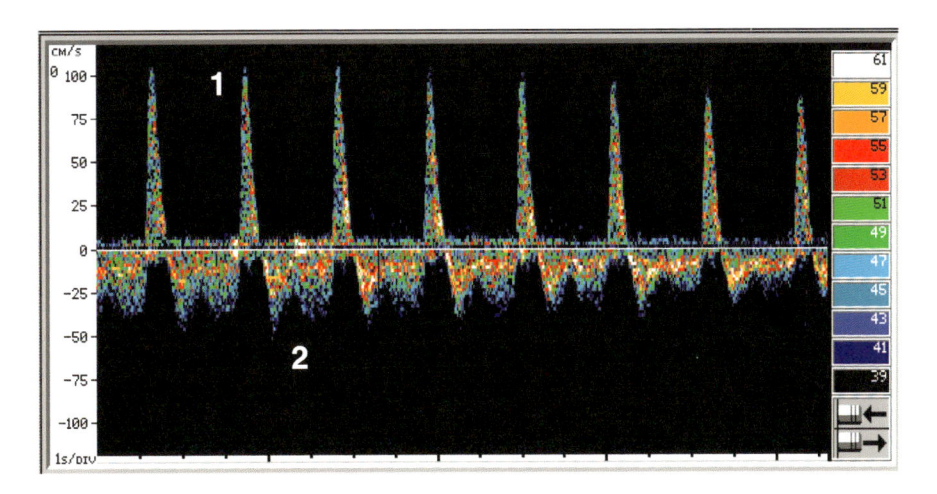

Figure 5.23 An oscillating or reverberating flow signal.

In this case, an extremely high resistance to flow precludes brain perfusion [32–34]. This waveform was observed in a patient who developed massive brain swelling with progression into cerebral circulatory arrest. If reverberating flow is found in both proximal MCAs and the basilar artery, it predicts the absence of brain perfusion that can be demonstrated by nuclear cerebral blood flow studies. Hemodynamically, this waveform indicates that all blood that passed through the sample volume towards the brain in systole was pushed out of the distal vasculature in diastole, resulting in no flow passage to brain parenchyma.

References

1. von Reutern GM, Budingen HJ. *Ultrasound Diagnosis of Cerebrovascular Disease*. Stuttgart: Georg Thieme, 1993.
2. Liepsch D. Principles and models of hemodynamics. In: Hennerici M, Mearis S, eds. *Cerebrovascular Ultrasound: Theory, Practice and Future Developments*. Cambridge: Cambridge University Press, 2001: 27–8.
3. Spencer MP, Reid JM. Quantitation of carotid stenosis with continuous wave Doppler ultrasound. *Stroke* 1979;**10**:326–30.
4. Alexandrov AV. The Spencer's curve: clinical implications of a classic hemodynamic model. *J Neuroimaging* 2007;**17**:6–10.
5. Giller CA, Bowman G, Dyer H, et al. Cerebral arterial diameters during changes in blood pressure and carbon dioxide during craniotomy. *Neurosurgery* 1993;**32**:737–42.
6. Kontos HA. Validity of cerebral arterial blood flow calculations from velocity measurements. *Stroke* 1989;**20**:1–3.
7. Newell DW, Aaslid R, Lam A, et al. Comparison of flow and velocity during dynamic autoregulation in humans. *Stroke* 1994;**25**:793–7.
8. Hoffman JIE, Spaan JAE. Pressure–flow relations in the coronary circulation. *Physiol Rev* 1990;**70**:331–89.
9. Early CB, Dewey RC, et al. Dynamic pressure-flow relationships of brain blood flow in the monkey. *J Neurosurg* 1974;**41**:590–6.
10. Aaslid R. Hemodynamics of cerebrovascular spasm. *Acta Neurochir (Suppl)* 1999;**72**:47–57.
11. Markus HS, Harrison MJ. Estimation of cerebrovascular reactivity using transcranial Doppler, including the use of breath-holding as the vasodialtory stimulus. *Stroke* 1992;**23**:668–73.
12. Silvestrini M, Vernieri F, Pasqualetti P, et al. Impaired cerebral vasoreactivity and risk of stroke in patients with asymptomatic carotid stenosis. *JAMA* 2000;**283**:2122–7.
13. Vernieri F, Pasqualetti P, Matteis M, et al. Effect of collateral blood flow and cerebral vasomotor reactivity on the outcome of carotid artery occlusion. *Stroke* 2001;**32**:1552–8.
14. Alexandrov AV, Sharma VK, Lao AY, et al. Reversed Robin Hood syndrome in acute ischemic stroke patients. *Stroke* 2007;**38**:3045–8.
15. Alexandrov AV, Ngyuen TH, Rubiera M, et al. Prevalence and risk factors associated with reversed Robin Hood syndrome in acute ischemic stroke. *Stroke* 2009;**40**:2738–42.
16. Guyton AC. *Textbook of Medical Physiology*, 7th edn. Philadelphia, PA: W.B. Saunders, 1986: 230–43.
17. Ringelstein EB, Weiller C, Weckesser M, et al. Cerebral vasomotor reactivity is significantly reduced in low-flow as compared to thrombo-embolic infarctions: the key role of the circle of Willis. *J Neurol Sci* 1994;**121**:103–9.
18. Demchuk AM, Burgin WS, Christou I, et al. Thrombolysis in brain ischemia (TIBI): transcranial Doppler flow grades predict clinical severity, early recovery and mortality in patients treated with tissue plasminogen activator. *Stroke* 2001;**32**:89–93.
19. von Reutern GM, Budingen HJ. *Ultrasound Diagnosis of Cerebrovascular Disease*. Stuttgart: Georg Thieme, 1993: 56–62.
20. Alexandrov AV, Sloan MA, Wong LKS, et al. Practice standards for transcranial Doppler (TCD) ultrasound. Part I. Test performance. *J Neuroimaging* 2007;**17**:11–8.
21. von Reutern GM, Budingen HJ. *Ultrasound Diagnosis of Cerebrovascular Disease*. Stuttgart: Georg Thieme, 1993: 52–63.
22. Kidwell CS, el-Saden S, Livshits Z, et al. Transcranial Doppler indicies as a measure of diffuse small-vessel disease. *J Neuroimaging* 2001;**11**:229–35.
23. Harders A. *Neurosurgical Applications of Transcranial Doppler Sonography*. Vienna: Springer, 1986:117.
24. Giller CA, Mathews D, Purdy P, et al. The transcranial Doppler appearance of acute carotid occlusion. *Ann Neurol* 1992;**31**:101–3.
25. Edelman SK. *Understanding Ultrasound Physics*, 2nd edn. The Woodlands, TX: ESP, 1997;135.
26. Felberg RA, Christou I, Demchuk AM, et al. Screening for intracranial stenosis with transcranial Doppler: the accuracy of mean flow velocity thresholds. *J Neuroimaging* 2002;**12**:9–14.
27. Sharma VK, Tsivgoulis G, Lao AY, et al. Noninvasive detection of diffuse intracranial disease. *Stroke* 2007;**38**:3175–85.
28. Ratanakorn D, Kremkau FM, Myers LG, et al. Mirror-image artifact can affect trasncranial Doppler interpretation. *J Neuroimaging* 1998;**8**:175–7.
29. Lindegaard KF, Nornes H, Bakke SJ, et al. Cerebral vasospasm diagnosis by means of angiography and blood velocity measurements. *Acta Neurochir (Wien)* 1989;**100**(1–2):12–24.
30. Moehring MA, Spencer MP. Power M-mode Doppler (PMD) for observing cerebral blood flow and tracking emboli. *Ultrasound Med Biol* 2002;**28**:49–57.
31. Ries F, Honisch C, Lambertz M, et al. A transpulmonary contrast medium enhances the transcranial Doppler signal in humans. *Stroke* 1993;**24**:1903–9.
32. Ropper AH, Kehne SM, Wechsler L. Transcranial Doppler in brain death. *Neurology* 1987;**37**:1733–5.
33. Petty GW, Mohr JP, Pedley TA, et al. The role of transcranial Doppler in confirming brain death: sensitivity, specificity and suggestions for performance and interpretation. *Neurology* 1990;**40**:300–3.
34. Ducrorq X, Hassler W, Moritake K, et al. Consensus opinion on diagnosis of cerebral circulatory arrest using Doppler-sonography. Task Force Group on Cerebral Death of the Neurosonology Research Group of the World Federation of Neurology. *J Neurol Sci* 1998;**159**:145–50.

III Criteria for Interpretation

6 Diagnostic Criteria for Cerebrovascular Ultrasound

Georgios Tsivgoulis[1], Marsha M. Neumyer[2] & Andrei V. Alexandrov[3]
[1]University of Alabama Hospital, Birmingham, AL, USA and Democritus University of Thrace, Alexandroupolis, Greece
[2]Vascular Diagnostic Educational Services, Harrisburg, PA, USA
[3]University of Alabama Hospital, Birmingham, AL, USA

Introduction

Laboratory accreditation, such as offered by the Intersocietal Commission for the Accreditation of Vascular Laboratories (ICAVL, www.icavl.org), requires documentation and consistent application of the diagnostic criteria for interpretation of cerebrovascular studies [1]. The diagnostic criteria in this chapter represent those currently used by the University of Alabama at Birmingham Neurovascular Ultrasound Laboratory based on a summary of previously published criteria for extra- and intracranial ultrasound and those developed at the STAT Neurosonology Service, UT-Stroke Treatment Team and the Vascular Laboratory, PennState University College of Medicine, Milton S. Hershey Medical Center. These criteria can be used as a template to establish and accredit a vascular laboratory; however, any ultrasound laboratory should perform local validation of the accepted criteria [1]. We also review pertinent correlative imaging tests and their clinical applicability.

The required *diagnostic criteria for cerebrovascular ultrasound* include [1, 2]:
1 normal extra- and intracranial findings
2 carotid stenosis and plaque formation
3 carotid occlusion and dissection
4 vertebral artery stenosis or occlusion
5 intracranial arterial stenosis
6 arterial spasm
7 hyperemia
8 collateral flow patterns and flow directions
9 cerebral embolization
10 increased intracranial pressure
11 cerebral circulatory arrest
12 intracranial arterial occlusion
13 subclavian steal syndrome.

Cerebrovascular Ultrasound in Stroke Prevention and Treatment, 2nd edition. Edited by Andrei V. Alexandrov. © 2011 Blackwell Publishing Ltd.

In addition, we added the following criteria due to recent developments in our hemodynamic understanding of ischemic stroke and related conditions:
14 intracranial steal and reversed Robin Hood syndrome
15 grading right-to-left shunts
16 arterial recanalization and re-occlusion.

The last two will be discussed in detail in separate sections that deal with these subjects.

Normal extracranial and intracranial findings

Laminar flow

Under normal conditions, when blood flows a steady rate through a long, smooth vessel, it flows in streamlines, i.e. laminae or layers, with the fastest moving cells flowing in the center of blood stream [3] (Figure 6.1, upper left inset). Cells adjacent to the arterial wall experience inertial pull and shear stresses [4] as they rub against the wall and cells moving in neighboring layers. Endothelial lining and its functions aim to reduce this stress and aid regulation of blood flow. The resulting blood flow velocities will be fairly slow adjacent to the wall and both forward and reverse flow can be seen. This velocity gradient and low-frequency spectrum are detected when the Doppler sample volume is placed near the vessel wall (Figure 6.1, right upper inset). Therefore, a sample volume comparable to or larger than the vessel diameter can display *spectral broadening* in a normal vessel with laminar and undisturbed flow because the velocity gradient through the entire vessel lumen is sampled. For example, all normal transcranial Doppler recordings have spectral broadening since even a small sample volume of <3 mm on a duplex image is comparable with the dimensions of the entire middle cerebral artery stem (Figure 6.2). Therefore, we no longer use the term "spectral broadening" as an independent diagnostic criterion for disease without other direct imaging findings.

PART III Criteria for Interpretation

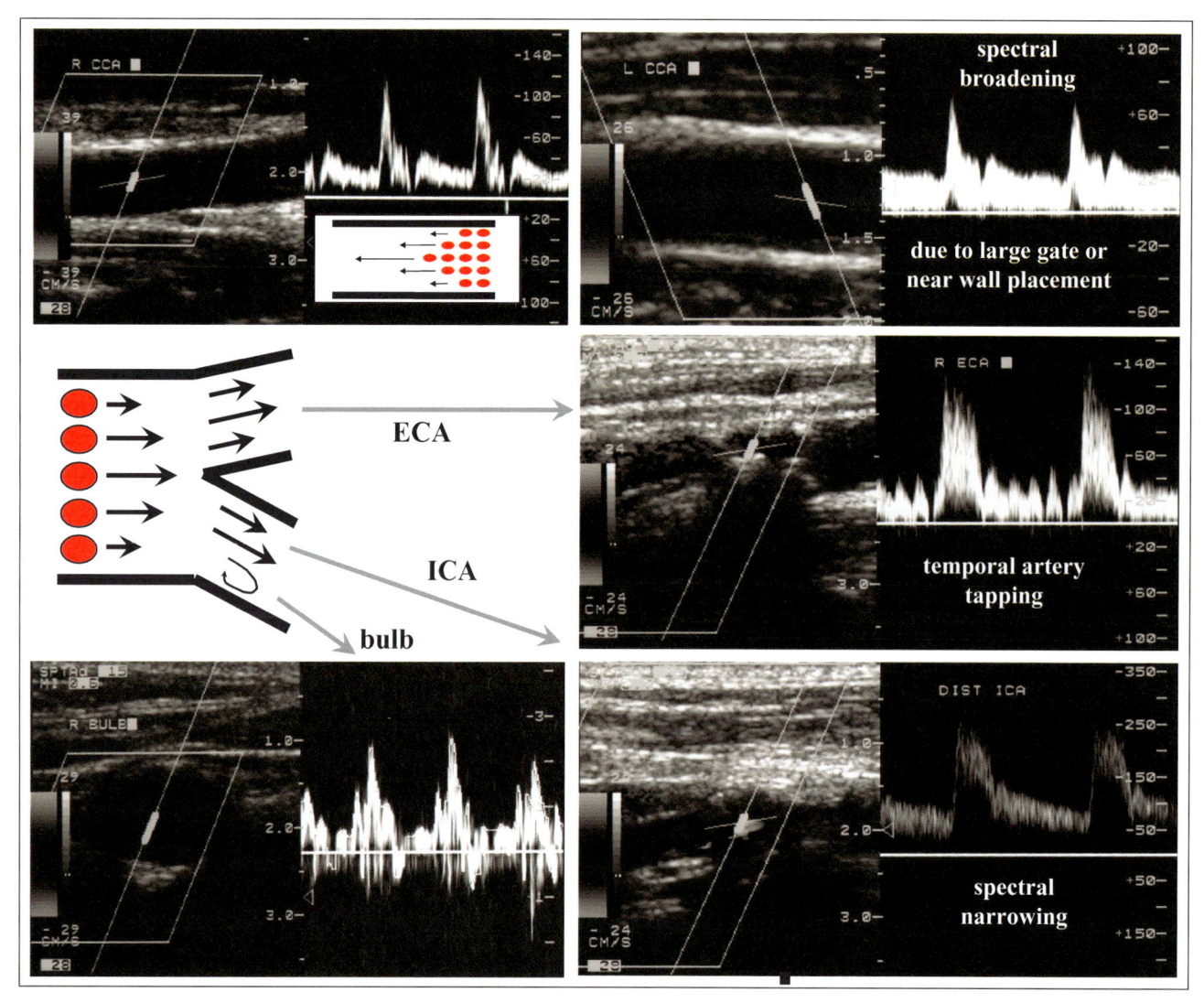

Figure 6.1 Sampling blood flow in the carotid arteries with a duplex scanner. Arrows represent velocity vectors. Faster moving blood is present in the mid-stream of parabolic flow or laminar flow. Spectral broadening is depicted with a larger Doppler gate and near-wall sampling. Spectral narrowing can be seen with a small gate positioned in the middle of the vessel as well at the point of maximum flow acceleration across a severe stenosis.

Arterial wall pulsation

Systolic ejection of blood delivers the highest blood pressure and the arterial wall moves outward during this phase of the cardiac cycle. This expansion of the vessel lumen occurs due to compliance of the vessel wall and the energy stored in the vessel wall determines the so-called compliance flow [5]. During the deceleration phase of systole, the arterial wall moves inwards, forcing the layers closer together. This inward movement and crowding of the cell layers cause the cells to move at a narrow range of velocities in the center stream. During diastole, the resting phase of the cardiac cycle with the lowest blood pressure values, the cells are spinning around, with their movement between layers expressed as a spectrum of low flow velocities. The pressure gradient along the vessel length determines the so-called resistance flow.

Therefore, during outward vessel wall pulsation, the laminae move apart, allowing forward flow to occur with little or no disruption. Thus, arterial flow waveforms represent the sum of resistance and compliance flow [5]. Note the difference in waveforms from the common to the internal and external carotid arteries (Figure 6.1). Accurate depiction of a disturbance of the arterial wall pulsation on a real-time B-mode image may be the first indirect sign of an arterial obstruction.

Normal flow in the CCA

Approximately 80% of the blood flow from the common carotid artery (CCA) will enter the low-resistance vascular circulation of the brain and eye, resulting in 300–400 ml being delivered to the brain via each internal carotid every

CHAPTER 6 Diagnostic Criteria for Cerebrovascular Ultrasound

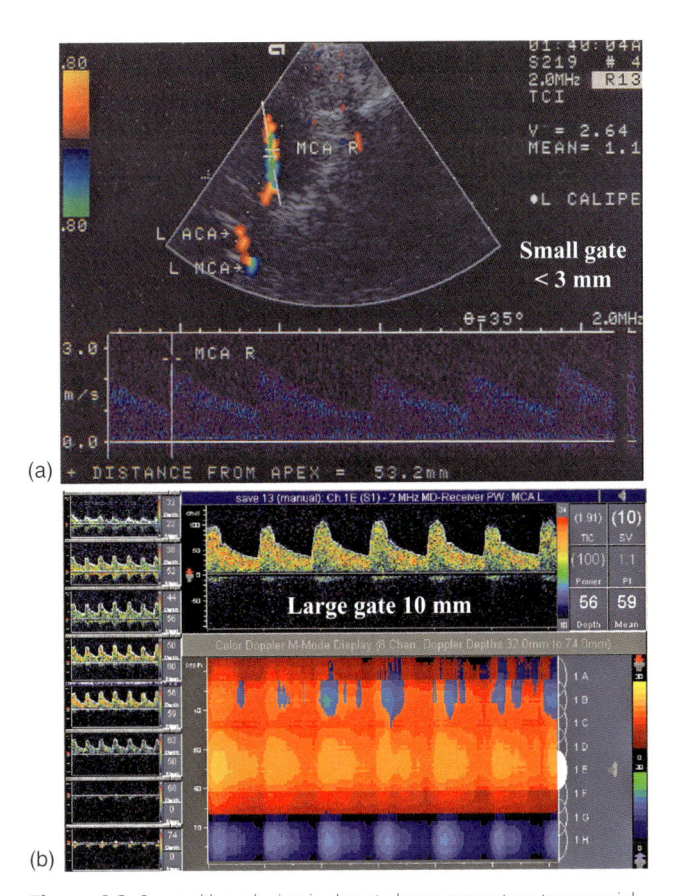

Figure 6.2 Spectral broadening is almost always present on transcranial duplex (a) and transcranial Doppler (b) examinations since the gates of insonation are comparable (duplex) or exceeding (TCD) the dimensions of a proximal intracranial artery.

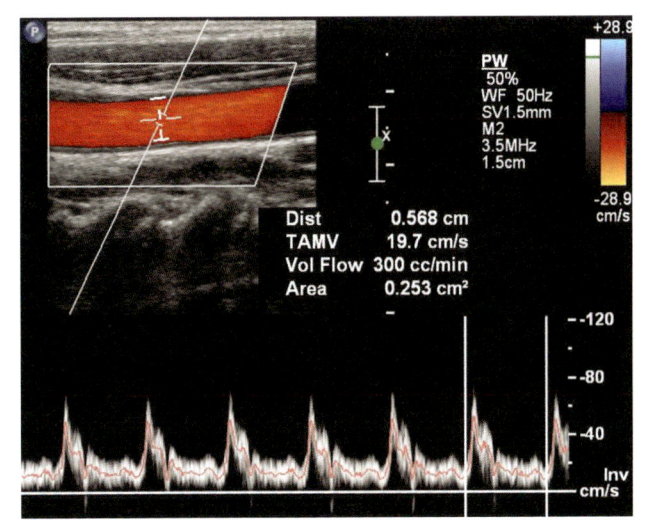

Figure 6.3 Flow volume measurements in a normal CCA are done in a longitudinal plane when a vessel with parallel walls has a consistently measurable diameter to estimate a cross-section area. Flow volume = velocity × cross-sectional area = 300 cm^3 min^{-1} in this normal volunteer.

minute [6] (Figure 6.3). For this reason, the CCA waveform will largely mimic the flow patterns in the ICA, yet it represents a sum of low- and high-resistance waveforms (Figure 6.1). This is evidenced by positive diastolic flow (above the zero baseline) associated with flow to the low-resistance circulation of the internal carotid artery (ICA). Like the external carotid artery (ECA), the common carotid artery will demonstrate the sharp systolic peak, rapid systolic deceleration and relatively low diastolic flow typical of the high-resistance external carotid artery flow pattern (Figure 6.1).

Normal flow in the ICA

Due to cerebral autoregulation and low vascular resistance in the brain, the Doppler spectral waveforms from the ICA show a quasi-steady flow pattern with constant forward diastolic flow, also described as a low-resistance flow pattern (Figure 6.1). There is rapid systolic upstroke, often with a somewhat rounded peak at systole and continuous deceleration during diastolic runoff. If the blood pressure drops, the brain vessels dilate to maintain flow through it low-resistance channels whereas vessels constrict in the body's high-resistance systems to raise the blood pressure in response to its fall. This low-resistance flow pattern in the ICA can be present even with a high-grade carotid stenosis when the end-diastolic velocities are artificially elevated despite an increase in focal resistance across the lesion.

Each ICA carries approximately 40% of the total cerebral blood flow volume [6]. The ICA flow stream adjacent to the flow divider will accelerate faster than ECA and move cephalad throughout the cardiac cycle to meet the demands imposed by cerebral autoregulation. The geometry of the ICA origin, or so-called "bulb," results in retrograde movement of cells towards the opposite wall and oscillatory forward and reverse flow patterns, leading to separation of the flow stream [7] (Figure 6.1). Flow is slower on the wall opposite the flow divider and, therefore, the blood particle resident time may be increased, one of the theories supporting the pathophysiology of atherogenesis on the posterolateral wall of the bulb [8].

Normal flow in the ECA

The external carotid artery feeds the high-resistance vascular bed of the muscles of the face, forehead and scalp. This high resistance is expressed by the classic signature waveform demonstrating rapid systolic upstroke, rapid deceleration, sometimes with a brief flow reversal during aortic valve closure and a low diastolic flow velocity (Figure 6.1). Note that younger individuals may have relatively low-resistance flow signatures in the ECA. The ECA flow waveform changes with rhythmic tapping on the pre-auricular branch of the temporal artery in most individuals [9]. However, we do *not* recommend the routine use of carotid compression to differentiate between the ICA and ECA, or to determine collateral

PART III Criteria for Interpretation

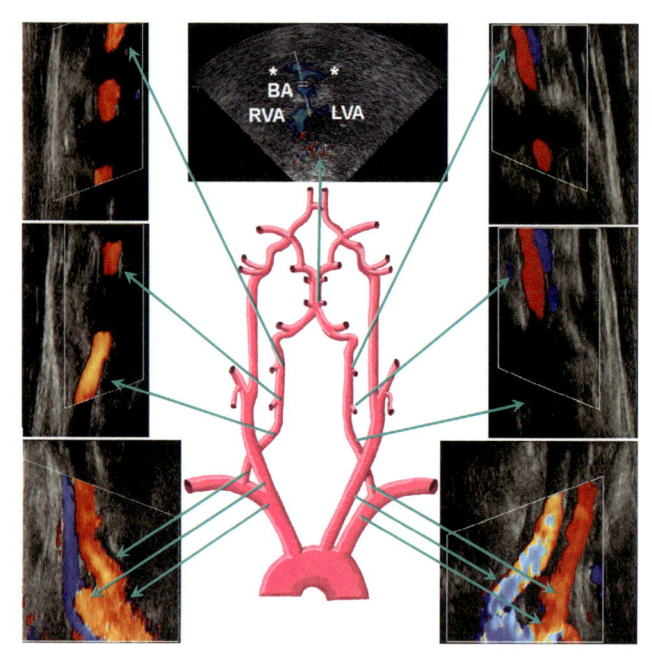

Figure 6.4 Color flow visualization of a normal course of the vertebral arteries at origin, along the neck and intracranially.

channels with intracranial examination. The reasons for this include a small chance of complications and lack of measurable efficacy of compression efforts to produce a complete obstruction of the CCA flow during this maneuver.

Normal flow in the VA

The vertebral artery (VA) supplies a low-resistance system of the brainstem and the vessels of posterior cerebral circulation. Both vertebral arteries deliver approximately 20% of a total cerebral blood flow [6]. VAs can be imaged at their origins (the left VA normally originates from the subclavian artery and the right from the brachio-cephalic trunk) and along their course between transverse processes finally ending in VA junction intracranially to form the basilar artery (Figure 6.4). Similarly to the ICAs, the vertebrals also have a low-resistance waveform profile; however, blood flow velocities in the VA are generally lower than in the anterior circulation vessels [6].

Often, there is a marked difference in flow velocities between the two vertebral arteries that may be attributable to dominance and/or hypoplasia of one of the vessels. An atretic vertebral artery may have a more pulsatile waveform with lower flow velocities. It is important to measure arterial blood pressure on both arms and under normal conditions the difference between arms should not exceed 10 mmHg.

Normal intracranial flow findings

Transcranial Doppler or duplex (Figure 6.2) examination may reveal a broad range of findings including different waveforms in the anterior and posterior circulation vessels, flow pulsatility and velocities. This variety can be attributed to a number of factors including the anatomy of the circle of Willis, side differences in the angle of insonation, velocity modulation with breathing cycles and autoregulatory responses as well as cardiac output and effects of chronic hypertension. Therefore, the absolute velocity values have less significance compared with the abnormal waveform recognition, asymmetry of intracranial findings and interrelationship of flow findings between the vessels. When we perform and interpret transcranial examinations, we first pay attention to:

1 sound
2 waveform (and power motion Doppler flow signature appearance, if available)
3 flow direction and (only then)
4 actual velocity and pulsatility measurements.

Previous studies have established normal ranges for TCD measurements and analyzed the value of different parameters and indices [10–22]. Based on this information, our laboratories adopted the following criteria for *normal transcranial Doppler examination* [2]:

1 Good windows of insonation, all proximal arterial segments found. "Not found" does not mean occluded since atresia of intracranial arterial segments is common in addition to suboptimal windows and angles of insonation.
2 Direction of flow and depths of insonation are as shown in Table 6.1 in adults.
3 The difference between flow velocities in the homologous arteries is less than 30%: 15% is attributable to the difference in angle of insonation and another 15% to breathing cycles. However, posterior cerebral and vertebral arteries may have a 50–100% difference due to dominance, hypoplasia and tortuous course. Similarly, M2 and M1 MCAs may have up to 100% variation in velocity depending on tortuousity.
4 A normal M1 MCA mean flow velocity (MFV) does not exceed 170 cm s^{-1} in children with sickle cell disease and 80 cm s^{-1} in adults free of anemia.
5 A normal velocity ratio: MCA ≥ ACA ≥ Siphon ≥ PCA ≥ BA ≥ VA. Velocity values can be equal between these arterial segments or sometimes exceed by 5–10 cm s^{-1}, i.e. ACA > MCA or BA > ICA, likely due to the angle of insonation or common anatomic variations.
6 Patients free of hypertension while breathing room air have a positive end-diastolic flow velocity (EDV) of approximately 25–50% of the peak systolic (PSV) values and a low resistance pulsatility index of Gosling and King (PI) of 0.6–1.1 in all intracranial arteries. A high-resistance flow pattern (PI ≥ 1.2 is seen in the OAs only (Figure 6.5).
7 High-resistance flows (PI ≥ 1.2) can be found in patent cerebral arteries with aging, chronic hypertension, increased cardiac output and during hyperventilation.

Normal intracranial waveforms were presented in detail in Chapter 4.

Table 6.1 Normal depth, direction and mean flow velocities at assumed zero degree angle of insonation of the arteries of the circle of Willis

Artery	Depth (mm, adults)	Direction	Mean flow velocity (cm s⁻¹) Children[a]	Adults
M2 MCA	30–45	Bidirectional	<170	<80
M1 MCA	45–65	Towards	<170	<80
A1 ACA	62–75	Away	<150	<80
A2 ACA[b]	45–65	Towards	N/A	<80
ICA siphon	60–65	Bidirectional	<130	<70
OA	40–60	Towards	Variable	Variable
PCA	55–70	Bidirectional	<100	<60
BA	80–100+	Away	<100	<60
VA	45–80	Away	<80	<50

[a]Values are given for children with sickle cell anemia.
[b]A2 ACA can be found through the frontal windows with TCCD in select patients [26].

Figure 6.5 illustrates the range of pulsatility index of Golsing and King [23] that can be found in the arteries supplying the brain. PI is calculated as follows:

$$PI = PSV - EDV/MFV$$

Note that wide variations in the velocity and pulsatility of flow can be found under normal and abnormal circulatory conditions.

Besides PI, the resistance to flow can be expressed using the resistance index (RI) described by Pourcellot [24]. This index is calculated as the ratio (PSV − EDV)/PSV with normal values below 0.75. There is controversy as to which index better describes the resistance to flow since PI may be more influenced by cardiac output whereas RI is more reflective of the distal resistance [25]. We prefer to use mostly the pulsatility index since in our laboratories we have validated our criteria for a broad range of PI values.

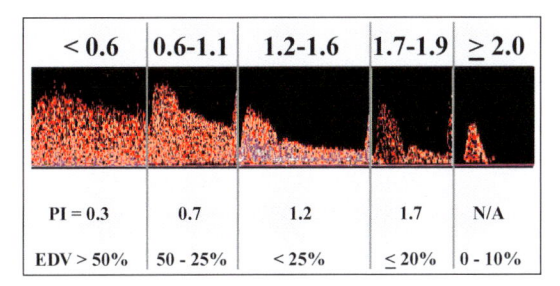

Figure 6.5 The range of pulsatility index (Gosling and King [23]) findings from very low resistance (left-most image) to extremely high (right-most image). PI = (PSV − EDV)/MFV. Normotensive individuals have PIs in the range 0.6–1.1 while breathing room air.

Carotid stenosis and plaque formation

The risk of ischemic stroke increases proportionately to the severity of carotid stenosis (Table 6.2) and randomized carotid endareterectomy (CEA) clinical trials showed that patients with severe carotid stenosis benefit from CEA combined with medical therapy compared to medical therapy alone [27–29].

Since surgery and interventions to prevent stroke such as stenting are not without risks [30], it is extremely important to apply the results of the clinical trials carefully into practice to minimize risks associated with CEA or stenting. These steps include risk factor assessment and application of the specific methods of measuring carotid stenosis in patient selection for surgery (Figure 6.6a). In clinical practice and

Table 6.2 The risk of stroke and the severity of carotid stenosis in symptomatic patients in the NASCET trial [20]

ICA stenosis (%)[a]	Medical group (%)[b]	Surgical group (%)[c]	NNT[d]
70–99	26.1	12.9	8
50–69	22.2	15.7	15
<50	18.7	14.9	26

[a]ICA stenosis is expressed as percentage diameter reduction of the residual lumen on digital subtraction angiography measured by the North American (N) method.
[b]Medical group received antiplatelet therapy to prevent stroke.
[c]Surgical group underwent CEA within 6 months after TIA or minor stroke.
[d]NNT is the number of patients needed to treat to prevent one stroke.

PART III Criteria for Interpretation

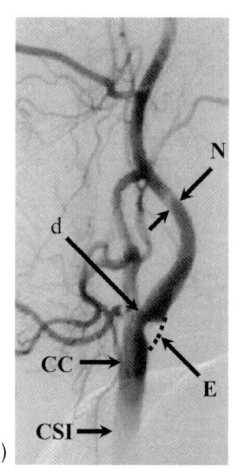

NASCET trial used the "N", or North American, or "distal" method

ECST trial used the "E", or European, or "local" method

CC and CSI are experimental methods that use CCA diameter as denominator

d – diameter of the tightest residual lumen

Stenosis = (1 − d/n) × 100%

Residual lumen S_1 Total vessel S_2

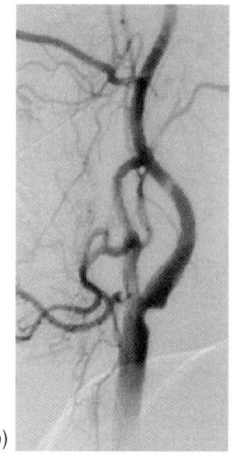

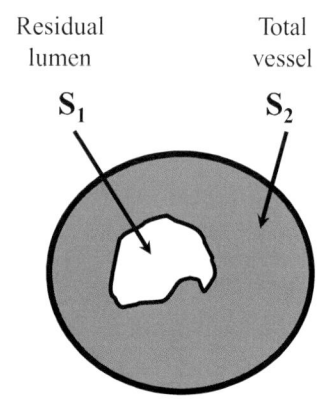

Figure 6.6 Methods of measuring carotid stenosis.

(S_2) are measured (Figure 6.6). The anatomic stenosis is calculated using the following equation:

Stenosis = (1 − S_1/S_2) × 100%

This method was employed in validation studies to assess the accuracy of digital subtraction angiography (DSA) and ultrasound for measuring carotid stenosis [32,33]. Overall, DSA tends to underestimate anatomic stenosis when diameter reduction measurements on angiography are compared with plaque planimetry [32,33].

The advantages of carotid plaque planimetry include accurate assessment of the *area* of anatomic stenosis and direct visualization of plaque surface configuration and its internal structure. To its disadvantage, the method is time consuming and it provides a *post factum* measurement of the stenosis.

Carotid stenosis measured by angiography

Randomized trials [27–29] used DSA as the diagnostic test to measure the degree of carotid stenosis expressed as the percentage *linear diameter* reduction of the vessel determined by strict and specific methods. To apply these methods, only one view of the tightest residual lumen (*d*) should be selected and the measurement sites (*n*) should be chosen differently for each method (Figure 6.6). The stenosis is calculated using the equation

ICA diameter reduction = (1 − d/n) × 100%

where *d* and *n* are the diameter measurements made on a hard copy in millimeters.

The *North American (N) method*, or the *"distal" degree of stenosis*, was used in the Asymptomatic Carotid Atherosclerosis Study (ACAS) and the North American Symptomatic Carotid Endarterectomy Trial (NASCET) trials and refers to the distal ICA as the denominator *n* [34]. The measurement is made using a jeweler's eye-piece and calipers at the segment of the far-distal ICA with parallel walls beyond poststenotic dilatation (Figure 6.6).

The advantages of the N method include its widespread use, the availability of validated diagnostic criteria for ultrasound screening and firm prognostic data regarding the risk of stroke and benefit of CEA [35]. It is now recommended by the National Quality Forum in the US as a mandatory component for reporting carotid angiographic studies. The disadvantages include the underestimation of the degree of carotid stenosis by 15–25% compared with other angiographic methods and area estimates, the inter-observer variability of up to 30% for the values determined for the same angiogram and the distal ICA disease or collapse and its obscuration with ECA branches in 10–20% of consecutive angiograms [35].

laboratory accreditation, angiography is used as a gold standard for evaluation of ultrasound performance and sonographers should be familiar with its methods and pitfalls.

In reality, surgeons may select patients based on carotid duplex results alone and without angiographic control [31]. These ultrasound laboratories have to rely on stenosis assessment by a surgeon who determines the residual lumen size during plaque removal and this information is often submitted for accreditation without standardized methods of measuring percent stenosis. In fact, the true standard for measuring anatomic arterial stenosis is the planimetry of an atherosclerotic plaque removed en block at surgery [32,33] (Figure 6.6b). Although impractical in the clinical setting, this standard is used as a research tool providing the measurement of carotid stenosis and plaque composition.

To perform carotid plaque planimetry [32], the specimen is placed in formalin, which decalcifies the plaque and induces uniform shrinkage by 11–13%. Then the plaque is fixed and sliced into transverse cuts to visualize the plaque internal structure and the residual lumen. The area of the tightest residual lumen (S_1) and the area of the entire lumen

The *European (E) method*, or the *"local" degree of stenosis*, was employed in the European Carotid Surgery Trial (ECST) and requires drawing an imaginary outline of the ICA bulb to estimate the normal dimensions of the vessel at the site of the tightest narrowing [28]. Although there is no objective way to decide where exactly the normal vessel wall is supposed to be on the DSA image, the E method has good reproducibility between the experienced observers and provides stenosis values closer to anatomic stenosis than the N method. For instance, a 70% N stenosis is equal to 84% E stenosis and 90% area stenosis [32]. This is largely due to the fact that ICA bulb diameter estimate is greater than the diameter of the distal ICA in the normal vessel and its segment beyond the stenosis (Figure 6.6).

The advantages of the E method include good reproducibility despite its subjective nature, estimation of the stenosis closer to area values, the widespread use and firm prognostic data regarding the risk of stroke and benefit of CEA [35]. The disadvantages include the subjective nature (guesswork) of the bulb diameter estimation and dependency on the interpreter's experience [35].

The *Common Carotid (C) method* was developed to avoid the subjective nature of the E measurement [36]. The denominator *n* is derived from the disease-free distal CCA diameter, which is usually well opacified and unobscured by arterial branches (Figure 6.6). In case the distal CCA is diseased, the CCA 3–5 cm proximal to the bifurcation may be used [37] to estimate the widest normal ICA bulb diameter (ICA bulb = 1.18 proximal CCA diameter) [38]. Both CCA sites [36,37] offer comparable diameter reduction estimates.

The advantages of the C method are the reliability of the CCA as the measurement site since it is rarely (<3%) affected by atherosclerosis, values close to the E method and area stenosis, the discrepancy between observers is the lowest (<15%) and it is applicable to most consecutive angiograms [35,37]. The disadvantages include infrequent use, fewer prognostic data available [36] and only a few correlations with ultrasound available [39]. Currently, it is not used or recommended for routine angiographic measurements.

These methods of measuring carotid stenosis represent indexes rather than a precise measurement of the disease severity since they are based on the diameter reduction estimates derived from only one angiographic projection. The residual lumen asymmetry is most common with mild-to-moderate carotid stenoses, which together with imaging artifacts and operator-dependency account for most of the discrepancies with other imaging modalities. The agreement between all three angiographic methods can be achieved [36] and the percent stenosis measurements are the closest for the high-grade carotid stenoses [40]. Before magnetic resonance angiography (MRA), contrast-enhanced CT angiography (CTA) and ultrasound can supplant DSA, these imaging modalities have to be compared against DSA [41–44] to ensure that a non-invasive workup allows prediction of the specific DSA stenosis measurements with a clinically acceptable level of accuracy relevant to the equipment and observers employed. It is necessary to perform this self-assessment validation study at each individual institution for MRA and CTA as well as for ultrasound.

Although the same methods of measuring carotid stenosis can be applied to non-invasive angiographic images, tight and tortuous residual lumen, turbulence, slow near-wall and post-stenotic flows can produce artifacts with MRA. MRA overestimates the degree of carotid stenosis compared to DSA when both are measured by the same method [41,42].

The discrepancy increases with moderate-to-mild carotid stenoses and arises from the differences in the residual lumen and turbulent flow visualization. The presence of a flow signal void due to turbulence or slow flow may lead to underestimation of the residual lumen with MRA, thus increasing the ratio with the local or distal denominator. However, a flow "gap" (which appears as a segment of the vessel completely free of signal with reappearance of the signal distally) indicates greater than 60% N stenosis with sensitivity of 91% and specificity of 97% [45]. Further improvement in image resolution is necessary for MRA to achieve the precision comparable to that of DSA in measuring the residual lumen and normal vessel diameters. Despite these shortcomings, the meta-analysis of published series [46] showed that MRA has sensitivities of 0.82–0.86, specificities of 0.89–0.94 and composite receiver–operator curve (ROC) curve areas of 0.91–0.92 similar to that of ultrasound when compared with DSA. MRA offers an advantage of a complete extra- and intracranial examination compared with ultrasound. A combination of carotid ultrasound and MRA is safe and it has sufficient accuracy compared with DSA in patient selection for CEA [47]. Since most outpatients with a history of transient ischemic attack undergo MRI/MRA, a combination of non-invasive screening with ultrasound and MRA appears the most common clinical pathway for patient selection. In laboratories with validated and accurate ultrasound screening, MRA offers minimal additional information for measuring the proximal ICA stenosis [48]. Some physicians reserve the use of DSA only for patients with discrepant ultrasound and MRA results.

The agreement between CTA and DSA in quantifying the degree of carotid stenosis was about 80–95% [49–52]. The limiting factors are plaque calcification, the thickness of tissue slices and imaging artifacts. Interpretation of CTA relies on good quality three-dimensional reconstruction and expertise in reading two-dimensional source images. In addition to MRA and CTA, ultrasound helps to determine the extent and composition of atheromatous plaque and offers a non-invasive real-time tool for patient follow-up. The advantages of both MRA and CTA include non-invasiveness, repeatability and lower costs compared with DSA. The disadvantages include imaging artifacts,

PART III Criteria for Interpretation

inapplicability in selected patients, inter-interpreter variability, overestimation of the carotid stenosis and lack of validation in randomized trials. With these shortcomings, a local validation of the non-invasive angiographic techniques is as desirable as the quality control for ultrasound screening. The caveats in measuring carotid stenosis are known [52] and strict requirements for research study analysis [53,54] and everyday measurement and reporting should be followed.

Carotid stenosis measured by ultrasound

B-mode imaging of carotid plaques

B-mode imaging was applied to evaluate patients with carotid disease to visualize plaque burden directly [55]. Using B-mode, a normal arterial wall can be visualized and early stages of carotid atherosclerosis can be detected, including the intimal–medial thickening (IMT), fatty streak or soft plaques and small non-stenosing plaques (Figure 6.7). Although IMT measurements are not required yet to be part of a carotid duplex report, we comment if a thick (i.e. ≥ 1 mm) IMT complex is seen at a routine examination (for more information, see Chapter 8).

As the plaque grows, it protrudes into the vessel lumen. The percentage diameter reduction of the vessel can be measured in the absence of shadowing and if the near-wall positioning of the sound beam is avoided (remember, "keep the ends of pipe open"). The percentage diameter reduction can be best measured on the longitudinal views and these measurements can be used to decide if a plaque causes less or greater than 50% diameter reduction (Figure 6.8). The longitudinal views have to be compared with cross-sectional views to avoid false-positive results with near-wall beam position and overestimation of plaque protrusion. Validation studies and the impact of B-mode measurements were summarized in a consensus statement [56].

When a plaque is detected, its morphology can be characterized from acoustic properties displayed on a B-mode image [57,58] (Figure 6.7). A *plaque description* in the report should include its:
1 location
2 length
3 composition and
4 surface of the lesion.

Plaque location and *length* are given in the context of the artery or segments affected including the length of the plaque in centimeters. Plaques longer that 2 cm particularly with extensive shadowing may lead to difficulties with grading severity of carotid stenosis since the velocity is inversely proportional to the lesion length. Most importantly, the report should state if the *distal end of the plaque* was clearly visualized. The reason is that the extent of the artery available to B-mode imaging is the part accessible to the surgeon

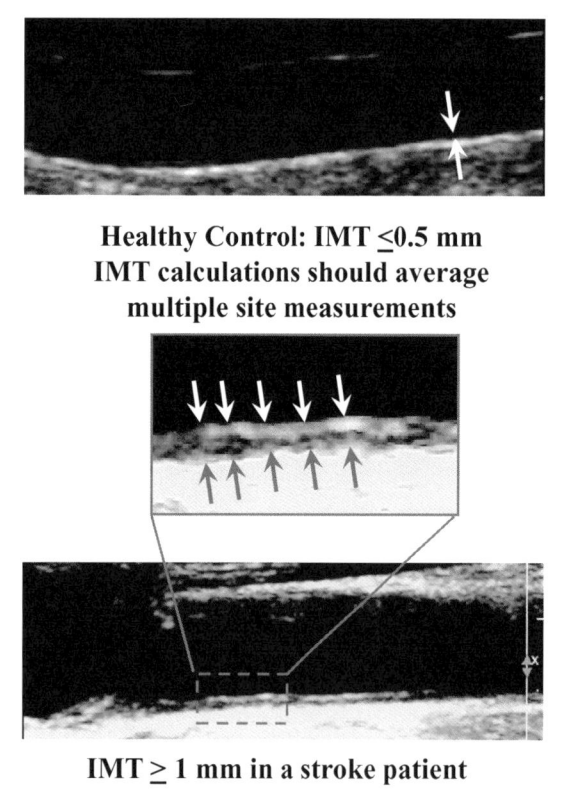

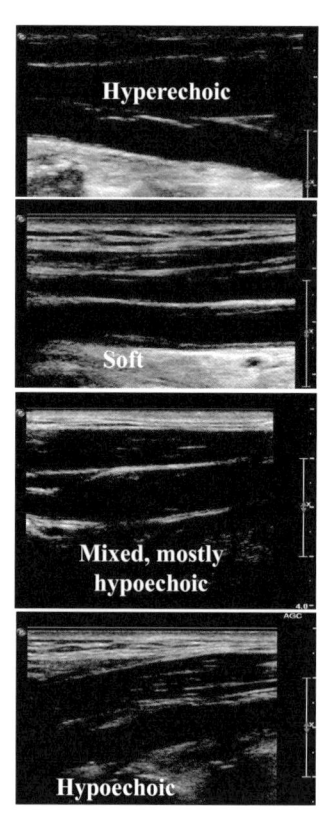

Figure 6.7 Intima-media thickness (IMT) and atheromatous plaques.

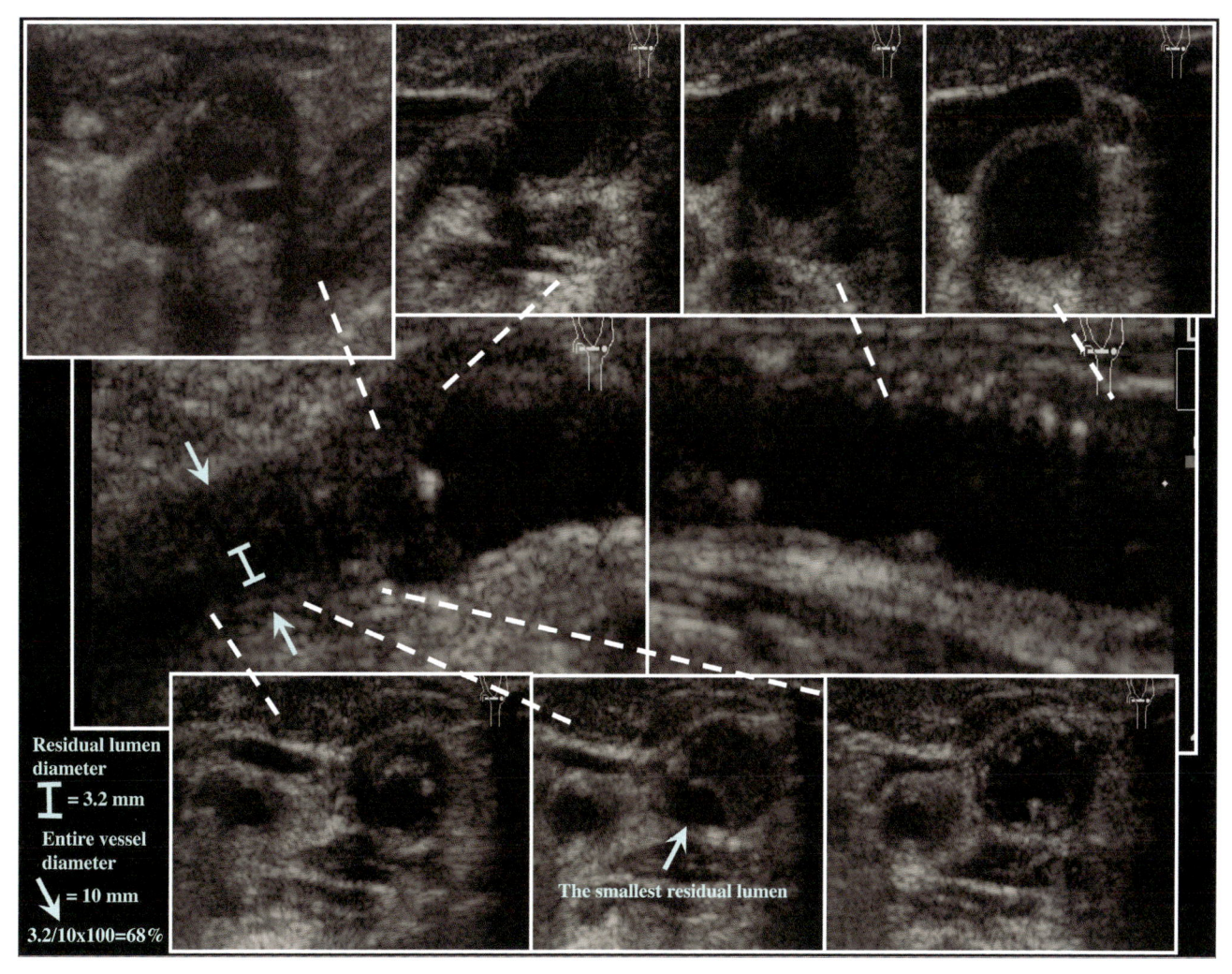

CHAPTER 6 Diagnostic Criteria for Cerebrovascular Ultrasound

Residual lumen diameter
$\mathbf{I}$ = 3.2 mm
Entire vessel diameter
$\downarrow$ = 10 mm
3.2/10x100=68%

The smallest residual lumen

Figure 6.8 Transverse and longitudinal visualization of a complex carotid plaque with a longitudinal diameter reduction measurement.

during endarterectomy. If the distal end is not visualized, the plaque likely extends beyond the jaw level and may be damaged during cross-clamping. This in turn can produce emboli to the brain and incomplete removal since surgical access will be limited by the cross-clamp.

Plaque composition is assessed for its:
1 echogenicity (brightness)
2 texture
3 extent and
4 edges.

Plaque echogenicity can be described using a variety of terms and, recently, computer-assisted techniques were tested to minimize inter-observer discrepancies [59–68]. To ensure consistent grading of plaque echogenicity, the B-mode image should be optimized so that the patent segment of the vessel that contains moving blood should be dark and have no reflections between the vessel walls. Due to B-mode/color trade-off, images should be analyzed first without color flow superimposition. Color flow imaging should be added later as it confirms the presence of the residual lumen and also sometimes helps to outline echolucent structures better. If the echoes are uniform throughout all regions of the plaque, it is considered to be acoustically homogeneous (Figure 6.7). A heterogeneous plaque has mixed areas of brightness and variations in texture (Figure 6.7). B-mode imaging is ideally suited to determine whether or not atherosclerotic plaques are acoustically homogeneous or heterogeneous.

Clearly, *homogeneous* plaques (Figure 6.7) are most likely to be purely cellular in nature with little evidence of becoming complex (when calcifications, significant cholesterol deposition or hemorrhage appear). Homogenous plaques are commonly associated with intimal hyperplasia.

The presence of an acoustically *heterogeneous* plaque, however, signifies that the atherosclerotic process has become complicated. The difficulty remains in determining the correlation between heterogeneous plaques as identified by B-mode ultrasound and their ability subsequently to produce

PART III Criteria for Interpretation

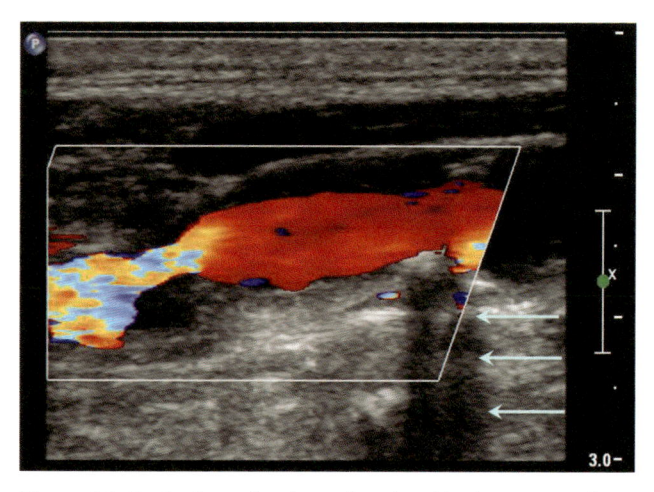

Figure 6.9 Shadowing artifact (arrows) produced by the presence of calcium in an atherosclerotic plaque.

stroke symptoms. A heterogeneous plaque, without acoustic shadowing, most commonly signifies a fibro-fatty lesion. The presence of calcifications usually leads to shadowing (Figure 6.9).

Fisher [68] described *pathological changes* that occur in carotid atherosclerotic plaques as:
1 neovascularity
2 calcification
3 intraplaque hemorrhage
4 ulceration and
5 thrombosis.

Ultrasound assessment of heterogeneous plaque provides evidence for some of these processes. As plaques age and organize, they may acquire calcium deposits that reflect ultrasound and produce acoustic shadowing. This may prevent visualization of the arterial segment lying beneath the shadow. Anechoic or hypoechoic regions within the plaque may represent hemorrhage, lipid deposits or necrotic regions [69] and a hypoechoic plaque may predict higher risk of stroke independently of the degree of carotid stenosis [58,60,62,64]. The higher the degree of carotid stenosis, the more likely the plaque will appear heterogeneous and almost all pathological changes can be present [68].

The *surface* of plaques can be characterized as smooth (Figure 6.7) or irregular (Figure 6.8). Surface irregularity on ultrasound may suggest potential ulceration [70] (Figure 6.10) and thrombogenic surface by exposing the lipid core to blood flow [68]. Characterization of the surface of lesions requires assessment at multiple image angles. It is difficult to visualize the plaque surface of a heterogeneous [71,72] and low echogenic plaque even using the edge-enhancing techniques or gray-scale median [73]. The application of color [74,75] or B-flow or power Doppler [76] may help to delineate the residual lumen, but a trade-off between the color flow and B-mode imaging may preclude precise measurements and may also fail to identify ulcerations [77] that often could be small or thrombosed. Another uncertainty arises when slow flow or flow reversal are seen along the distal edge of a plaque (Figure 6.11). This flow reversal may be seen in a post-stenotic increase in the lumen size and erroneously described as a large ulceration with a crater filled with moving blood. Therefore, there is little correlation between angiographic, ultrasonographic and pathomorphological definitions of plaque ulceration [69,71,78]. Several factors affect this agreement, including definitions and size of ulceration, superimposed thrombi and image projection. Although in certain circumstances B-mode ultrasound may also be useful for identifying areas of loss of endothelial integrity, the highly subjective nature of this observation renders it unsatisfactory for routine use. Future applications include multi-dimensional (≥3D) real-time ultrasound measurements of plaque mobility and flow interfaces [79,80].

The advantages of B-mode grading of the carotid stenosis include the quantification of early atherosclerotic changes, visualization of the plaque structure and extent and the

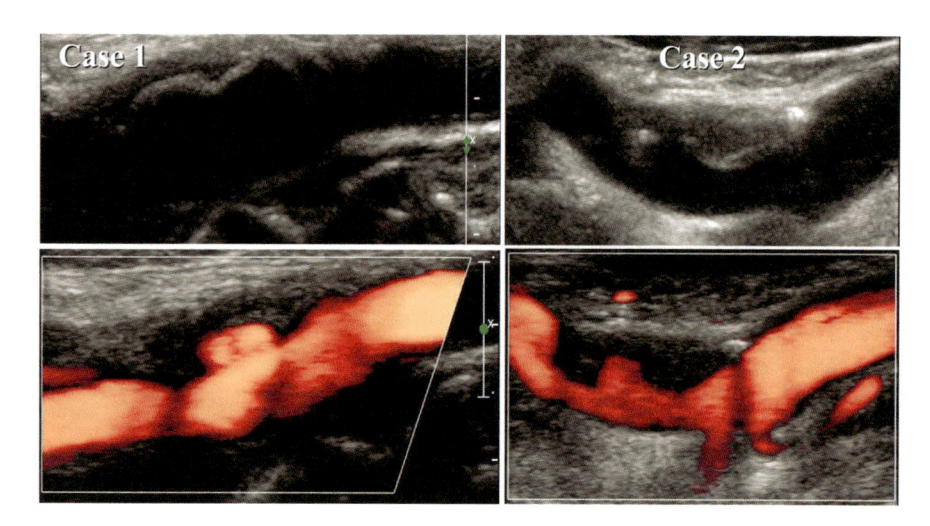

Figure 6.10 Irregular plaque surfaces with probable ulcerations depicted by B-mode and power mode imaging.

CHAPTER 6 Diagnostic Criteria for Cerebrovascular Ultrasound

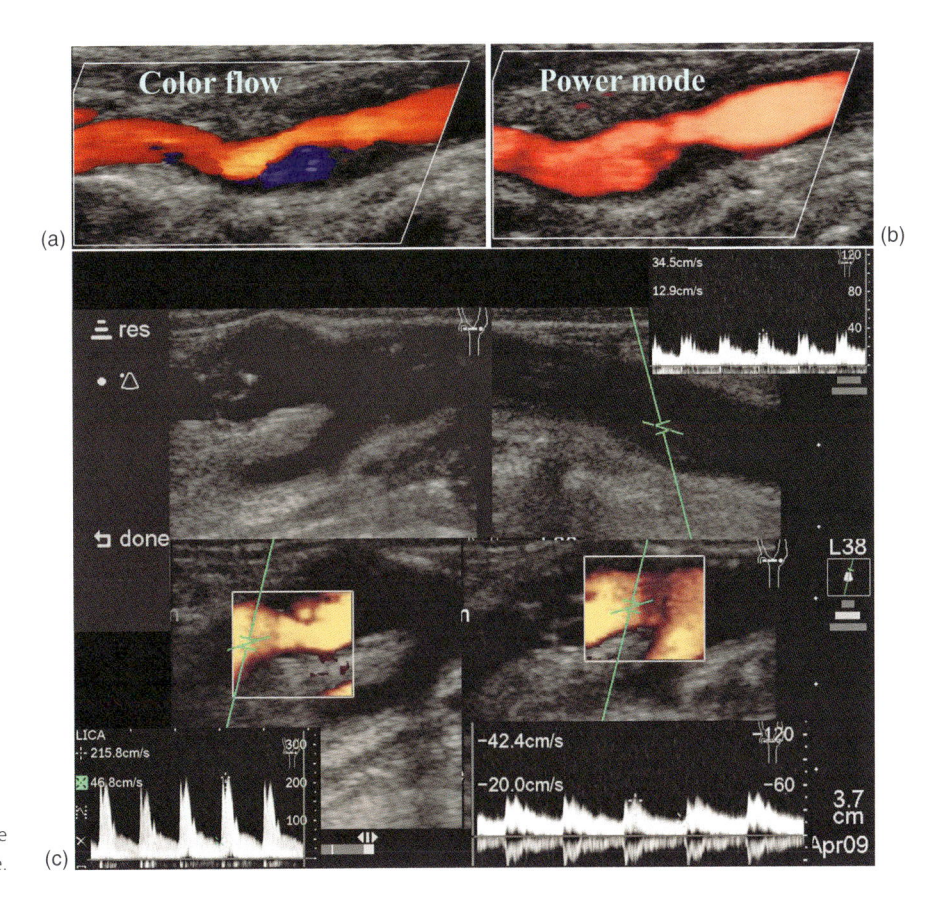

Figure 6.11 Color flow imaging (a) shows the flow direction with rainbow color scale whereas power mode imaging (b) shows the energy of any Doppler shift using a uni-color scale. Images in (c) represent evaluation of the carotid stenosis using power mode as a guide.

possibility of the "on-site" diameter reduction measurements (the site similar to the E method). The disadvantages include common imaging artifacts (inappropriate gain settings, shadowing due to calcium deposition and scattering) and the inability to differentiate fresh clot from moving blood.

Color-coded flow imaging of carotid stenosis

Color Doppler flow imaging (CDFI) can help to identify vascular structures and the residual lumen [81,82]. However, CDFI alone should *not* be used for grading carotid stenosis since it displays the mean frequency shift and is therefore more prone to aliasing with inappropriate velocity scale settings (Figure 6.12) compared with angle-corrected velocimetry. On transverse images, CDFI can also demonstrate the residual lumen and area stenosis [75,83], but precise measurements are difficult due to the same trade-off between the gray-scale and color flow imaging modes, sound scattering at vessel walls and brighter lumen filling during systoli compared with diastoli. Also, the lumen appearance can be greatly altered by gain and scale settings. The dimension of color flow residual lumen changes significantly between systoli and diastoli. CDFI is used to identify vessel abnormalities and the tightest residual lumen and to adjust the Doppler angle for pulse-wave velocimetry [81,84]. Power mode can also be used for the same purposes and may offer an advantage of flow display regardless of its direction and velocity values [85] (Figure 6.11).

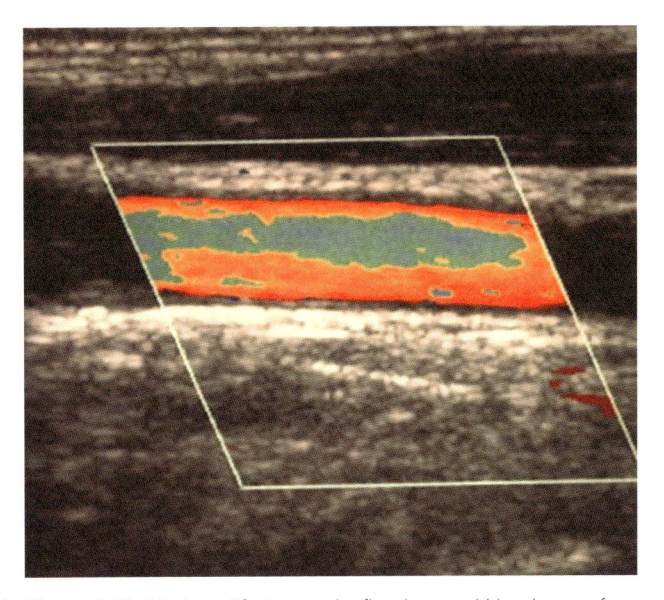

Figure 6.12 Aliasing artifact on a color flow image within a lumen of a normal vessel due to low-velocity scale settings.

PART III Criteria for Interpretation

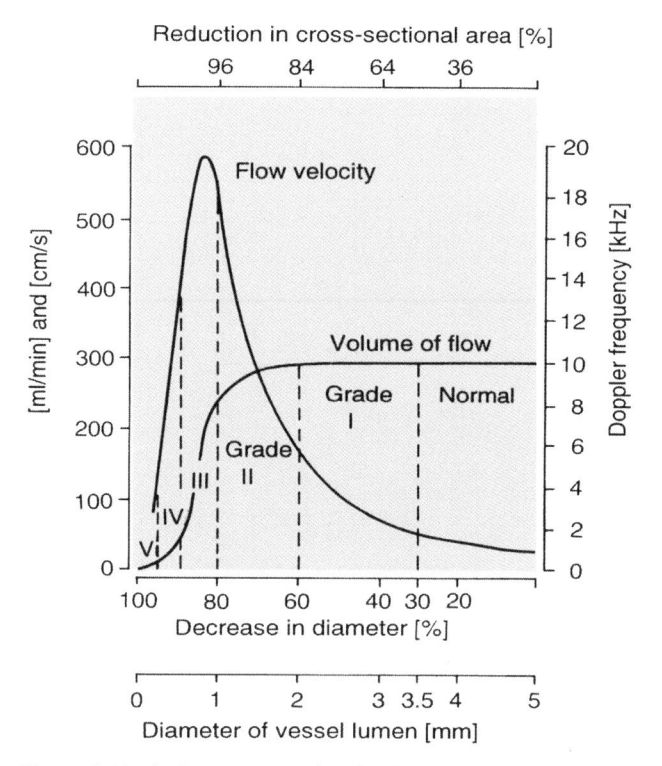

Figure 6.13 The Spencer's curve describes the relationship between flow velocity, flow volume and stenosis severity for an axis symmetric and short arterial lesion.

Angle-corrected Doppler velocimetry of the carotid stenosis

The velocity is inversely proportional to the radius of the residual lumen, stenosis length, blood viscosity and peripheral resistance [86,87]. The peak systolic velocity (PSV) is inversely proportionate to the linear, squared and cubic functions of the residual lumen radius [88], resulting in a complex polynomial curve of the third order which demonstrates this relationship (Figure 6.13). The ICA velocity starts to increase slowly when the carotid atheroma reduces the residual lumen diameter by 15–30% and the area by 30% or more [86–88]. However, only when atheroma results in a 50% diameter reduction of the ICA does the angle-corrected PSV double. In adult patients, it amounts to at least ≥125 cm s^{-1} (or frequency shift ≥4 kHz) [86] (Table 6.3). This frequency/velocity threshold is commonly used in various criteria for grading carotid stenosis and may be modified if collateralization of flow is present [89,90]. Most truly 50% diameter-reducing lesions produce PSV of 150 cm s^{-1} or greater. The consensus criteria also recommend looking for supportive evidence in the ICA/CCA PSV ratio that should be at least 2 for 50% stenosis [56].

Further velocity increase compensates for blood flow volume until it reaches approximately 60–80% diameter or 84–90% area stenosis (Figure 6.13). In addition to the diameter reduction, the axis-asymmetry and length of the stenosis will result in flow volume reduction along the path of the lesion and will determine the hemodynamic significance of the stenosis [86]. Therefore, although uncommon, the flow volume reduction may occur with elongated stenoses of less than 70% (diameter measurements). Decreasing flow volume through a long and resistant lesion is responsible for the secondary and indirect flow changes, such as velocity deceleration, blunting of a post-stenotic waveform and development of collaterals.

The advantages of Doppler velocimetry include the direct physiological measurement of flow acceleration at the stenosis site, its widespread use and the availability of validated diagnostic criteria. The disadvantages include operator dependency (angle of insonation, experience), velocity changes due to cardiac output, bilateral stenoses, flow volume reduction, etc., and equipment dependency (carrier frequency, beam geometry, etc.).

The *peak systolic velocity* (PSV) is mainly a function of the radius of the residual lumen and also length of the stenosis and cardiac output. These Doppler measurements proximal, at the site and distal to a stenotic lesion (Figure 6.14) form the basis of application of PSV and ratio criteria that will be presented below. A variety of circulatory conditions influence the flow volume and velocity in CCA and ICA. In practice, individual variations of PSV and their influence on

Table 6.3 The Society of Radiologists in Ultrasound Multidisciplinary Consensus Criteria for Carotid Stenosis [56]

Stenosis range (%)	ICA PSV (cm s^{-1})	ICA/CCA PSV ratio	ICA EDV (cm s^{-1})	Plaque
Normal	<125	<2.0	<40	None
<50	<125	<2.0	<40	<50% diameter reduction
50–69	125–230	2.0–4.0	40–100	≥ 50% diameter reduction
70–near occlusion	>230	>4.0	>100	≥ 50% diameter reduction
Near occlusion	May be low or undetectable	Variable	Variable	Significant, detectable lumen
Occlusion	Undetectable	Not applicable	Not applicable	Significant, no detectable lumen

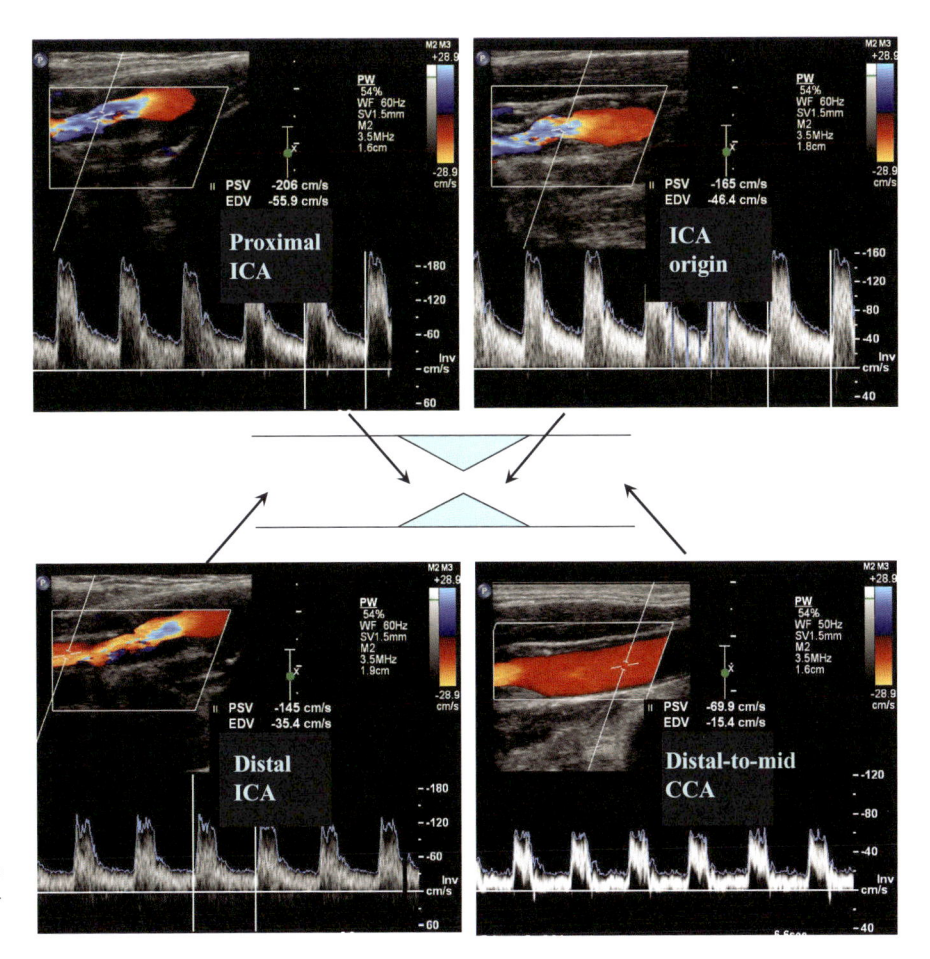

Figure 6.14 Flow velocity measurements proximal to, at and distal to a focal ICA stenosis 50–69% range by the Society of Radiologists in Ultrasound multi-disciplinary consensus criteria. The ICA PSV 205 cm s^{-1}, ICA/CCA ratio of 2.9 and imaging appearance of the lesion indicate that the stenosis is closer to a 50% diameter reduction.

grading carotid stenosis can be reduced if the highest peak systolic velocities in the ICA and CCA are used to calculate the ICA/CCA PSV ratio [91]. The highest PSV, color flow definition of the residual lumen and ICA/CCA ratio along with the B-mode findings form the basis for ultrasound grading of carotid stenosis [56,92–97].

Society of Radiologists in Ultrasound multidisciplinary Consensus Criteria for carotid stenosis measurements with duplex

A multi-disciplinary panel of experts was invited by the Society of Radiologists in Ultrasound to attend a 2002 consensus conference on diagnostic criteria to grade carotid stenosis with duplex ultrasound. The Consensus Panel determined a set of criteria most suitable for grading a focal (short and unilateral) stenosis in the proximal ICA (Table 6.3). It is recommended to use these criteria if a laboratory is new and seeking a set of most applicable criteria for prospective validation. If a laboratory has previously developed a set of their own criteria, validated them and continues to use them successfully in clinical practice, then there is no need to change the diagnostic criteria.

Validation of ultrasound measurements of carotid stenosis

The three validated criteria for greater than 50% N carotid stenosis are [56]:
1 maximum peak systolic velocity (PSV) or Doppler frequency shift
2 ICA/CCA ratio and
3 B-mode measurements of diameter reduction.

These criteria were validated in several studies with good and excellent accuracy parameters [56]. This fact may partly be attributable to a publication bias towards carefully evaluated series and the reported accuracies may not necessarily reflect the performance of these criteria in common practice. Nevertheless, the published validity of these criteria and the experience of many sonographers indicate that an accurate and consistent grading of the carotid stenosis is possible if both the operator and technical aspects of vascular imaging

PART III Criteria for Interpretation

are standardized through a prospectively established protocol and ongoing quality control.

In order *to apply locally any published criteria*, the following information should be available from the source:
1 type of equipment;
2 carrier frequency for Doppler velocimetry, i.e. 4–7 MHz;
3 scanning parameters such as pulse repetition frequency set at the highest value; sample volume of 1.5 mm; high pass filters used to detect slow post-stenotic flow and maximum frequencies in severe stenosis, i.e. 50 and 100 Hz; Doppler angle ≤60°;
4 angiographic method of imaging as gold standard, i.e. DSA, MRA or CTA;
5 measurement method employed, i.e. N, E or C methods; or residual lumen measurements during CEA.

To validate locally any diagnostic criteria, a comparison of the screening test (ultrasound) against the best available gold standard (i.e. DSA) must be made (Table 6.3) and the sensitivity, specificity, positive and negative predictive values should be calculated using the following equations:

$$\text{Sensitivity} = [A/(A+C)] \times 100\%$$

$$\text{Specificity} = [D/(D+B)] \times 100\%$$

$$\text{Positive predictive value} = [A/(A+B)] \times 100\%$$

$$\text{Negative predictive value} = [D/(D+C)] \times 100\%$$

$$\text{Accuracy} = [(A+D)/(A+B+C+D)] \times 100\%$$

where A, B, C and D are given in Table 6.4. As a rule, ultrasound and angiography should be performed closely in time to avoid the influence of the intraplaque hemorrhage, thrombosis or stenosis regression. The interpreters should be "blinded" to the results of another test and ideally a prospective data collection need to be employed.

A more precise validation may require a ROC analysis [93], which examines the trade-off between sensitivity and specificity for certain diagnostic thresholds. For example, a low PSV threshold of 4 kHz will have the best sensitivity of >95% but a poor specificity of <70% to predict >50% N stenosis. A high PSV threshold of >8 kHz for the same degree of stenosis will have moderate sensitivity of approximately 80% but the highest specificity exceeding 95%. Similar correlations are applicable to PSV thresholds expressed in cm s^{-1} [93]. Usually at least 100 observations (two measurements of the left and right carotids per patient) are required for this analysis and, to further avoid biases, measurements that represent mild, moderate and severe carotid stenoses are necessary. In landmark studies [93,94], the PSV and ICA/CCA ratio thresholds were determined for >70% N stenosis and, to translate the final results from the NASCET trial, additional ultrasound criteria for stenoses with >50% diameter reduction compared with the distal ICA should also be employed [56,96]. Note that the 50% N stenosis corresponds to 70–75% E or C stenosis.

Validation of ultrasound criteria for different scanners

This kind of validation study is particularly difficult since different scanners used in the same laboratory have different Doppler carrying frequencies and transducer configurations [98]. The steps to validate criteria for different scanners should include:
1 Identify the reference scanner (usually the most used or previously validated machine).
2 Establish the velocity difference between the scanners (use the same patient and normal controls).
3 Establish a consistent scanning protocol between users and scanners.
4 Prospectively compare several studies obtained on each scanner with angiography.
5 Make adjustments to local diagnostic criteria, if necessary. These validation steps are particularly important in laboratories with multiple sonographers and scanners. Technical supervision by a senior sonographer should provide ongoing quality control of scanning protocols and improvement of scanning techniques of new sonographers.

Since ultrasound results change with different equipment and variable circulatory conditions, diagnostic criteria should encompass prediction of the stenosis range, i.e. 50–69% NASCET stenosis as opposed to a "62.5% stenosis" measurement at ultrasound.

Additional difficulties in grading severity of carotid stenosis arise when a discrepancy is found between standard velocity criteria and B-mode and color flow findings. Note that velocities are a complex function of the entire residual lumen whereas B-mode and color images are at best two-dimensional estimates of the same structure. New imaging techniques allow a three-dimensional reconstruction of structural and flow images and the value of this technology is being tested [79,80]. The diagnostic criteria should also include definitions for hemodynamically significant lesions

Table 6.4 A, B, C and D[a]

Screening test	Diagnostic test	
	Disease +	Disease −
Disease +	A	B
Disease −	C	D

[a]The validity and predictive value of the screening test against the best available gold standard are calculated from true-positive (A), false-positive (B), false-negative (C) and true-negative (D) values (see the text for equations).

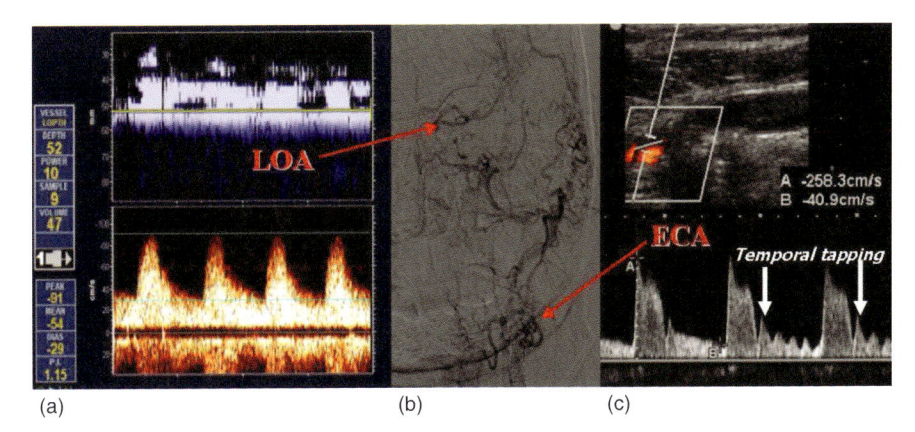

Figure 6.15 A reversed ophthalmic artery on power-motion Doppler (a) and angiography (b). Carotid duplex examination of a proximal external carotid artery shows positive diastolic flow and the waveform response to the temporal artery tapping.

as well as for grading bilateral and tandem lesions. These additional criteria are discussed below.

Hemodynamically significant ICA lesions can be present with or without significant PSV increase. They are termed "significant" since they cause a post-stenotic drop in flow volume equivalent to or greater than 80% diameter stenosis on the Spencer curve (developed for axis-symmetric and focal stenoses). The development of such a significant blood pressure gradient occurs with the lesions "on the other side of the Spencer's curve" (Figure 6.13) and it requires compensation via distal vasodilation and development of collaterals. In human carotid arteries, hemodynamically significant ICA lesions are usually in the 80–99% diameter reduction range by the NASCET method or appear as elongated stenoses of variable diameter reduction, tandem lesions, near-occlusions or occlusions. Note that flow volume starts to drop at 70% narrowing according to the Spencer's curve but it reaches a significant drop at 80% diameter reduction. Often, these lesions can only be discovered using indirect criteria for grading carotid stenosis. The *indirect criteria for hemodynamically significant carotid stenosis* include [99–108]:

1 decreased end-diastolic flow velocity in the CCA and/or ICA in the presence of a distal lesion;
2 color flow findings such as narrow and elongated residual lumen;
3 internalization of the external carotid artery (low-resistance and high-velocity flow in the extracranial ECA) and reversed flow direction in the ophthalmic artery (Figure 6.15);
4 anterior cross-filling via anterior communicating artery (Figure 6.16);
5 posterior communicating artery flow (presented below in the section on Collaterals);
6 increased flow pulsatility in the unilateral CCA;
7 decreased flow pulsatility in the unilateral MCA;
8 abnormal flow acceleration and pulsatility transmission index (unilateral MCA).

These findings can be accompanied by evidence of microembolism, particularly in the acute phase of cerebral ischemia when tandem ICA/MCA lesions and artery-to-artery embolization are common (Figure 6.17).

Criteria 4 and 5 are illustrated in subsequent sections of this chapter while blunting of the MCA waveform was discussed in Chapter 5. These indirect criteria may help to detect severe or hemodynamically significant carotid stenosis when the velocity and gray-scale findings are insufficient for diagnosis.

Post-carotid endarterectomy assessment and carotid stents

B-mode imaging of carotid arteries reconstructed after successful carotid endarterectomy [109] or stenting [110] shows changes in the vessel wall consistent with suture placement or stent material. Particular attention should be paid to inspection of the wall changes at the edges of carotid reconstruction where incomplete plaque removal and residual stenosis can be found. Color flow images demonstrate flow that fills the entire lumen. Angle-corrected velocity measurement may show values above normal through the reconstructed part of the vessel, likely due to flow remodeling [109–111].

Our criteria for *patent stents* (Figure 6.18) include:
1 The stented area shows no deformities and the vessel has parallel walls on transverse and longitudinal planes (when obtainable).
2 No hyperplastic tissue, plaque or intra-luminal thrombus protrusion into the vessel lumen is seen within and at the proximal and distal ends of the stent.
3 Color flow fills the entire stent lumen.
4 The peak systolic velocity throughout the stent area is ≤ 150 cm s^{-1} (other laboratories may have different velocity cut-offs).

Our criteria for *stent deformity* or *re-stenosis* that include some previously published findings [112–113] include:
1 B-mode evidence for $\geq 30\%$ narrowing of the stent/vessel lumen (note that if a calcified plaque is present outside the

PART III Criteria for Interpretation

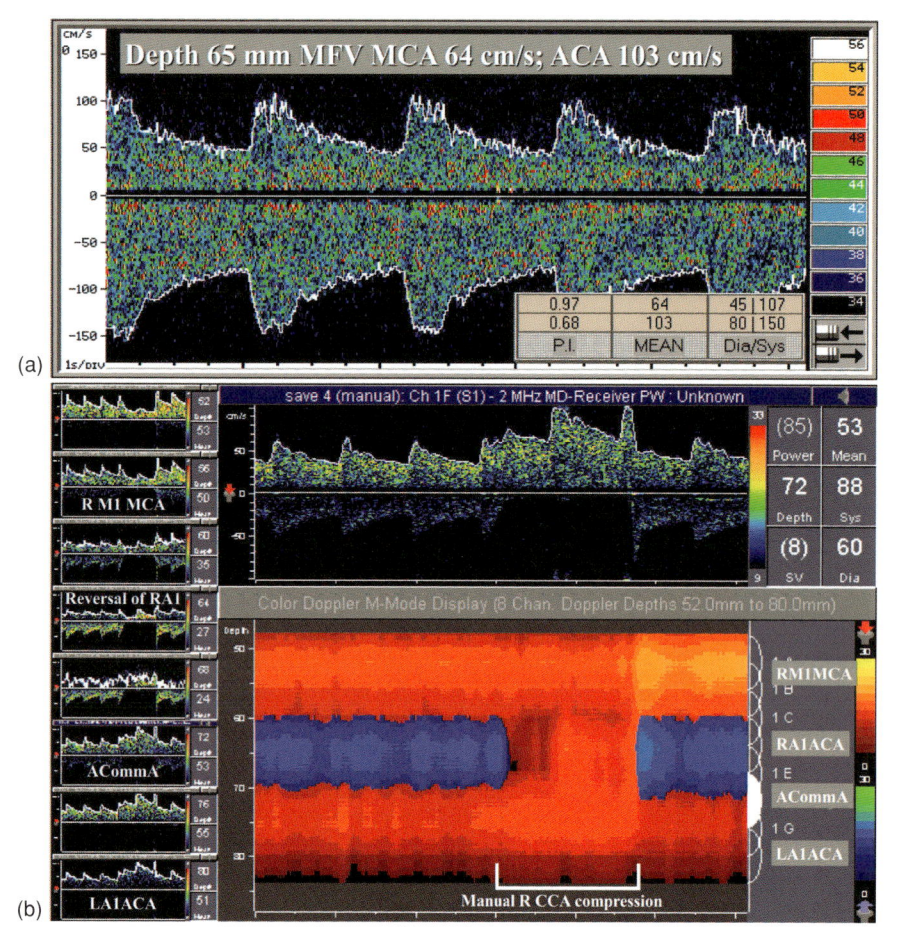

Figure 6.16 Anterior cross-filling via the anterior communicating artery (AComA). TCD examination of the donor side (a) via the temporal window shows MFV ACA > MCA with PIs ACA < MCA due to distal vasodilation that creates an incentive for collateral flow. TCD examination on the recipient side (b) shows the recruitment of AComA and the recipient ACA flow reversal during manual CCA compression.

stent with parallel walls, it may produce shadowing and false impression of vessel narrowing).

2 Focal velocity increase at the point of maximal narrowing >150 cm s^{-1} and pre-stenotic (or pre-stent) to stenotic segment PSV ratio of 1:≥2.

3 Additional evidence of plaque or thrombus formation at the site of stent deformity or at the proximal or distal ends of the stent (note that low velocities and high-resistance waveforms can be found with a subtotal obstruction of the stent). Of note, specific velocity cut-offs have recently been proposed by AbuRahma *et al.* [112,113] for detecting in-stent restenosis of ≥30%, ≥50% and ≥80% as PSVs of 154, 224 and 325 cm s^{-1}, respectively.

Our criteria for *stent or post-surgical thrombosis or occlusion* (Figures 6.18 and 6.19) include:

1 B-mode evidence of hypo- or hyperechoic filling of the reconstructed vessel lumen (A "crescent moon" appearance of an intraluminal thrombus without significant velocity and waveform changes could also be diagnostic and will be discussed in detail in the section **Carotid artery occlusion and dissection**).

2 An abnormal residual flow signal (i.e. stenotic, blunted, minimal or reverberating) is obtained at the longitudinal view of the reconstructed vessel or just proximal to flow void zone.

3 High-resistance pre-reconstructed vessel or CCA signals.

Grading bilateral carotid stenosis

The severity of bilateral disease is difficult to grade due to the compensatory flow increase in one of the carotid arteries or flow volume diversion into posterior circulation. The range of stenosis and relative contribution of compensatory flow should be mentioned for each artery. If both carotids have abnormally high peak systolic velocities, this may lead to overestimation of the stenosis if the velocity criterion is not adjusted to higher values [113] or it is used alone [114]. The following parameters may help to identify the more severely stenosed side:

1 high ICA/CCA ratio on the side of maximum stenosis;

2 low ICA/CCA ratio on the side of compensatory velocity increase;

3 collateralization of flow on TCD from the side with compensatory velocity increase towards the side with maximum narrowing;

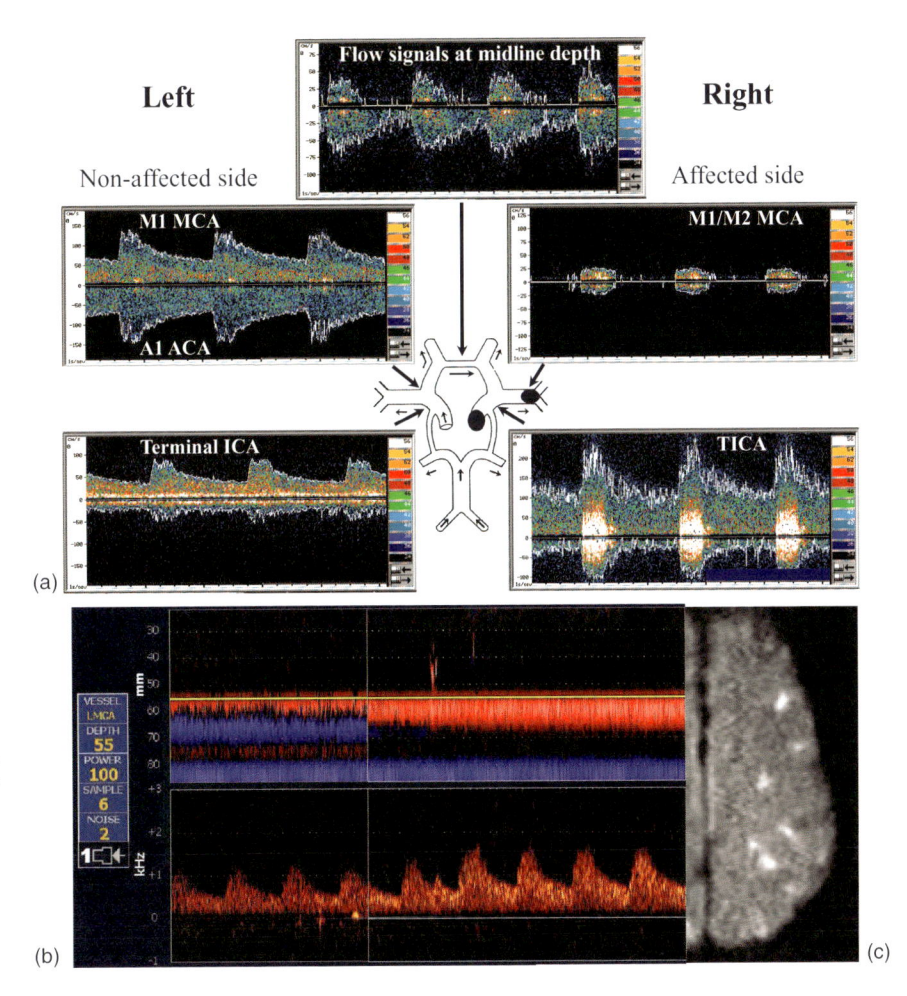

Figure 6.17 A tandem ICA/MCA occlusion in an acute stroke patient with the recruitment of partial anterior cross-filling via AComA (a) and a microembolic signal [(middle of power mode image in (b)) with subsequent flow velocity improvement on spectral Doppler. Image (c) represents diffusion-weighted MRI findings of an artery-to-artery embolic lesions.

4 reversed ophthalmic artery flow on the side of maximum stenosis;

5 abnormal post-stenotic waveforms (blunted waveform, extremely turbulent flow, dampening of flow);

6 ultrasound estimates of flow volume reduction on the side of maximum stenosis.

Tandem carotid lesions

Tandem lesions in the carotid artery can lead to increased risk of peri-operative stroke [115] and distal lesions may change after flow is reconstituted in the proximal ICA [116]. Recent analysis of published series suggested that tandem lesions do not affect hemodynamics as a simple summation of separate degrees of stenosis [117]. Ultrasound diagnosis of tandem lesions should therefore include careful evaluation of carotid duplex results for subtle signs of distal obstruction to flow. This may occur in the CCA if the first or the second lesion or a combination of the two is hemodynamically significant. Often, evaluation of peri-orbital flows and intracranial vasculature using transcranial Doppler is required to demonstrate hemodynamic significance of lesions distal to the field of extracranial duplex [99,101,105,107]. These tests are of particular value when only moderate ICA stenosis is found proximally and more severe distal lesion cannot be studied directly. The report should specify all arterial segments affected with the range of stenosis estimated for each lesion.

Our criteria for *tandem carotid lesions* (Figures 6.17 and 6.20) in an adult patient include [99]:

1 High-grade stenotic ICA PSV or relatively low ICA PSV despite the high grade of lesion severity estimated from color and B-mode findings.

2 Increased flow pulsatility in the CCA.

3 Contralateral ICA or posterior circulation compensatory velocity increase.

4 Stenotic flow signatures and MFV ≥ 100 cm s^{-1} or absent ICA siphon signal through the orbit unilateral to a proximal ICA lesion.

5 Stenotic flow signatures and MFV ≥ 100 cm s^{-1} in the terminal ICA through the transtemporal window.

6 Delayed systolic flow acceleration in the MCA or an abnormal residual flow waveform with or without anterior

PART III Criteria for Interpretation

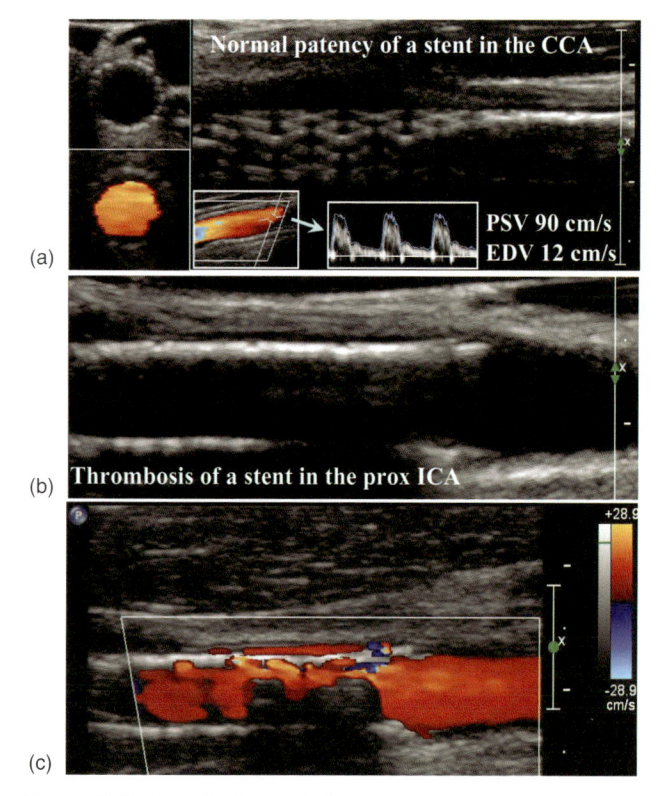

Figure 6.18 Image (a) shows a typical stent appearance on B-mode ultrasound and normal patency on transverse images as well as normal longitudinal assessment of intra-stent flow velocity. Images (b) and (c) show intra-stent thrombus of B-mode and color flow imaging.

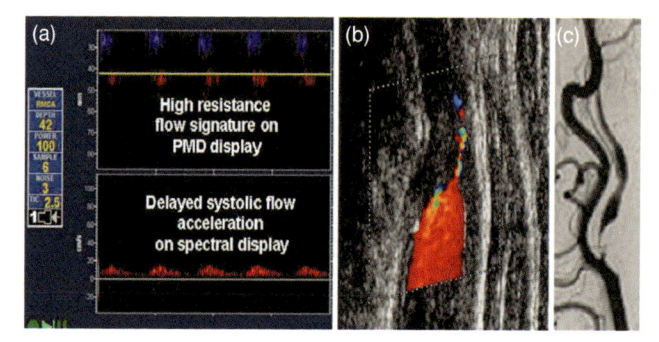

Figure 6.20 A tandem proximal ICA/MCA acute obstruction: (A) power motion Doppler findings of residual flow at the MCA occlusion level; (B) carotid duplex and angiographic findings of a proximal ICA lesion with a string sign appearance of the distal ICA flow.

cross-filling or detectable PComA flow (abnormal residual flow waveforms will be discussed in detail in the section **Carotid artery occlusion and dissection**).

The diagnosis of a hemodynamically significant, bilateral or tandem carotid lesion becomes more certain if more than one of the above-mentioned criteria are found. Sometimes, particularly in younger patients, these flow abnormalities can be very subtle and often the presence of just one abnormal finding raises suspicion. Since grading carotid stenosis with ultrasound is largely driven by velocity measurements, some discrepancy between anatomic degree of a stenosis and velocities can be expected as factors other than lumen diameter can influence the velocity. Furthermore, time delays between correlative tests can account for discrepancies, i.e. rapid progression to a complete occlusion. Therefore, different levels of certainty should be reflected in the report, i.e. possible, probable or definite presence of an ICA lesion and its severity.

The most confusing situation, i.e. a discrepancy between ultrasound and angiographic results, often occurs due to time delays between ultrasound and angiography. In our experience in stroke patients, the closer both tests are performed to the onset of symptoms, the greater is the agreement that can be expected between them. We repeat ultrasound on admission for scheduled surgery, if more than 3 days have elapsed since angiography.

Factors that can lead to *discrepant duplex/angio results* include:

A. *Patient:*
1 arterial occlusion, clot propagation and recanalization
2 intraplaque hemorrhage
3 growth of collaterals.

B. *Technique:*
1 use of different scanners
2 single projection measurements
3 time delays between tests.

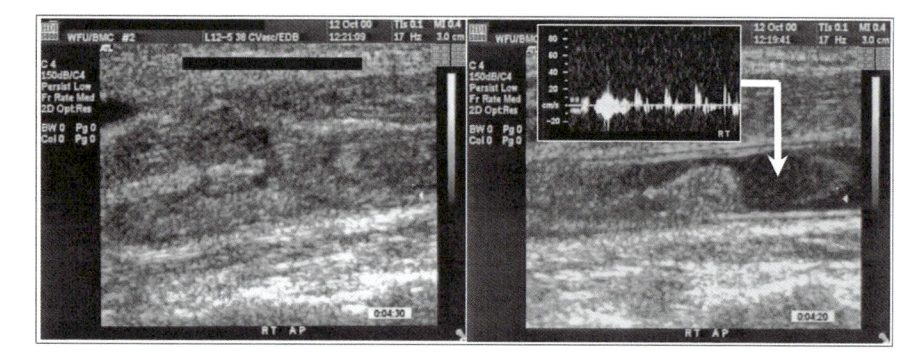

Figure 6.19 Intraluminal thrombosis following carotid endarterectomy. Images courtesy of Drs Disya Ratanakorn and Charles Tegeler.

CHAPTER 6 Diagnostic Criteria for Cerebrovascular Ultrasound

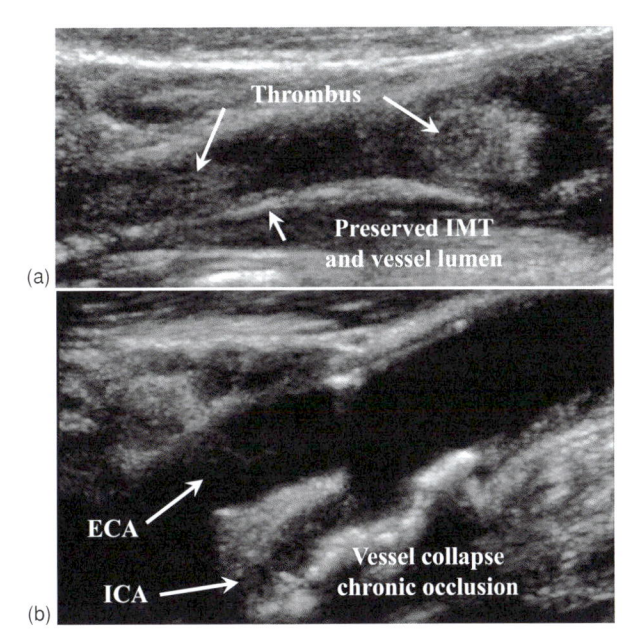

Figure 6.21 An acute (a) versus chronic (b) occlusion on B-mode imaging. ECA was identified by distal branches on color flow imaging and temporal tapping (images not shown). ICA in (b) has a smaller vessel diameter than ECA and its origin contains an atherosclerotic plaque.

C. Operator:
1 inconsistent scanning protocol
2 application of uniform criteria for different scanners without local validation
3 limited angiographic views and insufficient selective vessel studies.

Carotid artery occlusion and dissection

With current technologies, it is difficult to be certain of the diagnosis of a *complete* (particularly acute or "fresh") carotid artery occlusion based on ultrasound findings without invasive angiographic confirmation. In fact, when a patient appears to have complete occlusion at first-ever carotid ultrasound examination, a "benefit of the doubt" should be given by reporting occlusion *or* 99% stenosis. If there is a minimal residual lumen and flow in the distal ICA, this can change patient management, i.e. surgery or stenting may be possible. It is preferable to obtain angiographic confirmation for complete ICA occlusion. The diagnostic accuracy of ultrasound in the differentiation of complete occlusion from subtotal stenosis may be improved with contrast agents and sensitive flow imaging techniques [118–121]. The ultrasound diagnosis can become more certain with repeat assessments by experienced sonographers, optimized velocity scales to depict slow flow states and with the presence of a chronic occlusion with lumen fibrosis.

The following criteria for *carotid artery occlusion* were derived from multiple studies [89,122–135] and our own observations:

1 Absent flow signal in the distal ICA on flow imaging and spectral analysis.
2 High resistance "stump" waveform with absent or reversed end-diastolic flow just proximal to the flow void area or structural lesion in the ICA (Figures 6.19 and 6.20).
3 Drum-beat sounds of lesion motion and vessel wall co-vibration (usually systolic spikes of low frequency).
4 Decreased arterial wall pulsations on real time B-mode imaging compared with the contra-lateral side.
5 Delayed systolic flow acceleration, blunting of the MCA waveform or evidence of flow diversion to a branching vessel (i.e. ECA) and/or collateralization of flow via OA, AComA or PComA.

In the absence of a structural lesion in the proximal ICA and bifurcation, the absence or reversal of the diastolic flow in these segments should raise high suspicion of a distal ICA occlusion [136].

In a patient with new onset stroke symptoms or a recent TIA, ultrasound can detect an *acute thrombosis or an embolus in the ICA* [137–140] (Figures 6.19–6.22). This can be suspected when:

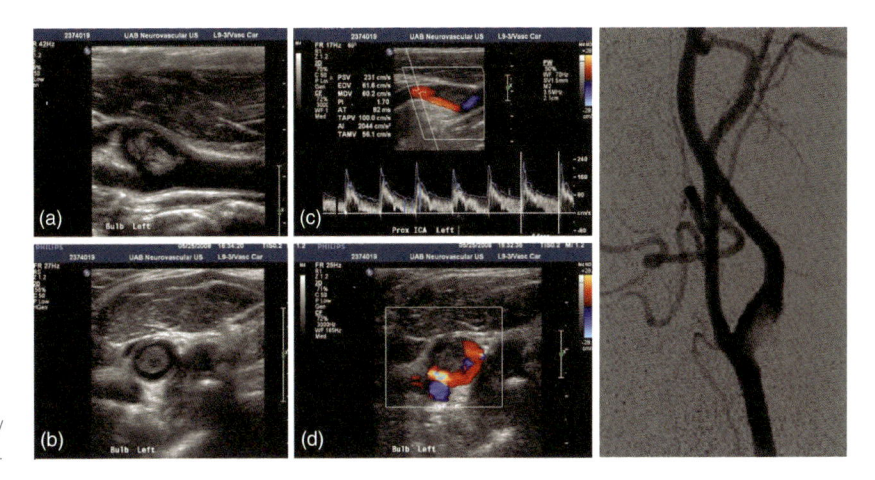

Figure 6.22 Thrombo-embolic obstruction in the proximal ICA from a cardiac source: (A) longitudinal view; (B) transverse view; (C) angle corrected velocity measurement; (D) transverse color flow visualization.

105

PART III Criteria for Interpretation

1 Flow signal void is found over a lesion with hypo- or anechoic intraluminal appearance (possible fresh clot on B-mode).
2 "Crescent moon" appearance of the residual lumen on color flow imaging indicating that the hypoechoic structure is an intraluminal inclusion.
3 High velocity in the ECA or contra-lateral vessels indicating flow diversion (in cases of flow limiting thrombi).
4 Presence of intracranial collaterals (in cases of flow limiting thrombi).
5 Microemboli found in the MCA unilateral to the ICA lesion and symptomatic brain side.

An acute thrombosis associated with carotid plaque usually shows an underlying atheroma that may be hyperechoic and have shadowing, whereas an acute embolus from the cardiac source may appear mostly hypoechoic and mobile (Figures 6.21 and 6.22) [137,138,140,141].

Carotid artery dissection can be detected sonographically directly in the CCA or proximal ICA or indirectly for the distal ICA due to its common location at the entrance to the skull. Sonographers should focus on finding an intimal flap and hemodynamic effects of an upstream lesion [142–157]. Carotid dissection can be suspected when (Figure 6.23):

1 Intimal flap is visualized in the carotid artery with abnormal flow waveforms (differentiate B-mode artifacts caused by jugular vein walls, its valves or other bright reflectors).
2 High-resistance pulsatile flow signals are found proximal to hemodynamically significant dissections without evidence for an atheromatous lesion.
3 Two waveforms are identified reflecting flow through the true and false lumens.
4 Reversed OA or other intracranial collaterals could be found.
5 Microemboli could be found in the MCA unilateral to a suspected carotid lesion.
6 If a dissection is found in the CCA, suspect its origin in the aortic arch and check other proximal pre-cerebral vessels.

Non-invasive diagnosis of ICA dissection is difficult since most of these lesions have variable locations often involving distal ICA at the entrance to the skull [158,159]. The diagnosis is often based on indirect evidence of the distal ICA lesion and may be impossible until the dissection becomes hemodynamically significant or descends to the field of insonation. Patient history often points to trauma, neck manipulation, neck pain, episodes of excessive coughing or sneezing with respiratory infection, etc. [160–162].

ICA dissections can recanalize and this process can be documented angiographically and monitored with ultrasound [144,148,163–166]. Ultrasound criteria for *recanalization of previously dissected carotid artery* include:

1 recovery of end-diastolic flow in the distal ICA (low resistance flow) or proximal to the lesion;

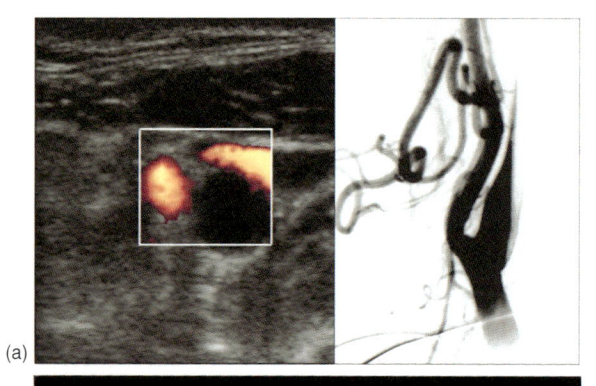

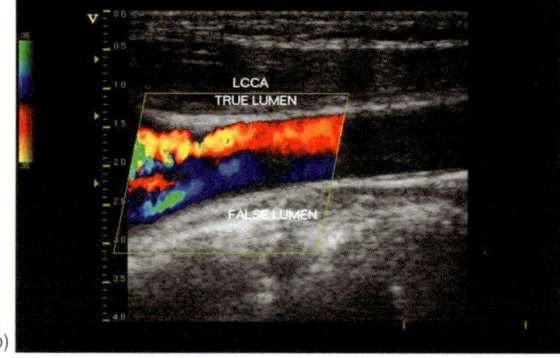

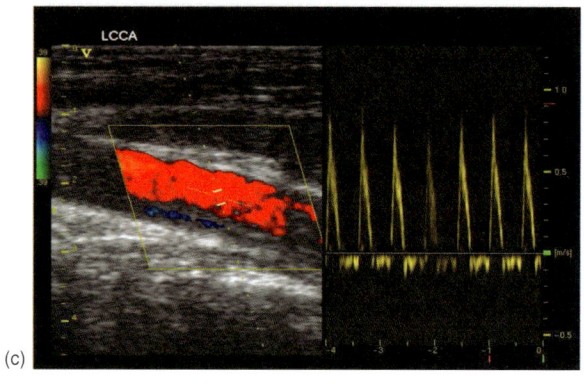

Figure 6.23 Arterial dissection: (a) ICA at the entrance to the skull; (b) and (c) an aortic arch dissection extending into the CCA.

2 return of normal systolic flow acceleration in the MCA without collateralization of flow;
3 return of normal siphon and OA signals.

Note that recanalization of dissected vessels may be only partial with persistent findings of the proximal high-resistance flow signatures, distal delay in systolic acceleration and retained collaterals. The only change could be the appearance or augmentation of the diastolic flow to and through the lesion.

Vertebral artery stenosis or occlusion

Most vascular laboratories simply determine the presence and direction of blood flow in the mid-cervical vertebral artery (VA) without an extensive exploration of the VA origin and its terminal portion. To see the extent of VA segments available for duplex and TCD interrogation, refer to the first two chapters, that detail complete scanning protocols. Compared with carotid imaging, fewer validation studies are available for detection and quantification of the VA lesions [167–183]. However, VA stenoses, occlusions and dissections are increasingly being recognized as potential causes or risk factors for the posterior circulation ischemia [167,177,188]. VA stenosis occurs more often in V_3–V_4 segments followed by the origin of the vertebral artery (V_0) and mid-cervical section (V_1–V_2) [185]. Direct assessment of the V_3 segment with ultrasound is not possible [185]. Therefore, the diagnosis of vertebral obstruction at this level is based on finding indirect proximal signs (i.e. increased flow pulsatility and different waveforms between two sides) or distal signs (post-stenotic turbulence, blunted waveform). Diagnostic criteria for direct assessment of the V_4 segment are presented below in the section **Intracranial stenosis**.

During extracranial duplex examination, the assessment of the vertebral artery should include scanning the mid-cervical portion and attempts to visualize the proximal VA and its origin whenever possible. Diagnostic criteria for *VA stenosis* derived from previous studies [167–183] and our own experience include:

1 Focal significant PSV velocity increase with the ratio between pre- or post-stenotic and stenotic segments of 1:≥2 (usually the highest PSV exceeds 100 cm s^{-1} to reach any significance of this finding).

2 When detectable, the presence of a structural lesion on B-mode or turbulence, spectral narrowing or additional abnormal waveforms on Doppler at the site of the lesion.

3 Indirect pre- or post-stenotic signs (abnormal pulsatility and waveforms).

Our criteria for VA stenoses do not include a PSV cutoff since tortuosity of the proximal VA segment, compensatory velocity increase with ICA lesions [186] and VA dominance may produce relatively high velocities. The keys to diagnosis of the VA stenosis with ≥50% diameter reduction are the terms "focal" and "significant." The velocity increase should be found over a relatively short (usually 1–2 cm) segment of the VA with normal or decreased pre- and post-stenotic velocities. This increased velocity should at least double the velocities found in other segment of the same VA. A hypoplastic VA is more likely to have low velocity and greater pulsatility over longer a arterial segment, particularly with changes in hemorheology [187].

Derived from previous studies [167–185], diagnostic criteria for **VA occlusion** include:

1 flow void area and absent pulsed Doppler signals in a segment or entire VA stem;

2 hypoechoic vessel lumen (acute and subacute occlusion);

3 hyperechoic vessel lumen (chronic occlusion);

4 abnormal residual flow waveforms on TCD with intracranial VA occlusion (Figure 6.24).

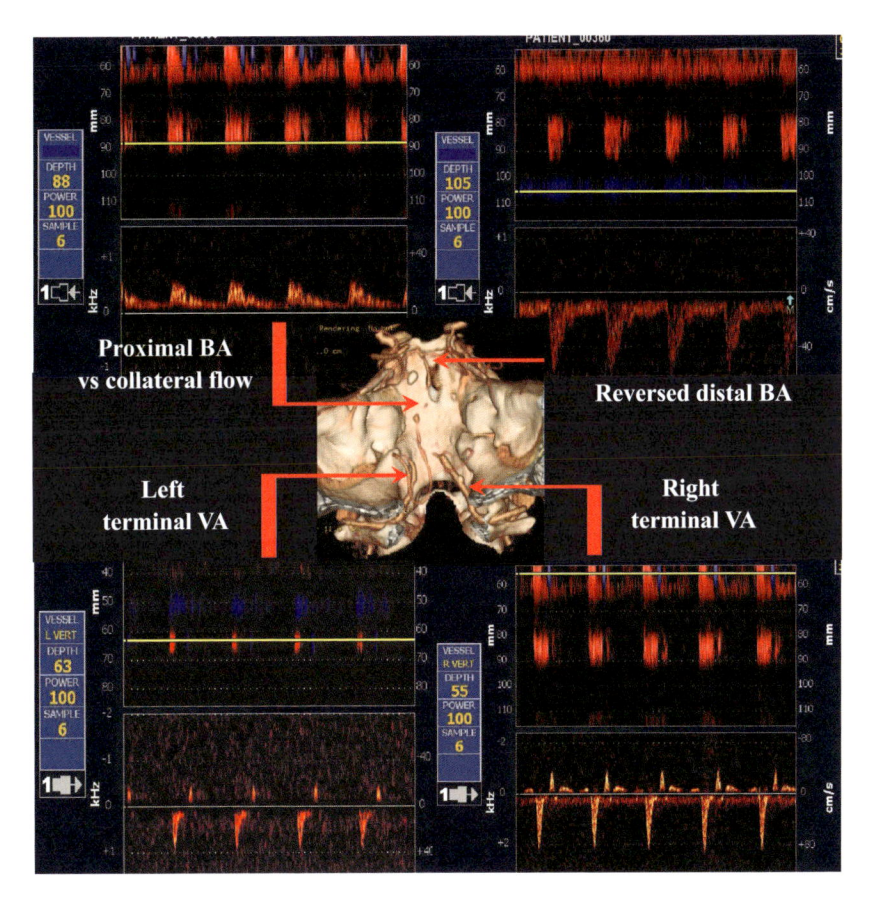

Figure 6.24 Bilateral terminal vertebral artery and the proximal basilar artery occlusions with the retrograde filling of the distal basilar artery.

PART III Criteria for Interpretation

Occasionally, a *segmental VA occlusion* can be found [188] due to the tremendous capacity of the vertebral artery to compensate via muscular collaterals. In these cases, patent distal and particularly terminal VA segments are found carrying antegrade low-resistance flow, often with delayed systolic upstroke. The latter should be differentiated with a proximal lesion in the subclavian artery. Therefore, incomplete assessment of the VA stem can miss a short segmental occlusion.

Intracranial stenosis

Intracranial stenosis is now recognized as a serious risk factor with severe and multiple lesions carrying the highest risk of stroke recurrence. Recent emphasis on identification of ≥50% and ≥70% stenoses (Figure 6.25) prompted re-evaluation of the previous criteria and development of new ones.

Middle cerebral artery (MCA) stenosis

Primary findings for any significant MCA stenosis (i.e. ≥50% diameter reduction) include a focal significant mean flow velocity increase (MFV ≥100 cm s^{-1}) or peak systolic velocity increase (PSV ≥140 cm s^{-1}) or inter-hemispheric MFV difference of 1:2 in adults free of abnormal circulatory conditions [14,19,99,189–201] (Figure 6.26). A ≥70% stenosis in the MCA could produce higher velocities and in our laboratory we use MFV cut-off ≥128 cm s^{-1} (L. Zhao *et al.*, unpublished data). This velocity increase should further be associated with a ratio to a homologous segment of 1:4 or higher. With MCA stenoses "on the other side" of the Spencer's curve, a paradoxical flow velocity decrease can be found in the presence of findings such as flow diversion that indicate hemodynamic significance of a lesion.

A proximal M2–distal M1 MCA stenosis is present if the velocity increase is found at 30–45 mm [202]. A proximal M1 MCA stenosis is usually found at 45–65 mm depths in adults [203]. Chimowitz *et al.* in the prospective part of the Warfarin Aspirin Stroke and Intracranial Disease (WASID) Study [204] adopted criterion that the MCA MFV ≥100 cm/−1s indicates ≥50% M1 MCA diameter reduction. An algorithm was developed to measure intracranial stenosis on digital subtraction angiograms (Figure 6.25). A recent meta-analysis of available studies indicated that the 100 cm s^{-1} cut-off yielded a mean weighted average sensitivity of 100% and specificity of 97% [201]. Figure 6.25 also illustrates a false-positive TCD finding of 125 cm s^{-1} velocity in the M1 MCA that was measured at 40% diameter reduction on an angiogram. To improve the predictive value of any chosen velocity threshold, we use the ratio with a homologous or proximal MCA segment [198]. There is increased interest in defining the most severe intracranial stenoses as these patients have the highest risk of stroke recurrence and novel stenting technology (Wingspan™) is now being tested as an adjunct to the best medical therapy for secondary stroke prevention.

If anemia, congestive heart failure and other circulatory conditions associated with elevated or decreased velocities are present, then a focal MFV difference ≥30% between neighboring or homologous arterial segments should be applied to see if the velocity increase reaches any

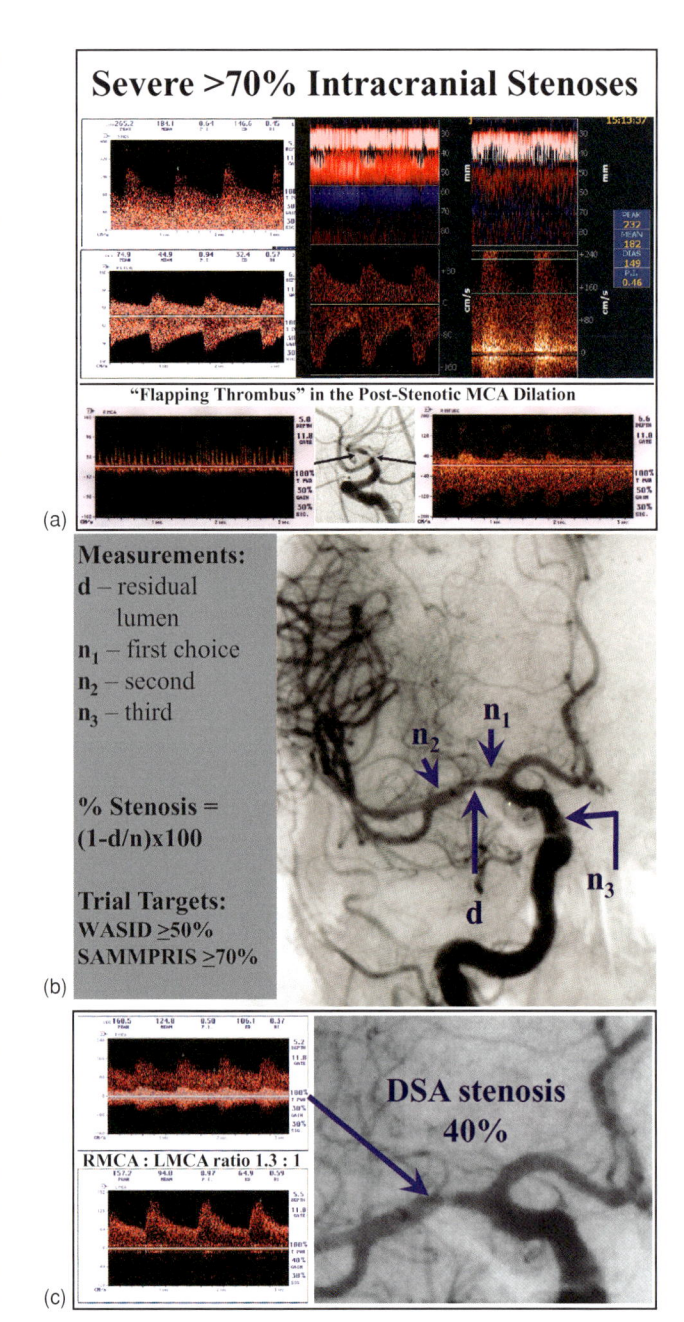

Figure 6.25 Intracranial stenoses on TCD and angiography. (a) Focal flow velocity increases and signs of flow diversion with severe ≥70% stenoses. (b) Measurement of the intracranial diameter reduction of the vessel. (c) A false-positive TCD result to predict a >50% MCA stenosis if a ratio to a homologous or pre-stentic to stenotic segment is not taken into account.

108

CHAPTER 6 Diagnostic Criteria for Cerebrovascular Ultrasound

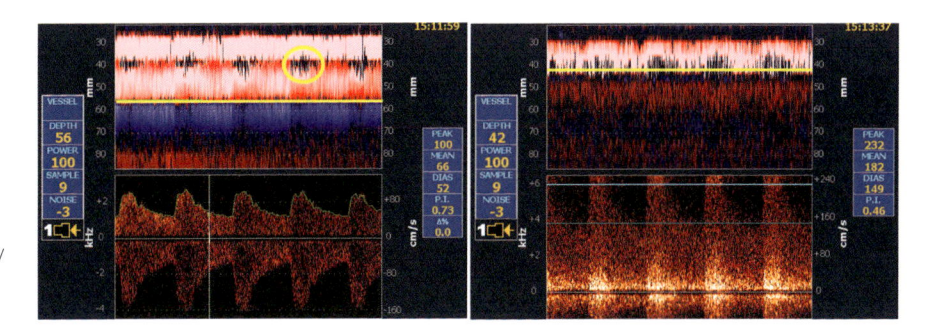

Figure 6.26 Systolic "holes" artifact on power motion Doppler due to turbulence and bruit at the site of a severe MCA stenosis: MFV MCA 182 cm s^{-1}, MFV ACA > proximal MCA, indicating compensatory flow diversion.

significance. Adult patients with anemia or hyperthyroidism often have MCA mean flow velocities in the range 60–110 cm s^{-1}. In children with sickle cell disease, an MCA MFV up to 170 cm s^{-1} is considered normal [12,205] (see Chapter 7).

A stenosis in the middle cerebral artery may be also suspected if indirect flow disturbances are detected by TCD. These important *additional findings* may include:

1 Turbulence or disturbed flow distal to the stenosis or presence of characteristic flow voids on Power Motion Mode display indicating a low-frequency bi-directional turbulent flow during systole (Figure 6.26).
2 An increased unilateral anterior cerebral artery (ACA) MFV indicating compensatory flow diversion [199,200]. This finding may also indicate A1 ACA or an ICA bifurcation stenosis with a side-to-side ACA MFV ratio 1:≥1.2.
3 A low-frequency noise produced by non-harmonic co-vibrations of the vessel wall and musical murmurs due to harmonic co-vibrations producing pure tones.
4 Microembolic signals found in the distal MCA.

If FVs are increased throughout the M1 MCA stem, the differential diagnosis includes MCA stenosis, terminal ICA or siphon stenosis, hyperemia or compensatory flow increase in the presence of contralateral ICA stenosis, ACA occlusion or incorrect vessel identification.

MCA sub-total stenosis or near-occlusion

A critical stenosis or obstruction with near-occlusive thrombus or an embolus can produce a focal FV decrease or a "blunted" MCA waveform with slow or delayed systolic acceleration, slow later-systolic flow deceleration, low velocities and MFV MCA < ACA or any other intracranial artery [19,99,206,207].

Decreased or minimal flow velocities with slow systolic acceleration can be found due to a tight elongated MCA stenosis or thrombus causing near-occlusion. These focal lesions should be differentiated from a proximal ICA obstruction that can also produce delayed flow acceleration in the MCA [100,101,103]. The minimal, blunted or dampened waveforms are common in patients with acute ischemic stroke, particularly in those presenting with a hyperdense MCA signs on non-contrast CT scan or a flow gap on MRA (Figure 6.27) (see also the criteria for *Arterial occlusion*).

A false-positive diagnosis of MCA sub-total stenosis can occur because of problems with vessel identification and a suboptimal angle of insonation. Incorrect probe angulation and shallow insonation usually lead to these errors. To confirm the presence of a flow-limiting lesion, branching vessels need to be evaluated. Note that an M1–M2 MCA sub-total stenosis is usually accompanied by flow diversion to the ACA and/or compensatory flow increase in the PCA, indicating transcortical collateralization of flow [206,207].

Anterior cerebral artery (ACA)

Primary findings in an ACA stenosis include a focal significant ACA FV increase (ACA > MCA) and/or ACA MFV ≥80 cm s^{-1} (Figure 6.28), and/or a ≥30% difference between the proximal and distal ACA segments, and/or a ≥30% difference compared with the contralateral ACA [14,19,206]. Collateralization via the anterior communicating artery (AComA) can be excluded by a normal contralateral ACA flow direction and the absence of stenotic signals at 75 mm (i.e. midline). Usually, an A1 ACA stenosis can be detected at 60–75 mm.

The differential diagnosis includes anterior cross-filling due to a proximal carotid artery disease [128,130,134]. Additional findings may include turbulence and flow diversion into the MCA and/or compensatory flow increase in the contralateral ACA.

Decreased or minimal flow velocities at the A1 ACA origin may indicate a suboptimal angle of insonation from the unilateral temporal window, an atretic or tortuous A1 ACA segment and A1 ACA near-occlusion. Since the A2 ACA segment cannot be assessed directly by TCD, its obstruction can be suspected only if a high-resistance flow is found in the distal dominant A1 ACA segment (70–75 mm).

Common errors include incorrect vessel identification (terminal ICA versus ACA), velocity underestimation (suboptimal angle of insonation, poor window, weak signals) and inability to differentiate a collateral flow from the stenosis.

PART III Criteria for Interpretation

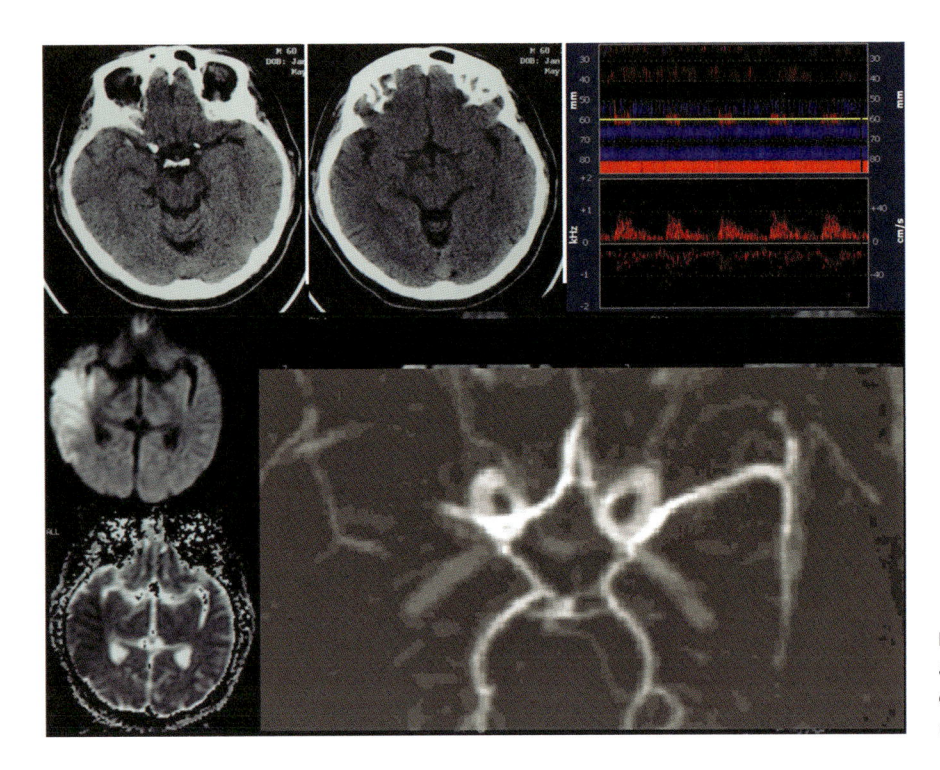

Figure 6.27 A typical appearance of an acute MCA occlusion: hyperdense MCA sign on CT, flow void on MRA and an abnormal residual flow signal on power motion Doppler.

Terminal ICA and ICA siphon

The ICA siphon and paracellar and supraclinoid ICA segments are difficult to examine in their entirety since they navigate through bones. An orbital examination may reveal stenotic flow directed towards or away from the probe at 55–65 mm in adults with signals often traceable to 70 mm. The terminal ICA bifurcation is located at 60–75 mm from the transtemporal window. A terminal ICA/siphon stenosis produces a focal significant MFV increase ICA > MCA, and/or an ICA MFV ≥ 70 cm s^{-1}, and/or a ≥30% difference between arterial segments [14,19,99,208]. The higher the focal velocity increase, the more likely are TCD findings to be confirmed by other imaging modalities. However, TCD velocity is more sensitive to mild and moderate degrees of intracranial stenosis and correlative angiograms may still be negative for a significant disease.

The differential diagnosis includes moderate proximal ICA stenosis and/or a compensatory flow increase with contralateral ICA stenosis. Additional findings in the presence of an ICA stenosis may include turbulence, blunted unilateral MCA, OA MFV increase and/or flow reversal with low pulsatility. The ICA siphon MFVs may decrease due to siphon near-occlusion (a blunted siphon signal) or distal obstruction (i.e. MCA occlusion or increased ICP).

Common errors include vessel identification such as MCA versus TICA via transtemporal approach or ACA versus ICA with deep (>65 mm) transorbital insonation and consequently collateralization of flow via the anterior cross-filling

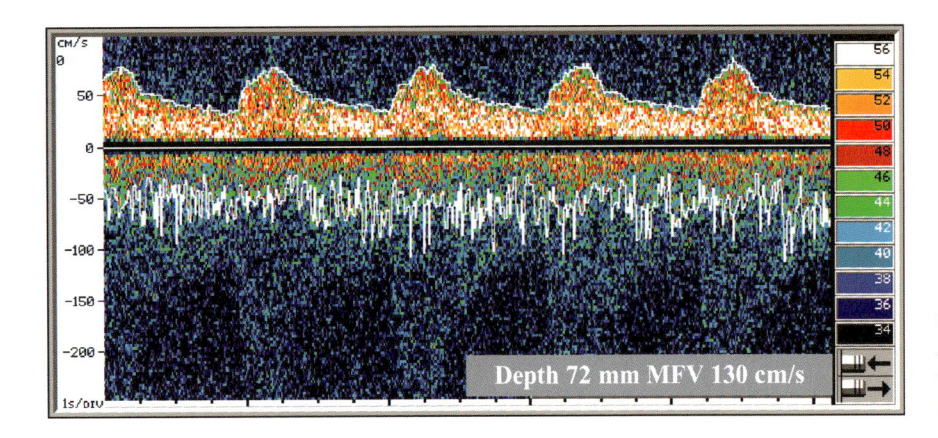

Figure 6.28 A focal velocity increase with A1 ACA stenosis on TCD: the signal is weak and the envelope cannot follow it below the baseline even at high gain settings.

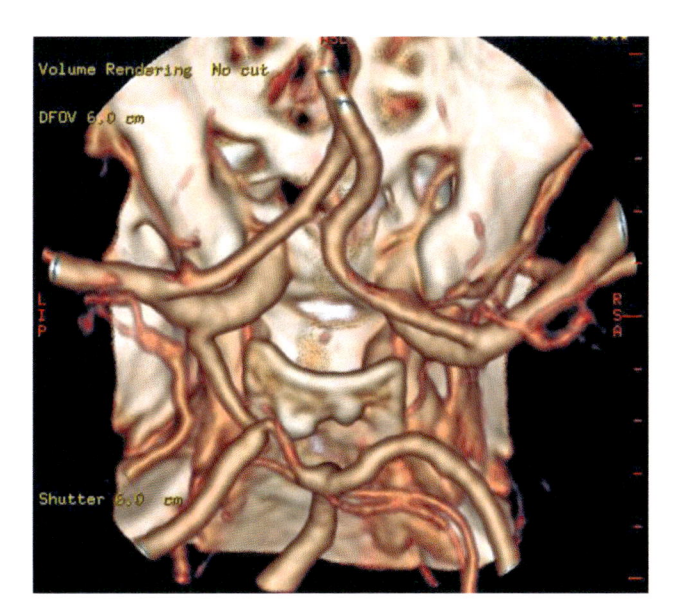

Figure 6.29 PCA stenosis versus P1 hypoplasia.

misinterpreted as an arterial stenosis. In the absence of temporal windows, these findings may be the only yet confusing indicators of a significant carotid disease.

Posterior cerebral artery (PCA)

A PCA stenosis produces a focal significant FV increase resulting in a PCA MFV > ACA or ICA, and/or a PCA MFV $\geq$50 cm s^{-1} in adults [14,18,209–212] (Figure 6.29). The PCA signals are usually located at 55–65 mm; the top-of-the-basilar can be found at 70–80 mm; the P1 segment is directed towards the probe, the contralateral P1 and unilateral P2 segments are directed away from the probe [18, 99]. Additional findings may include turbulence and a compensatory flow increase in the MCA.

The differential diagnosis includes collateral flow via the posterior communicating artery (PComA) either towards the posterior circulation in case of basilar artery occlusion or towards the anterior circulation in case of MCA, TICA or tandem extracranial ICA/MCA occlusions and siphon stenosis. Of note, PComA is a tortuous artery and its flow direction on TCD does not necessarily indicate where the lesion is that requires collateralization. Using transcranial duplex imaging, it may be possible to differentiate PCA stenosis from collateralization of flow using the peak systolic velocity [212].

Common sources of error include unreliable vessel identification, the presence of an arterial occlusion and a top of the basilar stenosis.

Basilar artery (BA)

Primary findings in the presence of a BA stenosis include a focal significant velocity increase where a BA MFV > MCA or ACA or ICA, and/or MFV BA $\geq$60 cm s^{-1} in adults, and/or $\geq$30% difference between arterial segments [14,18,99,213–215] (Figure 6.30). The findings of a recent study indicated that a BA stenosis of $\geq$50% can be more reliably identified when BA MFV exceeds 80 cm s^{-1} and when the stenotic-to-normal MFV ratio is $\geq$2 [18]. To detect >70% intracranial vertebro-basilar stenosis, we use MFV > 119 cm s^{-1} and a ratio of 4 (L. Zhao *et al.*, unpublished data).

Although the depth range for basilar segments varied between previous studies [213,214], it is also dependent on the size of the neck and skull and the technical skills. Insonation of the distal basilar artery should be accomplished with failure rates far less than 30% [215]. In our laboratory, we aim to detect the distal basilar artery in practically all subjects using the following depth criteria. The proximal basilar artery is located at $\geq$75 mm, the mid-BA segment is located at 90 mm and the distal BA is found at 100+ mm in most adults [18,206,215].

The differential diagnosis includes a terminal VA stenosis if elevated velocities are found proximally, i.e. 70–80 mm. If elevated velocities are found throughout the BA stem, the differential diagnosis includes a compensatory flow velocity increase. With the latter velocities at least one of the VAs are also elevated.

Basilar artery sub-total stenosis or near-occlusion produces a focal FV decrease ($\leq$30% difference between arterial segments and/or BA < VA), resulting in a blunted waveform [18]. The differential diagnosis includes a fusiform (dolicho-ectatic) basilar artery with or without thrombus since an enlarged vessel diameter may reduce flow velocities. If the end-diastolic flow is absent, the differential diagnosis includes BA occlusion or tortuousity with branch insonation at a suboptimal angle.

Additional findings may include:
1 turbulence and disturbed signals distal to the stenosis;
2 compensatory flow increase in VAs and PICAs, indicating cerebellar collateralization;
3 collateral supply via PComA to PCA and reversed distal basilar artery (see the section on Collaterals).

Common sources of error include tortuous basilar ("not found" does not always mean obstructed), elongated BA obstruction and distal BA lesions that were not reached by TCD insonation or identified due to flow presence to the superior cerebellar arteries (SCA) producing false-negative results. In cases of distal BA occlusions, transtemporal insonation of the top of the basilar using characteristic PMD flow signatures may be a valuable alternative for the identification of distal BA pathology and monitoring of recanalization [18]. Application of power Doppler, ultrasound contrast and duplex imaging may help the detection of the distal basilar segment, tortuousity and distal branches [18,99,216,217]. Also, a collateral flow from the posterior to anterior circulation in the presence of carotid lesions may increase flow velocity changes associated with mild stenosis and/or tortuosity. In the case of flow collateralization, the dominant vertebral artery velocities are

PART III Criteria for Interpretation

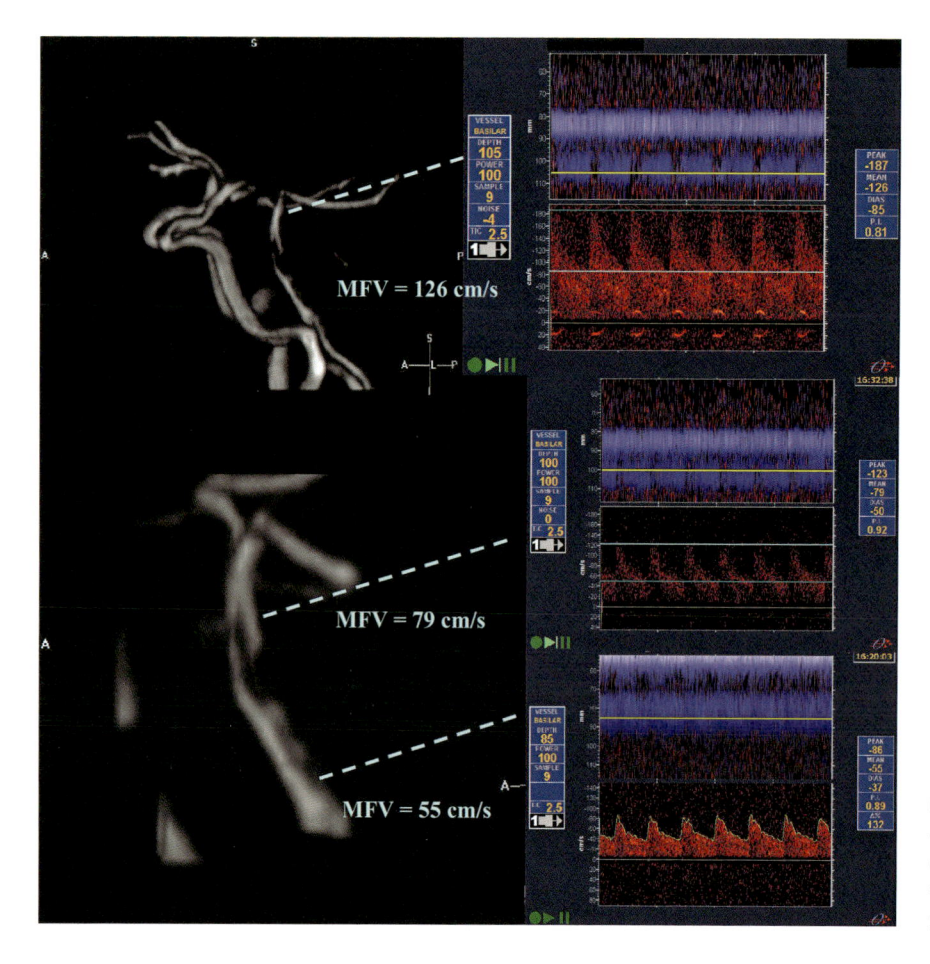

Figure 6.30 A focal velocity increase in the distal basilar with an intraluminal thrombus (possible dissection or dissecting atheroma of the basilar artery). Images courtesy of Dr Vijay Sharma.

also increased [186]. Finally, reversed flow in basilar artery (low-resistance flow moving towards the flow at depths of 80–100 mm in the absence of antegrade basilar flow signals during suboccipital insonation (Figure 6.24) is diagnostic of the proximal BA occlusion with retro-filling the distal BA through the PComA [18,218]. The origin of the collateral flow in the anterior circulation can be confirmed with carotid artery tapping that can be transmitted to the reversed BA flow.

Terminal vertebral artery (VA)

Primary findings with intracranial VA stenosis include a focal significant velocity increase [99,180] where MFV VA > BA, and/or MFV VA ≥ 50 cm s^{-1} in adults (Figure 6.31), and/or $\geq 30\%$ difference between VAs or its segments [2,14]. Similarly with BA stenoses, the higher the focal velocity increase, the greater is the chance that angiography will show a significant stenosis. This correlation may be less optimal if angiography is performed days later after stroke symptom onset and TCD, since the degree of a stenosis could be less on angio due to continuing recanalization (Figure 6.31). The main problem with detecting and grading VA stenoses with TCD is that these vessels are often affected by multiple, diffuse or elongated lesions and the resulting velocity may not necessarily be high.

An occlusion of the terminal VA may also present as a high-resistance (PI ≥ 1.2) flow in one of the vertebral arteries proximal to the obstruction, and/or a blunted or minimal flow signal including those with reverberating pattern [99,209] (Figure 6.24). The terminal VA is found through the suboccipital window at 40–75 mm depending on the size of neck and skull. To detect $\geq 50\%$ intracranial stenoses, the peak systolic velocity criteria were also developed for angle-corrected duplex ultrasound of the vertebral and other intracranial arteries [219]. The findings of a recent study have indicated that a $\geq 50\%$ VA stenosis can be more reliably identified when VA MFV exceeds 80 cm s^{-1} and when the stenotic-to-normal MFV ratio is ≥ 2 [18]. The cut-off of 80 cm s^{-1} for detecting >50% stenosis in the vertebrobasilar system was also adopted by the investigators of the Stroke Outcomes and Neuroimaging of Intracranial Atherosclerosis (SONIA) trial [220].

The differential diagnosis includes proximal BA or contralateral terminal VA stenoses and a compensatory flow increase in the presence of a contralateral VA occlusion or carotid stenosis [187].

CHAPTER 6 Diagnostic Criteria for Cerebrovascular Ultrasound

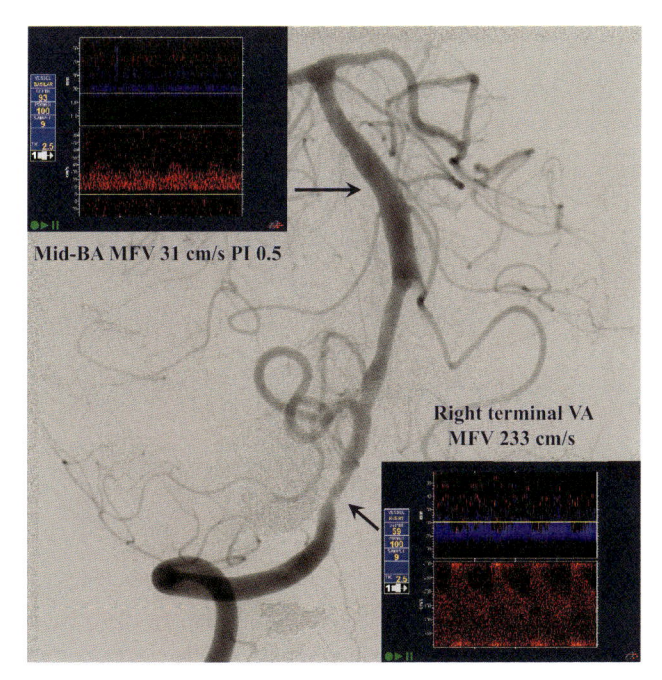

Figure 6.31 A focal velocity increase with the terminal vertebral artery stenosis. A less than anticipated stenosis severity on an angiogram is due to over 24 h delay between TCD and angiography and continuing recanalization of the lesions (frequent micro-emboli on TCD, images not shown). Images courtesy of Dr Vijay Sharma.

Additional findings may include:
1 turbulence or disturbed flow signal distal to the stenosis;
2 a compensatory flow increase in the contralateral vertebral artery or its branches (cerebellar collaterals);
3 low BA flow velocities (hemodynamically significant lesion, hypoplastic contralateral VA) and low-resistance flow distal to stenoses (compensatory vasodilation);
4 the presence of distal embolization in BA or cerebellar collaterals (detectable elevated velocity in PICA or other cerebellar arteries).

Common sources of error include a compensatory flow increase due to hypoplastic contralateral VA, low velocities in both VAs due to suboptimal angle of insonation, extracranial VA stenosis or occlusion with well-developed muscular collaterals, elongated VA stenosis/hypoplasia and incorrect vessel identification, i.e. posterior inferior cerebellar artery.

Arterial stenosis and near-occlusions: summary

An intracranial stenosis should be suspected when the normal hierarchy of flow velocities is disrupted, i.e. MCA ≥ ACA ≥ ICA ≥ PCA ≥ BA ≥ VA by the mean flow velocity difference greater than 20%, i.e. BA > MCA and focal velocity elevation (Table 6.5). Remember, however, that not all focal velocity increases represent a stenosis or predict a significant stenosis. As a rule, one needs to think of an explanation when testing patients older than 60 years reveals mean velocities greater than patients' age. Fairly often mild velocity elevations may represent hemodynamic changes other than those due to a significant stenosis and should not be over-interpreted.

TCD can reliably detect stenoses located in the M1 MCA, detectable portions of TICA and ICA siphon, terminal vertebral, proximal basilar arteries and P1 PCA. The reported sensitivity ranges are 85–90%, specificity 90–95%, PPV 85% and NPV 98% with lower accuracy parameters for the posterior circulation. TCD sensitivity to measure velocity without aliasing is limited in patients with deep (>65 mm) stenoses due to the low pulse repetition frequency of TCD instruments [14,221,222]. If velocities cannot be displayed without aliasing, use end-diastolic velocity to document a significant increase since MFV will exceed EDV (i.e. if EDV of 90 cm s^{-1} is found with flow of normal pulsatility, MFV will be greater than 100 cm s^{-1}). Stenoses of M2, A2, P2 segments are difficult to find due to a suboptimal angle of insonation or less predictable location. Intracranial collaterals and hyperemia may mimic a stenotic flow.

Finally, the recently published results of the Stroke Outcomes and Neuroimaging of Intracranial Atherosclerosis (SONIA) trial [223] along with recent studies from our group [18,19] comparing the accuracy of TCD [single-channel or Power Motion Mode (PMD) Doppler] to angiography (CTA or DSA) for detecting steno-occlusive disease in the setting of acute arterial ischemia have indicated that TCD is superior for ruling out than ruling in intracranial stenotic arterial disease (higher NPV than PPV for all studied arterial segments). In addition, there is increasing evidence that PMD

Table 6.5 Maximum mean flow velocity thresholds at assumed zero angle of insonation for a focal (≥50%) intracranial arterial stenosis on TCD

Artery	Depth (mm)	MFV (cm s^{-1})	MFV ≥50% stenosis (cm s^{-1})	MFV ≥70% stenosis (cm s^{-1})
M1–M2 MCA	30–65	≥80	≥100 (use 1:2 ratio)	≥128 (1:4 ratio)
A1 ACA	60–75	≥80	N/A	N/A
ICA siphon	60–65	≥70	≥90 (use 1:2 ratio)	≥128 (1:4 ratio)
PCA	60–72	≥50	N/A	N/A
BA	80–100+	≥60	≥80 (use 1:2 ratio)	≥119 (1:4 ratio)
VA	40–80	≥50	≥80 (use 1:2 ratio)	≥119 (1:4 ratio)

PART III Criteria for Interpretation

display permits better interrogation of the affected and non-affected vessel segments because it simultaneously shows vessel segments with turbulent and laminar flow over a wide range of depths [18,19,99]. This, in turn, facilitates a more detailed insonation of the affected segments, prompting better estimation of stenotic-to-normal MFV ratios. Moreover, in our series PMD display depicted diagnostic flow signatures that were complementary to the information provided by the spectral display in the majority of the true-positive cases [18,19,99]. The presence of reverberating or high-resistance flow signatures on PMD can facilitate the rapid diagnosis and localization of vertebrobasilar [18] or middle cerebral [19] artery occlusions. This observation is in keeping with the findings by Saqqur et al., who reported that absent or high-resistance PMD flow signatures can reliably diagnose 87% of angiographic-proven proximal middle cerebral artery occlusions [22]. Arterial stenoses and near-occlusions may present with a broad range of velocity findings and it is very important to refer to the Spencer's curve during interpretation as the most severe stenotic or pre-occlusive lesions may present with low velocity/variable pulsatility (i.e. findings on the "other side" of the Spencer's curve).

Also, the PMD display can show embolic flow signatures and yield a greater embolic count compared with the single-gate spectral display since PMD allows simultaneous display of flow over long arterial segments as well as more than one vessel [16]. In our series, we noted PMD embolic tracks in the cerebellar arteries (depicted as red bands on PMD display over different depths), whereas our sample volume interrogation was set in depths corresponding to VA or BA. Because the cerebellar arteries are not routinely insonated during the assessment of posterior circulation vessels with single-gate TCD, the presence of embolization distal to an extracranial or intracranial steno-occlusive arterial lesion may have not been identified without PMD–TCD. Embolic signals on TCD may sometimes be the only sign of artery-to-artery embolization from a proximal lesion that could be an arterial stenosis.

Arterial vasospasm and hyperemia

Arterial vasospasm is a complication of subarachnoid hemorrhage (SAH), which becomes symptomatic in more than 25% of patients leading to a delayed ischemic deficit (DID) [224]. DID usually occurs when vasospasm results in severe ($\leq$1 mm) intracranial arterial narrowing producing flow depletion with extremely high velocities [225]. Vasospasm may affect proximal stems and distal branches of intracranial arteries with the most common locations being:
1 MCA/TICA ± ACA
2 bilateral ACAs
3 basilar ± terminal vertebral artery and
4 distal branches [226].

Vasospasm may coexist with hydrocephalus, edema and cerebral infarction. The differential diagnosis with TCD should always consider the hyperdynamic state that we will refer to as *hyperemia*. Hyperemia may be induced by spontaneous cardiovascular responses to SAH or induced by the hypertension–hemodilution–hypervolemia (HHH) therapy [227]. Although inadequate, the term "hyperemia" is used to describe increased velocity changes on TCD that are not related to vasospasm. The flow velocity measured by TCD is not a direct measurement of cerebral blood flow volume [228]. However, focal or global velocity changes can help differentiate between spasm and hyperemia. Both conditions may coexist since most SAH patients with spasm routinely receive HHH therapy.

Although quantitative criteria have been studied extensively, grading vasospasm severity remains difficult and the interpretation of TCD findings should be individualized, perhaps even age adjusted in the future. TCD in patients with SAH is performed to:
1 detect early development of vasospasm;
2 monitor its progression to severe stage (often despite nimodipine and triple-H therapies);
3 identify those with severe or recurrent vasospasm prior to or after day 7 post-SAH (since angiographic control may be limited by a number of contrast studies to certain days); and
4 determine vasospasm resolution (findings often observed after successful interventional treatment or during the second week after SAH).

Daily TCDs may detect considerable flow velocity and pulsatility changes that should be related to the patient clinical condition, medications, blood pressure, time after day 0 (usually onset of the worst headache of patient's life) and intracranial pressure (ICP) findings.

Proximal vasospasm in any intracranial artery results in a focal (or present along one or two branching segments) elevation of mean flow velocities without a parallel velocity increase in feeding extracranial arteries (intracranial/extracranial vessel ratio $\geq$3).

Distal vasospasm in any intracranial artery may produce a focal pulsatile flow (PI $\geq$1.2) indicating increased resistance distal to the site of insonation. No MFV increase may be found since vasospasm is located distal to the site of insonation [229]. Additional findings may include daily changes in velocities, ratio's and PIs during the first 2 weeks but particularly pronounced during the critical days 3–7 after the onset of SAH.

For *MCA-specific criteria*, see Table 6.6 and Figure 6.32.

The MCA findings on TCD were most rigorously validated and correlated with the diameter of the residual lumen on DSA [225,230–233]. According to Lindegaard et al., the MCA MFV $\geq$200 cm s^{-1} predict residual lumen of 1 mm or less [225]. A representative angiogram and velocity findings are shown in Figure 6.32. The differential diagnosis includes hyperemia, combination of vasospasm and hyperemia in

CHAPTER 6 Diagnostic Criteria for Cerebrovascular Ultrasound

Table 6.6 TCD criteria for grading the proximal MCA vasospasm

Mean flow velocity (cm s⁻¹)	MCA/ICA MFV ratio	Interpretation
<120	≤3	Hyperemia
≥120	3–4	Development of mild spasm + hyperemia
≥120	4–5	Moderate spasm + hyperemia
≥120	5–6	Moderate spasm
≥180	6	Moderate-to-severe spasm
≥200	≥6	Severe spasm
>200	4–6	Moderate spasm + hyperemia
>200	3–4	Hyperemia + mild (often residual) spasm
>200	<3	Hyperemia

Table 6.7 Predictors of adverse outcomes in patients with SAH: TCD findings indicating vasospasm progression and ICP changes

Parameter	Values
Velocity	Early appearance of MCA MFV ?180 cm s⁻¹
	Rapid (>20% or + >65 cm s⁻¹) daily MFV rise during critical days 3–7
Ratio	MCA/ICA ratio ≥6
Pulsatility	Abrupt appearance of high-resistance PI ≥1.2 due to increased ICP (hydrocephalus)
	Appearance of PI ≥1.2 due to distal spasm

the same vessel, residual vasospasm and hyperemia. Unlike focal atherosclerotic lesions, vasospasm may affect longer segments of the terminal ICA and MCA. Vasospasm may be unequally distributed along the MCA stem and branches. However, the presence of hyperdynamic cardiovascular state and HHH-therapy may promote high velocities even in the presence of moderate or severe spasm affecting multiple segments.

Prognostically unfavorable findings on TCD are summarized in Table 6.7. These criteria were modified from a review by Sloan [224].

Criteria for vasospasm in other intracranial arteries

Grading vasospasm severity in the arteries other than the MCA is difficult [224,234]. Sloan *et al.* suggested reporting vasospasm in these arteries as possible, probable and definite [224,235] (Table 6.8). The key indicator of a significant vasospasm is a focal, asymmetric and disproportionate velocity increase (Figure 6.33) that may occur in an artery distant from the aneurysm site or blood clot collection on CT (Figure 6.34). The differential diagnosis includes hyperemia and its combination with vasospasm in these arteries.

Soustiel *et al.* have shown that the BA/EVA (extracranial VA assessed at the first cervical level at depths ranging from 45 to 55 mm) ratio (termed Soustiel's ratio) may contribute to an improved discrimination between BA vasospasm and vertebrobasilar hyperemia and enhance the accuracy and reliability of TCD in the diagnosis of BA vasospasm [236]. Their data further suggested that the BA/EVA ratio may provide an approximation of vasospasm severity and help in identifying patients who are likely to suffer from hemodynamically significant vasospasm. Sviri and colleagues have independently validated the accuracy of Soustiel's ratio [237,238] and, after showing that this ratio improved the

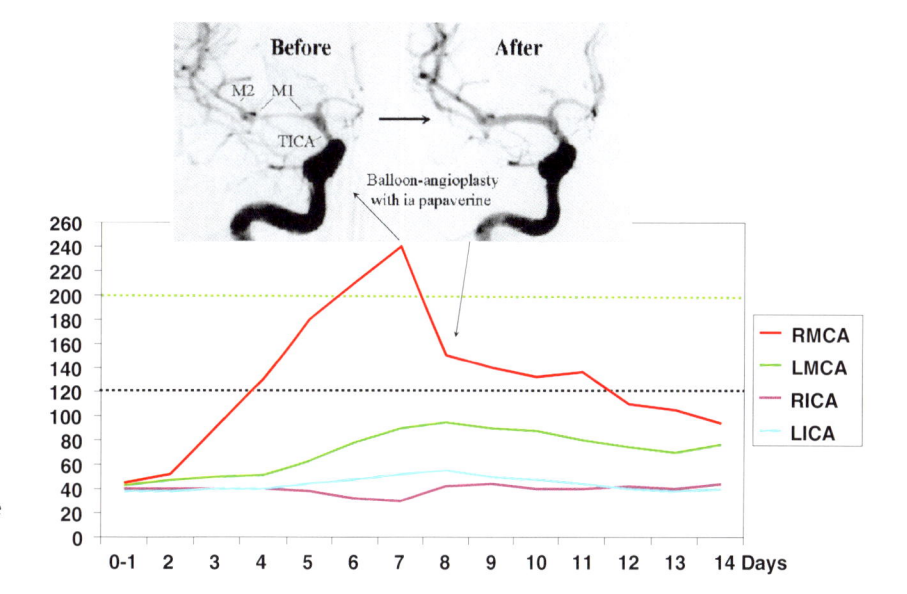

Figure 6.32 A typical course of velocity findings with a proximal vasospasm after SAH affecting the terminal ICA, MCA and ACA segments. An angiogram and intervention were done on day 7.

PART III Criteria for Interpretation

Table 6.8 Sloan's optimized criteria for grading vasospasm in intracranial arteries

Artery/MFV	Possible VSP[a]	Probable VSP[a]	Definite VSP[a]
ICA	>80	>110	>130
ACA	>90	>110	>120
PCA	>60	>80	>90
BA	>70	>90	>100
VA	>60	>80	>90

[a]After hyperemia has been mostly ruled out by the focal velocity increase and by the intracranial artery/extracranial ICA ratio ≥3 except for posterior circulation vessels. Optimized criteria were modified from the review by Sloan [224].

Table 6.9 Sviri's optimized criteria [238] for grading vasospasm in basilar artery using Soustiel's ratio [236]

	Soustiel's ratio	BA MFV velocity (cm s^{-1})	Sensitivity (%)	Specificity (%)
BA vasospasm	>2	>70	77	82
Moderate or severe BA vasospasm	>2.5	>85	86	97
Severe BA vasospasm	>3	>85	92	97

[a]Soustiel's ratio: MFV BA/MFV EXVA, where MFV = mean flow velocity, BA = basilar artery and EXVA = extracranial vertebral artery (at the first cervical level, depth 45–55 mm).

sensitivity and specificity of TCD detection of BA vasospasm, they introduced new TCD grading criteria for BA vasospasm (Table 6.9).

An ongoing individual correlation of digital subtraction angiography with same-day TCD findings may improve the accuracy of TCD to detect vasospasm onset. A focal and disproportionate to therapy increase in flow velocities indicates the development of vasospasm. For example, an MCA MFV increase by 50 cm s^{-1} may indicate a 20% diameter reduction of the vessel, and since FV is inversely proportional to the vessel radius, a 50% diameter reduction usually doubles the velocity on TCD [239]. Therefore, TCD may be more sensitive to intracranial artery diameter changes than angiography particularly at the early phases of spasm development. Since TCD is a screening tool, the criteria should be adjusted to a higher sensitivity to detect any degree of vasospasm in order to institute HHH therapy. At the same time, a higher specificity threshold should be used for severe vasospasm to minimize the number of false-negative angiograms, particularly if TCD is used to select patients for angioplasty.

In our experience, vasospasm that affects basilar artery stem, PCAs or ACAs may cause a compensatory velocity increase in the MCAs with low Lindegaard ratios. Therefore, a complete daily TCD examination may reveal more significant hemodynamic changes that can be used to identify patients with spasm in arteries other than MCA.

Hyperemia

Hyperemia is suspected with elevated velocities in the intracranial and often in the feeding extracranial vessels (Table 6.5). Hyperemic changes on TCD are common in patients with SAH receiving HHH therapy (see also Vasospasm criteria above). The use of the Lindegaard ratio [232] and new flow and area indices [240] may help to minimize false-positive TCD results and predict better the diameter of the residual lumen on angiography.

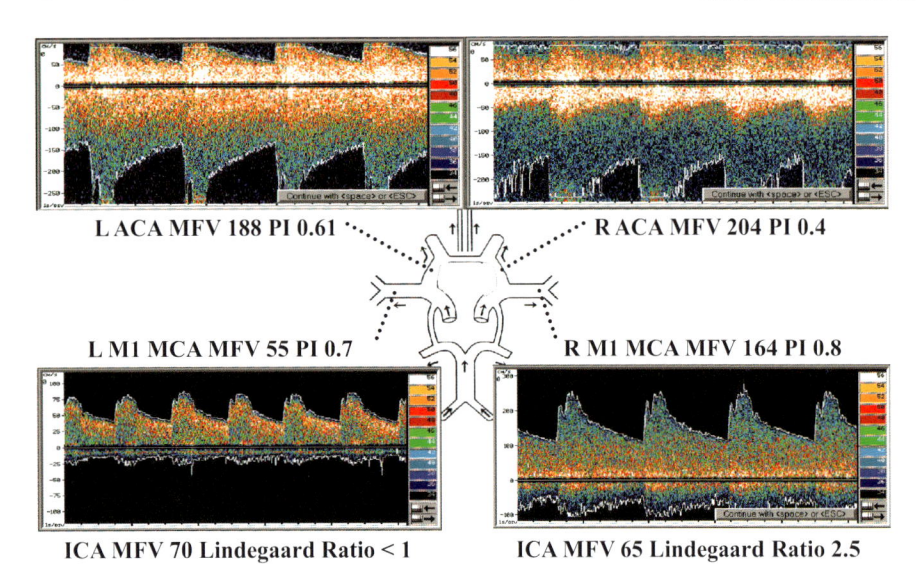

L ACA MFV 188 PI 0.61   R ACA MFV 204 PI 0.4
L M1 MCA MFV 55 PI 0.7   R M1 MCA MFV 164 PI 0.8
ICA MFV 70 Lindegaard Ratio < 1   ICA MFV 65 Lindegaard Ratio 2.5

Figure 6.33 Bilateral "spear-headed" A1 ACA vasospasm on TCD.

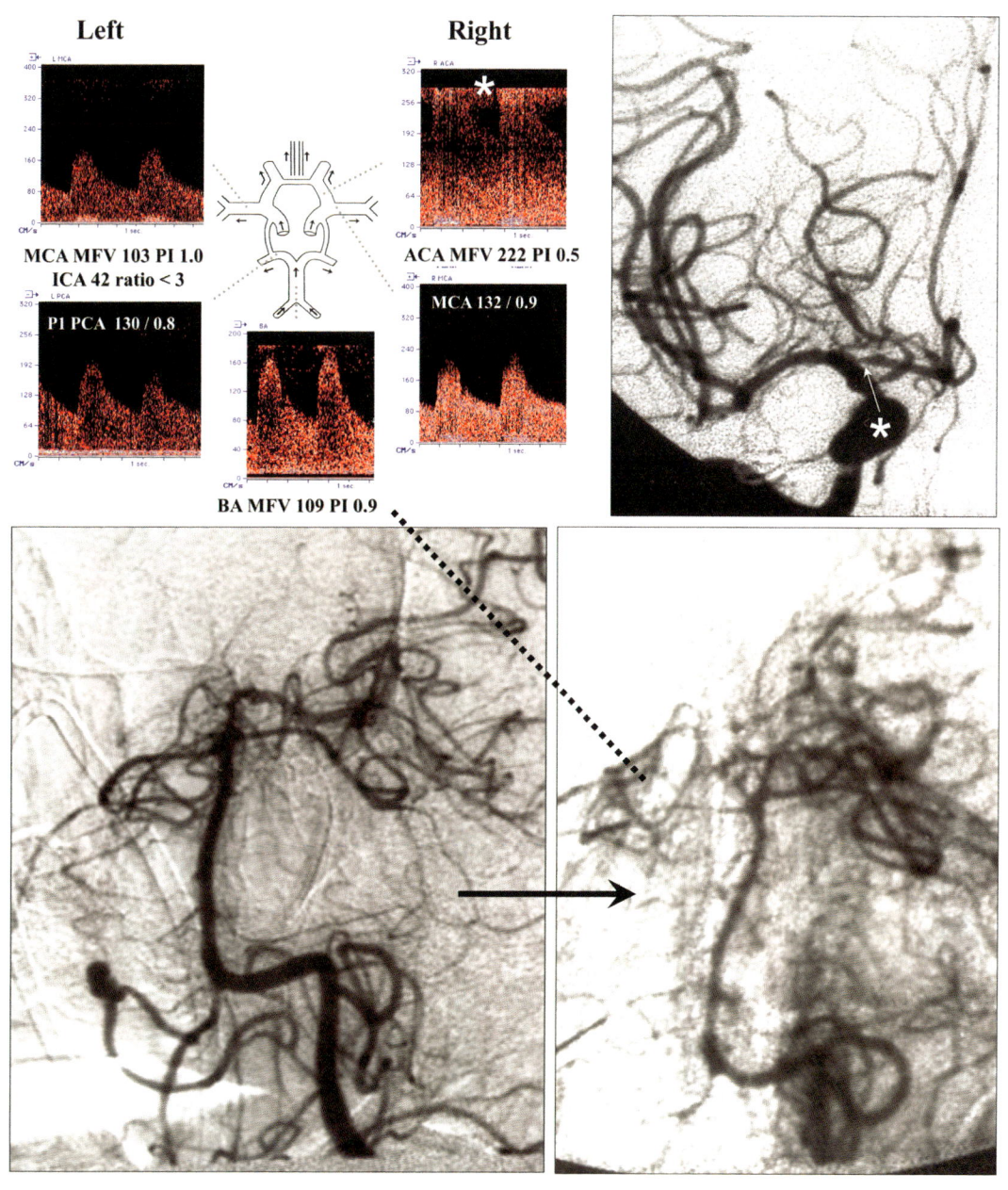

CHAPTER 6 Diagnostic Criteria for Cerebrovascular Ultrasound

Figure 6.34 Vertebro-basilar and remote A1 ACA vasospasm in a patient with SAH and the right posterior inferior cerebellar artery aneurysm.

Otherwise, hyperperfusion syndrome may develop after carotid endarterectomy or angioplasty due to limited or impaired capacity of the brain to regulate restored blood flow volume [241–244]. Patients with post-revascularization hyperemia frequently experience headache and seizures. TCD often shows a ≥30% increase in MCA MFV unilateral to the reconstructed carotid artery and low-pulsatility waveforms compared with the contralateral side, indicating decreased capacity of distal vasculature to regulate the re-established flow volume. The pulsatility index may decrease by >20% compared with the contralateral side. These changes can often be found during surgery immediately after cross-clamp release. Spencer diagnosed hyperperfusion when the MCA MFV is 1.5 times the pre-cross-clamp values and persists at that level without corrective measures [245].

Hyperemic reperfusion can also be observed with systemic thrombolytic therapy (Figure 6.35) and intra-arterial revascularization procedures for acute ischemic stroke [99]. These findings may precede hemorrhagic transformation and may require tight blood pressure control to avoid complications of reperfusion.

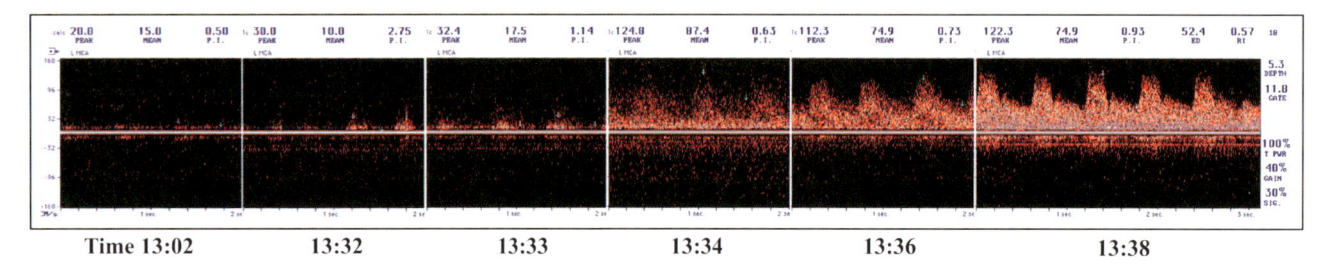

Figure 6.35 Hyperemic reperfusion during the tissue plasminogen activator (tPA) infusion in an acute ischemic stroke patient.

Collateral Patterns and Flow Direction

TCD can directly detect the following collateral channels [18,19,246–250]:

1 anterior cross-filling via the anterior communicating artery (Figure 6.16)
2 posterior communicating artery (Figure 6.36)
3 reversed ophthalmic artery (Figure 6.15) and
4 reversed BA (Figures 6.36 and 6.37).

The intracranial collateral channels are "dormant" under normal circulatory conditions. A collateral channel opens when a pressure gradient develops between the two anastomosing arterial systems. TCD can detect some of these collateral pathways: reversed OA, anterior cross-filling via AComA and PComA flow either to or from the anterior circulation [18,19,99,246–250]. Collateral flow is directed from the donor to the recipient vessels; however, its depiction by ultrasound may be affected by the angle at which the flow was intercepted. When present, collateral flow patterns rarely imply anatomic variants. Most often, detection of a collateral implies the presence of a flow-limiting (i.e. "hemodynamically significant") lesion or an anatomic variant proximal to the recipient arterial system and the origin of the collateral channel.

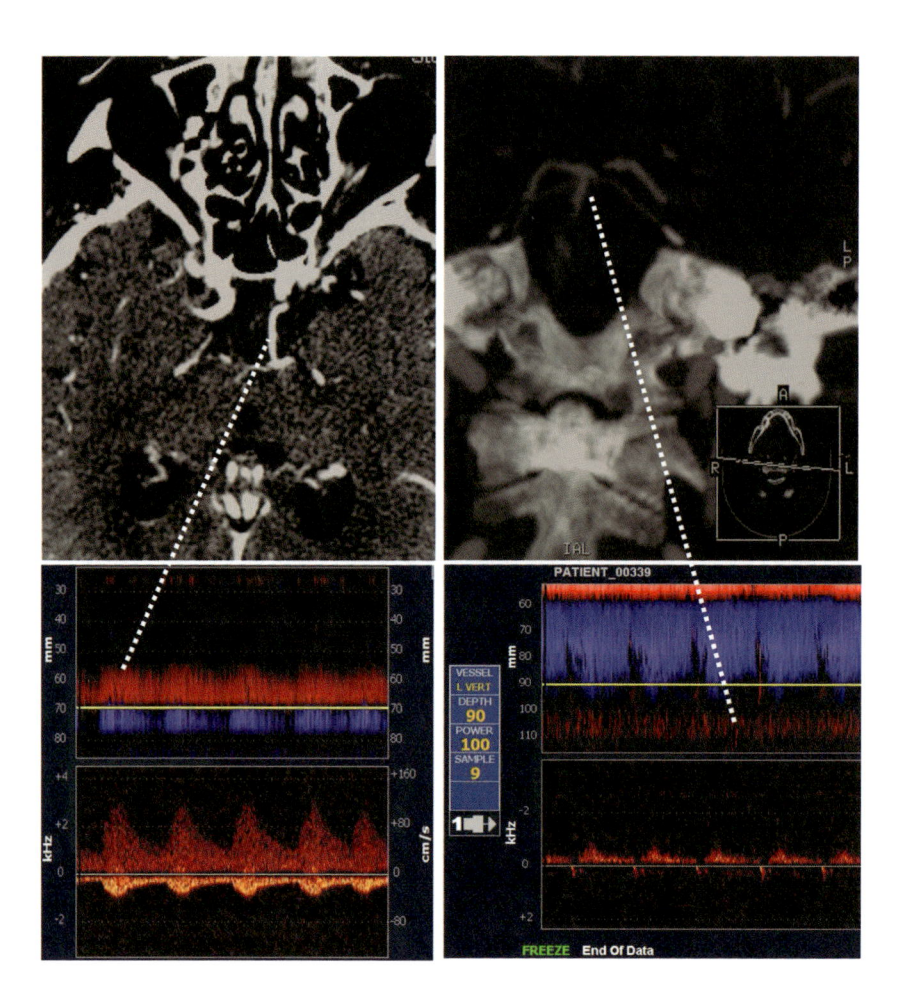

Figure 6.36 The posterior communicating artery (PComA) and the reversed basilar artery on CT–angiography and power motion Doppler.

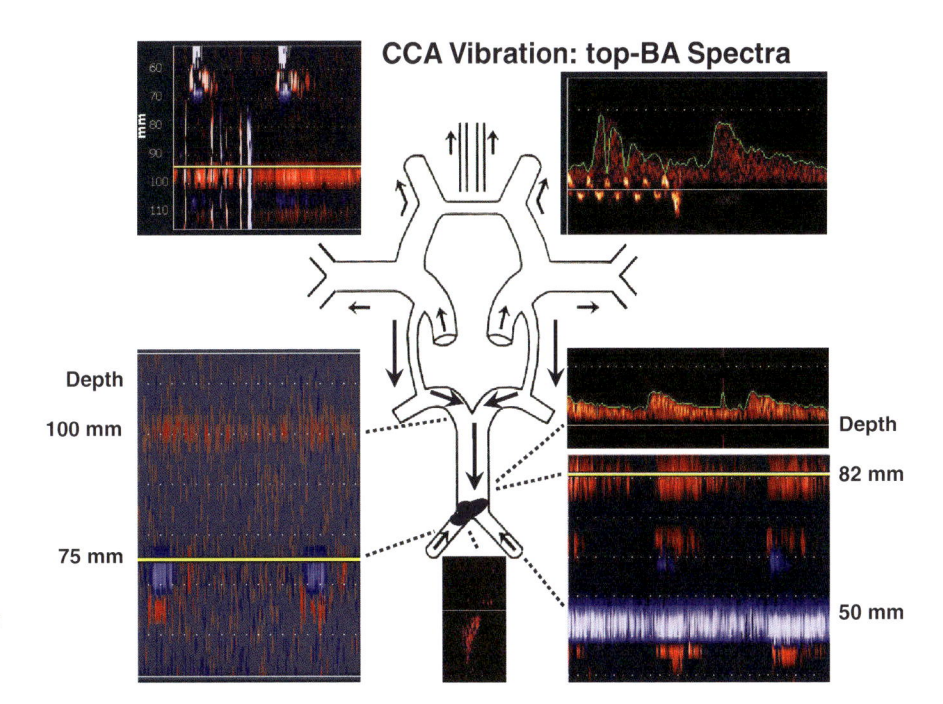

CHAPTER 6 Diagnostic Criteria for Cerebrovascular Ultrasound

Figure 6.37 The reversed basilar artery with the terminal vertebral/proximal basilar occlusion on power motion Doppler.

The direction of flow indicates which arterial system is the *donor* (the source of flow) and which is the *recipient* (the collateral flow destination) [14,99]. TCD provides information on functioning collateral channels and direction of collateral flow. An expanded battery of TCD parameters may be used to refine the evaluation of the severity of ICA lesions, particularly when multiple lesions are found or the applicability of other tests is limited due to the presence of the distal ICA lesions [18–22,99,251–253].

Reversed ophthalmic artery

Primary findings: an abnormal OA signal includes low-pulsatility flow directed primarily away from the probe via transorbital window at 40–60 mm depth (Figure 6.15). Check the vessel identification since an ICA siphon flow signal can be taken in the presence of low velocity OA signals.

Additional findings may include no substantial difference in MFVs detected in the OA and siphon, high velocities in the ICA siphon, suggesting either a high-grade proximal ICA and/or siphon stenosis, and no flow signals at depths ≥60 mm, suggesting an ICA occlusion proximal to OA origin.

Interpretation: If the reversed OA is the only abnormal finding, this indicates possible proximal ICA occlusion or severe stenosis. Occasionally, this may be the only sign of an ICA dissection or occlusion. If a reversed OA is found with a delayed systolic flow acceleration in the unilateral MCA, there is a probable proximal ICA occlusion or severe stenosis and collateralization capacities through the circle of Willis are likely suboptimal (i.e. atretic A1 ACA or absent PComA). If a reversed OA is found with at least one other collateral channel (i.e. partial anterior cross-filling or PComA), there is a definite proximal ICA occlusion or a high-grade stenosis.

Common sources of error include shallow or deep OA insonation, vessel identification problems (vein, branching and anastomosing arteries in the orbit), ICA dissection with considerable residual flow, terminal ICA occlusion distal to the OA origin and retrograde filling of the ICA siphon with normal OA direction. Furthermore, a normal OA direction does not rule out the proximal ICA stenosis.

Anterior communicating artery

Collateral flow through AComA cannot be reliably distinguished from the neighboring A1 and A2 ACA segments due to the smaller AComA length and diameter compared with a large sample volume with which ultrasound intercepts this area. Therefore, we report findings consistent with the anterior cross-filling via AComA as opposed to the velocity and direction of flow in the AComA itself. Sometimes a high-velocity jet with bruit can be found at midline depth, highly suggestive of flow interception through AComA. Even under these circumstances, other flow findings pointing to collateralization of flow should be found since focal velocity elevations can be present with an arterial stenosis as well as collaterals.

Anterior cross-filling:

1 elevated A1 ACA MFVs on the donor side presenting as ACA > MCA and/or donor ACA MFVs >1.2 times greater than contralateral ACA (Figure 6.16);
2 possible stenotic-like flow at 72–78 mm directed away from the donor side;
3 a normal or low MFV in A1 ACA of the recipient side with or without A1 flow reversal.

The *differential diagnosis* includes distal A1 ACA stenosis and compensatory flow increase if one of the A1 segments is atretic. Identification of the reversed A1 segment depends on the skill of the operator. With retrograde filling of the ICA siphon, the terminal ICA can have bi-directional flow. Hence the flow away from the probe (i.e. towards the siphon) may be mistaken for a normal A1 ACA flow direction. A clue to differential diagnosis is that flow velocities tend to be higher the closer one insonates to the donor site. Some advocate common carotid artery compression or vibration to aid decision making (Figure 6.16).

Interpretation: if only elevated donor ACA velocities are found, the differential diagnosis includes A1 ACA stenosis and atresia of the contralateral A1 segment. With the latter, the donor A1 segment supplies both A2 segments (may be present in normal individuals due to anatomic variations of the circle of Willis and also in patients with ICA or MCA obstructive lesions).

1 If an elevated donor ACA velocity is found with stenotic flow at midline depths, the differential diagnosis includes distal A1 stenosis, ICA siphon stenosis and cross-filling via AComA.

2 If an elevated donor ACA MFV is found with a reversed contralateral A1, this indicates probable proximal ICA stenosis.

3 If an elevated donor ACA MFV is found with stenotic-like flow at midline depths and a reversed contralateral A1 ACA, there is a definite proximal ICA stenosis or occlusion.

Posterior communicating artery

PComA connects the posterior and anterior cerebral arterial systems and can be detected by TCD since it usually has a considerable length of >5 mm and a favorable angle of insonation. When functioning, it may be detected as a flow signal consistently present at varying depths from 55 to 70 mm via the transtemporal approach (Figure 6.36). Under normal conditions, this area has no detectable flow when the sonographer switches from the ICA bifurcation posteriorly to locate the PCA (with depth usually set around 60–64 mm). The direction of flow in PComA corresponds to collateralization (Figure 6.36): anterior to posterior collateral flow is directed away from the probe, whereas the posterior to anterior collateral flow is directed towards the probe. Flow direction, however, can be misleading due to the tortuosity of PComA. Without imaging, vessel identification is difficult since the PComA and PCA are prone to anatomic variations.

Collateralization via PComA

Flow signals directed either away from or towards the probe with posterior angulation of the transducer over temporal window are consistently found at 55–70 mm (Figure 6.36). The velocity range is similar to or higher than those detected in the M1 MCA and ICA bifurcation (anterior to posterior collateral flow) or basilar artery (posterior to anterior collateral flow). A possible stenotic-like flow signal may be found at 55–70 mm with similar probe angulation. Elevated velocities can also be found all the way to the top of the basilar (up to 75–80 mm via the trans-temporal approach) and in the P2 PCA segment (usually with an additional transcortical collateralization of flow). The differential diagnosis includes the terminal ICA or PCA stenoses.

Of note, collateralization of flow via PComA carries the systolic flow acceleration signature from the donor site. The posterior-to-anterior circulation flow could have a slight delay in systolic flow acceleration similar to that seen the vertebral arteries, whereas anterior-to-posterior collaterals often have more vertical upstroke similar to that in the ICAs.

Reversed basilar artery

With advantages in transcranial imaging and also power motion Doppler, it became possible to perform more detailed bedside studies of the distal basilar artery in patients with acute posterior circulation strokes. The finding of reversed basilar artery arises from either functional PComA or cerebellar collaterals and could explain often less devastating patient symptoms with the proximal basilar artery occlusion and also better prognosis [18,218]. We use the following criteria to identify the reversed BA (Figures 6.24, 6.36 and 6.37):

1 Detectable flow towards the probe in the basilar artery (low-resistance flow at depths of 80–110 mm).

2 Absence of the antegrade low-resistance basilar flow signals during suboccipital insonation except abnormal TIBI flow grades 0–3 indicating a proximal basilar artery obstruction.

3 Anterior circulation flow origin at the top of the basilar demonstrated by vertical systolic flow acceleration similar to that in the ICAs and also a response to the common carotid tapping (Figure 6.37). Of note, carotid tapping should be performed with caution, preferably after the extracranial ultrasound examination has confirmed the absence of significant stenosis or hypoechoic plaques in the carotid arteries.

Cerebral embolization and detection of right to left shunts

Ultrasound can detect, quantify and localize embolism in real time [254] and TCD can document this process in the cerebral vessels [255–257]. TCD has an established clinical value to monitor stroke patients with presumed cardiac, arterial or paradoxical sources for brain embolization. It can also be used to monitor carotid and cardiac surgery, angioplasty/stenting and intra-arterial rescue procedures in acute stroke. Some institutions use TCD as an established monitoring tool and some still regard this application as investigational.

Most microembolic signals (MES) detected by TCD are asymptomatic since the size of the particles producing them is usually comparable to or even smaller than the diameter of brain capillaries [258]. However, the MES cumulative count is related to the incidence of neuropsychological deficits after cardio-pulmonary bypass [256,259,260], stroke after carotid endarterectomy [257,261–263] and the significance of MES as a risk factor for ischemic stroke is emerging. MES detected with hypoperfusion may be particularly harmful.

It is important to know how to detect and identify MES. Occasionally, a sonographer may be the only witness to cerebral microembolization during a routine examination and this finding may suggest a vascular origin of the neurological event and point to potential sources of embolism (heart chambers and septum, aortic arch, arterial stenosis or dissection, circulating emboli with infection or fat embolism, etc.) [264–271].

Strict standards should be followed when an interpreter documents and reports microemboli on TCD [272]. The gold standard for MES identification still remains the on-line interpretation of real-time, video-taped or digitally stored flow signals [272–274]. The spectral recording should be obtained with minimal gain at a fixed angle of insonation with a small (<10 mm) sample volume. The probe should be maintained with a fixation device during at least 0.5–1 h monitoring. The use of a two-channel simultaneous registration and a prolonged monitoring period may improve the yield of the procedure. Multigated or multiranged registration at different insonation depths may improve differentiation of embolic signals from artifacts. As in fishing, using multiple lines may yield a better catch during the same period of time (Figure 6.38).

According to the International Cerebral Hemodynamics Society definition [275], the microembolic signals (MES) have the following characteristics (Figure 6.38):
1 random occurrence during the cardiac cycle
2 brief duration (usually <0.1 s)
3 high intensity (>3 dB over background)
4 primarily unidirectional signals (if fast Fourier transformation is used)
5 audible component (chirp, pop).

According to Ringelstein and the international panel of experts [272], quality control of studies that report microemboli should include documentation of the following 14 parameters: ultrasound device, transducer frequency, type, size, insonated artery, insonation depth, algorithms for signal intensity measurement, scale settings, detection threshold, axial length of sample volume, fast Fourier transform (FFT) size (number of points used), FFT length (time), FFT overlap, transmitted ultrasound frequency, high-pass filter settings and the recording time. There is an agreement that no current system of automated embolus detection has the required sensitivity and specificity for clinical use. Therefore, the interpreting physician has to review every stored signal, listen to the sound characteristics, determine the difference between the signal and background (dB) and attempt to determine the source of microemboli.

Moehring and Spencer, in their pivotal paper describing the development of PMD, highlighted its potential superiority compared with single-channel TCD in the detection of microembolic flow signatures [276]. Independent prospective studies conducted in neurosonology laboratories of academic centers provided further evidence for this hypothesis. Saqqur *et al.* [277] have developed stringent criteria for tracking embolic flow signatures on PMD track (Table 6.10, Figure 6.38). Their study showed that when compared with spectral TCD, transcranial PMD detected more microbubbles, thereby improving the diagnostic accuracy of PMD in detecting cardiac right-to-left shunts. The reason for the increased yield of microbubble counts with PMD is greater spatial sampling with simultaneous insonation of both MCA and ACA, allowing detection of emboli traveling in either artery before and after the Valsalva maneuver. Interestingly, in a *post hoc* analysis, transcranial PMD continued to show improved microbubble detection when only the MCA counts were assessed.

The potential of PMD to improve emboli counts was also shown in another report where the utility of submandibular extracranial internal carotid artery (ecICA) recording using the PMD was evaluated in comparison with standard MCA insonation [278]. The authors concluded that contrast PMD with cervical ICA recording is at least as sensitive and specific as the traditional MCA method in detecting right-to-left shunts (RLS). Furthermore, this method seemed to be more sensitive for low-volume RLS because of air microbubble decay (9.2%) and entry into

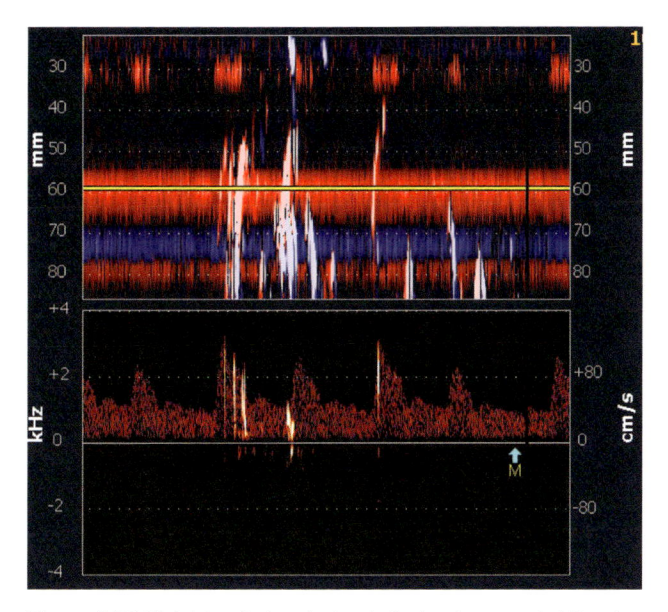

Figure 6.38 High-intensity transient embolic signals on spectral Doppler and power motion Doppler.

Table 6.10 Criteria for counting emboli signals on spectral display of a single-channel TCD [275] and on M-mode display of power motion-mode Doppler (PMD) [277]

Criterion	TCD	PMD
1	Transient, lasting 0.3 s	"Embolic signature" visible at least 3 dB higher than the highest spontaneous PMD display of background blood flow signal
2	≥3 dB higher intensity than that of the highest background flow signal	"Embolic signature" reflects motion in one direction at a minimum spatial extent of 7.5 mm and a minimum temporal extent of 30 ms. An MCA embolic signature is required to move toward the probe, with a positively sloped track (Figure 6.41). An ACA embolic signature moves away from the probe, with a negatively sloped track (Figure 6.41)
3	Uni-directional	The "embolic signature" must tranverse a specific depth determined by the highest intensity of the insonated artery in order to avoid repeated counting of the same embolus
4	Accompanied by snap, chip or moan on the audible output	Not applicable

the ipsilateral ACA (34.2%). This resulted in an increase in detection of RLS grades observed in 32.7% of patients with echocardiography-documented RLS. Based on these striking findings, the authors therefore suggested the incorporation of ecICA PMD not only in patients with poor ultrasonic bone windows but also in every patient being evaluated for suspected RLS. The findings of the former study are in line with an elegant study performed by Spencer *et al.* that compared the sensitivity of PMD TCD and single-gate TCD (sgTCD) to detect contrast bubble emboli through RLS during transcatheter PFO closure [279]. The authors documented that significantly more emboli were detected using PMD than with sgTCD. Based on their findings, they developed a six-level logarithmic scale (Spencer's Logarithmic Scale, SLS) for the grading of RLS (Table 6.11).

SLS grades 3–5 were shown to be highly sensitive and specific in predicting whether a functional PFO was present on transesophageal echocardiography and whether it can be determined with catheterization. Their findings showed that Spencer's grade III–V criteria have a higher positive predictive value in detecting large and functional RLS as compared with ICC (60% vs 32%). Our group has recently prospectively compared the SLS with the International Consensus Criteria (ICC) for the grading of RLS [280]. Our findings confirmed advantages of using SLS criteria since they offer a broader range for grading shunt conductance while being equally sensitive to ICC but more specific to detect large shunts. In our study, the use of SLS grade III or higher for quantification of RLS decreased by more than 50% the number of false-positive TCD diagnoses to predict large RLS on TEE.

Increased intracranial pressure (ICP)

A normal intracranial waveform on TCD reflects the brain being a low-resistance vascular system with low ICP values. When ICP increases up to the diastolic pressure in the resistance vessels, EDV is being affected first as it decreases and flow deceleration occurs more rapidly (Figure 6.39). These changes on TCD are often noted with ICP values of 20 mmHg or higher [281–291]. The following changes can be observed on TCD with increasing ICP:
1 end-diastolic velocity decrease
2 pulsatility index increase (PI ≥ 1.2 for previously normotensive young individuals)
3 resistance index of Pourcellot increase
4 shortening of the trans-systolic time
5 decrease in peak and mean flow velocities
6 abolishment of the end-diastolic flow
7 appearance of reverberating or oscillating flow signals and
8 disappearance of detectable blood flow signals.

When ICP becomes greater than diastolic blood pressure but less than systolic pressure, the result is either a tri-phasic

Table 6.11 Spencer's logarithmic scale for grading right-to-left shunt during bilateral middle cerebral artery (MCA) monitoring [279]

Grade	No. of embolic tracks[a]
0	0
I	1–10
II	11–30
III	31–100
IV	100–300
V	>300

[a]Count of embolic tracks is performed on the PMD display during bilateral MCA monitoring.

CHAPTER 6 Diagnostic Criteria for Cerebrovascular Ultrasound

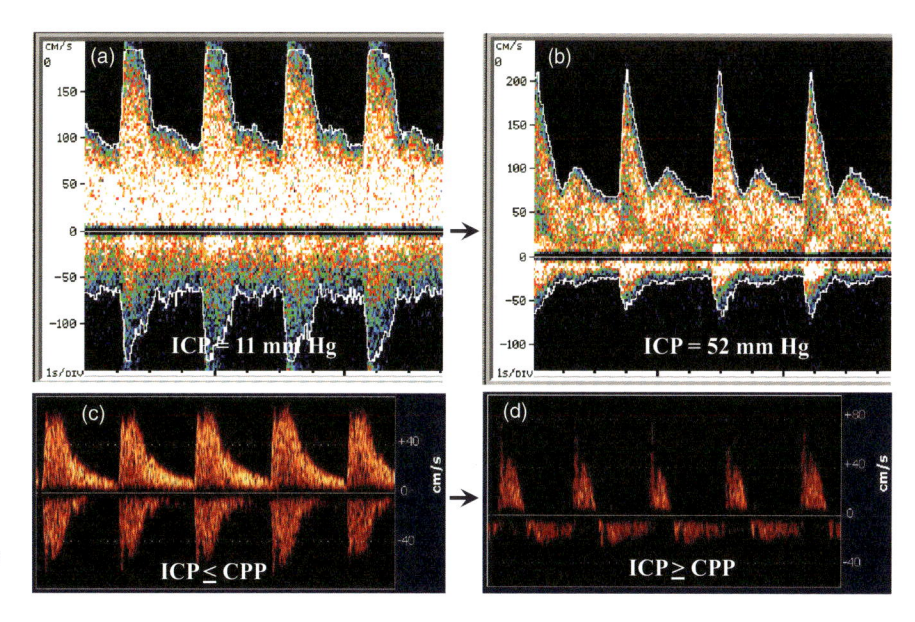

Figure 6.39 Spectral waveform changes with intracranial pressure (ICP).

waveform as seen in the peripheral arteries or a sharply peaked systolic signal and an absent end-diastolic component. Further increase in ICP may lead to cerebral circulatory arrest (this will be discussed in detail below).

Increased ICP may result in high-resistance waveforms: PI ≥ 1.2, decreased or absent EDV, tri-phasic or reverberating flow (Figure 6.39). We use the following algorithm that may help to differentiate among the mechanisms of increased resistance to flow:

If PI ≥ 1.2 and positive end-diastolic flow is present in:

  A. All arteries: hyperventilation; increased cardiac output, hypertension; increased ICP.
  B. Unilateral: compartmental ICP increase; stenoses distal to the site of insonation.
  C. One artery: distal obstruction (spasm, stenosis, edema).

If PI ≥ 2.0 and end-diastolic flow is absent in:

  A. All arteries: distal arterial occlusions; extremely high ICP; possible arrest of cerebral circulation.
  B. Unilateral: compartmental ICP increase, occlusion distal to the site of insonation.
  C. One artery: distal obstruction (occlusion, severe spasm, edema).

Cerebral circulatory arrest

Progressive elevation of ICP due to brain edema or mass effect produces stepwise compression of small and large intracranial arteries, eventually leading to cerebral circulatory arrest (Figure 6.40). A prolonged absence of brain perfusion can be detected using an oscillating (reverberating) flow pattern, systolic spike or absent flow signals [292–305], and this process will lead to brain death [304]. Hence there is a difference in terms of cerebral circulatory arrest (that can be shown by TCD or a nuclear flow scanning) and brain death. The latter is a clinical term with specific diagnostic criteria [304,305].

TCD is a reliable tool to confirm cerebral circulatory arrest with accuracy parameters close to 100% at experienced centers [292–305]. Recently, de Freitas and Andre [306] performed a systematic review of previous studies of TCD in patients with the clinical diagnosis of brain death. The overall sensitivity was 88% and the overall specificity was 98%. The cause of false negatives was attributed to a lack of signal in 7% of cases and persistence of some antegrade flow in the remaining 5%. However, it should be noted that the criteria for brain death were also variable, with only seven groups assessing the vertebrobasilar arteries as part of their TCD scanning protocol and some authors accepting the absence of flow in only one artery as a confirmatory finding.

Based on previous published studies, reviews and criteria [291–306] and our own clinical experience, we developed the following scanning protocol and algorithm if cerebral circulatory arrest is suspected:

1 Document arterial blood pressure at the time of TCD examination.
2 Assess both MCAs (starting depth 50 mm) and BA (80 mm).
3 If positive MCA or BA end-diastolic flow is found = no cerebral circulatory arrest.
4 Absent end-diastolic flow = uncertain cerebral circulatory arrest (too early or too late).

PART III Criteria for Interpretation

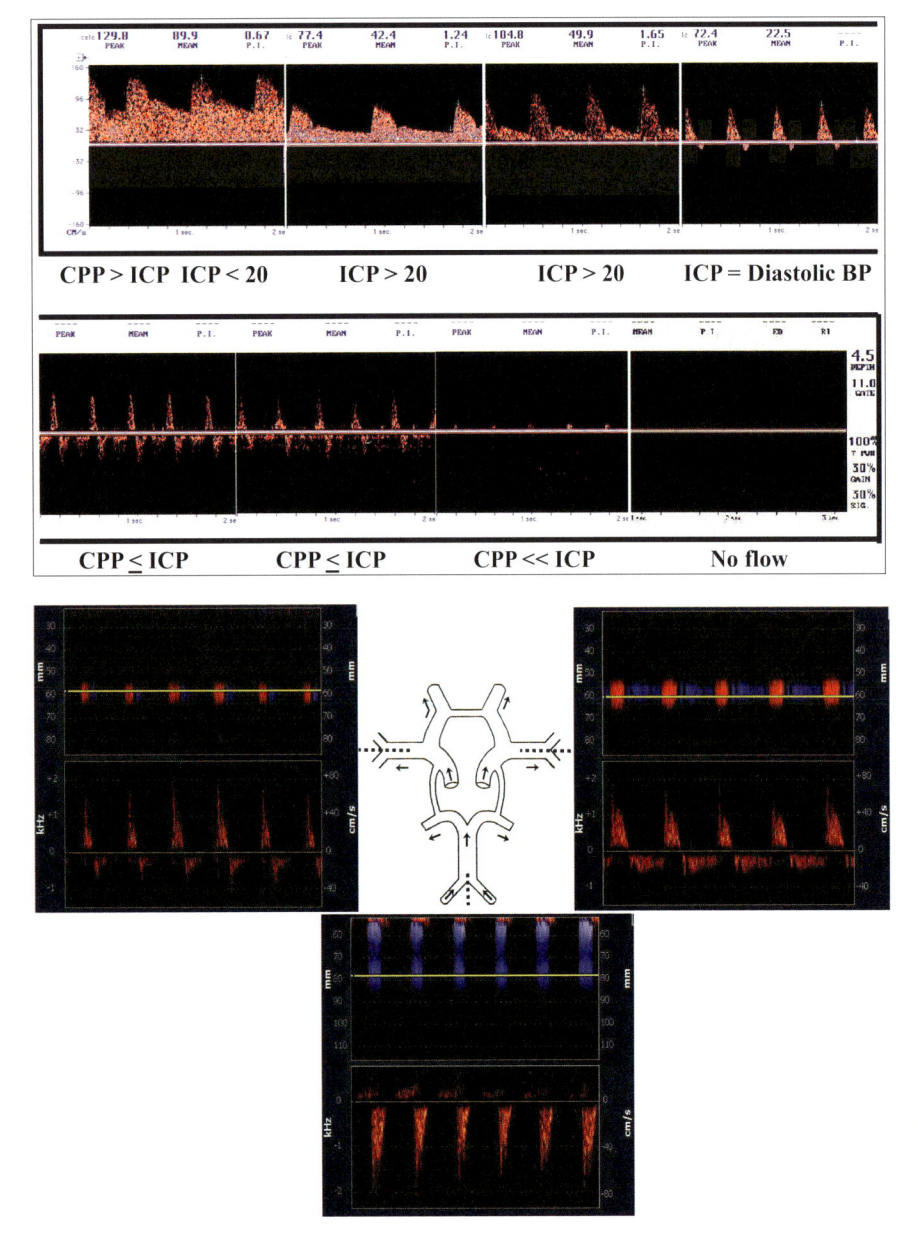

Figure 6.40 TCD findings with progression to cerebral circulatory arrest (upper panel) and a representative case of a complete cerebral circulatory arrest (lower panel).

5 Reversed minimal end-diastolic flow = possible cerebral circulatory arrest (continue monitoring, document diastolic BP ≥50 mmHg).
6 Reverberating flow = probable cerebral circulatory arrest (confirm in both MCAs at 50–60 mm and BA at 80–90 mm, then monitor arrest for 30 min if TCD is used as a sole confirmatory test).

An example of true-positive TCD findings of a complete cerebral circulatory arrest in a patient with clinical examination consistent with brain death is shown in Figure 6.40. TCD can *not* be used to diagnose brain death since this is a clinical diagnosis [305]. TCD can be used to confirm cerebral circulatory arrest in adults and children *except* in infants younger than 6 months [291–303]. TCD can be used to monitor progressive flow changes towards cerebral circulatory arrest. Once a reverberating signal is found, it should be monitored for at least 30 min in the both MCAs and BA to avoid false-positive findings. Also, avoid insonation of bifurcations, i.e. MCA/ACA, since bidirectional reverberating signals may overlap, creating an illusion of positive EDV.

A transient cerebral circulatory arrest can occur in patients with SAH and head trauma due to A-waves of ICP or in other critically ill patients who cannot sustain their cardiac function and diastolic blood pressure drops below 50 mmHg. The latter could lead to absent diastolic flow or reverberating flow signals that would be rapidly replaced by low-resistance flow once BP raises spontaneously or on pressors.

TCD can also be used to determine the appropriate time for other confirmatory tests (i.e. to minimize nuclear flow studies with residual CBF) and to discuss the consequent issues with the patient's family.

Arterial occlusion, recanalization and re-occlusion

The diagnosis of an acute intracranial arterial occlusion with TCD is complex for beginners and may present considerable challenges even to experienced sonographers. TCD yields more information about intracranial thrombus than described in previously published criteria [16,18,19,99,250–252,307–312] and our understanding of the significance of the residual flow around acute occlusion as well as flow diversion and re-modeling is still evolving. Despite this, a good-to-excellent correlation with urgent invasive angiography can be achieved for diagnosis of an acute occlusion at bedside [250–252].

The operator must be experienced and the best results are usually obtained for the M1 MCA, terminal ICA/siphon and basilar artery. The main requirement for confidence in TCD findings is a good window of insonation (or the ability to use imaging or contrast agents) whereby other patent arteries should be identified through the same approach. Initial criteria included no detectable signals at the site of a proximal intracranial occlusion or velocity asymmetry between the homologous segments on TCD in acute ischemic stroke [16,18,19,250–251,306–313].

Since then, ongoing studies showed that a variety of flow signals around the thrombus can be detected [314,315]. To determine the presence of an acute arterial occlusion, it is extremely important to depart from a simplistic concept of asymmetry in flow velocities between affected and non-affected sides (that could largely be attributed to tortuosity, differences in angles of interception and respiratory variations). An acute lesion may represent a complete occlusion, subtotal stenosis or partial, yet hemodynamically significant flow obstruction or near-wall thrombus with the only signs being marginal elevation of velocities and occasional distal microemboli. Instead of relying on velocity measurements in detectable segments, the TCD examiner should pay attention to flow waveforms and signs of flow diversion, collateralization and embolization. This approach leads to a greater yield of abnormal TCD findings that are highly predictive of the presence of a thrombus at urgent angiography [251,314,315].

To achieve better sensitivity to slow and weak flow, a single-gate spectral TCD system should be set at maximum allowed power and large (12–15 mm) sample volume. A PMD/TCD system should be set at a depth range of presumed arterial occlusion and a small (3 mm) spectral TCD sample volume as it allows a higher power output compared with a large (9 mm) PMD/TCD gate.

In at least 75% of cases with acute intracranial occlusions, some residual flow signals can be detected from presumed clot location [314,315]. Waveform morphology discloses more information about clot location, hemodynamic significance of obstruction and resistance in the distal vasculature than velocity difference by itself. Moreover, if the affected MCA has MFV 30% or less than non-affected side and it also has delayed systolic flow acceleration, these findings could point to a proximal ICA obstruction and not necessarily an isolated MCA lesion [16,19,99,316]. As a rule, if any unilateral ICA segment gets involved in a steno-occlusive process or acute thrombo-embolism, there is an incentive to collateralize flow through AComA or PComA and stenotic-range velocities can be found on the contralateral side or posteriorly to the blunted MCA signal [316].

Further waveform analysis of the MCA is required to establish the presence of an additional lesion in the MCA. If diastolic flow disappears at any depth along the MCA course, this strongly suggests the presence of a tandem acute obstruction (Figure 6.20). The presence of the diastolic flow at 65–45 mm depth range could imply patency of small perforating arteries arising from the M1 MCA stem [315]. This finding is often helpful in explaining the distribution of the neurological deficits in the acute stroke patient. Andrew Demchuk with our group developed the Thrombolysis in Brain Infarction (TIBI) flow grading system (Figures 6.41 and 6.42) to predict success of intracranial clot lysis and short-term improvement after ischemic stroke [313]. Detailed TIBI flow definitions are provided in Figure 6.42. For more information, see also Chapter 15.

Both acute and chronic intracranial occlusions can present with TIBI flow grades 0–3 and accurate differentiation may not be possible without imaging of the vessel lumen. An acute occlusion is more likely to be found with recent stroke symptoms or fluctuating neurological deficits and signs of flow diversion and elevated velocities in the branching vessels. A chronic occlusion is often associated with well-developed major collateral channels and absent flow or lower velocities (less flow diversion to branches).

Based on the previous studies [306–312] and our own correlations with invasive angiography, our group described detailed criteria for intracranial occlusions on TCD [209,314–316]. For the diagnosis of the *MCA occlusion*, the abnormal TIBI waveforms 0–3 have to be found between 30 and 65 mm via the transtemporal approach (Figures 6.43–6.45). The presence of positive end-diastolic flow (TIBI grades 2 and 3) implies flow to the nearest branching vessels to the depth at which these were located such as perforators, anterior temporal artery or M2 MCA. Variable anatomy of MCA bifurcations and length of the M1 segment preclude precise definition without imaging which branch(es) could be open.

PART III Criteria for Interpretation

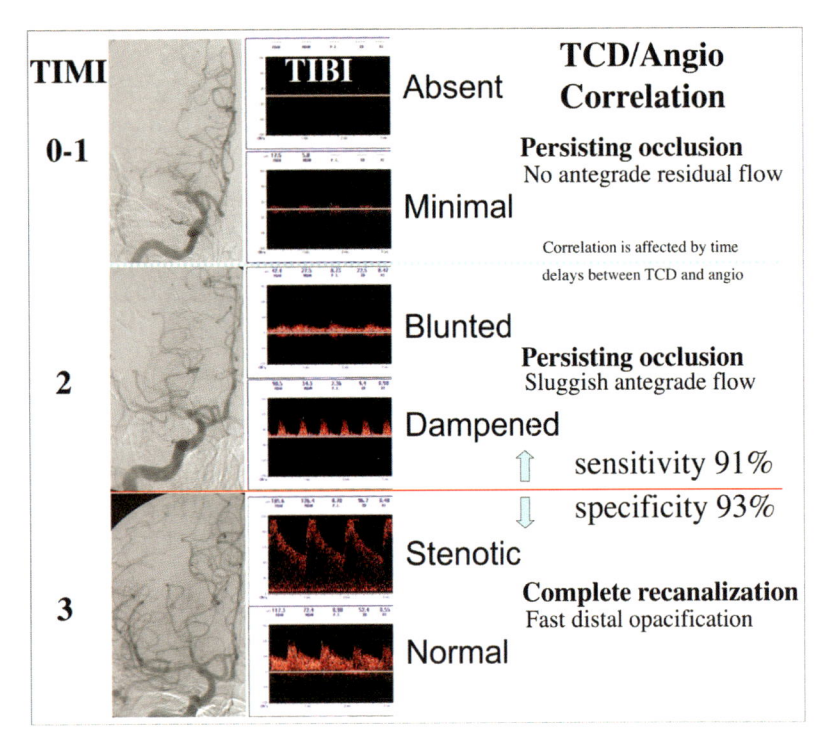

Figure 6.41 Thrombolysis in brain ischemia (TIBI) and thrombolysis in myocardial infarction (TIMI) correlation.

Secondary findings are:
1 a flow diversion/compensatory velocity increase in the unilateral ACA and/or PCA;
2 no flow signals from the ACA and ICA with PCA flow identified (possible "T"-type terminal ICA occlusion);
3 a diastolic flow and overall velocity decrease from the TICA to the distal MCA.

With the *intracranial or terminal ICA occlusion*, TCD findings are dependent on collateralization and the extent of collusion into the MCA such as "T" or "L" types (Figure 6.46). If an extension into the MCA is present, TIBI flow grades 0–2 are usually found with MCA velocities below 20 cm s^{-1} for a TIBI grade 2 blunted flow [316]. If collateralization via AComA is present, there is either partial or complete anterior cross-filling with A1 ACA reversal and retrograde filling of the siphon (Figure 6.47) (see the section on Collaterals).

Besides abnormal TIBI waveforms at 60–70 mm and recruitment of collaterals and contralateral compensatory velocity increases, ICA occlusions above the origin of the ophthalmic artery can also produce a high resistance or dampened ICA siphon signals transorbitally and velocity reduction and pulsatility increase in the proximal ICA on carotid duplex examination. The hallmark of an isolated distal ICA occlusion is the presence of patent proximal ICA on duplex and traceable MCA signals (often blunted with insufficient collaterals) throughout M1–proximal M2 stems and the presence of collateralization of flow indicating a hemodynamically significant lesion in the ICA.

With a *proximal ICA occlusion*, the most common findings include a blunted MCA signal and reversed OA (Figure 6.15) or absent orbital signals from the OA and ICA siphon. TCD by itself cannot differentiate complete ICA occlusion from hemodynamically significant proximal high-grade stenosis and direct carotid examination should be used to answer this question. TCD can help to determine an extension of the proximal ICA occlusion into supraclinoid siphon or terminal ICA, tandem MCA/ICA lesions and the presence of collateral channels.

Secondary findings for an ICA occlusion at any level include:
1 collateral flow in the PComA and/or cross-filling via AComA;
2 contra-lateral ICA compensatory velocity increase;
3 flat MCA waveform (in case of failing collaterals, "trapped" MCA); and
4 possible frequent microemboli in the unilateral TICA or MCA.

TCD is most accurate in the diagnosis of the anterior circulation vessels such as MCA and ICA. The diagnosis of an arterial occlusion at other locations is more difficult and may result in more frequent false-positive and false-negative studies. Using imaging or power motion Doppler can improve the accuracy of ultrasound diagnosis of arterial occlusion beyond MCA or ICA.

With an *occlusion of the basilar artery*, the abnormal waveforms are found either at the distal end of the dominant terminal vertebral artery or at 80–100+ mm via the

TIBI Flow Grade Definitions

For credentialing purposes, interpret flow signals above the baseline. Supporting flow information may be gained from the entire image. For interpretation, assume all images are optimized (i.e. appropriate gain, power, window, angle, sample volume, depth).

0. **Absent**
Absent flow signals are defined by the lack of regular pulsatile flow signals despite varying degree of background noise.

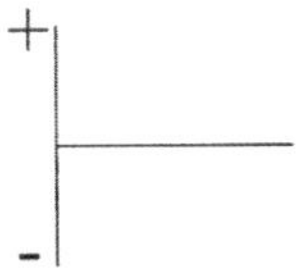

1. **Minimal**
   A- systolic spikes of variable velocity and duration
   B- absent diastolic flow during all cardiac cycles based on a visual interpretation of periods of no flow during end diastoli (ED). Reverberating flow is a type of minimal flow.
   Caution: Despite absent ED flow by visual interpretation, TCD equipment may erroneously report end diastolic (ED) velocity figures due to noise artifacts. Do not rely on machine ED velocity measurements to determine the presence or absence of end diastolic flow.

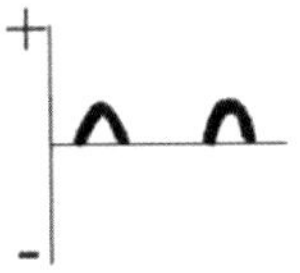

2. **Blunted**
   A- flattened or delayed systolic flow acceleration of variable duration compared to control
   B- positive end diastolic (ED) velocity
   C- a pulsatility index (PI) < 1.2.
   Caution: Flow velocities are usually >20% lower than those in the comparison side.
   Caution: With low velocities, blunted versus minimal signals may be hard to differentiate. Blunted is distinguished by the visual presence of end-diastolic flow.

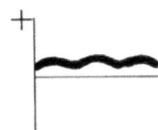

3. **Dampened**
   A- normal systolic flow acceleration
   B- positive end diastolic (ED) velocity
   C- decreased mean velocities by ≥30% compared to control (please calculate if close)
   Caution: With subtle velocity / PI difference, look for dampened waveforms to have a more pulsatile shape
   Caution: Dampened versus blunted signals can be differentiated by dampened having a clear peak systolic complex (initially sharp systolic upstroke without flattening).
   Caution: Dampened versus normal signals can be distinguished by dampened having a more abrupt down-slope of late systoli and early diastoli and other signs of obstruction, i.e. flow diversion (flow velocity ACA > MCA – where flow velocities below the baseline are greater than those above the baseline).

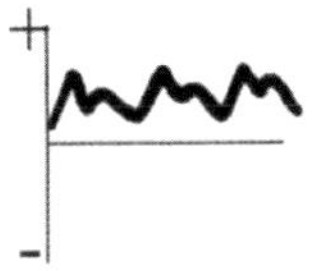

4. **Stenotic**
   A- mean flow velocities of ≥80 cm/s AND velocity difference of ≥30% compared to the control side (please calculate if close); if velocity difference is less than 30%, look for additional signs of stenosis, i.e. turbulence, spectral narrowing
   OR
   B- if both affected and comparison sides have MFV <80 cm/s due to low end-diastolic velocities, mean flow velocities ≥30% compared to the control side (please calculate if close) AND signs of turbulence.

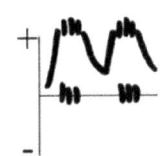

5. **Normal**
   A- <30% mean velocity difference compared to control (please calculate if close)
   B- similar waveform shapes compared to control
   Caution: Hypertensive individuals may have symmetric, high resistance signals with PI ≥ 1.2 and low end-diastolic velocities.
   Caution: Normal versus blunted signals can be differentiated by normal waveforms having initial sharp systolic upstrokse even if the rest of the waveform shows slow deceleration (note slower heart rate).

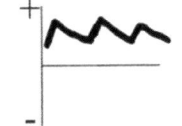

© 2000 Health Outcomes Institute, Inc.

Figure 6.42 Detailed TIBI flow grades definitions.

PART III Criteria for Interpretation

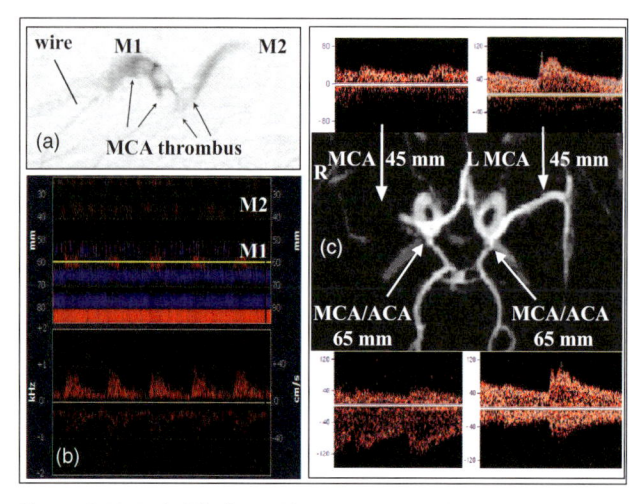

Figure 6.43 Typical findings with an M1 MCA occlusion on TCD, MRA and catheter angiography.

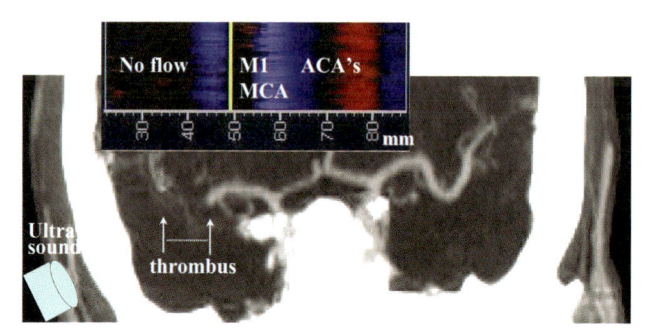

Figure 6.44 A comparison of thrombus location on coronal CT angiogram and residual flow signals on power motion Doppler relative to a trans-temporal aiming of a TCD transducer.

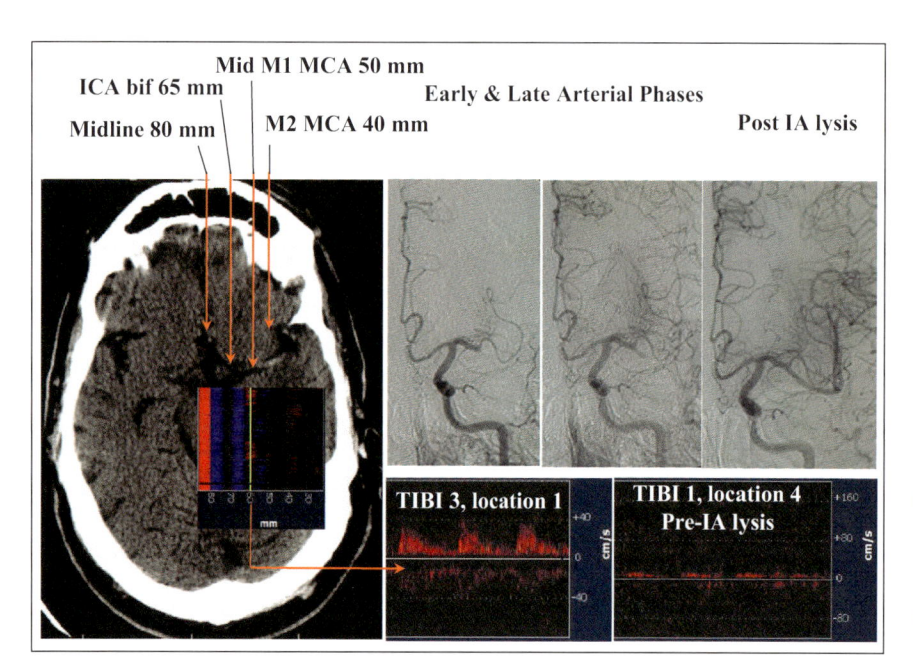

Figure 6.45 A comparison of the MCA thrombus location on non-contrast head CT (hyperdense artery sign), catheter angiography (flow to perforators, distal M1 occlusion) and TIBI waveforms including a positive diastolic flow at the MCA origin.

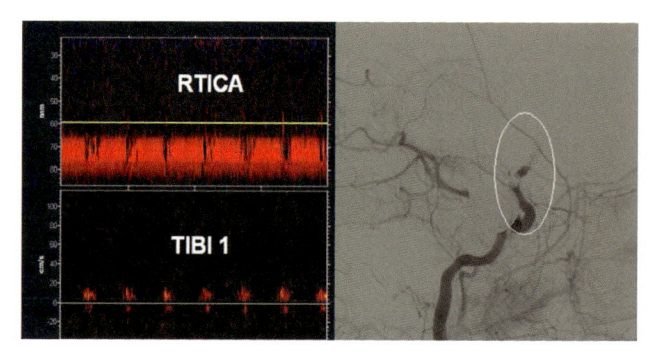

Figure 6.46 Right terminal ICA occlusion on power motion Doppler and catheter angiography. Bottom images courtesy of Dr Disya Ratanakorn.

transforaminal approach (Figures 6.24, 6.36, 6.37 and 6.48). Arbitrarily, proximal BA is located at 80 mm, mid-basilar at 90 mm and distal BA at 100+ mm depth. Typical findings with the mid to distal basilar artery occlusion are shown in Figures 6.36, 6.37 and 6.48.

Secondary findings may include [18,99]:

1 a flow velocity increase in one or both VAs or PICAs, indicating cerebellar collateral flow;
2 a high-resistance flow signal in one or both VAs, indicating proximal BA occlusion;
3 a high-resistance flow signal at the origin of the BA, indicating distal BA occlusion;
4 retrograde (low-resistance, stenotic) flow towards the probe at the top of the BA (proximal BA occlusion collateralized via PComAs);
5 functional PComA(s) with flow directed away from the probe via the temporal window;
6 low distal BA velocities or loss of end-diastolic flow with the top-of-the basilar occlusion.

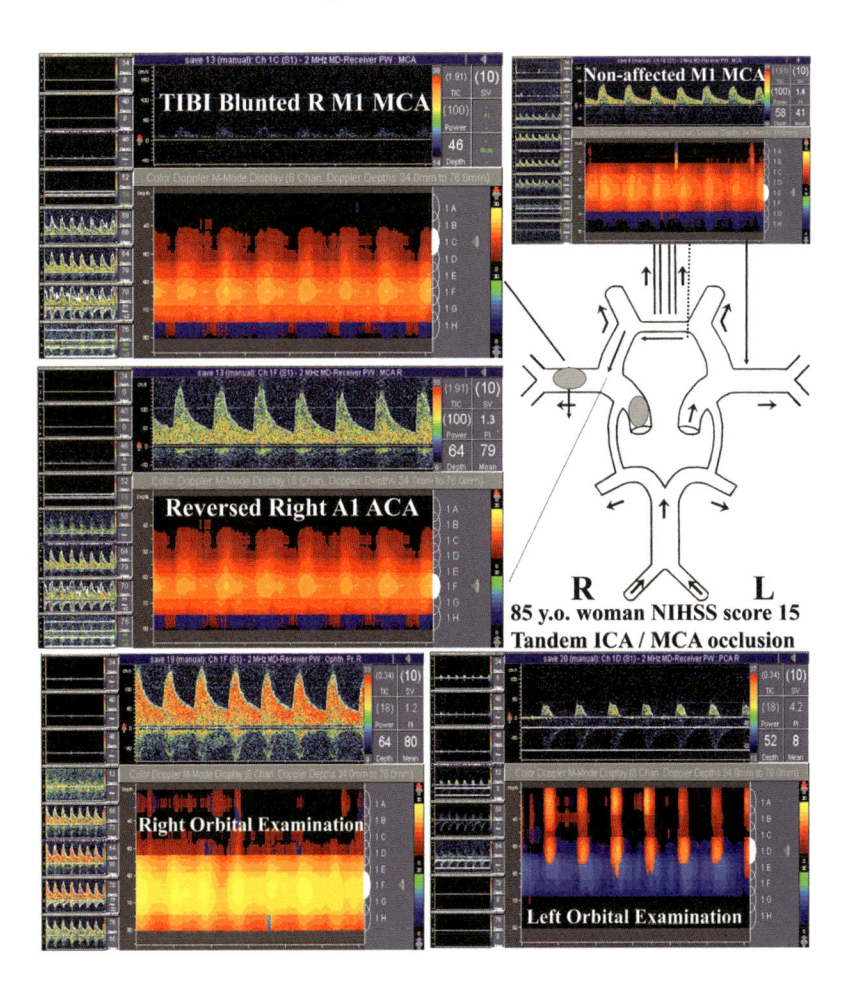

CHAPTER 6 Diagnostic Criteria for Cerebrovascular Ultrasound

Figure 6.47 TCD and motion mode findings in a tandem ICA/MCA acute occlusion.

The TCD diagnosis of the distal basilar occlusion or subtotal stenosis without obvious PComA or flow diversion indicating cross-cerebellar collateral flow is particularly challenging [317,318]. CT–angiography or three-dimensional contrast-enhanced transcranial Doppler or duplex imaging with color and power modes may be techniques of choice if distal basilar occlusion is suspected [317–319]. Special caution must be paid to the situation when only relatively low distal BA velocities are found without any other abnormal findings. In these cases, assessment of the top of the basilar (that can be easily identified on PMD display) using the transtemporal approach may be especially useful in making the correct diagnosis.

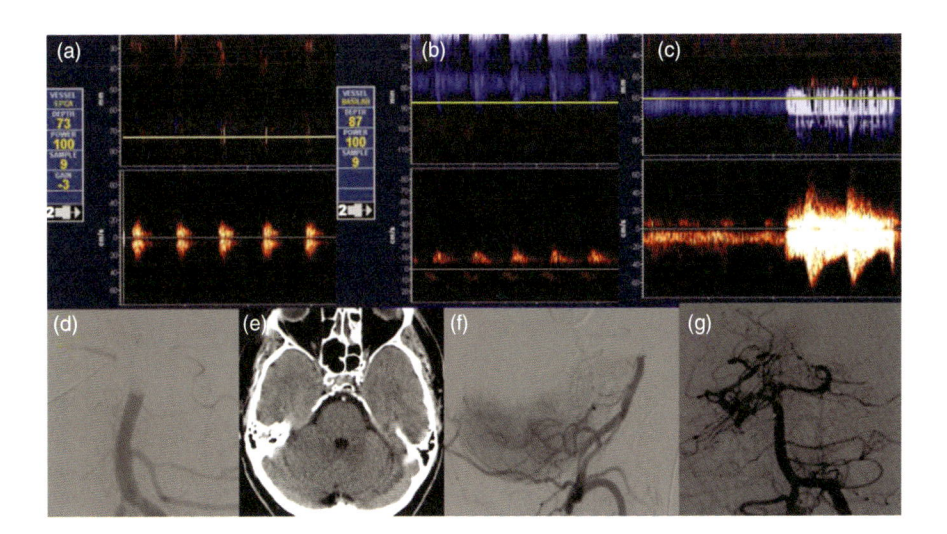

Figure 6.48 Distal basilar artery occlusion and recanalization during intra-arterial thrombolysis.

PART III Criteria for Interpretation

The diagnosis of the intracranial *vertebral artery (VA) occlusion* is difficult to establish using TCD alone, since it:
1 has to be differentiated with atretic terminal VA segment that could be present distal to PICA origin;
2 may present as a short and collateralized occluded segment; and
3 an extracranial segmental VA occlusion may also be present [320].

The most accurate diagnosis with TCD can be made for a terminal VA occlusion [171]; however, the sensitivity of abnormal flow findings is only about 60% [316,320,321]. Normal intracranial TCD examination cannot completely rule out VA occlusion, particularly with a proximal location of a segmental and collateralized VA occlusion or hypoplasia [322]. Secondary findings may include normal flow signals directed towards the probe on the side of occlusion, indicating collateralization of flow from the other side and filling of posterior inferior cerebellar arteries (PICA) as well as distal embolization in the PICA [18]. TCD findings with the vertebral artery occlusion at the skull entrance due to arterial dissection will be considered in the corresponding section.

Any arterial *recanalization* is diagnosed when the residual flow improves by at least one flow grade (i.e. TIBI 1 to TIBI 2) [314,315]. Complete recanalization with or without residual stenosis is diagnosed when the residual flow signals improve to TIBI flow grade 4 or 5. Arterial *re-occlusion* is diagnosed when the TIBI flow grade worsened to 3 or less [323]. Both recanalization and re-occlusion are dynamic processes that can present with transient changes in flow velocity, flow spectral intensity and micro-embolic signals [207,323,324]. Additional findings could include changes in flow pulsatility and velocity in branching vessels [324]. These processes are further discussed in Chapter 15.

Subclavian steal syndrome

Subclavian steal is a hemodynamic condition of reversed flow in one vertebral artery to compensate for a proximal hemodynamic lesion in the unilateral subclavian artery [325,326]. Thus, blood flow is diverted or "stolen" from the brain to feed the arm (Figure 6.49). Subclavian steal is usually an accidental finding since it rarely produces neurological symptoms. If the patient is asymptomatic, it is called the "subclavian steal phenomenon," and it usually indicates a widespread atherosclerosis in aortic branches. If symptoms

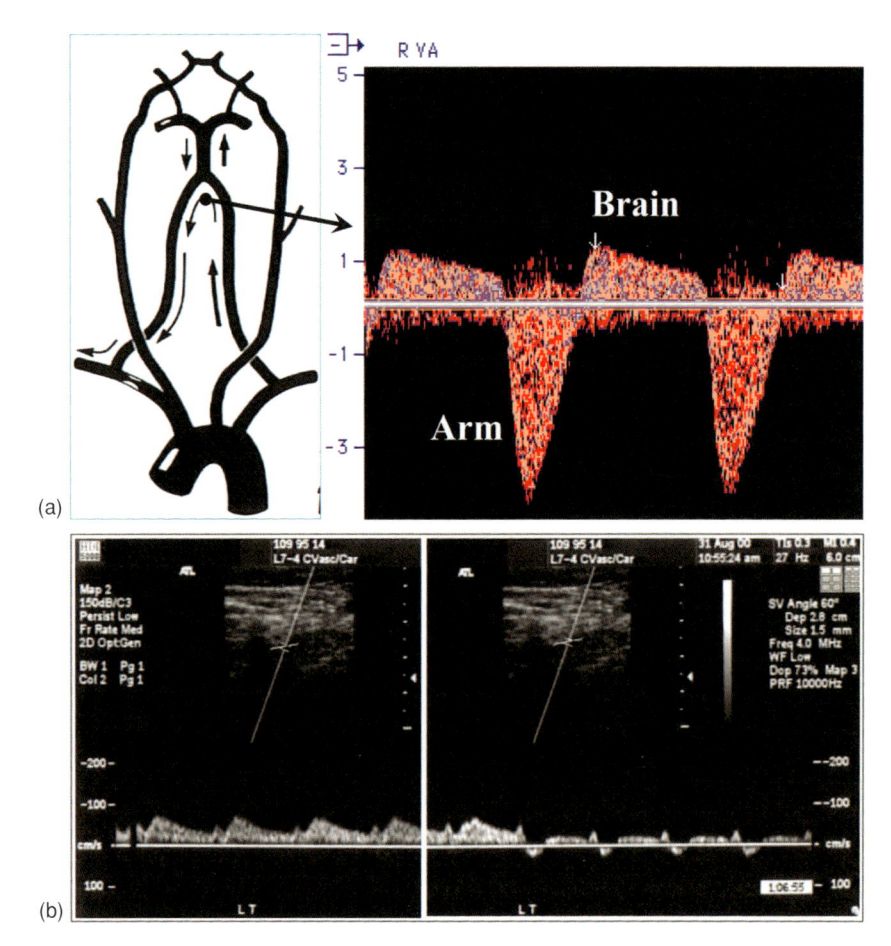

Figure 6.49 Subclavian steal at rest (a) and augmentation with hyperemia cuff test in a patient with latent subclavian steal (b).

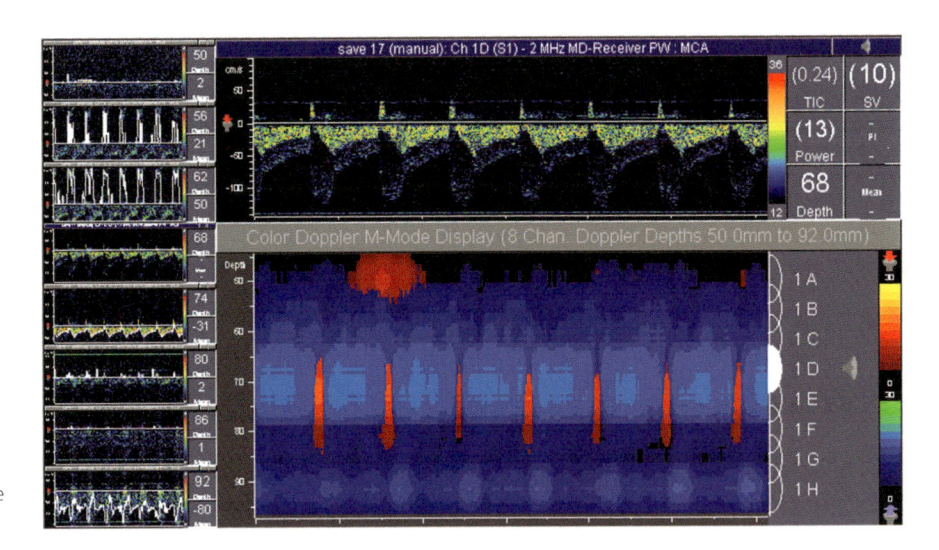

Figure 6.50 Spectral TCD and motion mode findings in subclavian steal.

of vertebro-basilar ischemia are present, it is called "subclavian steal syndrome" [325].

Subclavian steal is well studied with ultrasound [325–346]. When steal is present at rest, the main findings include a difference in blood pressure between arms of ≥20 mmHg and, usually, systolic flow reversal (alternating flow signal or absent diastolic flow) in the "stealing" vertebral artery as well as a low resistance flow in the donor artery. Right to left subclavian steal is found in 85% of cases due to the anatomic differences in the origin of these arteries.

If the BP difference between the arms is 10–20 mmHg and the steal waveforms are not present at rest or flow reversal is incomplete, the hyperemia test should be performed to provoke the steal and to augment flow reversal (Figure 6.49b). The cuff should be inflated to over-systolic BP values and flow reduction to the arm should be maintained about 1–1.5 min (maximum 3 min, if tolerated by patient). This duration of arterial compression produces ischemia in the arm. The cuff should be quickly released and any augmentation of flow should be monitored by TCD. Once the cuff has been released, the blood flow enters tissues with increased metabolic demand produced by a short period of ischemia. Greater demand for blood flow augments the steal and alternating flow can be visualized for a short period of time in the recipient vertebral artery. Recent studies [18,19] have shown that the subclavian steal phenomenon can be easily identified by alternating flow signatures on a motion mode display (Figure 6.50). Of note, however, a differential diagnosis that needs to be kept in mind is dissection of intracranial VA (Figure 6.51).

Reversed Robin Hood syndrome

Neurological deterioration can occur in about 15% of acute stroke patients [347–349]. Several mechanisms can lead to ischemic lesion extension and subsequent neurological worsening, including re-occlusion, edema progression and cardiovascular instability [323,350–352]. However, these long-recognized mechanisms do not account for all cases of neurological deterioration or symptom recurrence. Changes in cerebral hemodynamics can be detected in real time using TCD and several groups, including ours, have deployed this modality to determine predictors of neurological deterioration [348,350–352].

We observed paradoxical decreases in flow velocity during episodes of hypercapnia in vessels supplying ischemic areas of the brain at the time of expected velocity increase in non-affected vessels [353]. Hypercapnia triggered vasodilation more effectively in normal vessels, thus producing arterial blood flow steal towards the path of least resistance (Figure 6.52). The steal magnitude was linked to severity of neurological worsening in acute stroke patients [353,354]. We termed this "reversed Robin Hood" by analogy with "rob the poor to feed the rich" [353]. In the first documented cases of the reversed Robin Hood syndrome, neurological worsening was also more pronounced in patients with sleep apnea [353], a condition that can trigger a perfect storm in an acute stroke patient, while apnea correction can reduce the chances of new vascular events.

Our recently developed criterion for detection of this *hemodynamic steal phenomenon* with TCD [353,354] is as follows:

- MFV decrease in the affected vessel at the time of hypercapnia-induced velocity increase in the normal MCA (Figure 6.52).

The *steal magnitude* (SM, %) is quantified as the maximum negative percentage velocity reduction during breath-holding:

$$SM = [(MFV_m - MFV_b)/MFV_b] \times 100$$

where MFV_m = minimum and MFV_b = baseline MFVs (Figure 6.50).

PART III Criteria for Interpretation

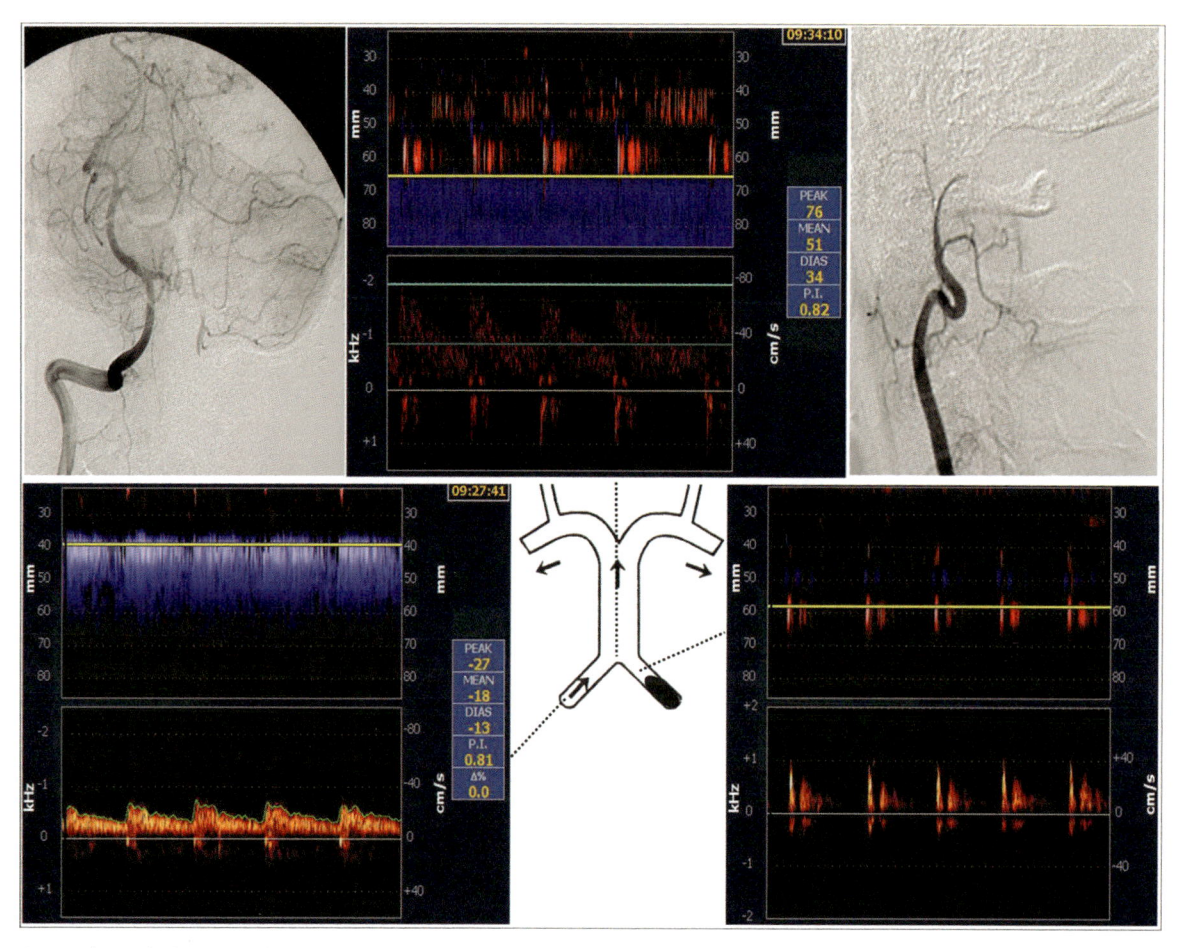

Figure 6.51 Left vertebral artery occlusion due to dissection at the entrance to the skull. Power motion Doppler shows normal patency of the right vertebral and basilar artery and a high resistance signal with absent diastolic flow in the reversed terminal left vertebral artery.

Steal is considered present when SM is negative, i.e. SM < 0, in the affected vessel. After the steal is documented on TCD, reversed Robin Hood syndrome is suspected if new or recurrent neurological worsening by ≥2 National Institutes of Health Stroke Scale (NIHSS) points are observed without concurrent changes in blood pressure (BP) or arterial patency.

Our group recently studied the prevalence of RRHS in a consecutive series of patients with acute cerebral ischemia using the previously developed set of ultrasonographic and clinical criteria. Interestingly, we documented that RRHS and the hemodynamic steal in vessels detectable by TCD can be found in 7 and 14%, respectively, of consecutive patients with stroke without other known causes of deterioration [355]. Patients with persisting arterial occlusions and excessive daytime sleepiness were particularly vulnerable to the steal phenomenon.

The presence of detectable collaterals such as AComA, PComA and reversed OA were also more common in patients with reversed Robin Hood syndrome. This is counterintuitive, at first: collaterals are supposed to protect the brain. However, since the blood follows the path of least resistance, disproportionately large vasodilation on the normal side can diminish flow through collaterals. The more proximal collaterals are, the easier it is to detect the steal. If one is able to assess flow at bifurcations distal to these collaterals in the cerebral vasculature using multi-gate technology (Figure 6.52b), findings of the hemodynamic steal would probably be more common. Figure 6.52b shows spontaneous velocity fluctuations in a patient with the distal M1 MCA occlusion and flow diversion to ACA. If cardiac output or blood pressure decreases, MFV also decreases. In a vessel with normal patency (ACA), this decrease is associated with compensatory vasodilation, as evident from a concurrent PI decrease: MFV 21 to 18 cm s^{-1}; PI 0.82 to 0.67. The residual flow in an acutely obstructed vessel shows an opposite trend in PI: MFV 15 to 11 cm s^{-1}; PI 1.38 to 1.47. In the future, we hope to explore this intracranial steal phenomenon and associated reversed Robin Hood syndrome as the missing links between systemic hemodynamics, ventilation and the fate of ischemic tissue.

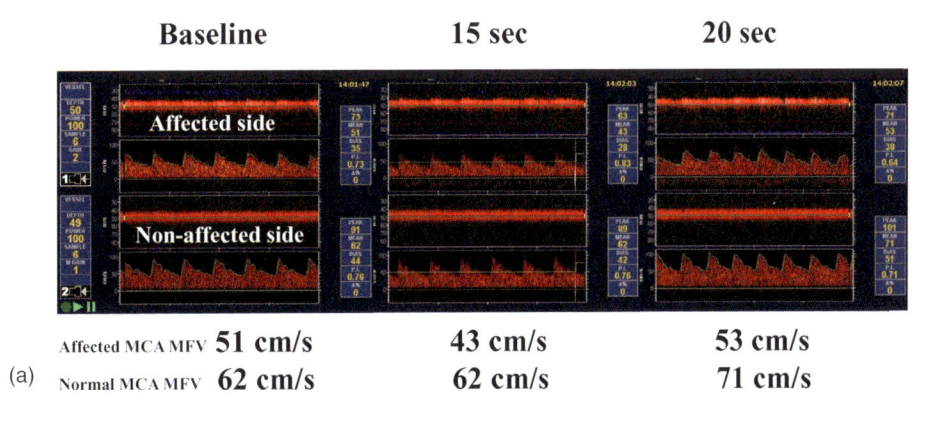

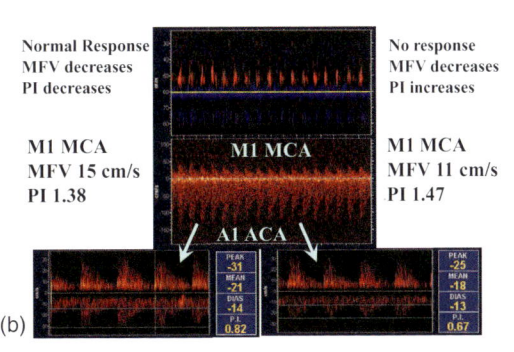

Figure 6.52 Velocity changes with an intracranial steal. Upper panel shows a paradoxical velocity decrease at 15 s of breath-holding in the MCA on the affected side in a patient with reversed Robin Hood syndrome. Normal vasculature responds with velocity increase (bilateral simultaneous MCA monitoring). Lower panel shows flow diversion to ACA in a patient with M1 MCA occlusion. Spontaneous changes in the MCA and ACA velocities can be seen either due to changes in the cardiac output or breathing cycles. When the residual flow velocity in the acutely obstructed MCA decreases from 15 to 11 cm s^{-1}, flow pulsatility remains high, PIs 1.38 to 1.47, respectively. At the same time ACA velocity decreased from 21 to 18 cm s^{-1} and pulsatility also decreased from 0.82 to 0.67. The latter indicates a normal vasomotor response to either a decrease in the cardiac output or a vasodilatory stimulus. This response is absent in the affected MCA and thus preserved vasomotor reactivity in the ACA may augment the impact of transient velocity reductions on the residual flow through the MCA.

Summary of technical findings

After each ultrasound examination, our technologists provide a summary of technical findings that includes key imaging and specific parameter measurements such as velocity and embolic signals. This is an important part of making ultrasound findings available to referring clinicians and, to maximize the agreement between this summary and a subsequent final interpretation by a reading physician, we consistently apply our predefined diagnostic criteria described in this chapter.

The final interpretation

The final interpretation of a non-invasive ultrasound examination should contain, at the minimum:

1 date of the examination
2 clinical indications
3 a description of the test that was performed
4 a statement of the data obtained
5 reasons for limited evaluation (if not complete)
6 interpretation of the ultrasound examination data
7 a comparison with results from previous examinations and
8 clinical implications of this study.

References

1 Intersocietal Commission for the Accreditation of Vascular Laboratories. *Accreditation Material*. Columbia, MD: ICAVL, 2009.
2 Alexandrov AV, Tegeler CH. Diagnostic criteria for transcranial Doppler sonography: a model for quality assurance and laboratory accreditation. *Vasc Ultrasound Today* 1999;**4**:1–24.
3 Guyton AC. *Textbook of Medical Physiology*, 7th edn. Philadelphia, PA: W.B. Saunders, 1986: 209–10.
4 Liepsch D. Principles and models of hemodynamics. In: Hennerici M, Mearis S, eds. *Cerebrovascular Ultrasound: Theory, Practice and Future Developments*. Cambridge: Cambridge University Press, 2001: 27–8.

5 von Reutern GM, Budingen HJ. *Ultrasound Diagnosis of Cerebrovascular Disease*. Stuttgart: Georg Thieme, 1993: 56–62.
6 Toole JF. *Cerebrovascular Disorders*, 4th edn. New York: Raven Press, 1990: 28–49.
7 Perktold K, Karner G. Computational principles and models of hemodynamics. In: Hennerici M, Mearis S, eds. *Cerebrovascular Ultrasound: Theory, Practice and Future Developments*. Cambridge: Cambridge University Press, 2001: 63–76.
8 Glagov S, Bassiouny HS, Zarins CK, *et al*. Morphogenesis of the atherosclerotic plaque. In: Hennerici M, Mearis S, eds. *Cerebrovascular Ultrasound: Theory, Practice and Future Developments*. Cambridge: Cambridge University Press, 2001: 117–33.
9 von Reutern GM, Budingen HJ. *Ultrasound Diagnosis of Cerebrovascular Disease*. Stuttgart: Georg Thieme, 1993: 76–80.
10 Lindegaard KF, Bakke SJ, Grolimund P, *et al*. Assessment of intracranial hemodynamics in carotid artery disease by trasncranial Doppler ultrasound. *J Neurosurg* 1985;**63**:890–898.
11 Hennerici M, Rautenberg W, Schwartz A. Transcranial Doppler ultrasound for the assessment of intracranial arterial flow velocity - Part I. Examination technique and normal values. *Surg Neurol* 1987;**27**:439–48.
12 Adams RJ, Nichols FT, Figueroa R, *et al*. Transcranial Doppler correlation with cerebral angiography in sickle cell disease. *Stroke* 1992;**23**:1073–7.
13 Otis SM, Ringelstein EB. The transcranial Doppler examination: principles and applications of transcranial Doppler sonography. In: Tegeler CH, Babikian VL, Gomez CR, eds. *Neurosonology*. St. Louis, MO: Mosby, 1996: 140–55.
14 Babikian V, Sloan MA, Tegeler CH, *et al*. Transcranial Doppler validation pilot study. *J Neuroimaging* 1993;**3**:242–249.
15 Bragoni M, Feldmann E. *Transcranial Doppler indicies of intracranial hemodynamics*. In: Tegeler CH, Babikian VL, Gomez CR, eds. St. Louis, MO: Mosby, 1996: 129–39.
16 Alexandrov AV, Sloan MA, Wong LK, *et al*.; American Society of Neuroimaging Practice Guidelines Committee. Practice standards for transcranial Doppler ultrasound: Part I – test performance. *J Neuroimaging* 2007;**17**:11–8.
17 Sharma VK, Tsivgoulis G, Lao AY, *et al*. Role of transcranial Doppler ultrasonography in evaluation of patients with cerebrovascular disease. *Curr Neurol Neurosci Rep* 2007;**7**:8–20.
18 Tsivgoulis G, Sharma VK, Hoover SL, *et al*. Applications and advantages of power motion-mode Doppler in acute posterior circulation cerebral ischemia. *Stroke* 2008;**39**:1197–204.
19 Tsivgoulis G, Sharma VK, Lao AY, *et al*. Validation of transcranial Doppler with computed tomography angiography in acute cerebral ischemia. *Stroke* 2007;**38**:1245–9.
20 Tsivgoulis G, Saqqur M, Sharma VK, *et al*.; CLOTBUST Investigators. Association of pretreatment ASPECTS scores with tPA-induced arterial recanalization in acute middle cerebral artery occlusion. *J Neuroimaging* 2008;**18**:56–61.
21 Tsivgoulis G, Saqqur M, Sharma VK, *et al*.; CLOTBUST Investigators. Association of pretreatment blood pressure with tissue plasminogen activator-induced arterial recanalization in acute ischemic stroke. *Stroke* 2007;**38**:961–6.
22 Saqqur M, Hill MD, Alexandrov AV, *et al*. Derivation of power M-mode transcranial Doppler criteria for angiographic proven MCA occlusion. *J Neuroimaging* 2006;**16**:323–8.
23 Gosling RG, King DH. Arterial assessment by Doppler-shift ultrasound. *Proc R Soc Med* 1974;**67**:447–9.
24 Pourcellot L. Applications cliniques de l'examen Doppler transcutane. Les colloques de l'Institut National de la Santé et de la Recherche Medicale. *INSERM* 1974; 213–40.
25 Michel E, Zernikow B. Gosling's pulsatility index revisited. *Ultrasound Med Biol* 1998;**24**:597–9.
26 Stolz E, Kaps M, Kern A, *et al*. Frontal bone windows for transcranial color-coded duplex sonography. *Stroke* 1999;**30**:814–20.
27 North American Symptomatic Carotid Endarterectomy Trial Collaborators. Beneficial effect of carotid endarterectomy in symptomatic patients with high-grade carotid stenosis. *N Engl J Med* 1991;**325**:445–53.
28 European Carotid *Surgery* Trialists' Collaborative Group. Randomised trial of endarterectomy for recently symptomatic carotid stenosis: final results of the MRC European Carotid Surgery Trial (ECST). *Lancet* 1998;**351**:1379–87.
29 Executive Committee of the Asymptomatic Carotid Atherosclerosis Study. Endarterctomy for asymptomatic carotid artery stenosis. *JAMA* 1995;**273**:1421–8.
30 Gomez CR. Carotid angioplasty and stenting: new horizons. *Curr Atheroscler Rep* 2000;**2**:151–9.
31 Gertler JP, Cambria RP, Kistler JP, *et al*. Carotid surgery without arteriography: non-invasive selection of patients. *Ann Vasc Surg* 1991;**5**:253–256.
32 Alexandrov AV, Bladin CF, Maggisano R, *et al*. Measuring carotid stenosis: time for a re-appraisal. *Stroke* 1993;**24**:1292–6.
33 Pan XM, Saloner D, Reilly LM, *et al*. Assessment of carotid artery stenosis by ultrasonography, conventional angiography and magnetic resonance angiography: correlation with ex vivo measurement of plaque stenosis. *J Vasc Surg* 1995;**21**:82–8.
34 Fox AJ. How to measure carotid stenosis? *Radiology* 1993;**186**:316–8.
35 Alexandrov AV, Bladin CF, Murphy J, *et al*. Clinical applicability of methods to measure carotid stenosis. *J Stroke Cerebrovasc Dis* 1994;**4**:258–61.
36 Rothwell PM, Gibson RJ, Slattery J, *et al*. Equivalence of measurements of carotid stenosis. A comparison of three methods on 1001 angiograms. European Carotid Surgery Trialists' Collaborative Group. *Stroke* 1994;**25**:2435–9.
37 Bladin CF, Alexandrov AV, Murphy J, *et al*. Carotid Stenosis Index: a new method of measuring carotid stenosis. *Stroke* 1995;**26**:230–4.
38 Williams MA, Nicolaides AN. Predicting the normal dimensions of the internal and external carotid arteries from the diameter of the common carotid artery. *Eur J Vasc Surg* 1986;**1**:91–6.
39 Alexandrov AV, Brodie DS, McLean A, *et al*. Correlation of peak systolic velocity and angiographic measurement of carotid stenosis revisited. *Stroke* 1997;**28**:339–42.
40 Bladin CF, Alexandrova NA, Murphy J, *et al*. The clinical value of methods to measure carotid stenosis. *Int Angiol* 1996;**16**:252–9.
41 Vanninen RL, Manninen HI, Partanen PK, *et al*. How should we estimate carotid stenosis using magnetic resonance angiography? *Neuroradiology* 1996;**38**:299–305.
42 Fox AJ. How should we estimate carotid stenosis using magnetic resonance angiography? *Neuroradiology* 1997;**39**:532–3.

43 Cumming MJ, Morrow IM. Carotid artery stenosis: a prospective comparison of CT angiography and conventional angiography. *AJR Am J Roentgenol* 1994;**163**:517–523.
44 Bladin C, Alexandrov AV, Norris J. Comparison of the carotid stenosis index with CT angiography. *Stroke* 2007;**38**(10): e100–1.
45 Heiserman JE, Zabramnski JM, Drayer BP, et al. Clinical significance of the flow gap in carotid magnetic resonance angiography. *J Neurosurg* 1996;**85**:384–7.
46 Blakely DD, Oddone EZ, Hasselbad V, et al. Noninvasive carotid artery testing. A meta-analytic review. *Ann Intern Med* 1995;**122**:360–7.
47 Kent KC, Kuntz KM, Patel MR, et al. Perioperative imaging strategies for carotid endarterectomy. An anlysis of morbidity and cost-effectiveness in symptomatic patients. *JAMA* 1995;**274**:888–93.
48 Erdoes LS, Marek JM, Mills JL, et al. The relative contributions of carotid duplex scanning, magnetic resonance angiography and cerebral arteriography to clinical decision making: a prospective study in patients with carotid occlusive disease. *J Vasc Surg* 1996;**23**:950–6.
49 Leclerc X, Godefroy O, Pruvo JP, et al. Computed tomographic angiography for the evaluation of carotid artery disease. *Stroke* 1995;**26**:1577–81.
50 Post K, Eckstein HH, Hoffmann E, et al. The accuracy of angiography and CT angiography of the carotid bifurcation compared with macro-morphological correlation [German]. *Rofo Fortschr Geb Roentgenstr Neuen Bildgeb Verfahr* 1996;**164**:196–200.
51 Link J, Brossman J, Panselin V, et al. Common carotid bifurcation: preliminary results of CT angiography and color-coded duplex sonography compared with digital subtraction angiography. *AJR Am J Roentgenol* 1997;**168**:361–365.
52 Bousser MG. Benefits from carotid surgery? Yes, but ... *Cerebrovasc Dis* 1992;**2**:122–6.
53 Rothwell PM, Pendlebury ST, Wardlaw J, et al. Critical appraisal of the design and reporting of studies of imaging and measurement of carotid stenosis. *Stroke* 2000;**31**:1444–50.
54 Qureshi AI, Alexandrov AV, Tegeler CH, et al.; American Society of Neuroimaging; Society of Vascular and Interventional Neurology. Guidelines for screening of extracranial carotid artery disease: a statement for healthcare professionals from the multidisciplinary practice guidelines committee of the American Society of Neuroimaging; cosponsored by the Society of Vascular and Interventional Neurology. *J Neuroimaging* 2007;**17**:19–47.
55 Comerota AJ, Cranley JJ, Cook SE. Real-time B-mode carotid imaging in diagnosis of cerebrovascular disease. *Surgery* 1981;**89**:718–29.
56 Grant EG, Benson, CB, Moneta, GL, et al. Carotid artery stenosis: gray-scale and Doppler US diagnosis - Society of Radiologists in Ultrasound Consensus Conference. *Radiology* 2003;**229**:340–6.
57 Paivansalo M. Ultrasound terminology. *Eur Med Ultrason* 1984;**6**:3–4.
58 Johnson JM, Kennely M, Decesare D, et al. Natural history of asymptomatic carotid plaque. *Arch Surg* 1985;**120**:1010–2.
59 Ruthlein VM, Spengel FA. Diagnosis of symptomatic plaque in the carotid arteries of patients with neurologic ischemia symptoms [German]. *Bildebung* 1987-9;**56**:19–22.
60 Sterpetti AV, Schultz RD, Feldhaus RJ, et al. Ultrasonic features of carotid plaque and the risk of subsequent neurologic deficits. *Surgery* 1988;**104**:652–60.
61 Gray-Weale AC, Graham JC, Burnett JR, et al. Carotid artery atheroma: comparison of pre-operative B-mode ultrasound appearance with carotid endarterectomy specimen pathology. *J Cardiovasc Surg (Torino)* 1988;**29**:676–81.
62 Widder B, Paulat K, Hackspacher J, et al. Morphological characterization of carotid artery stenoses by duplex scanning. *Ultrasound Med Biol* 1990;**16**:349–354.
63 Geroulakos G, Ramaswami G, Nicolaides A, et al. Characterization of symptomatic and asymptomatic carotid plaques using high-resolution real-time ultrasonography. *Br J Surg* 1993;**80**:1274–7.
64 Polak JF, Shemanski L, O'Leary DH. Hypoechoic plaque at US of the carotid artery: an independent risk factor for incident stroke in adults aged 65 years or older. Cardiovascular Health Study. *Radiology* 1998;**208**:649–54.
65 Sabetai MM, Tegos TJ, Nicolaides AN, et al. Hemispheric symptoms and carotid plaque echomorphology. *J Vasc Surg* 2000;**31**:39–49.
66 el-Barghouty N, Geroulakos G, Nicolaides A, et al. Computer-assisted carotid plaque characterization. *Eur J Vasc Endovasc Surg* 1995;**9**:389–93.
67 Pedro LM, Pedro MM, Goncalves I, et al. Computer-assisted carotid plaque analysis: characteristics of plaques associated with cerebrovascular symptoms and cerebral infarction. *Eur J Vasc Endovasc Surg* 2000;**19**:118–23.
68 Fisher M. Carotid plaque morphology in symptomatic and asymptomatic patients. In: Caplan LR, Shifrin EG, Nicolaides AN, Moore WS, eds. *Cerebrovascular Ischemia: Investigation and Management.* London: Med-Orion, 1996: 19–24.
69 Schulte-Altendorneburg G, Droste DW, Haas N, et al. Preoperative B-mode ultrasound plaque appearance compared with carotid endarterectomy specimen histology. *Acta Neurol Scand* 2000;**101**:188–94.
70 Wolverson MK, Bashiti HM, Peterson GJ. Ultrasonic tissue characterization of atheromatous plaques using a high resolution real time scanner. *Ultrasound Med Biol* 1983;**9**:599–609.
71 O'Leary DH, Holen J, Ricotta JJ, et al. Carotid bifurcation disease: prediction of ulceration with B-mode US. *Radiology* 1987;**162**:523–5.
72 Bluth EI, McVay LV, Merritt CR, et al. The identification of ulcerative plaque with high resolution duplex carotid scanning. *J Ultrasound Med* 1988;**7**:73–6.
73 Tegos TJ, Kalomiris KJ, Sabetai MM, et al. Significance of sonographic tissue and surface characteristics of carotid plaques. *AJNR Am J Neuroradiol* 2001;**22**:1605–12.
74 Steinke W, Els T, Hennerici M. Comparison of flow disturbances in small carotid atheroma using a multi-gate pulsed Doppler and Doppler color flow imaging. *Ultrasound Med Biol* 1992;**18**:11–8.
75 Steinke W, Hennerici M, Rautenberg W, et al. Symptomatic and asymptomatic high-grade carotid stenoses in Doppler color-flow imaging. *Neurology* 1992;**42**:131–8.

76 Steinke W, Mearis S, Reis S, et al. Sonographic assessment of carotid artery stenosis. Comparison of power Doppler imaging and color Doppler flow imaging. Stroke 1996;27:91–4.

77 Sitzer M, Muller W, Rademacher J, et al. Color-flow Doppler-assisted duplex imaging fails to detect ulceration in high grade internal carotid artery stenosis. J Vasc Surg 1996;23:461–5.

78 Droste DW, Karl M, Bohle RM, et al. Comparison of ultrasonic and histopathological features of carotid artery stenosis. Neurol Res 1997;19:380–4.

79 Schminke U, Motsch L, Hilker L, et al. Three-dimensional ultrasound observation of carotid artery plaque ulceration. Stroke 2000;31:1651–5.

80 Mearis S, Hennerici M. Four-dimensional ultrasonographic characterization of plaque surface motion in patients with symptomatic and asymptomatic carotid artery stenosis. Stroke 1999;30:1807–13.

81 Sliwka U, Rother J, Steinke W, et al. The value of duplex sonography in cerebral ischemia [German]. Bildebung 1991;58:182–91.

82 Tschammler A, Landwehr P, Hohmann M, et al. Color-coded duplex sonography of the extracranial arteries supplying the brain: diagnostic significance and sources of error compared in comparison with i.a. DSA. Rofo Fortschr Geb Roentgenstr Neuen Bildgeb Verfahr 1991;155:452–9.

83 Bray JM, Galland F, Lhoste P, et al. Colour Doppler and duplex sonography and angiography of the carotid bifurcations. Prospective, double-blind study. Neuroradiology 1995;37:219–24.

84 Hetzel A, Eckenweber B, Trummer B, et al. Color-coded duplex ultrasound in pre-occlusive stenoses of the internal carotid artery [German]. Ultraschall Med 1993;14:240–6.

85 Steinke W, Reis S, Artemius N, et al. Power Doppler imaging of carotid stenosis. Comparison with color Doppler flow imaging and angiography. Stroke 1997;28:1981–7.

86 Spencer MP, Reid JM. Quantitation of carotid stenosis with continuous wave (C-W) Doppler ultrasound. Stroke 1979;10:793–8.

87 Bendick PJ. Hemodynamics of arterial narrowing and occlusion. J Vasc Tech 1994;18:235–40.

88 Alexandrov AV, Brodie DS, McLean A, et al. Correlation of peak systolic velocity and angiographic measurement of carotid stenosis revisited. Stroke 1997;28:339–42.

89 Widder B, von Reutern GM, Neuerburg-Heusler D. Morphologic and Doppler sonographic criteria for determining the degree of stenosis of the internal carotid artery [German]. Ultraschall Med 1986;7:70–5.

90 AbuRhama AF, Richmond BK, Robinson PA, et al. Effect of contra-lateral severe stenosis or carotid occlusion on duplex criteria of ipsilateral stenoses: comparative study of various duplex parameters. J Vasc Surg 1995;22:751–61.

91 Blackshear WM, Phillips DJ, Chikos PM, et al. Carotid artery velocity patterns in normal and stenotic vessels. Stroke 1980;11:67–71.

92 Moneta GL, Edwards JM, Chitwood RW, et al. Correlation of North American Symptomatic Carotid Endarterectomy Trial (NASCET) angiographic definiton of 70–99% internal carotid stenosis with duplex scanning. J Vasc Surg 1993;17:152–7.

93 Hunink MG, Polak JF, Barlan MM, et al. Detection and quantification of carotid artery stenosis: efficacy of various Doppler velocity parameters. AJR Am J Roentgenol 1993;160:619–25.

94 Soulez G, Therasse E, Robillard P, et al. The value of internal carotid systolic velocity ratio for assessing carotid artery stenosis with Doppler sonography. AJR Am J Roentgenol 1999;172:207–12.

95 Paivansalo M, Leinonen S, Turunen J, et al. Quantification of carotid artery stenosis with various Doppler velocity parameters. Rofo Fortschr Geb Rontgenstr Neuen Bildgeb Verfahr 1996;164:108–13.

96 Neschis DG, Lexa FJ, Davis JT, et al. Duplex criteria for determination of 50% or greater carotid stenosis. J Ultrasound Med. 2001;20:207–15.

97 Ray SA, Lockhart SJ, Dourado R, et al. Effect of contralateral disease on duplex measurements of internal carotid artery stenosis. Br J Surg 2000;87:1057–62.

98 Daigle RJ, Stavros AT, Lee RM. Overestimation of velocity and frequency values by multielement linear array Dopplers. J Vasc Tech 1990;14:206–13.

99 Tsivgoulis G, Alexandrov AV, Sloan MA. Advances in transcranial Doppler sonography. Curr Neurol Neurosci Rep 2009;9:46–54.

100 Blackshear WM, Lamb SL, Kollipara VS, et al. Correlation of hemodynamically significant internal carotid stenosis with pulsed Doppler frequency analysis. Ann Surg 1984;199:475–481.

101 Lindegaard K, Bakke S, Grolimund P, et al. Assessment of intracranial hemodynamics in carotid artery disease by transcranial Doppler ultrasound. J Neurosurg 1985;63:890–8.

102 Schneider P, Rossman M, Bernstein E, et al. Effect of internal carotid artery occlusion on intracranial hemodynamics: transcranial Doppler evaluation and clinical correlation. Stroke 1988;19:589–93.

103 Cantelmo N, Babikian V, Johnson W, et al. Correlation of transcranial Doppler and non-invasive tests with angiography in the evaluation of extracranial carotid disease. J Vasc Surg 1990;11:786–92.

104 Giller CA, Mathews D, Purdy P, et al. The transcranial Doppler appearance of acute carotid artery occlusion. Ann Neurol 1992;31:101–3.

105 Wilterdink JL, Feldmann E, Furie KL, et al. Transcranial Doppler ultrasound battery reliably identifies severe internal carotid artery stenosis. Stroke 1997;28:133–6.

106 Can U, Furie KL, Suwanwela N, et al. Transcranial Doppler ultrasound criteria for hemodynamically significant internal carotid artery stenosis based on residual lumen diameter calculated from en bloc endarterectomy specimens. Stroke 1997;28:1966–71.

107 Christou I, Felberg RA, Demchuk AM, et al. Accuracy parameters of a broad diagnostic battery for bedside transcranial Doppler to detect flow changes with internal carotid artery stenosis or occlusion. J Neuroimaging 2001;11:236–42.

108 Reynolds PS, Greenberg JP, Lien LM, et al. Ophthalmic artery flow direction on color flow duplex imaging is highly specific for sever carotid stenosis. J Neuroimaging 2002;12:5–8.

109 Roederer GO, Langlois Y, Chan AT, *et al.* Post-endarterectomy carotid ultrasonic duplex scanning concordance with contrast angiography. *Ultrasound Med Biol* 1983;**9**:73–8.

110 Robbin ML, Lockhart ME, Weber TM, *et al.* Carotid artery stents: early and intermediate follow-up with Doppler US. *Radiology* 1997;**205**:749–56.

111 AbuRahma AF, Maxwell D, Eads K, *et al.* Carotid duplex velocity criteria revisited for the diagnosis of carotid in-stent restenosis. *Vascular* 2007;**15**:119–25.

112 AbuRahma AF, Abu-Halimah S, Bensenhaver J, *et al.* Optimal carotid duplex velocity criteria for defining the severity of carotid in-stent restenosis. *J Vasc Surg* 2008;**48**:589–94.

113 AbuRahma AF, Richmond BK, Robinson PA, *et al.* Effect of contralateral severe stenosis or carotid occlusion on duplex criteria of ipsilateral stenoses: comparative study of various duplex parameters. *J Vasc Surg* 1995;**22**:751–61.

114 Ray SA, Lockhart SJ, Dourado R, *et al.* Effect of contralateral disease on duplex measurements of internal carotid artery stenosis. *Br J Surg* 2000;**87**:1057–62.

115 Rouleau PA, Huston J III, Gilbertson J, *et al.* Carotid artery tandem lesions: frequency of angiographic detection and consequences for endarterectomy. *AJNR Am J Neuroradiol* 1999;**20**:621–5.

116 Day AL, Rhoton AL, Quisling RG. Resolving siphon stenosis following endarterectomy. *Stroke* 1980;**11**:278–81.

117 Guppy KH, Charbel FT, Loth F, *et al.* Hemodynamics of in-tandem stenosis of the internal carotid artery: when is carotid endarterectomy indicated? *Surg Neurol* 2000;**54**: 145–52.

118 Sitzer M, Furst G, Siebler M, *et al.* Usefulness of an intravenous contrast medium in the characterization of high-grade internal carotid stenosis with color Doppler-assisted duplex imaging. *Stroke* 1994;**25**:385–9.

119 Furst G, Saleh A, Wenserski F, *et al.* Reliability and validity of non-invasive imaging of internal carotid artery pseudo-occlusion. *Stroke* 1999;**30**:1444–9.

120 Ferrer JM, Samso JJ, Serrando JR, *et al.* Use of ultrasound contrast in the diagnosis of carotid artery occlusion. *J Vasc Surg* 2000;**31**:736–41.

121 Jung EM, Kubale R, Clevert DA, *et al.* B-flow and contrast medium-enhanced power Doppler (Optison(R)) – preoperative diagnosis of high-grade stenosis of the internal carotid artery [German]. *Rofo Fortschr Geb Rontgenstr Neuen Bildgeb Verfahr* 2002;**174**:62–9.

122 Maroon JC, Campbell RL, Dyken ML. Internal carotid artery occlusion diagnosed by Doppler ultrasound. *Stroke* 1970;**1**:122–7.

123 Muller HR. The diagnosis of internal carotid artery occlusion by directional Doppler sonography of the ophthalmic artery. *Neurology* 1972;**22**:816–23.

124 Hill SL, Christie A, McDannald ER, *et al.* Noninvasive differentiation of carotid artery occlusion from high-grade stenosis. *Am Surg* 1987;**53**:84–93.

125 Bodily KC, Phillips DJ, Thiele BL, *et al.* Noninvasive detection of internal carotid artery occlusion. *Angiology* 1981;**32**: 517–21.

126 Ringelstein EB, Zeumer H, Angelou D. The pathogenesis of strokes from internal carotid artery occlusion. Diagnostic and therapeutic implications. *Stroke* 1983;**14**:867–75.

127 Bishop CC, Powell S, Insall M, *et al.* Effect of internal carotid artery occlusion on middle cerebral artery blood flow at rest and in response to hypercapnia. *Lancet* 1986;**i**:710–2.

128 Schneider PA, Rossman ME, Bernstein EF, *et al.* Effect of internal carotid artery occlusion on intracranial hemodynamics. Transcranial Doppler evaluation and clinical correlation. *Stroke* 1988;**19**:589–93.

129 Giller CA, Steig P, Batjer HH, *et al.* Transcranial Doppler ultrasound as a guide to graded therapeutic occlusion of the carotid artery. *Neurosurgery* 1990;**26**:307–11.

130 Kuwert T, Hennerici M, Langen KJ, *et al.* Compensatory mechanisms in patients with asymptomatic carotid artery occlusion. *Neurol Res* 1990;**12**:89–93.

131 Yasaka M, Omae T, Tsuchiya T, *et al.* Ultrasonic evaluation of the site of carotid axis occlusion in patients with acute cardioembolic stroke. *Stroke* 1992;**23**:420–2.

132 Lee TH, Ryu SJ, Chen ST, *et al.* Comparison between carotid duplex sonography and angiography in the diagnosis of extracranial internal carotid artery occlusion. *J Formos Med Assoc* 1992;**91**:575–9.

133 Hetzel A, Eckenweber B, Trummer B, *et al.* Color-coded duplex ultrasound in pre-occlusive stenoses of the internal carotid artery [German]. *Ultraschall Med* 1993;**14**(5): 240–6.

134 Muller M, Hermes M, Bruckmann H, *et al.* Transcranial Doppler ultrasound in the evaluation of collateral blood flow in patients with internal carotid artery occlusion: correlation with cerebral angiography. *AJNR Am J Neuroradiol* 1995;**16**:195–202.

135 AbuRahma AF, Pollack JA, Robinson PA, *et al.* The reliability of color duplex ultrasound in diagnosing total carotid artery occlusion. *Am J Surg* 1997;**174**:185–7.

136 Lee TH, Ryu SJ, Chen ST, *et al.* Carotid ultrasonographic findings in intracranial internal carotid artery occlusion. *Angiology* 1993;**44**:607–13.

137 Kimura K, Yonemura K, Terasaki T, *et al.* Duplex carotid sonography in distinguishing acute unilateral atherothrombotic from cardioembolic carotid artery occlusion. *AJNR Am J Neuroradiol* 1997;**18**:1447–52.

138 Delcker A, Diener HC, Wilhelm H. Source of cerebral microembolic signals in occlusion of the internal carotid artery. *J Neurol* 1997;**244**:312–7.

139 Kimura K, Yasaka M, Minematsu K, *et al.* Oscillating thromboemboli within the extracranial internal carotid artery demonstrated by ultrasonography in patients with acute cardioembolic stroke. *Ultrasound Med Biol* 1998;**24**:1121–4.

140 Eudo M, de Bray JM. Floating thrombus in the carotid [French]. *J Radiol* 2000;**81**:1713–4.

141 Sharma VK, Tsivgoulis G, Lao AY, *et al.* Thrombotic occlusion of the common carotid artery (CCA) in acute ischemic stroke treated with intravenous tissue plasminogen activator (TPA). *Eur J Neurol* 2007;**14**:237–40.

142 de Bray JM, Dubas F, Joseph PA, *et al.* Ultrasonic study of 22 cases of carotid artery dissection. *Rev Neurol (Paris)* 1989;**145**(10): 702–9.

143 Hennerici M, Steinke W, Rautenberg W. High-resistance Doppler flow pattern in extracranial carotid dissection. *Arch Neurol* 1989;**46**:670–2.

144 Kaps M, Dorndorf W, Damian MS, *et al.* Intracranial haemodynamics in patients with spontaneous carotid dissection.

Transcranial Doppler ultrasound follow-up studies. *Eur Arch Psychiatry Neurol Sci* 1990;**239**:246–56.

145 Steinke W, Schwartz A, Hennerici M. Doppler color flow imaging of common carotid artery dissection. *Neuroradiology* 1990;**32**:502–5.

146 Sturzenegger M. Ultrasound findings in spontaneous carotid artery dissection. The value of duplex sonography. *Arch Neurol* 1991;**48**:1057–63.

147 de Bray JM, Lhoste P, Dubas F, et al. Ultrasonic features of extracranial carotid dissections: 47 cases studied by angiography. *J Ultrasound Med* 1994;**13**:659–64.

148 Steinke W, Rautenberg W, Schwartz A, et al. Noninvasive monitoring of internal carotid artery dissection. *Stroke* 1994;**25**:998–1005.

149 Desfontaines P, Despland PA. Dissection of the internal carotid artery: aetiology, symptomatology, clinical and neurosonological follow-up and treatment in 60 consecutive cases. *Acta Neurol Belg* 1995;**95**(4): 226–34.

150 Sturzenegger M, Mattle HP, Rivoir A, et al. Ultrasound findings in carotid artery dissection: analysis of 43 patients. *Neurology* 1995;**45**:691–8.

151 Babikian VL, Forteza AM, Gavrilescu T, et al. Cerebral microembolism and extracranial internal carotid artery dissection. *J Ultrasound Med* 1996;**15**:863–6.

152 Srinivasan J, Newell DW, Sturzenegger M, et al. Transcranial Doppler in the evaluation of internal carotid artery dissection. *Stroke* 1996;**27**:1226–30.

153 Bassetti C, Carruzzo A, Sturzenegger M, et al. Recurrence of cervical artery dissection. A prospective study of 81 patients. *Stroke* 1996;**27**:1804–7.

154 Koennecke HC, Trocio SH Jr, Mast H, et al. Microemboli on transcranial Doppler in patients with spontaneous carotid artery dissection. *J Neuroimaging* 1997;**7**:217–20.

155 Giroud M, Lemesle M, Madinier G, et al. Stroke in children under 16 years of age. Clinical and etiological difference with adults. *Acta Neurol Scand* 1997;**96**:401–6.

156 Rommel O, Niedeggen A, Tegenthoff M, et al. Carotid and vertebral artery injury following severe head or cervical spine trauma. *Cerebrovasc Dis* 1999;**9**:202–9.

157 Sidhu PS, Chauduri KR, Khaw KT. Moyamoya disease mimicking a spontaneous internal carotid artery dissection on Doppler ultrasound. *Eur Radiol* 2000;**10**:149–53.

158 O'Dwyer JA, Moscow N, Trevor R, et al. Spontaneous dissection of the carotid artery. *Radiology* 1980;**137**:379–85.

159 Houser OW, Mokri B, Sundt TM Jr, et al. Spontaneous cervical cephalic arterial dissection and its residuum: angiographic spectrum. *AJNR Am J Neuroradiol* 1984;**5**:27–34.

160 Mokri B, Sundt TM Jr, Houser OW, et al. Spontaneous dissection of the cervical internal carotid artery. *Ann Neurol* 1986;**19**:126–38.

161 Baumgartner RW, Arnold M, Baumgartner I, et al. Carotid dissection with and without ischemic events: local symptoms and cerebral artery findings. *Neurology* 2001;**57**:827–32.

162 Beletsky V, Norris JW. Spontaneous dissection of the carotid and vertebral arteries. *N Engl J Med* 2001;**345**:467.

163 Markwalder TM, Starrett RW, Mumenthaler M. Spontaneous bilateral recanalization in bilateral internal carotid artery occlusion. *Stroke* 1980;**11**:95–8.

164 Bogousslavsky J, Regli F, Despland PA. Spontaneous dissecting aneurysms of the internal carotid artery. Prospective evaluation of the prognosis and arterial repermeation in 14 cases [French]. *Rev Neurol* 1984;**140**:625–36.

165 Kasner SE, Hankins LL, Bratina P, et al. Magnetic resonance angiography demonstrates vascular healing of carotid and vertebral artery dissections. *Stroke* 1997;**28**:1993–7.

166 Engelter ST, Lyrer PA, Kirsch EC, et al. Long-term follow-up after extracranial internal carotid artery dissection. *Eur Neurol* 2000;**44**:199–204.

167 Ringelstein EB, Zeumer H, Hundgen R, et al. Angiologic and prognostic evaluation of brain stem injuries. Clinical, Doppler-sonographic and neuroradiological findings [German]. *Dtsch Med Wochenschr* 1983;**108**:1625–31.

168 Davis PC, Nilsen B, Braun IF, et al. A prospective comparison of duplex sonography vs angiography of the vertebral arteries. *AJNR Am J Neuroradiol* 1986;**7**:1059–64.

169 Winter R, Biedert S, Staudacher T, et al. Vertebral artery Doppler sonography. *Eur Arch Psychiatry Neurol Sci* 1987; **237**:21–8.

170 Touboul PJ, Mas JL, Bousser MG, et al. Duplex scanning in extracranial vertebral artery dissection. *Stroke* 1988;**19**:116–21.

171 De Bray JM, Blard JM, Tachot C, et al. Transcranial Doppler ultrasonic examination in vertebro-basilar circulatory pathology [French]. *Mal Vasc* 1989;**14**:202–5.

172 Delcker A, Diener HC. The value of color duplex for sonography of the vertebral artery [German]. *Vasa Suppl* 1991; **33**:204–5.

173 Bartels E. Duplex sonography of the vertebral arteries. 2. Clinical application [German]. *Ultraschall Med* 1991;**12**(2): 63–9.

174 Trattnig S, Schwaighofer B, Hubsch P, et al. Color-coded Doppler sonography of vertebral arteries. *J Ultrasound Med* 1991;**10**:221–6.

175 Schneider PA, Rossman ME, Bernstein EF, et al. Noninvasive evaluation of vertebrobasilar insufficiency. *J Ultrasound Med* 1991;**10**:373–9.

176 Bartels E, Fuchs HH, Flugel KA. Duplex ultrasonography of vertebral arteries: examination, technique, normal values and clinical applications. *Angiology* 1992;**43**(3 Pt 1): 169–80.

177 Delcker A, Diener HC, Timmann D, et al. The role of vertebral and internal carotid artery disease in the pathogenesis of vertebrobasilar transient ischemic attacks. *Eur Arch Psychiatry Clin Neurosci* 1993;**242**:179–83.

178 Sturzenegger M, Mattle HP, Rivoir A, et al. Ultrasound findings in spontaneous extracranial vertebral artery dissection. *Stroke* 1993;**24**:1910–21.

179 Bartels E, Flugel KA. Evaluation of extracranial vertebral artery dissection with duplex color-flow imaging. *Stroke* 1996; **27**:290–5.

180 de Bray JM, Missoum A, Dubas F, et al. Detection of vertebrobasilar intracranial stenoses: transcranial Doppler sonography versus angiography. *J Ultrasound Med* 1997;**16**:213–8.

181 de Bray JM, Penisson-Besnier I, Dubas F, et al. Extracranial and intracranial vertebrobasilar dissections: diagnosis and prognosis. *J Neurol Neurosurg Psychiatry* 1997;**63**:46–51.

182 de Bray JM, Pasco A, Tranquart F, et al. Accuracy of color-Doppler in the quantification of proximal vertebral artery stenoses. *Cerebrovasc Dis* 2001;**11**:335–40.

183 Droste DW, Junker K, Stogbauer F, et al. Clinically silent circulating microemboli in 20 patients with carotid or vertebral artery dissection. *Cerebrovasc Dis* 2001;**12**:181–5.

184 Caplan LR, Amarenco P, Rosengart A, et al. Embolism from vertebral artery origin occlusive disease. *Neurology* 1992;**42**:1505–12.

185 Bartels E. *Color-Coded Duplex Ultrasonography of the Cerebral Vessels*. Stuttgart: Schattauer; 1999: 118.

186 Nicolau C, Gilabert R, Garcia A, et al. Effect of internal carotid artery occlusion on vertebral artery blood flow: a duplex ultrasonographic evaluation. *Ultrasound Med* 2001;**20**:105–11.

187 Oder B, Oder W, Lang W, et al. Hypoplasia, stenosis and other alterations of the vertebral artery: does impaired blood rheology manifest a hidden disease? *Acta Neurol Scand* 1998;**97**:398–403.

188 Besson G, Vallee B, Mimassi N, et al. Disabling segmental occlusion of the vertebral artery. Surgical treatment using a venous by pass from the external carotid to the C1-C2 portion if the vertebral artery (2 cases) [French]. *Neurochirurgie* 1981;**27**:59–64.

189 Lindegaard KF, Bakke SJ, Aaslid R, et al. Doppler diagnosis of intracranial artery occlusive disorders. *J Neurol Neurosurg Psychiatry* 1986;**49**:510–8.

190 de Bray JM, Joseph PA, Jeanvoine H, et al. Transcranial Doppler evaluation of middle cerebral artery stenosis. *J Ultrasound Med* 1988;**7**:611–6.

191 Ley-Pozo J, Ringelstein EB. Noninvasive detection of occlusive disease of the carotid siphon and middle cerebral artery. *Ann Neurol* 1990;**28**:640–7.

192 Schwarze JJ, Babikian V, DeWitt LD, et al. Longitudinal monitoring of intracranial arterial stenoses with transcranial Doppler ultrasonography. *J Neuroimaging* 1994;**4**:182–7.

193 Rother J, Schwartz A, Rautenberg W, et al. Middle cerebral artery stenoses: assessment by magnetic resonance angiography and transcranial Doppler ultrasound. *Cerebrovasc Dis* 1994;**4**:273–9.

194 Alexandrov AV, Bladin CF, Norris JW. Intracranial blood flow velocities in acute ischemic stroke. *Stroke* 1994;**25**:1378–83.

195 Wong KS, Li H, Lam WW, et al. Progression of middle cerebral artery occlusive disease and its relationship with further vascular events after stroke. *Stroke* 2002;**33**(2): 532–6.

196 Segura T, Serena J, Castellanos M, et al. Embolism in acute middle cerebral artery stenosis. *Neurology* 2001;**56**:497–501.

197 Arenillas JF, Molina CA, Montaner J, et al. Progression and clinical recurrence of symptomatic middle cerebral artery stenosis: a long-term follow-up transcranial Doppler ultrasound study. *Stroke* 2001;**32**:2898–904.

198 Felberg RA, Christou I, Demchuk AM, et al. Screening for intracranial stenosis with transcranial Doppler: the accuracy of mean flow velocity thresholds. *J Neuroimaging* 2002;**12**:9–14.

199 Mattle H, Grolimund P, Huber P, et al. Transcranial Doppler sonographic findings in middle cerebral artery disease. *Arch Neurol* 1988;**45**:289–95.

200 Brass LM, Duterte DL, Mohr JP. Anterior cerebral artery velocity changes in disease of the middle cerebral artery stem. *Stroke* 1989;**20**:1737–40.

201 Navarro JC, Lao AY, Sharma VK, et al. The accuracy of transcranial Doppler in the diagnosis of middle cerebral artery stenosis. *Cerebrovasc Dis* 2007;**23**:325–30.

202 Monsein LH, Razumovsky AY, Ackerman SJ, et al. Validation of transcranial Doppler ultrasound with a stereotactic neurosurgical technique. *J Neurosurg* 1995;**82**:972–5.

203 Aaslid R. *Transcranial Doppler Sonography*. Vienna: Springer, 1986: 39–59.

204 Chimowitz MI, Kokkinos J, Strong J, et al. The Warfarin-Aspirin Symptomatic Intracranial Disease Study. *Neurology* 1995;**45**:1488–93.

205 Adams RJ, McKie V, Nichols F, et al. The use of transcranial ultrasonography to predict stroke in sickle cell disease. *N Engl J Med* 1992;**326**:605–10.

206 Alexandrov AV, Demchuk AM, et al. Yield of transcranial Doppler in acute cerebral ischemia. *Stroke* 1999;**30**:1604–9.

207 Alexandrov AV, Demchuk AM, Felberg RA, et al. Intracranial clot dissolution is associated with embolic signals on transcranial Doppler. *J Neuroimaging* 2000;**10**:27–32.

208 Hennerici M, Rautenberg W, Schwartz A. Transcranial Doppler ultrasound for the assessment of intracranial arterial flow velocity – Part 2. Evaluation of intracranial arterial disease. *Surg Neurol* 1987;**27**:523–32.

209 Demchuk AM, Christou I, Wein TH, et al. Specific transcranial Doppler flow findings related to the presence and site of arterial occlusion with transcranial Doppler. *Stroke* 2000;**31**:140–6.

210 Steinke W, Mangold J, Schwartz A, et al. Mechanisms of infarction in the superficial posterior cerebral artery territory. *J Neurol* 1997;**244**:571–8.

211 Kimura K, Minematsu K, Yasaka M, et al. Evaluation of posterior cerebral artery flow velocity by transcranial color-coded real-time sonography. *Ultrasound Med Biol* 2000;**26**:195–9.

212 Ringelstein EB. Ultrasonic diagnosis of the vertebrobasilar system. II. Transnuchal diagnosis of intracranial vertebrobasilar stenoses using a novel pulsed Doppler system [German]. *Ultraschall Med* 1985;**6**:60–67.

213 Budingen HJ, Staudacher T. Identification of the basilar artery with transcranial Doppler sonography [German]. *Ultraschall Med* 1987;**8**:95–101.

214 Volc D, Possnigg G, Grisold W, et al. Transcranial Doppler sonography of the vertebro-basilar system. *Acta Neurochir (Wien)* 1988;**90**:136–8.

215 Alexandrov AV. Transcranial Doppler sonography: principles, examination technique and normal values. *Vasc Ultrasound Today* 1998;**3**:141–60.

216 Droste DW, Nabavi DG, Kemeny V, et al. Echocontrast enhanced transcranial colour-coded duplex offers improved visualization of the vertebrobasilar system. *Acta Neurol Scand* 1998;**98**:193–9.

217 Postert T, Federlein J, Przuntek H, et al. Power-based versus conventional transcranial color-coded duplex sonography in the assessment of the vertebrobasilar-posterior system. *J Stroke Cerebrovasc Dis* 1997;**6**:398–404.

218 Ribo M, Garami Z, Uchino K, et al. Detection of reversed basilar flow with power-motion Doppler after acute occlusion predicts favorable outcome. *Stroke* 2004;**35**:79–82.

219 Baumgartner RW, Mattle HP, Schroth G. Assessment of ≥50% and <50% intracranial stenoses by transcranial color-coded duplex sonography. *Stroke* 1999;**30**:87–92.

220 Stroke Outcomes and Neuroimaging of Intracranial Atherosclerosis (SONIA) Trial Investigators. Stroke outcome and neuroimaging of intracranial atherosclerosis (SONIA): design of a prospective, multicenter trial of diagnostic tests. *Neuroepidemiology* 2004;**23**:23–32.

221 Otis SM, Ringelstein EB. The transcranial Doppler examination: principles and applications of transcranial Doppler sonography. In: Tegeler CH, Babikian VL, Gomez CR, eds. *Neurosonology*. St. Louis, MO: Mosby, 1996: 140–55.

222 Hennerici M, Neuerburg-Heusler D. *Vascular Diagnosis With Ultrasound: Clinical References with Case Studies*. Stuttgart: Georg Thieme, 1998: 96.

223 Feldmann E, Wilterdink JL, Kosinski A, et al.; The Stroke Outcomes and Neuroimaging of Intracranial Atherosclerosis (SONIA) Trial Investigators. The Stroke Outcomes and Neuroimaging of Intracranial Atherosclerosis (SONIA) trial. *Neurology* 2007;**68**:2099–106.

224 Sloan MA. Transcranial Doppler monitoring of vasospasm after subarachnoid hemorrhage. In: Tegeler CH, Babikian VL, Gomez CR, eds. *Neurosonology*. St. Louis, MO: Mosby, 1996: 156–71.

225 Lindegaard KF, Nornes H, Bakke SJ, et al. Cerebral vasospasm after subarachnoid haemorrhage investigated by means of transcranial Doppler ultrasound. *Acta Neurochir (Wien)* 1988; **42**(Suppl): P81–4.

226 Newell DW, Grady MS, Eskridge JM, et al. Distribution of angiographic vasospasm after subarachnoid hemorrhage: implications for diagnosis by transcranial Doppler ultrasonography. *Neurosurgery* 1990;**27**:574–7.

227 Awad IA, Carter LP, Spetzler RF, et al. Clinical vasospasm after subarachnoid hemorrhage: response to hypervolemic hemodilution and arterial hypertension. *Stroke* 1987;**18**:365–72.

228 Kontos HA. Validity of cerebral arterial blood flow calculations from velocity measurements. *Stroke* 1989; **20**:1–3.

229 Mizuno M, Nakajima S, Sampei T, et al. Serial transcranial Doppler flow velocity and cerebral blood flow measurements for evaluation of cerebral vasospasm after subarachnoid hemorrhage. *Neurol Med Chir (Tokyo)* 1994;**34**:164–71.

230 Sloan MA, Haley EC Jr, Kassell NF, et al. Sensitivity and specificity of transcranial Doppler ultrasonography in the diagnosis of vasospasm following subarachnoid hemorrhage. *Neurology* 1989;**39**:1514–8.

231 Newell DW, Winn HR. Transcranial Doppler in cerebral vasospasm. *Neurosurg Clin N Am* 1990;**1**:319–28.

232 Lindegaard KF. The role of transcranial Doppler in the management of patients with subarachnoid haemorrhage: a review. *Acta Neurochir Suppl* 1999;**72**:59–71.

233 Lysakowski C, Walder B, Costanza MC, et al. Transcranial Doppler versus angiography in patients with vasospasm due to a ruptured cerebral aneurysm: a systematic review. *Stroke* 2001;**32**:2292–8.

234 Wozniak MA, Sloan MA, Rothman MI, et al. Detection of vasospasm by transcranial Doppler sonography. The challenges of the anterior and posterior cerebral arteries. *J Neuroimaging* 1996;**6**:87–93.

235 Sloan MA, Alexandrov AV, Tegeler CH, et al. Therapeutics and Technology Assessment Subcommittee of the American Academy of Neurology. Assessment: transcranial Doppler ultrasonography: report of the Therapeutics and Technology Assessment Subcommittee of the American Academy of Neurology. *Neurology* 2004;**62**:1468–81.

236 Soustiel JF, Shik V, Shreiber R, et al. Basilar vasospasm diagnosis: investigation of a modified Lindegaard Index based on imaging studies and blood velocity measurements of the basilar artery. *Stroke* 2002;**33**:72–7.

237 Sviri GE, Lewis DH, Correa R, et al. Basilar artery vasospasm and delayed posterior circulation ischemia after aneurysmal subarachnoid hemorrhage. *Stroke* 2004;**35**:1867–72.

238 Sviri GE, Ghodke B, Britz GW, et al. Transcranial Doppler grading criteria for basilar artery vasospasm. *Neurosurgery* 2006;**59**:360–6.

239 Piepgras A, Hagen T, Schmiadek P. Reliable prediction of grade of angiographic vasospasm by transcranial Doppler sonography. *Stroke* 1994;**25**:260 [Abstract].

240 Giller CA, Hatab MR, Giller AM. Estimation of vessel flow and diameter during cerebral vasospasm using transcranial Doppler indices. *Neurosurgery* 1998;**42**:1076–81.

241 Reigel MM, Hollier LH, Sundt TM Jr, et al. Cerebral hyperperfusion syndrome: a cause of neurologic dysfunction after carotid endarterectomy. *J Vasc Surg* 1987;**5**:628–34.

242 Powers AD, Smith RR. Hyperperfusion syndrome after carotid endarterectomy: a transcranial Doppler evaluation. *Neurosurgery* 1990;**26**:56–9.

243 Schoser BG, Heesen C, Eckert B, et al. Cerebral hyperperfusion injury after percutaneous transluminal angioplasty of extracranial arteries. *J Neurol* 1997;**244**:101–4.

244 Dalman JE, Beenakkers IC, Moll FL, et al. Transcranial Doppler monitoring during carotid endarterectomy helps to identify patients at risk of postoperative hyperperfusion. *Eur J Vasc Endovasc Surg* 1999;**18**:222–7.

245 Spencer MP. Transcranial Doppler monitoring and causes of stroke from carotid endarterectomy. *Stroke* 1997;**28**:685–91.

246 Padayachee TS, Kirkham FJ, Lewis RR, et al. Transcranial measurement of blood velocities in the basal cerebral arteries using pulsed Doppler ultrasound: a method of assessing the circle of Willis. *Ultrasound Med Biol* 1986;**12**:5–14.

247 Bass A, Krupski WC, Dilley RB, et al. Comparison of transcranial and cervical continuous-wave Doppler in the evaluation of intracranial collateral circulation. *Stroke* 1990;**21**:1584–8.

248 Byrd S, Wolfe J, Nicolaides A, et al. Vascular surgical society of Great Britain and Ireland: transcranial doppler ultrasonography as a predictor of haemodynamically significant carotid stenosis. *Br J Surg* 1999;**86**:692–3.

249 Schneider PA, Rossman ME, Bernstein EF, et al. Noninvasive assessment of cerebral collateral blood supply through the ophthalmic artery. *Stroke* 1991;**22**:31–6.

250 Rutgers DR, Klijn CJ, Kappelle LJ, et al. A longitudinal study of collateral flow patterns in the circle of Willis and the ophthalmic artery in patients with a symptomatic internal carotid artery occlusion. *Stroke* 2000;**31**:1913–20.

251 Chernyshev OY, Garami Z, Calleja S, et al. Yield and accuracy of urgent combined carotid/transcranial ultrasound testing in acute cerebral ischemia. *Stroke* 2005;**36**:32–7.

252 Saqqur M, Tsivgoulis G, Molina CA, et al.; CLOTBUST Investigators. Symptomatic intracerebral hemorrhage and recanalization after IV rt-PA: a multicenter study. *Neurology* 2008;**71**:1304–12.

253 Saqqur M, Tsivgoulis G, Molina CA, et al.; CLOTBUST-PRO Investigators. Design of a PROspective multi-national CLOTBUST collaboration on reperfusion therapies for stroke (CLOTBUST-PRO). *Int J Stroke* 2008;**3**(1): 66–72.

254 Spencer MP, Campbell SD, Sealey JL, et al. Experiments on decompression bubbles in the circulation using ultrasonic and electromagnetic flowmeters. *J Occup Med* 1969;**11**:238–44.

255 Padayachee TS, Gosling RG, Bishop CC, et al. Transcranial measurement of blood velocities in the basal cerebral arteries using pulsed Doppler ultrasound: a method of assessing the circle of Willis. *Ultrasound Med Biol* 1986;**12**:5–14.

256 Deverall PB, Padayachee TS, Parsons S, et al. Ultrasound detection of micro-emboli in the middle cerebral artery during cardiopulmonary bypass surgery. *Eur J Cardiothorac Surg* 1988;**2**:256–60.

257 Spencer MP, Thomas GI, Nicholls SC, et al. Detection of middle cerebral artery emboli during carotid endarterectomy using transcranial Doppler ultrasonography. *Stroke* 1990;**21**:415–23.

258 Russell D. The detection of cerebral emboli using Doppler ultrasound. In: Newell DW, Aaslid R, eds. *Transcranial Doppler*. New York: Raven Press, 1992: 52–8.

259 Clark RE, Brillman J, Davis DA, et al. Microemboli during coronary artery bypass grafting. Genesis and effect on outcome. *J Thorac Cardiovasc Surg* 1995;**109**:249–57.

260 Diegeler A, Hirsch R, Schneider F, et al. Neuromonitoring and neurocognitive outcome in off-pump versus conventional coronary bypass operation. *Ann Thorac Surg* 2000;**69**: 1162–6.

261 Jansen C, Moll FL, Vermeulen FE, et al. Continuous transcranial Doppler ultrasonography and electroencephalography during carotid endarterectomy: a multimodal monitoring system to detect intraoperative ischemia. *Ann Vasc Surg* 1993;**7**:95–101.

262 Ackerstaff RG, Jansen C, Moll FL, et al. The significance of microemboli detection by means of transcranial Doppler ultrasonography monitoring in carotid endarterectomy. *J Vasc Surg* 1995;**21**:963–9.

263 Ackerstaff RG, Moons KG, van de Vlasakker CJ, et al. Association of intraoperative transcranial Doppler monitoring variables with stroke from carotid endarterectomy. *Stroke* 2000;**31**:1817–23.

264 Georgiadis D, Grosset DG, Kelman A, et al. Prevalence and characteristics of intracranial microemboli signals in patients with different types of prosthetic cardiac valves. *Stroke* 1994;**25**:587–92.

265 Tong DC, Bolger A, Albers GW. Incidence of transcranial Doppler-detected cerebral microemboli in patients referred for echocardiography. *Stroke* 1994;**25**:2138–41.

266 Tong DC, Albers GW. Transcranial Doppler-detected microemboli in patients with acute stroke. *Stroke* 1995;**26**:1588–92.

267 Nabavi DG, Georgiadis D, Mumme T, et al. Clinical relevance of intracranial microembolic signals in patients with left ventricular assist devices. A prospective study. *Stroke* 1996;**27**: 891–6.

268 Sliwka U, Lingnau A, Stohlmann WD, et al. Prevalence and time course of microembolic signals in patients with acute stroke. A prospective study. *Stroke* 1997;**28**:358–63.

269 Koennecke HC, Mast H, Trocio SS Jr, et al. Microemboli in patients with vertebrobasilar ischemia: association with vertebrobasilar and cardiac lesions. *Stroke* 1997;**28**:593–6.

270 Nadareishvili ZG, Choudary Z, Joyner C, et al. Cerebral microembolism in acute myocardial infarction. *Stroke* 1999;**30**:2679–82.

271 Rundek T, Di Tullio MR, Sciacca RR, et al. Association between large aortic arch atheromas and high-intensity transient signals in elderly stroke patients. *Stroke* 1999;**30**:2683–6.

272 Ringelstein EB, Droste DW, Babikian VL, et al. Consensus on microembolus detection by TCD. International Consensus Group on Microembolus Detection. *Stroke* 1998;**29**:725–9.

273 Cullinane M, Reid G, Dittrich R, et al. Evaluation of new online automated embolic signal detection algorithm, including comparison with panel of international experts. *Stroke* 2000;**31**:1335–41.

274 Markus HS. Transcranial Doppler ultrasound. *Br Med Bull* 2000;**56**:378–88.

275 International Cerebral Hemodynamics Society. The International Cerebral Hemodynamics Society Consensus Statement. *Stroke* 1995;**26**:1123.

276 Moehring MA, Spencer MP. Power M-mode Doppler (PMD) for observing cerebral blood flow and tracking emboli. *Ultrasound Med Biol.* 2002;**28**:49–57.

277 Saqqur M, Dean N, Schebel M, et al. Improved detection of microbubble signals using power M-mode Doppler. *Stroke* 2004;**35**:e14–7.

278 Topcuoglu MA, Palacios IF, Buonanno FS. Contrast M-mode power Doppler ultrasound in the detection of right-to-left shunts: utility of submandibular internal carotid artery recording. *J Neuroimaging* 2003;**13**:315–23.

279 Spencer MP, Moehring MA, Jesurum J, et al. Power m-mode transcranial Doppler for diagnosis of patent foramen ovale and assessing transcatheter closure. *J Neuroimaging* 2004;**14**: 342–9.

280 Lao AY, Sharma VK, Tsivgoulis G, et al. Detection of right-to-left shunts: comparison between the international consensus and Spencer logarithmic scale criteria. *J Neuroimaging* 2008;**18**:402–6.

281 Nornes H, Angelsen B, Lindegaard KF. Precerebral arterial blood flow pattern in intracranial hypertension with cerebral blood flow arrest. *Acta Neurochir* 1977;**38**:187–94.

282 Harders A. *Neurosurgical Applications of Transcranial Doppler Sonography*. Vienna: Springer, 1986: 45.

283 Fischer AQ, Livingstone JN. Transcranial Doppler and real-time cranial sonography in neonatal hydrocephalus. *J Child Neurol* 1989;**4**:64–9.

284 Homburg AM, Jakobsen M, Enevoldsen E. Transcranial Doppler recordings in raised intracranial pressure. *Acta Neurol Scand* 1993;**87**:488–93.

285 Hanlo PW, Peters RJ, Gooskens RH, et al. Monitoring intracranial dynamics by transcranial Doppler – a new Doppler index: trans systolic time. *Ultrasound Med Biol* 1995;**21**:613–21.

286 Mayer SA, Thomas CE, Diamond BE. Asymmetry of intracranial hemodynamics as an indicator of mass effect in acute

intracerebral hemorrhage. A transcranial Doppler study. *Stroke* 1996;**27**:1788–92.

287 Lewis S, Wong M, Myburgh J, *et al*. Determining cerebral perfusion pressure thresholds in severe head trauma. *Acta Neurochir Suppl* 1998;**71**:174–6.

288 Richards HK, Czosnyka M, Whitehouse H, *et al*. Increase in transcranial Doppler pulsatility index does not indicate the lower limit of cerebral autoregulation. *Acta Neurochir Suppl* 1998;**71**:229–32.

289 Treib J, Becker SC, Grauer M, *et al*. Transcranial Doppler monitoring of intracranial pressure therapy with mannitol, sorbitol and glycerol in patients with acute stroke. *Eur Neurol* 1998;**40**:212–9.

290 Czosnyka M, Smielewski P, *et al*. Hemodynamic characterization of intracranial pressure plateau waves in head-injury patients. *J Neurosurg* 1999;**91**:11–9.

291 Rainov NG, Weise JB, Burkert W. Transcranial Doppler sonography in adult hydrocephalic patients. *Neurosurg Rev* 2000;**23**:34–8.

292 Grolimund P, Seiler RW, Mattle H. Possibilities and limits of transcranial Doppler sonography [German]. *Ultraschall Med* 1987;**8**:87–94.

293 Klingelhofer J, Conrad B, Benecke R, *et al*. Intracranial flow patterns at increasing intracranial pressure. *Klin Wochenschr* 1987;**65**:542–5.

294 Kirkham FJ, Levin SD, Padayachee TS, *et al*. Transcranial pulsed Doppler ultrasound findings in brain stem death. *J Neurol Neurosurg Psychiatry* 1987;**50**:1504–13.

295 Ropper AH, Kehne SM, Wechsler L. Transcranial Doppler in brain death. *Neurology* 1987;**37**:1733–5.

296 Hassler W, Steinmetz H, Gawlowski J. Transcranial Doppler ultrasonography in raised intracranial pressure and in intracranial circulatory arrest. *J Neurosurg* 1988;**68**:745–51.

297 Bode H, Sauer M, Pringsheim W. Diagnosis of brain death by transcranial Doppler sonography. *Arch Dis Child* 1988;**63**:1474–8.

298 Newell DW, Grady MS, Sirotta P, *et al*. Evaluation of brain death using transcranial Doppler. *Neurosurgery* 1989;**24**:509–13.

299 Petty GW, Mohr JP, Pedley TA, *et al*. The role of transcranial Doppler in confirming brain death: sensitivity, specificity and suggestions for performance and interpretation. *Neurology* 1990;**40**:300–3.

300 van der Naalt J, Baker AJ. Influence of the intra-aortic balloon pump on the transcranial Doppler flow pattern in a brain-dead patient. *Stroke* 1996;**27**:140–2.

301 Hennerici M, Neuerburg-Heusler D. *Vascular Diagnosis With Ultrasound: Clinical References with Case Studies*. Stuttgart: Georg Thieme, 1998: 120.

302 Ducrocq X, Hassler W, Moritake K, *et al*. Consensus opinion on diagnosis of cerebral circulatory arrest using Doppler-sonography: Task Force Group on Cerebral Death of the Neurosonology Research Group of the World Federation of Neurology. *J Neurol Sci* 1998;**159**:145–50.

303 Ducrocq X, Braun M, Debouverie M, *et al*. Brain death and transcranial Doppler: experience in 130 cases of brain dead patients. *J Neurol Sci* 1998;**160**:41–6.

304 Hadani M, Bruk B, Ram Z, *et al*. Application of transcranial Doppler ultrasonography for the diagnosis of brain death. *Intensive Care Med* 1999;**25**:822–8.

305 Wijdicks EF. The diagnosis of brain death. *N Engl J Med* 2001;**344**:1215–21.

306 de Freitas GR, Andre C. Sensitivity of transcranial Doppler for confirming brain death: a prospective study of 270 cases. *Acta Neurol Scand* 2006;**113**:426–32.

307 Lindegaard K-F, Bakke SJ, Aaslid R, *et al*. Doppler diagnosis of intracranial occlusive disorders. *J Neurol Neurosurg Psychiatry* 1986;**49**:510–8.

308 Grolimund P, Seiler RW, Aaslid R, *et al*. Evaluation of cerebrovascular disease by combined extracranial and transcranial Doppler sonography. Experience in 1,039 patients. *Stroke* 1987;**18**:1018–24.

309 Halsey J. Prognosis of acute hemiplegia estimated by transcranial Doppler sonography. *Stroke* 1988;**19**:648–9.

310 Zanette EM, Fieschi C, Bozzao L, *et al*. Comparison of cerebral angiography and transcranial Doppler sonography in acute stroke. *Stroke* 1989;**20**; 899–903.

311 Kaps M, Damian MS, Teschendorf U, *et al*. Transcranial Doppler ultrasound findings in the middle cerebral artery occlusion. *Stroke* 1990;**21**:532–7.

312 Carmelingo M, Casto L, Censori B, *et al*. Transcranial Doppler in acute ischemic stroke of the middle cerebral artery territories. *Acta Neurol Scand* 1993;**88**:108–11.

313 Razumovsky AY, Gillard JH, Bryan RN, *et al*. TCD, MRA and MRI in acute cerebral ischemia. *Acta Neurol Scand* 1999;**99**:65–76.

314 Demchuk AM, Burgin WS, Christou I, *et al*. Thrombolysis in Brain Ischemia (TIBI) transcranial Doppler flow grades predict clinical severity, early recovery and mortality in patients treated with tissue plasminogen activator. *Stroke* 2001;**32**:89–93.

315 Burgin WS, Malkoff M, Felberg RA, *et al*. Transcranial Doppler ultrasound criteria for recanalization after thrombolysis for middle cerebral artery stroke. *Stroke* 2000;**31**:1128–32.

316 El-Mitwalli A, Saad M, Christou I, *et al*. Clinical and sonographic patterns of tandem ICA/MCA occlusion in TPA treated patients. *Stroke* 2002;**33**:99–102.

317 Demchuk AM, Christou I, Wein TH, *et al*. Accuracy and criteria for localizing arterial occlusion with transcranial Doppler. *J Neuroimaging* 2000;**10**:1–12.

318 Brandt T, Knauth M, Wildermuth S, *et al*. CT angiography and Doppler sonography for emergency assessment in acute basilar artery ischemia. *Stroke* 1999;**30**:606–12.

319 Klotzsch C, Bozzato A, Lammers G, *et al*. Contrast-enhanced three-dimensional transcranial color-coded sonography of intracranial stenoses. *AJNR Am J Neuroradiol* 2002;**23**:208–12.

320 Niederkorn K, Myers LG, Nunn CL, *et al*. Three-dimensional transcranial Doppler blood flow mapping in patients with cerebrovascular disorders. *Stroke* 1988;**19**:1335–44.

321 Bartels E. *Color-Coded Duplex Ultrasonography of the Cerebral Vessels*. Stuttgart: Schattauer, 1999: 123–4.

322 Delcker A, Diener HC. Various ultrasound methods for studying the vertebral artery – a comparative evaluation [German]. *Ultraschall Med* 1992;**13**:213–20.

323 Alexandrov AV, Grotta JC. Arterial re-occlusion in stroke patients treated with intravenous tissue plasminogen activator. *Neurology* 2002;**59**:862–7.

324 Alexandrov AV, Burgin WS, Demchuk AM, *et al*. Speed of intracranial clot lysis with intravenous TPA therapy: sonographic classification and short term improvement. *Circulation* 2001;**103**:2897–902.

325 Toole JF. *Cerebrovascular Disorders*, 4th edn. New York: Raven Press, 1990: 199–223.

326 Voigt K, Kendel K, Sauer M. Subclavian steal syndrome. Bloodless diagnosis of the syndrome using ultrasonic pulse echo and vertebral artery compression [German]. *Fortschr Neurol Psychiatr Grenzgeb* 1970;**38**:20–33.

327 Grossman BL, Brisman R, Wood EH. Ultrasound and the subclavian steal syndrome. *Radiology* 1970;**94**:1–6.

328 Reutern GM, Budingen HJ, Freund HJ. The diagnosis of obstructions of the vertebral and subclavian arteries by means of directional Doppler sonography [German]. *Arch Psychiatr Nervenkr* 1976;**222**:209–22.

329 von Reutern GM, Budingen HJ. Doppler sonographic study of the vertebral artery in subclavian steal syndrome [German]. *Dtsch Med Wochenschr* 1977;**102**:140–1.

330 Yoneda S, Nukada T, Tada K, *et al*. Subclavian steal in Takayasu's arteritis. A hemodynamic study by means of ultrasonic Doppler flowmetry. *Stroke* 1977;**8**:264–8.

331 Pourcelot L, Ribadeau-Dumas JL, Fagret D, *et al*. Contribution of the Doppler examination to the diagnosis of subclavian steal syndrome [French]. *Rev Neurol (Paris)* 1977;**133**:309–23.

332 Walker DW, Acker JD, Cole CA. Subclavian steal syndrome detected with duplex pulsed Doppler sonography. *AJNR Am J Neuroradiol* 1982;**3**:615–8.

333 Ringelstein EB, Zeumer H. Delayed reversal of vertebral artery blood flow following percutaneous transluminal angioplasty for subclavian steal syndrome. *Neuroradiology* 1984;**26**:189–98.

334 Ackerstaff RG, Hoeneveld H, Slowikowski JM, *et al*. Ultrasonic duplex scanning in atherosclerotic disease of the innominate, subclavian and vertebral arteries. A comparative study with angiography. *Ultrasound Med Biol* 1984;**10**:409–18.

335 Pokrovskii AV, Volynskii YuD, Kuntsevich GI, *et al*. Ultrasonic angiography in the diagnosis of lesions of the brachiocephalic branches of the aorta. *Kardiologiia* 1985;**25**:82–6.

336 Kuperberg EB, Grozovskii YuL, Agadzhanova LP. Functional test of reactive hyperemia in the diagnosis of the vertebrosubclavian steal syndrome using ultrasonic dopplerography. *Zh Nevropatol Psikhiatr Im S S Korsakova* 1986;**86**:28–34.

337 Bornstein NM, Norris JW. Subclavian steal: a harmless haemodynamic phenomenon? *Lancet* 1986;**ii**:303–5.

338 Ackermann H, Diener HC, Dichgans J. Stenosis and occlusion of the subclavian artery: ultrasonographic and clinical findings. *J Neurol* 1987;**234**:396–400.

339 Ackermann H, Diener HC, Seboldt H, *et al*. Ultrasonographic follow-up of subclavian stenosis and occlusion: natural history and surgical treatment. *Stroke* 1988;**19**:431–5.

340 Klingelhofer J, Conrad B, Benecke R, *et al*. Transcranial Doppler ultrasonography of carotid-basilar collateral circulation in subclavian steal. *Stroke* 1988;**19**:1036–42.

341 Bornstein NM, Krajewski A, Norris JW. Basilar artery blood flow in subclavian steal. *Can J Neurol Sci* 1988;**15**:417–9.

342 Lunev DK, Pokrovskii AV, Nikitin YuM, *et al*. Cerebrovascular disorders in various types of the subclavian steal syndrome [Russian]. *Zh Nevropatol Psikhiatr Im S S Korsakova* 1991;**91**:10–4.

343 Nicholls SC, Koutlas TC, Strandness DE. Clinical significance of retrograde flow in the vertebral artery. *Ann Vasc Surg* 1991;**5**:331–6.

344 de Bray JM, Zenglein JP, Laroche JP, *et al*. Effect of subclavian syndrome on the basilar artery. *Acta Neurol Scand* 1994;**90**:174–8.

345 Rossum AC, Steel SR, Hartshorne MF. Evaluation of coronary subclavian steal syndrome using sestamibi imaging and duplex scanning with observed vertebral subclavian steal. *Clin Cardiol* 2000;**23**:226–9.

346 Mukhtar OM, Miller AP, Nanda NC, *et al*. Transesophageal echocardiographic identification of left subclavian artery stenosis with steal phenomenon. *Echocardiography* 2000;**17**:197–200.

347 Toni D, Fiorelli M, Gentile M, *et al*. Progressing neurological deficit secondary to acute ischemic stroke: a study on predictability, pathogenesis and prognosis. *Arch Neurol* 1995;**52**:670–5.

348 Dávalos A, Toni D, Iweins F, *et al*. Neurological deterioration in acute ischemic stroke: potential predictors and associated factors in the European Cooperative Acute Stroke Study (ECASS) I. *Stroke* 1999;**30**:2631–6.

349 Grotta JC, Welch KM, Fagan SC, *et al*. Clinical deterioration following improvement in the NINDS rt-PA Stroke Trial. *Stroke* 2001;**32**:661–8.

350 Kasner SE, Demchuk AM, Berrouschot J, *et al*. Predictors of fatal brain edema in massive hemispheric ischemic stroke. *Stroke* 2001;**32**:2117–23.

351 Toni D, Fiorelli M, Zanette EM, Sacchetti ML, *et al*. Early spontaneous improvement and deterioration of ischemic stroke patients. A serial study with transcranial Doppler ultrasonography. *Stroke* 1998;**29**:1144–8.

352 Baracchini C, Manara R, Ermani M, *et al*. The quest for early predictors of stroke evolution: can TCD be a guiding light? *Stroke* 2000;**31**:2942–7.

353 Alexandrov AV, Sharma VK, Lao AY, *et al*. Reversed Robin Hood syndrome in acute ischemic stroke patients. *Stroke* 2007;**38**:3045–8.

354 Tsivgoulis G, Sharma VK, Ardelt AA, *et al*. Reversed Robin Hood syndrome: correlation of neurological deterioration with intracerebral steal magnitude. *Stroke* 2008;**39**:725 [Abstract].

355 Alexandrov AV, Ngyuen TH, Rubiera M, *et al*. Prevalence and risk factors associated with reversed Robin Hood syndrome in acute ischemic stroke. *Stroke* 2009;**40**:2738–42.

IV Ultrasound in Stroke Prevention and Treatment

7 Ultrasound in Stroke Prevention: TCD and Sickle Cell Disease

Fenwick T. Nichols III[1], Robert J Adams[2] & Anne M. Jones[3]
[1]Medical College of Georgia, Augusta, GAS, USA
[2]Medical University of South Carolina, Charleston, SC, USA
[3]Wake Forrest University Medical Center, Winston-Salem, NC, USA

Introduction

Children with sickle cell disease (hemoglobin HbSS) have a significant stroke risk, with 11% of all HbSS patients developing ischemic stroke before the age of 20 years [1]. These strokes primarily result from stenosis or occlusion of the distal intracranial internal carotid arteries (ICA, Figure 7.1A) and/or proximal middle cerebral arteries (MCA, Figure 7.1B). Many of these patients develop moya-moya phenomenon (Figure 7.1C) or a network of small collateral vessels to compensate for the ICA occlusive disease. In Japanese, "moya-moya" means "a puff of smoke." This is how these small arteries appear on a digital subtraction angiography in most advanced cases.

It is logical to suspect that as the proximal intracranial vessel narrowing increases or blood's ability to deliver oxygen decreases or hematocrit drops, the resulting flow velocity will increase. Thus, not surprisingly, several studies have demonstrated that TCD velocity measurements in the proximal cerebral vessels can identify those children with sickle cell disease who are at increased risk of stroke [2,3]. Based upon these data, the Stroke Prevention in Sickle Cell Disease (STOP) trial was undertaken to identify children at high risk of stroke with the goal to institute primary stroke prevention [4]. A total of 130 children were entered into the trial who had a time-averaged mean of the maximum (TAMM) velocities of >200 cm s^{-1} in one or both of the MCAs or terminal ICAs at baseline TCD.

Two points must be emphasized:

1 Entry criteria for STOP required that children with HbSS have TAMM (*not* peak systolic, Figure 7.2) velocities >200 cm s^{-1} in the MCA, and/or TICA recorded on *two* separate occasions separated by at least 2 weeks. A non-image-guided 2 MHz TCD was used with assumed 0° angle of insonation. The decision to require an initial examination and a subsequent confirmatory examination was made to avoid many transient physiologic variables affecting flow velocity.

2 Stroke risk was determined by velocities >200 cm s^{-1} in the terminal ICA and/or MCA. There are no data on the stroke risk for high velocities in other vessels [anterior (ACA) or posterior (PCA) cerebral arteries]; however, high velocities in these vessels are usually associated with stenosis in the terminal ICA or MCA. Therefore, discovery of high ACA or PCA velocities should prompt earlier repeat examinations in an effort to identify a missed terminal ICA and/or MCA stenosis.

Children who met these entry criteria were randomized to receive either transfusion or standard care. Over an average follow-up of about 20 months, there was one stroke in the 63 children randomized to transfusion and 11 strokes in the 67 children randomized to standard care. These results indicate a greater than 90% relative risk reduction in stroke incidence in the treated population [5]. As a result of these findings, the National Institutes of Health released a clinical alert on September 18, 1997, which stated: "The STOP Trial confirmed that TCD can identify children with sickle cell anemia at high risk for first time stroke. Since the greatest risk of stroke occurs in early childhood, it is recommended that children ages 2–16 receive TCD screening. Screening should be conducted at a site where clinicians have been trained to provide TCDs of comparable quality and information content to those used in the STOP trial and to read them in a manner consistent with what was done in STOP . . . It is recommended that centers that wish to start screening children with sickle cell anemia for stroke risk do studies to compare their current equipment with STOP trial TCD equipment."

Since then, STOP collaborators have performed subsequent studies. For instance, if a child started to receive blood transfusions, should he or she continue to receive transfusions? The STOP-2 trial provided an answer [6]. Once blood transfusion has been given, TCD velocities are likely to decrease. Therefore, children with sickle cell disease receiving transfusions and normal TCD velocities were eligible for the trial. Randomization was to either no subsequent transfusions or to continue periodic blood

Cerebrovascular Ultrasound in Stroke Prevention and Treatment, 2nd edition.
Edited by Andrei V. Alexandrov. © 2011 Blackwell Publishing Ltd.

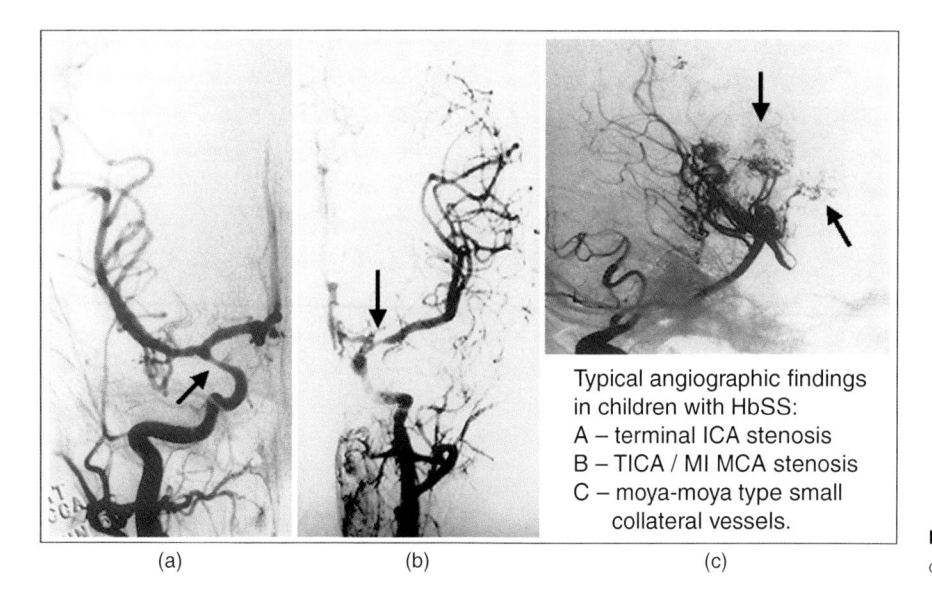

PART IV Ultrasound in Stroke Prevention and Treatment

Figure 7.1 Arterial lesions and collaterals in children with sickle cell disease.

Typical angiographic findings in children with HbSS:
A – terminal ICA stenosis
B – TICA / MI MCA stenosis
C – moya-moya type small collateral vessels.

transfusions. Primary end-points were either reversion to high stroke risk TCD velocities or stroke. Among 42 children who stopped transfusions, 14 reversed to TAMM > 200 cm s^{-1} and two had strokes, whereas none had the primary end-points out of 38 children who continued to receive transfusions. The average length of follow-up was 4.5 months [6]. The trialists concluded that those children with sickle cell disease who once qualified for blood transfusions should continue to receive transfusions to sustain the primary stroke prevention benefit.

STOP TCD protocol

The STOP TCD scanning protocol is slightly different from that used for routine clinical TCD examinations. This chapter describes the STOP scanning and reading technique and discusses the rationale for its modifications. Readers interested in additional background information on TCD use in sickle cell disease are referred to the references at the end of this chapter.

How to perform TCD in children

The TCD technique used to examine children is similar to that used on adults [7]. However, there are several important differences that must be recognized in order to perform and interpret TCD examinations properly. Children have smaller head diameters and higher normal flow velocities than adults. Those with HbSS have even higher flow velocities secondary to anemia. The TCDs performed as part of the STOP trial were very focused examinations specifically adapted for children. A brief overview is presented below to provide some background as to why certain modifications were made in the examinations for these children.

TCD is a non-image-guided vascular examination in that there is no B-mode or color flow map to identify the insonated vessel and its location. Therefore, it is important to pay attention to the relative position and angulation of the probe, the depth of insonation and the direction of flow. Failure to do so can result in misinterpretation of the examination.

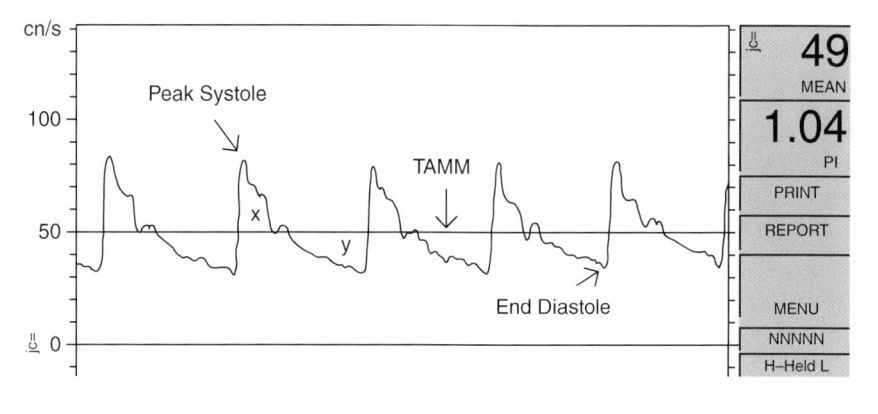

Figure 7.2 TAMM line placement. This is the spectral outline as traced by the V_{max} or waveform follower. The TAMM line is placed so that the area under the V_{max} trace above the TAMM line (labeled "x") is equal to the area below the TAMM line above the V_{max} trace (labeled "y").

Children generally have thinner skulls than adults, so rather than the usual small and difficult to find ultrasonic window of the adult, the examiner may be faced with a plethora of windows. In general, the windows that lie closer to the ear, in the posterior portion of the temporal window, are preferable to those that lie more anteriorly. If the probe is placed in the more anterior portion of the trans-temporal windows, it has to be angled further posteriorly to insonate any vessel. The circle of Willis is not large and it is easy to insonate either more posteriorly or more anteriorly than intended when an unfamiliar window is used.

Since the circle of Willis is small and the windows are usually good, it is better to use a small sample volume to avoid recording flow in adjacent vessels. The signal displayed on the screen represents any flow signal within the sample volume and is not necessarily located at the exact depth displayed on the screen. The depth displayed on the screen is the depth at the mid-portion of the sample volume length. The sample volume width varies with the depth of insonation, being narrowest at the focal zone of the probe and being somewhat wider at greater or lesser depths. With a 10 mm sample volume (length), the depth of insonation extends from 5 mm shallower to 5 mm deeper than the depth indicated. In a child's small circle of Willis, a 10 mm sample volume may result in unintended insonation of other arteries. This may be a particular problem when the anterior trans-temporal window is used and the probe is angled posteriorly to evaluate the PCA. A 10 mm sample volume may cross both the MCA and the PCA, making it difficult to ascertain the source of the Doppler signal. The STOP protocol specified a sample volume of 6 mm to increase confidence of the site of insonation. Decreasing the sample volume length does reduce the power, but this usually is not a problem in children since less power is needed to penetrate their thinner skulls.

Children have smaller heads than adults and consequently the depths at which vessels are identified differ (Table 7.1). If adult depth measurements are used as a basis for vessel determination, serious errors may occur. Measuring the bi-temporal diameter is helpful. The examiner can use either obstetric calipers or the instrument used by optometrists to determine head width when fitting eye glasses. The bi-temporal skull diameter is taken by measuring the distance between the two posterior trans-temporal windows. If the child's bi-temporal head diameter is 13 cm, then the midline is at 65 mm and the ICA bifurcation will be found at a depth of about 55 mm. If the probe is angled posteriorly, a bi-directional signal at 65 mm would represent the top of the basilar with flow into both PCAs; if the probe is angled anteriorly, a bi-directional signal at the midline could also represent both ACAs. For comparison, in a patient with a bi-temporal diameter of 15 cm, a bi-directional signal at 65 mm would be identified as the ICA bifurcation.

In smaller head diameters, the ICA bifurcation generally lies 5–15 mm off the midline (usually about 8–10 mm). In a patient with a 13 cm bi-temporal diameter, the ICA bifurcation will be found at a depth of 52–60 mm. The P-1 PCA segment can be insonated from the midline depth (65 mm) to a depth of at least 50 mm and frequently to a depth of 45 mm. This leads to potential vessel identification problems, in that flow towards the probe at a depth of 55 mm could be in either the MCA or PCA. In order to verify that the flow towards the probe arises from the MCA, it is crucial to insonate to as shallow a depth as possible. In a 13 cm diameter head, the MCA should be able to be tracked to depths of 30–35 mm and should always be tracked to at least a depth of less than 40 mm. If flow towards the probe can be insonated from a depth of 30 mm and tracked in 2 mm increments to a bi-directional signal at 55 mm depth, then the examiner can be confident that the vessel is the MCA. In addition, once the ICA bifurcation is identified, it is important that the examiner then angles the probe posteriorly and insonates the PCA. The PCA can then be tracked to the midline, with detection of bi-directional flow at the top of the basilar. If all of the above can be carried out, then the examiner can be confident of an accurate examination.

There is another source of bi-directional signals that is occasionally misidentified as the ICA bifurcation. These bi-directional signals can be found at MCA branch sites, either the anterior temporal artery or an early MCA bifurcation. If the head diameter nomogram is used (Table 7.1), the depth of the bi-directional signal from an MCA branch will be shallower than that expected for the ICA bifurcation.

The STOP protocol requires that the MCA signal be tracked and recorded in 2 mm steps from its shallowest depth to the ICA bifurcation. The signal should be optimized at each site of insonation. The ACA signal is recorded ~4 mm deeper than the ICA bifurcation. The distal ICA signal is recorded ~4 mm deeper than the ICA bifurcation or with a slightly downward probe angulation at the depths of ICA bifurcation. Then the probe is angled posteriorly and the PCA is recorded at 2 mm increments from its shallowest depth to the top of the basilar (Table 7.1).

Table 7.1 Expected arterial depths for different head diameters[a]

Head diameter (cm)	MCA	MCA-1	ICA Bif	ACA	PCA
12	30–54	30–36	50–54	50–58	40–60
13	30–58	30–36	52–58	52–62	42–66
14	34–62	34–40	56–64	56–68	46–70
15	40–66	40–46	56–66	56–72	50–70

[a]Depths of insonation are given for ipsi-lateral trans-temporal window of insonation.

Due to collateral flow patterns established in response to hemodynamically significant stenoses in children with HbSS, it is particularly crucial to differentiate the MCA from the PCA. With progressive stenosis of the distal ICA, proximal ACA and/or MCA, PCA flow becomes one of the major collateral sources to leptomeningeal collaterals, which then supply the distal MCA and/or ACA. In this situation, the PCA is readily insonated because of its high flow volume. The MCA may not be as easily detectable due to a high-grade stenosis or occlusion; therefore, it can be easy to misidentify the PCA as the MCA unless a thorough detailed examination is performed.

Early in our use of TCD (before development of the STOP protocol), we examined a child with HbSS and moya-moya phenomenon. The PCA's strong signal was misidentified as the MCA and we assumed that the PCA could not be insonated. Angiography revealed a virtually absent MCA, with high volume flow through the PCA. With subsequent modification and close adherence to our scanning protocol, we developed very reproducible examinations, which correlate well with angiographic findings.

Factors influencing cerebral blood flow velocities

The STOP protocol is driven to determine the highest TAMM velocity (*not* peak systolic) in the MCA or terminal ICA. Because the absolute TAMM velocity is important for study classification, it is also important to recognize the physiologic, anatomic, technique and equipment variables that may affect CBF and flow velocities (Table 7.2).

Physiologic factors

TCD measures the velocity of blood flow, which is determined by the volume of flow over time and the luminal area of the artery. There are a number of factors that influence the volume of flow, the primary determinants being tissue requirements for oxygen and glucose delivery. Listed below is a brief overview of the various factors influencing cerebral blood flow volume:

1 *Age:* Cerebral blood flow is highest around the age of 4 years (about 85 cm^3 per 100 g of tissue per minute) and then declines to approximately 65 cm^3 per 100 g of tissue per minute at age 20 years and to about 35 cm^3 per 100 g of tissue per minute at age 85 years. In addition to this gradual decline in cerebral blood flow with increasing age, there is a slight increase in arterial diameter with increasing age. The net effect is that blood flow velocities are highest around age 4 years and decrease thereafter.

2 *Hematocrit:* This is a major determinant of oxygen delivery. Mild degrees of anemia do not have any significant impact on CBF, but more severe anemia causes a measurable increase in total CBF. In order to maintain adequate oxygen delivery as the hematocrit decreases, the CBF must increase. Once the hematocrit is below 30, there is a reliably detectable increase in CBF and consequently in blood flow velocity. Sickle cell patients typically have hematocrit of 18–25, so their CBF is higher than that of age-comparable children with normal hematocrit. The TAMM for an otherwise normal 8-year-old HbSS patient with a hemoglobin of 7 and a hematocrit of 21 is approximately 140 cm s^{-1}. In those unusual situations of elevated hematocrit there may be a decrease in CBF, sometimes due to excessive oxygen delivery or hyperviscosity.

3 *Carbon dioxide:* Arterioles on the brain surface are the resistance vessels and are important in cerebral blood flow regulation. These arterioles respond to changes in CO_2. They dilate in response to increases in carbon dioxide, allowing blood to flow more easily, thus enhancing cerebral blood flow. *For every 1 mm increase in CO_2, there is a 2–4% rise in CBF.* Carbon dioxide plasma concentration increases in several situations, including lung disease, breath-holding or carbon dioxide administration. If the patient goes to sleep there may be a 2–5 mm rise in CO_2, resulting in an increase in CBF and blood flow velocity. Because of this potential

Table 7.2 Physiological variables affecting CBF and TAMM

Variable	Alteration	Effect on TAMM	Causes of alteration from baseline
Age	Increase	Decrease	Normal aging; decrease in CBF
Hematocrit	Decrease	Increase	Bone marrow failure; hemolysis; splenic sequestration; blood loss
	Increase	Decrease	Blood transfusion
Oxygen	Decrease	Increase	Sickle chest syndrome; pneumonia
	Increase	Minimal decrease	Oxygen administration
CO_2	Increase	Increase	Sleep; breath-holding; sedation
	Decrease	Decrease	Hyperventilation; crying
Body temperature	Increase	Increase	Fever of any cause
Glucose	Decrease	Increase	Hypoglycemia

Table 7.3 TCD optimization

1. Focused examination, meticulous tracking of the MCA course and terminal ICA
2. Probe manipulation, angling or sliding, to optimize angle of insonation
3. Careful attention to audible cues of high velocity: "hissing", turbulence (prompts a more detailed search for high velocity)
4. Correct scale settings
5. Sharpest waveforms
6. Best signal-to-noise ratio
7. Careful examination for the highest velocity

sleep-induced velocity increase, children should not be allowed to sleep during the examination. The arterioles decrease in diameter with lowering of carbon dioxide, causing an increased resistance to flow and decreased CBF and TAMM. As CO_2 decreases occur with hyperventilation and crying, TCD examinations should be avoided in these situations.

4 *Oxygen:* Hypoxia produces an increase in CBF in order to maintain oxygen delivery. Patients with pneumonia or other causes of lowered oxygen levels will have a compensatory increase in their cerebral blood flow.

5 *Hypoglycemia:* Patients who are hypoglycemic will have a compensatory increase in CBF to increase glucose delivery to the brain. Usually, this is only a minor phenomenon and does not cause a CBF increase unless the glucose is less than 40 mg%.

6 *Fever:* Fever increases CBF by about 10% for every 1 C temperature increase, so febrile patients will have elevated CBF and TCD velocities relative to their baseline.

7 *Blood pressure:* Within a broad range, the cerebral arterioles respond to changes in blood pressure to maintain a constant CBF volume. This phenomenon, referred to as autoregulation, generally prevents minor changes in blood pressure from affecting CBF. However, there are limits to autoregulation. This mechanism will fail when the blood pressure is severely elevated or depressed in acutely ill patients, significantly altering CBF.

8 *Cardiac output:* Under normal physiologic conditions, cardiac output is stable and is not a factor in CBF. However, in states of severely decreased cardiac output, such as cardiomyopathies or severe aortic stenosis, the CBF may fall. Cardiac arrhythmias may also decrease cardiac output, so third-degree heart block or supra-ventricular or ventricular tachycardias may result in decreased CBF. Aortic valvular insufficiency may also alter cardiac output, resulting in altered waveforms and possibly decreased CBF.

9 *Proximal arterial obstruction:* If there is a severe stenosis ($\geq 80\%$) affecting the source of blood to the artery being evaluated (e.g. an arterial stenosis proximal to the point of insonation), there may be a decrease in volume flow through the artery being evaluated. The severe stenosis prevents adequate flow volume delivery (resulting in lower velocity) with a low-resistance waveform. With more severe proximal stenosis, the upstroke of the waveform will become rounded.

10 *Distal arterial stenosis:* Severe arterial stenosis distal to the point of insonation causes decreased volume flow through the artery. Flow at the site of insonation will likely have decreased velocity with a high-resistance waveform. Increased intracranial pressure will have an effect similar to distal arterial stenosis, producing increased resistance to flow at the arteriolar level.

11 *Rhythmic oscillations:* Normal individuals have periodic variations in MCA velocity occurring every 30–180 s, producing up to a 15% increase in velocity.

12 *Arterio-venous malformations (AVM):* AVMs have no capillary bed and cause minimal resistance to flow. Insonation of a feeding artery to an AVM will demonstrate a high velocity (because of high volume flow) with a very low-resistance signal.

The STOP TCD examinations should be carried out when the child is at a "steady state." Although it is frequently easier to study the patients when they are in the hospital, many of the reasons prompting admission alter CBF. To apply STOP trial results, we do not recommend examining a child who is acutely ill, as fever, hypoxia, hypocarbia and worsened anemia may all transiently increase the TAMM, possibly resulting in a TAMM >200 cm s^{-1}. (STOP study randomization required two TCD examinations >200 cm s^{-1}, separated by at least 2 weeks, to avoid such problems.) Transfusion will decrease TAMM for several weeks, until the hematocrit returns towards its usual level.

Anatomic variables

1 The arteries may be very tortuous, making it difficult to obtain an optimal angle of insonation in these arteries. This may be partly addressed by probe manipulation.

2 Multiple trans-temporal windows may be present and used, making examination difficult and operator dependent.

Technique and equipment variables

In general, routine clinical TCD examinations are used to detect and roughly quantify areas of stenosis. The sonographer's efforts are directed at the recognition of an abnormal area and not necessarily the precise quantification of its severity (except in broad terms). There are several differences between routine clinical TCD examinations and the STOP protocol-based TCD examination. The STOP study used an exacting TCD scanning protocol to create a very focused reproducible examination because, based upon the Medical College of Georgia (MCG) patient cohort and STOP data, patients with TAMM velocities >200 cm s^{-1} had a significantly increased stroke risk, which could be decreased by transfusion. Therefore, the goal of the STOP TCD examination is to obtain the highest possible TAMM velocity in the MCA and/or terminal ICA and allow its reproducible measurement at follow-up. To help sonographers obtain these velocities, several modifications were made to the routine clinical TCD examination. The section below deals in detail with these variables.

Optimizing the angle of insonation

Since TCD is a non-image-guided technique, no correction to the angle of insonation can be applied to the kHz Doppler frequency shift detected during this study. As is well known, when the angle of insonation becomes larger than 15°, the kHz shift for a given velocity begins to decrease. In duplex Doppler examinations, the angle of insonation can be registered by the sonographer, so that the computer can calculate the actual velocity of flow. In TCD, the computer assumes that the angle of insonation is ideal, so that TCD cannot overestimate the velocity of flow. If the angle of insonation is 0°, the TCD-calculated velocity is accurate. If the angle of insonation is >30°, the calculated velocity will be falsely low. In order to obtain the highest TCD velocity possible, it is necessary to attempt to optimize the angle of insonation by aiming the ultrasound beam directly down the barrel of the artery being insonated. Because the proximal MCA may have one or more curves, the examiner may have to angle (or even move) the probe as the depth of insonation is changed in order to align the ultrasound beam optimally with the vessel as the MCA stem is tracked. Children generally have generous or large acoustic windows, making it easier to make these adjustments. We have found that when the sonographer uses the STOP TCD protocol, the velocities recorded are typically higher than those recorded as part of a routine clinical examination.

Optimization of the Doppler signal

This includes recognition of the audible and visual clues indicating local high-velocity flow, as well as making appropriate scale and gain settings. As noted above, part of signal optimization is accomplished by proper transducer positioning and minor probe manipulation to achieve the best angle of insonation. STOP TCD sonographers were trained to recognize visual clues of local high-velocity flow, such as turbulence and sudden cut-off of the waveform, plus audible clues of high velocity that may not be displayed visually on the TCD monitor. The sonographer should be able to identify characteristics of a high-velocity signal and recognize high frequencies in the background of the audible signal that may not be displayed on screen. Turbulence (high-amplitude, low-frequency/velocity, bi-directional signal that occurs at peak systole) is another audible clue to local stenosis. If the examiner hears either a high-frequency Doppler signal and/or significant turbulence, a very careful search for high velocities should be performed. It is possible to have a well-defined waveform displayed on the screen, but to hear a higher velocity in the background that is not displayed. In this situation, with probe manipulation, the higher velocity signal can almost always be identified and displayed.

Visual display of the waveform

The examiner should also pay close attention to the visual image of the Doppler waveform. The goal is to obtain the "cleanest," sharpest and highest velocity signal. The examiner must locate the area of the highest velocity and then make every effort to obtain a well-defined waveform with a sharp upstroke and a sharp systolic peak. Then the examiner must focus on making the minuscule movement necessary to obtain the highest velocity at the depth being evaluated. It is a common occurrence to identify a region of high velocity, but to fail to obtain the highest velocity at the site because not enough time was spent optimizing the signal.

In clinical TCD studies, once a pathologically high velocity has been identified, most sonographers tend not to spend much time attempting to optimize the waveform and peak velocity further as it does not matter to clinical decision-making if a child has a TAMM velocity of 150 or 190 cm s^{-1}, i.e. normal and conditional STOP values.

Waveform follower

The function of the waveform follower, or envelope, is closely tied to signal strength, optimization and gain settings. Most TCD equipment has been designed so that there is a waveform follower that will track the highest velocity displayed (V_{max}) that is above the zero line (or baseline). This waveform follower is the bright white outline that tracks the top of each of the waveforms. Some of the TCD units will also track the highest velocity signals below the zero line. The waveform follower tracks the highest velocities, which are then used to determine the TAMM. If there is too much noise in the background or a signal that is not strong enough for the waveform follower to recognize, the strongest signals with highest and lowest velocity amplitude will be tracked, resulting in either too high or too low mean velocity measurements. As the velocities measured by the waveform follower are used to compute the peak systolic, mean, end diastolic velocities, as well as the pulsatility and resistance indexes, it is important that the displayed signal be of adequate quality for accurate tracking by the waveform follower. If the signal-to-noise ratio is poor, the computer velocity measurements may be inaccurate and these cannot be used to apply STOP trial criteria. hence it is important to obtain as high a signal-to-noise ratio as possible.

Instrument settings

If the gain is set too high, there will be too much background noise and the V_{max} waveform follower will not be able to separate the actual waveform from the noise. In addition, it may sometimes result in the development of a "mirror image" display of the waveform. Simply decreasing the gain will usually resolve these problems.

The velocity scale should be set so that the waveform fills about half to three-quarters of the scale to avoid aliasing. On occasion this is not possible, but every effort should be made to achieve it. In otherwise normal pediatric sickle cell patients, the TAMM velocity for the MCA is usually around 140 cm s^{-1}, so as a starting point the velocity scale should be set to display at least 200–250 cm s^{-1} peak values in one direction. If the scale is set too low, "wrap around" will occur and accurate velocity measurements cannot be made. If the scale is set much too low, the velocities will completely fill the screen and no measurable signal will be recognized.

STOP TCD scanning protocol steps

1 Trans-temporal head diameter is measured and recorded.
2 Nomogram for expected depths for patients head diameter is reviewed (Table 7.1).
3 Sample volume is set to 6 mm.
4 Velocity scale is set to 200–250 cm s^{-1}.
5 Anterior TCD examination begins:
  a Anterior temporal window is identified.
  b MCA signal is acquired.
  c MCA is tracked to as shallow a depth as possible; for most children, this should be to a depth less than 40 mm (in STOP this depth was referred to as M1 MCA, indicating the shallowest depth of the MCA that could be recorded).
  d TCD signal is optimized and recorded.
  e MCA stem is then "tracked" by advancing the sample volume by 2 mm increments, optimizing and recording the signal.
  f The MCA is "tracked" (recording in 2 mm increments of depth) to the internal carotid bifurcation (ICA) where there is a bi-directional signal (flow towards the probe is the MCA and away is ACA). This signal is recorded as BIF.
  g The anterior cerebral artery (ACA) is tracked to 4–6 mm deeper than the ICA bifurcation and recorded as ACA.
  h The sample volume depth is then returned to the ICA bifurcation, the probe is angled slightly inferiorly, the depth is increased by 4–6 mm and the Doppler flow velocity waveforms in the distal ICA are recorded, labeled as dICA.
  i The sample depth is then returned to the ICA bifurcation, the probe is angled slightly posteriorly until the posterior cerebral artery (PCA) is detected. The sample volume depth is then decreased to the shallowest depth at which signal can be detected.
  j This PCA waveform is then recorded as PCA. The PCA is tracked (like the MCA in 2 mm increments and labeled as PCA) to the midline, where bi-directional flow is identified and recorded as the top of the basilar (TOB).
  k The opposite side is then examined (through the trans-temporal window) and recorded using this same technique.
6 Posterior examination was performed as per the standard TCD scanning protocol. As stenoses only very rarely affect the vertebro-basilar system in children with sickle cell disease, high velocities here were generally secondary to increased volume flow (collateralization of flow).
7 Ophthalmic TCD was not part of the STOP protocol, as small children will not generally lie quietly for a trans-orbital examination, however infrequently some abnormalities that can be identified by this examination (see below).

Reading STOP TCD

The TCD unit used at participating centers in the STOP trial was Nicolet TC 2000 model that can perform post-processing, including adjustments of the gain settings and zero line. Reading of the STOP TCDs was standardized so that all readers set the gain and zero line to the same levels before reading the velocities. The computer-generated waveform follower (V_{max}) was used to help adjust the gain. The gain was increased or decreased until the waveform follower accurately tracked the highest identifiable velocity profile, but did not identify background noise as signal and "spike" off the waveform. If there was signal that had aliasing, the baseline was adjusted to minimize the aliasing.

Most modern TCD equipment has software that will permit measurement of the TAMM and post-processing of the digitally stored audio signal (i.e. soundtracks). The computer calculates TAMM from the velocities registered by the waveform follower (V_{max}) that tracks the highest velocities over time. If the waveform follower is accurately tracking the highest velocities, then the computer-calculated TAMM may be used.

Unfortunately, when there is a poor signal-to-noise ratio, the waveform follower may not accurately track the highest velocities, resulting in over- or underestimation of the TAMM. For STOP, the TAMM was measured using a visually guided technique. The gain was adjusted, usually by increasing the gain, to the point that the waveform follower began to misidentify background noise as signal (the waveform follower would "spike" off the waveform to noise that was misidentified as signal). The gain was then decreased to the level just below the development of "spiking." A cursor was then brought up on to the screen and the TAMM measured by visual placement of the cursor.

Visual determination of the TAMM can be done reproducibly and accurately after some practice. The easiest way to explain this is to look at the waveform as if it were a

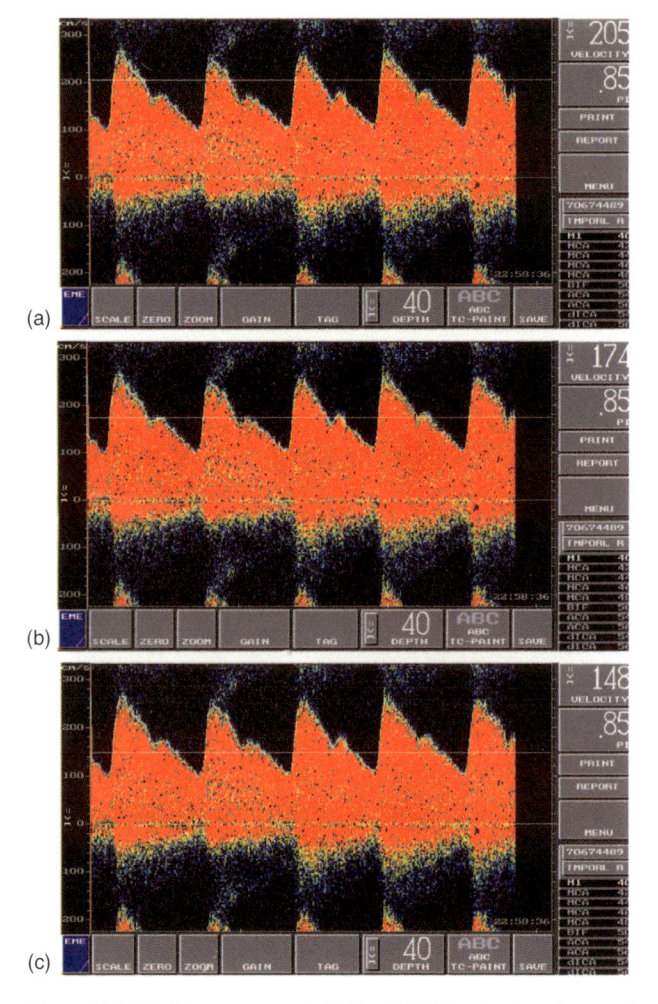

PART IV Ultrasound in Stroke Prevention and Treatment

Figure 7.3 TAMM measurements. (a) The TAMM line has been incorrectly placed resulting in too high a velocity (205 cm s^{-1}); (b) the TAMM line has been correctly placed, with correct measurement of velocity (174 cm s^{-1}); (c) the TAMM line has been incorrectly placed, resulting in too low velocity measurement (148 cm s^{-1}).

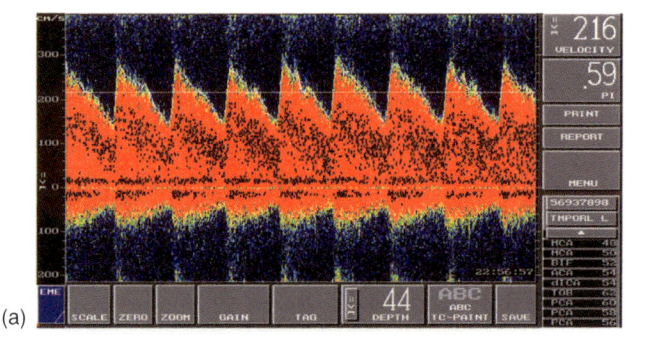

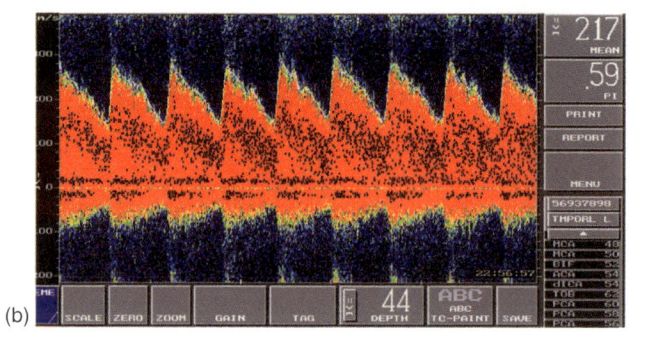

Figure 7.4 This is a well-defined waveform, with gain appropriately set. This demonstrates the correlation of computer measured TAMM with the TAMM line. (a) Abnormal TCD study of the MCA at 44 mm depth; (b) the TAMM line has been correctly placed, measuring 216 cm s^{-1}. Same study measured by the computer using the waveform follower, with 217 cm s^{-1}.

mountain range with peaks (systolic) and valleys (diastolic). If you wanted to level the mountains you would draw a line across the waveforms so that if the peaks (the areas under the curve, above the line) were pushed over they would fill the valleys (the area below the line and above spectral outline, Figure 7.2). A reader can rapidly acquire the skill to make this reading accurately by doing direct comparisons between the computer-generated TAMM and the visually determined TAMM. In general, the TAMM lies at the "shoulder" of the waveform. To minimize the effects of minor changes in velocity from irregular heart rhythm, the reader should attempt to read the TAMM across at least three waveforms. Correct and incorrect TAMM placements are given in Figures 7.3–7.6.

Using this visually guided technique, blinded repeat readings were within <5% of the original velocities. As noted above, all STOP velocity criteria are based on TAMM. There are a number of other possible mean velocities that can be calculated. None of them are the same as TAMM. These other mean velocities include (but are not limited to) the instantaneous mean, the time average of the mean and the intensity-weighted mean. Some centers have used the following rapid calculation to arrive at the mean: add one-third the peak systolic velocity and two-thirds the end diastolic velocity. We compared this calculation with the measured TAMM and found that this calculated mean velocity dose not match the TAMM and is almost always lower than the TAMM.

STOP criteria and the risk of stroke in children with HbSS

The TCD examination as performed by the STOP protocol is driven to obtain the highest absolute TAMM velocity. Using the STOP TCD protocol, it was found that children with HbSS with TAMM >200 cm s^{-1} in the terminal ICA and/or MCA were at significantly increased risk of ischemic stroke and that blood transfusions decreased this risk. The TAMM velocity cut-point of 200 cm s^{-1} was based on the Medical College of Georgia (MCG) Cohort Stroke Risk Model described by Robert Adams in 1992–96. This cut-off was also employed in 5000 screening TCD examinations performed

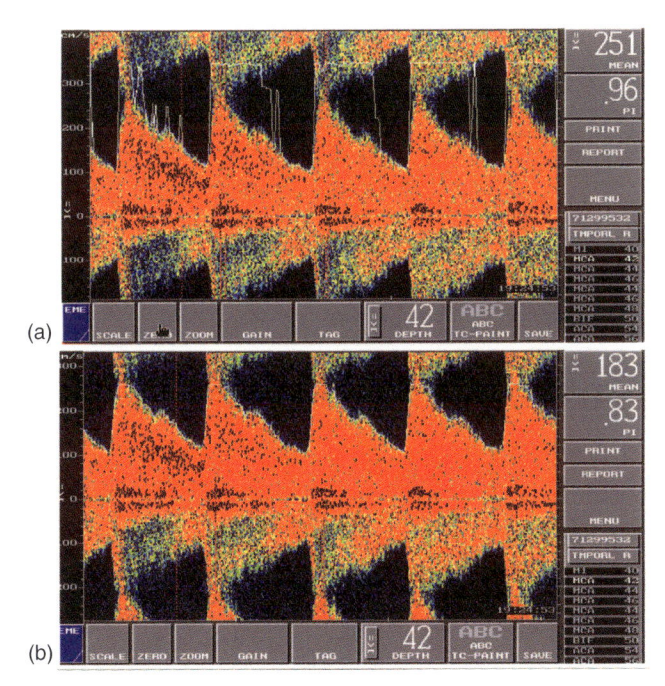

CHAPTER 7 Ultrasound in Stroke Prevention: TCD and Sickle Cell Disease

Figure 7.5 Incorrect computer-based TAMM measurement was obtained in the MCA at 42 mm depth (a). The waveform follower (V_{max}) is not tracking the velocity profile; it is incorrectly registering the "wrapped around" signal as part of the waveform, resulting in a computer measured velocity that is too high (251 cm s^{-1}) and incorrectly classifying this study as abnormal. Spectrum (b) shows correct baseline adjustment for the same Doppler signal presented above. On this measurement, the baseline has been adjusted so that the aliasing no longer interferes with computer measurements. The waveform follower now accurately tracks the highest velocity of the velocity profile and correctly measures velocity at 183 cm s^{-1}.

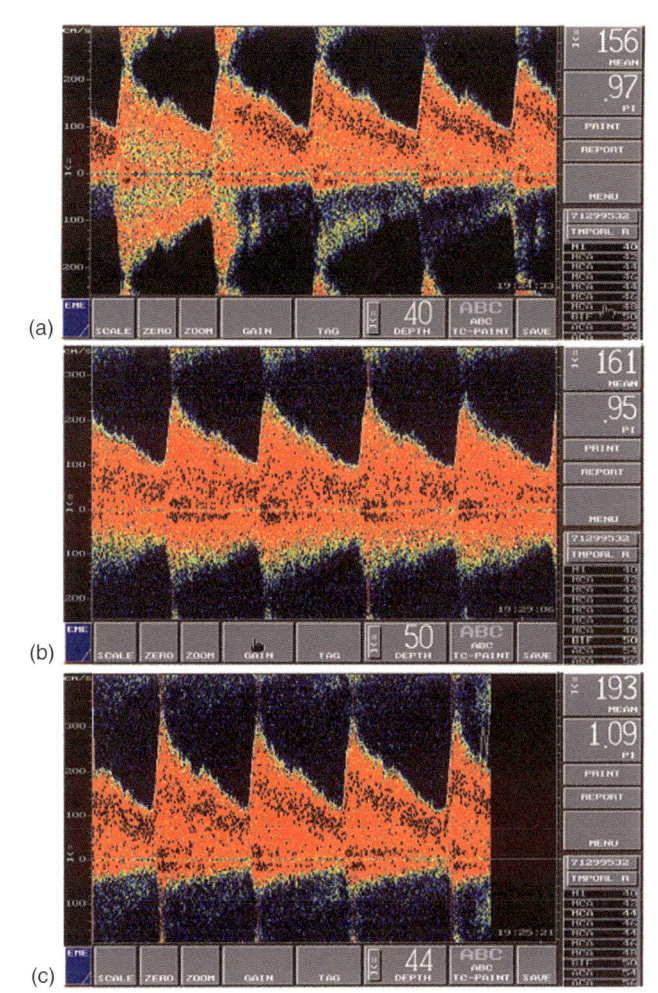

Figure 7.6 Spectra (a) and (b)s show incomplete sampling. These waveforms demonstrate how a thorough examination of the MCA is necessary to identify the highest velocity. In this patient. The velocities at 40 mm (a) and 50 mm (b) were in the normal range, i.e. 156 and 161 cm s^{-1}. A more detailed search using different aspects of the temporal window and probe manipulation demonstrated that at 44 mm there was a velocity more than 30 cm s^{-1} higher than measured at 40 or 50 mm. This measurement led to re-classification of TAMM as high conditional, i.e. 193 cm s^{-1}.

on the 1934 children in the during STOP screening phase [2,3].

In the MCG Cohort, children with TAMM velocities in the terminal ICA and/or proximal MCA of >200 cm s^{-1} had a 13% per year incidence of stroke. In the STOP trial, children with velocities >200 cm s^{-1} had a 10% per year incidence of stroke [8]. The Cooperative Study of Sickle Cell Disease collected data on 4082 sickle cell disease patients and demonstrated a risk of stroke in a pediatric sickle cell disease population of 0.5–1% per year [1]. The much higher incidence of stroke in the STOP study demonstrates that TCD can identify those at much greater risk of stroke. Stroke risk was looked at for all 1934 children screened for STOP: based on the first TCD results, with 36 months of follow-up, those with TAMM <170 cm s^{-1} (STOP "normal" velocities) had a 99% stroke-free survival. Those with 170–199 cm s^{-1} (STOP "conditional" velocities) had a 97% stroke free survival, and those with >200 cm s^{-1} (STOP "abnormal" velocities) had an 83% stroke-free survival.

However, not all strokes were predicted by TCD. This may be related to other mechanisms of stroke (dissection, embolism, hypercoagulable states, small artery infarction) or to timing of TCD performance in relation to stroke development or to failure to detect a stenosis by TCD. TCD has been demonstrated to be a very useful tool for identifying patients with HbSS at high risk for future development of stroke and can be used to identify those children who benefit from prophylactic transfusion.

Further guidelines on TCD performance using STOP study protocols were published in 2001 [9] and a modest underestimation of velocities by transcranial color Doppler imaging (TCDI) compared with TCD measurements was established [10,11]. If TCDI is used, scanning protocols should be modified to obtain comparable measurements to STOP TCD instruments [10,11].

Frequently asked questions about STOP

Q1. What are the indications for TCD use in children with sickle cell disease?
A1. TCD is used to screen children with HbSS between the ages of 2 and 16 years who have not suffered a stroke to identify those at risk for stroke.

Q2. What are the STOP criteria for classification of TCD examinations?
A2. STOP classification:

Normal:	TAMM velocity <170 cm s^{-1}
Conditional:	TAMM 170–200 cm s^{-1} in the MCA and/or terminal ICA
	TAMM >170 cm s^{-1} in the PCA or ACA
Abnormal:	TAMM >200 cm s^{-1} in the MCA and/or terminal ICA
Inadequate:	Absent/poor acoustic window.

All studies performed in the patient's baseline "steady state". Do not perform studies when the patient is acutely ill.

Q3. If a patient has one abnormal examination, when should a confirmatory (repeat) examination be performed?
A3. ≥2 weeks after the initial examination. This minimizes the risk of transient elevations of TCD-measured velocities.

Q4. If I have a child with one abnormal TCD examination, what are the chances that child will have a second abnormal examination?
A4. 85% of patients who had one abnormal TCD examination had a second examination that confirmed the abnormal velocity. Almost all of the children who had an initial examination with >220 cm s^{-1} had a second examination that was abnormal.

Q5. What should be done when a child has had two STOP TCD examinations with MCA or terminal ICA TAMM velocities >200 cm s^{-1}?
A5. Patients with two abnormal studies should be offered transfusion therapy to decrease their stroke risk.

Q6. What is the significance of the high velocities?
A6. Most of the abnormal velocities correlate with the presence of a local stenosis. Some children with abnormal velocities have normal MRAs of the intracranial circulation. These children are also at increased risk of stroke compared with the children with "normal" velocities. It may be that the high-velocity flow sets the stage for the subsequent development of stenosis or that it somehow is associated with the process that triggers the stenosis.

Q7. What should we expect if we screen our pediatric sickle cell population with TCD?
A7. STOP TCD examinations using the protocol described in this chapter were performed on children between the ages of 2 and 16 years with sickle cell disease in 13 centers in North America. The percentages of normal, conditional, abnormal and inadequate examinations were remarkably consistent across all sites: 70% of all the TCD examinations were classified as normal; 15% of all examinations were classified as conditional; and 10% of all examinations were abnormal. Only 5% were considered inadequate.

Q8. What about TCD in sickle cell patients who have had a stroke?
A8. All of the above STOP information relates to screening children who have not had a clinically recognized stroke to identify those who are at high risk for stroke development. Once stroke develops, TCD assumes less importance. Most hematologists will begin transfusion therapy in these children once they develop stroke. Children with HbSS who have suffered a stroke may have ICA or MCA occlusions, so that the MCA on the affected side may be absent or demonstrate very *low* velocities, rather than elevated velocities. There is not a precise cutoff, but TAMM velocities of less than 75 cm s^{-1} in non-transfused HbSS patients are very low and raise concerns about severe proximal stenosis.

Q9. What about TCD of the ophthalmic artery in children with sickle cell disease?
A9. TCD examination of the ophthalmic arteries was not part of the STOP protocol, so there are no STOP data to apply directly to this question. However, this examination may demonstrate several abnormalities:

(a) If the patient has developed transdural collaterals from the ophthalmic to the intracranial arteries (usually ACA branch), flow in the ACA will demonstrate a low-resistance pattern rather than its usual high-resistance pattern. This is usually a late phenomenon in the development of the moya-moya pattern.

(b) If the ICA distal to the takeoff of the ophthalmic is examined, abnormally high velocity flow may be detected, as this is a frequent site of stenosis of the ICA.

(c) Reversal of flow in the ophthalmic artery is almost never seen in these patients. The stenotic lesions are almost always distal to the takeoff of the ophthalmic artery, so that it cannot provide collateral flow.

Q10. Can you provide information about the incidence of high velocities by age?
A10. The highest velocities were found in younger children. Abnormal velocities by age are distributed as follows:

2–8 years   10.9%
9–12 years   9.7%
13–16 years 6.5%.

References

1 Ohene-Frempong K, Weiner SJ, *et al.* Cerebrovascular accidents in sickle cell disease: rates and risk factors. *Blood* 1998;**91**: 288–94.

2. Adams R, McKie V, Nichols F, et al. The use of transcranial ultrasonography to predict stroke in sickle cell disease. *N Engl J Med* 1992;**326**:605–10.

3. Adams RJ, McKie VC, Carl EM, et al. Long term risk of stroke in children with sickle cell disease screened with transcranial Doppler. *Ann Neurol* 1997;**42**:699–704.

4. Adams RJ, McKie VC, Brambilla D, et al. Stroke prevention trial in sickle cell anemia ("STOP"): study design. *Control Clin Trials* 1998;**9**:110–29.

5. Adams RJ, McKie VC, Hsu L, et al. Prevention of first stroke by transfusions in children with sickle cell anemia and abnormal results on transcranial Doppler ultrasonography. *N Engl J Med* 1998;**339**:5–11.

6. Adams RJ, Brambilla D. Optimizing Primary Stroke Prevention in Sickle Cell Anemia (STOP 2) Trial Investigators. Discontinuing prophylactic transfusions used to prevent stroke in sickle cell disease. *N Engl J Med* 2005;**353**:2769–78.

7. Aaslid R, ed. *Transcranial Doppler Sonography*. New York: Springer, 1986.

8. Adams RJ, Brambilla D, Vichinsky E, et al. Stroke prevention trial in sickle cell anemia (STOP Study). Risk of stroke in 1933 children screened with transcranial Doppler (TCD). *Stroke* 1999;**30**:238 [Abstract].

9. Nichols FT, Jones AM, Adams RJ. Stroke prevention in sickle cell disease (STOP) study guidelines for transcranial Doppler testing. *J Neuroimaging* 2001;**11**:354–62.

10. Jones AM, Seibert JJ, Nichols FT, et al. Comparison of transcranial color Doppler imaging (TCDI) and transcranial Doppler (TCD) in children with sickle-cell anemia. *Pediatr Radiol* 2001;**31**:461–9.

11. Bulas DJ, Jones A, Seibert JJ, et al. Transcranial Doppler (TCD) screening for stroke prevention in sickle cell anemia: pitfalls in technique variation. *Pediatr Radiol* 2000;**30**:733–8.

8 Cardiovascular Risk Factors and Carotid Ultrasound

Tatjana Rundek[1] & Joseph F. Polak[2]
[1]University of Miami, Miami, FL, USA
[2]Tufts University, Boston, MA, USA

Introduction

Carotid ultrasound is a non-invasive technology well suited to study atherosclerosis and its consequences. Carotid ultrasound is used to estimate the severity of carotid stenosis by evaluation of the extent of atherosclerotic changes on duplex ultrasound from the gray-scale images with the aid of Doppler waveform analysis. It is emerging as an important non-invasive imaging tool for evaluation of atherosclerotic lesions beyond percent stenosis among individuals without overt atherosclerotic disease. It can help in risk stratification for those individuals at moderate risk for stroke, myocardial infarction (MI) and other vascular events by evaluating small non-stenotic carotid plaques, their morphology including surface irregularity and echolucency and by measuring carotid intima-media thickness (IMT). The burden of subclinical atherosclerosis measured by ultrasound imaging markers such as carotid non-stenotic plaque and IMT in a given individual parallels the amount and extent of exposure to cardiovascular risk factors. The extent of atherosclerotic change seen on ultrasound images is associated with the likelihood of future stroke, MI or vascular mortality. These measures of subclinical and early manifestations of atherosclerosis, therefore, may help to target moderate- to high-risk individuals for more aggressive lifestyle and medical treatments and to monitor for the effects of these treatments.

This chapter briefly reviews the use of carotid ultrasound for evaluation of the presence of carotid artery disease in asymptomatic individuals. Other chapters review how carotid ultrasound measurements relate to the presence of clinically overt cerebrovascular disease and how this technology can help identify candidates for carotid endarterectomy. In this chapter, the carotid ultrasound imaging measures of subclinical atherosclerosis, carotid plaque and IMT are also presented and their relation to the risk of stroke and other vascular diseases is reviewed. This chapter shows how carotid ultrasound measurements of IMT can be used to quantify subclinical disease in the asymptomatic individual and to measure the response to therapeutic interventions aimed at reducing the risk of future stroke and cardiovascular events.

Doppler ultrasound and screening for carotid stenosis in asymptomatic individuals

Prevalence of asymptomatic carotid artery disease on carotid ultrasound

Carotid ultrasound is a non-invasive method to detect the presence of carotid atherosclerotic disease in asymptomatic individuals. Several carotid artery phenotypes of preclinical atherosclerosis can be identified on carotid ultrasound: carotid stenosis, carotid plaque without stenosis and carotid intima-media thickness (IMT). Traditionally, carotid ultrasound is used to assess presence and degree of carotid stenosis. Recently, carotid ultrasound is used to assess carotid IMT and non-stenotic carotid artery plaques as useful markers for vascular risk assessment and follow up of the anti-atherosclerotic therapies in individuals with moderate cardiovascular Framingham risk.

Carotid stenosis is usually defined as stenosis greater than 50% by carotid ultrasound criteria. Carotid ultrasound is accurate and reliable in the detection of carotid stenosis. Depending on the underlying population characteristics, the positive predictive value of carotid ultrasound in detecting carotid stenosis ranges from 82 to 97%. A recent meta-analysis of 17 studies comparing carotid ultrasound with carotid angiography demonstrated that carotid ultrasound had a pooled sensitivity of 86% [95% confidence interval (CI) 84 to 89] and a pooled specificity of 87% (95% CI 84 to 90) for carotid stenosis [1]. For recognizing occlusion, carotid ultrasound had a sensitivity of 96% (95% CI 94 to 100).

The prevalence of asymptomatic carotid stenosis in general population varies between 2 and 8%, depending on the

Cerebrovascular Ultrasound in Stroke Prevention and Treatment, 2nd edition. Edited by Andrei V. Alexandrov. © 2011 Blackwell Publishing Ltd.

characteristics of the studied population [2–12]. The prevalence of asymptomatic carotid stenosis is higher in individuals who already have established vascular disease. Asymptomatic carotid stenosis is more prevalent in patients with established coronary artery disease (CAD) or peripheral arterial disease (PAD). The prevalence of asymptomatic carotid stenosis by carotid ultrasound in patients with CAD ranges between 8 and 31% [13–18]. The prevalence of carotid stenosis increases with increase in the number of affected of coronary arteries. Carotid stenosis also is more frequent in patients referred for coronary artery bypass graft (CABG) surgery [19–25]. The prevalence of asymptomatic carotid stenosis on carotid ultrasound in patients with PAD ranges between 14 and 49% [5,26–31].

Risk factors for asymptomatic carotid artery disease

Most significant vascular risk factors for asymptomatic carotid stenosis are *age* and *male gender* [32–37]. Carotid stenosis is two to three times more frequent among individuals aged 75–85 years of age than among those aged 55–65 years [32,33]. In addition to the intrinsic process of aging, age affects many conditions and therefore in individuals with carotid stenosis most likely represents a combination of indirect expression of the continuous exposure to various risk factors and their complex interaction [37,38]. Carotid stenosis is twice as frequent in men than in women [37]. Other traditional vascular risk factors such as hypertension, diabetes, dyslipidemia, smoking and other lifestyle factors are associated with a higher prevalence of asymptomatic carotid stenosis, but the strength and consistency of this association vary between populations. The most potent vascular risk predictor of carotid stenosis is *diabetes*. Individuals with diabetes are three times more likely to develop carotid stenosis than non-diabetic persons [39]. In addition, the *metabolic syndrome* (a combination of three or more of risk factors of central obesity, impaired glucose metabolism, elevated blood pressure, low HDL cholesterol and hypertriglyceremia within individual) is associated with a more frequent incidence and progression of carotid stenosis [40]. *Smoking* is another potent risk factor for carotid stenosis [41–43]. Recently, a gene–environment interaction in smokers has been shown to promote the development of early carotid atherosclerosis [43]. *Hypertension* is also a potent risk factor associated with the severity of and progression of carotid atherosclerosis [8,9,11].

Asymptomatic carotid disease and risk of stroke and cardiovascular events

Carotid artery stenosis greater than 50% on carotid ultrasound is a well-established marker for ischemic stroke [44–46]. In the Cardiovascular Health Study [44], the presence of carotid stenosis was associated with a threefold increase in incidence of stroke irrespective of location and severity of plaque.

The risk of stroke or TIA is proportionally increased with the degree of asymptomatic carotid stenosis [46–48]. In the Asymptomatic Cervical Bruit Study [49] of individuals with asymptomatic carotid stenosis >50%, the annual rate of ipsilateral stroke was 1.4 and 4.2% for stroke and for stroke and TIA combined, respectively. This rate was greater, however, in the individuals with 80–99% stenosis, 2.8% for ipsilateral stroke and 7.5% for stroke and TIA combined. Severity of carotid stenosis was the most important predictor of vascular events. In the Asymptomatic Carotid Surgery Trial (ACST), the risk of stroke, however, did not differ significantly by the degree of carotid stenosis, most likely due to the selection criteria for enrollment in the trial [50]. In a series of 696 individuals with asymptomatic carotid stenosis referred to the Doppler laboratory and followed for a mean time of 41 months, the annual stroke rate was 1.3% in patients with carotid stenosis ≤75% and 3.3% in those with stenosis >75% [51]. In addition, the ipsilateral stroke rate was 2.5% in patients with carotid stenosis >75%. The rate of stroke and TIA combined was 10.5% per year among those with carotid stenosis >75%, and 75% of events were ipsilateral to carotid stenosis. The individuals in this study, however, were not representative of the general population. The convincing evidence regarding carotid stenosis and its associated risk of stroke came from the Asymptomatic Carotid Stenosis and Risk of Stroke (ACSRS) study, a large natural history observational study of 1101 patients with asymptomatic carotid stenosis who were followed up for up to 7 years [52]. The risk of ipsilateral ischemic stroke was dependent on the degree of carotid stenosis (Table 8.1). The three groups of individuals were identified according to their annual risk of ipsilateral stroke: (a) a low-risk group (carotid stenosis 50–69%) with a stroke risk of 1–2% per year; (b) a moderate-risk group (carotid stenosis 70–89%) with a risk of 2–4%; and (c) a high-risk group (carotid stenosis 90–99%) with a risk of 4–6% (Figure 8.1).

Individuals with asymptomatic carotid stenosis may be at high risk for cardiac events [53]. The risk of future ipsilateral ischemic stroke versus cardiac event in asymptomatic carotid stenosis will depend on the individual patient's risk factor profile. While some risk factors, such as smoking,

Table 8.1 Annual risk of ipsilateral stroke and transient ischemic attack (TIA) by the degree of asymptomatic carotid artery stenosis [52]

Carotid stenosis (%)	Stroke risk (%)	TIA risk (%)
50–69	1.5	2.1
70–89	3.9	4.2
90–99	6.1	4.6

PART IV Ultrasound in Stroke Prevention and Treatment

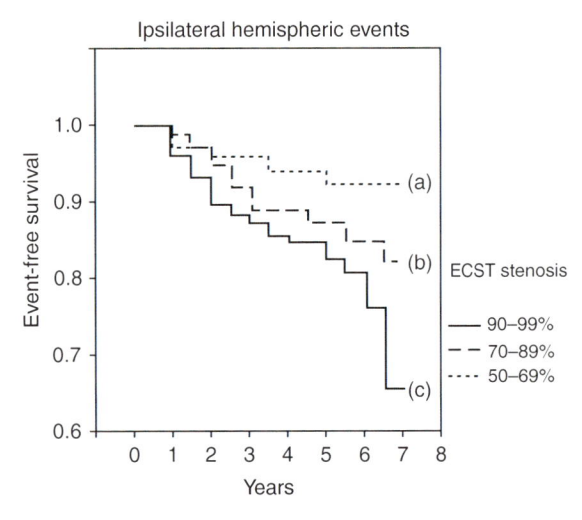

Figure 8.1 Kaplan–Meyer event-free curves of stroke and transient ischemic attack (TIA) by the three categories of asymptomatic carotid stenosis. Carotid stenosis: (a) 50–69% (b) 70–89% (c) 90–99% [52].

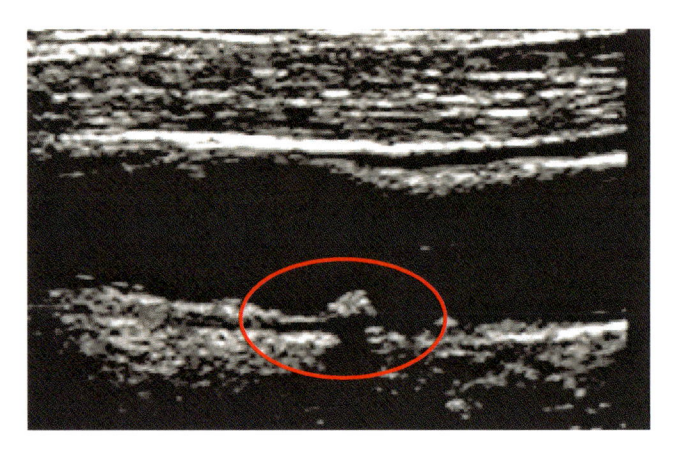

Figure 8.2 A small non-stenotic plaque in the carotid artery.

hypertension and diabetes in carotid stenosis, increase the risk for both stroke and cardiovascular events, other factors may be more important for one than another type of vascular event. Among patients with asymptomatic carotid stenosis, the presence of ischemic heart disease increases the risk of cardiac events more than that of stroke [54,55] as opposed to increased risk of stroke [56]. In the Veterans Affairs (VA) Cooperative study [57] among asymptomatic individuals with carotid stenosis, the 4-year risk of coronary events was significantly higher (40%) among those with a history of CAD than those without such a history (33%). In a study by Norris *et al.* [51], the annual cardiac event rate was 8.3% in patients with severe carotid stenosis and that risk was greater than the risk of ipsilateral stroke.

Patients with asymptomatic carotid stenosis also have a high mortality [51,54,58]. The average mortality risk in asymptomatic carotid stenosis is 5–7% per year, and it ranges between 1.5 and 12%. Cardiac death is, by far, the most common cause of death in these patients, followed by non-vascular and stroke-related deaths.

Accumulated evidence from the carotid ultrasound studies performed in selected series of asymptomatic individuals or from the population-based studies over three decades have shown that the degree of carotid artery stenosis is a significant predictor of an increased risk of ipsilateral stroke, coronary artery disease and vascular death. The vascular risk for individuals with asymptomatic carotid stenosis does not diminish with time [59]. In addition, progression of asymptomatic carotid stenosis can be found in up to 20% of patients with asymptomatic carotid stenosis. Progression of carotid stenosis to 80% or more considerably increases the risk of vascular events and death. Patients with asymptomatic carotid stenosis who progressed to stenosis >80%
have a three times greater risk of stroke or TIA than those without stenosis progression [59]. Although the majority of neurological events associated with carotid disease progression occur within 6 months of diagnosis, it remains controversial whether carotid disease progression precedes or occurs concurrently with neurological events [60]. In any instance, carotid stenosis greater than 80% or carotid stenosis progression beyond 80% is associated with a significant increased risk of ischemic ipsilateral stroke and these individuals should evaluated for possible revascularization treatments.

Carotid non-stenotic plaque is another ultrasound imaging phenotype of preclinical atherosclerosis. The presence of small non-stenotic carotid plaque (Figure 8.2) was associated with a 1.5-fold increased risk of ischemic stroke in the Northern Manhattan Study (NOMAS) [61], a 1.7-fold increased risk of stroke in the Cardiovascular Health Study (CHS) [62], a twofold increased risk of ischemic stroke in the Atherosclerosis Risk in Communities (ARIC) study [63] and a 1.5-fold increased risk in the Rotterdam Study [64].

In addition to the presence of small non-stenotic carotid plaques, the *carotid plaque size* or *plaque burden* among those individuals without evidence of carotid stenosis greater than 50% is an important predictor of future fatal and non-fatal vascular events. Carotid plaque size can be measured reliably by ultrasound as one of the following parameters: maximal carotid plaque thickness, plaque area or plaque volume. Although plaque size has a direct correlation with degree of stenosis, it is also an independent predictor of future vascular ischemic events (Figure 8.3) [61,64].

Large population-based studies have shown that *carotid plaque size* without significant carotid stenosis is an independent predictor of stroke, MI and vascular death [8,44,61,66]. Recent studies have proposed that *carotid plaque area* may be a better measure of subclinical atherosclerosis than plaque thickness [67,68], because plaque progresses along the carotid artery 2–3 times faster than it thickens [69,70]. The top quartile of carotid plaque area versus the lowest

CHAPTER 8 Cardiovascular Risk Factors and Carotid Ultrasound

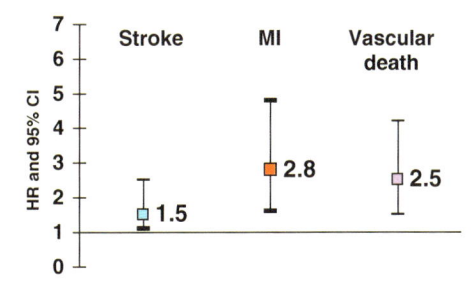

Figure 8.3 The presence of small non-stenotic carotid plaques is associated with an increased risk of stroke, MI and vascular death in the Northern Manhattan Study, population-based cohort of stroke-free individuals [61]. Hazard ratios (HR) are adjusted for age, gender, race–ethnicity, hypertension, diabetes, body-mass index, education, LDL and HDL cholesterol, alcohol, smoking and physical activity.

Carotid Doppler ultrasound in clinical trials

The use of carotid ultrasound to detect the presence of "significant" atherosclerotic disease in asymptomatic individuals is an example of a "screening" strategy. When used for this purpose, a carotid artery stenosis has to be defined by ultrasound criteria. Most commonly, carotid stenosis is defined by Doppler velocity parameters which are selected as lead parameters and their threshold is set in such a manner as to define a "significant" stenosis. Individuals are considered to have a significant carotid lesion if they have Doppler velocities above the selected threshold. The accuracy of such a diagnostic parameter, such as a peak systolic velocity above a certain value, is determined by its comparison with a gold-standard measurement technique that quantifies disease predicted by the ultrasound test. Conventional arteriography serves as this gold standard. Many studies have published imaging and ultrasound criteria for measurement of carotid stenosis that are discrepant with each other. Despite all this research, still there is no clear consensus about how best to image and measure carotid stenosis. Although ultrasound is a valid method, MRI and CT angiography are commonly used imaging modalities to determine the degree of carotid stenosis. The imaging criteria for the degree of carotid stenosis mostly rely on the results from the Asymptomatic Carotid Artery Surgery (ACAS) Trial and the North American Symptomatic Carotid Endarterectomy Trial (NASCET) [71–74]. Both methods calculated the percentage of stenosis from the residual lumen at a stenotic site with reference to the lumen of the non-affected artery as a reference from the angiographic images. Carotid ultrasound with B (brightness)-mode imaging and Doppler velocity profile is, however, an accurate and reliable technique for the detection of carotid stenosis. The positive predictive value (or the precision rate, i.e. the proportion of patients with a positive test who are correctly diagnosed) of carotid ultrasound

quartile or no plaque was associated with a 2–4-fold increased risk of stroke, MI or death [67]. In addition, carotid plaque area may be more sensitive and specific for defining patients without coronary artery stenosis than were CRP, coronary calcification or carotid IMT [68]. Measurement of carotid plaque by two-dimensional total plaque area may be a powerful new non-invasive tool for vascular risk estimation and evaluation of the effects of new therapies for stroke prevention (Figure 8.4).

In asymptomatic individuals with moderate vascular risk according to the Framingham risk factors, carotid ultrasound should be the first screening tool for further vascular risk assessment. If carotid artery plaque is detected but significant stenosis is not yet present, carotid plaque size should be measured by any of the available ultrasound parameters (plaque thickness, area or volume) and followed for progression because plaque size and its progression are important markers of subclinical atherosclerosis and a reliable predictor of stroke and cardiovascular events.

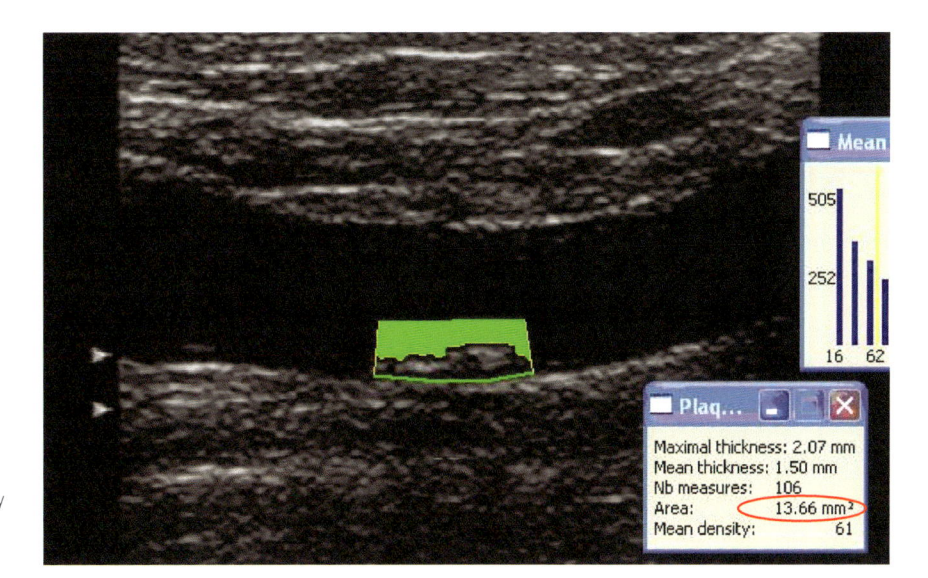

Figure 8.4 Measurement of carotid plaque by two-dimensional total plaque area (measured plaque area = 13.66 mm^2).

ranges from 82 to 97% depending on the underlying population characteristics [75].

The ACAS Trial was a multi-center trial that showed an advantage for surgical intervention compared with medical therapy for patients with at least a 60% stenosis of internal carotid artery stenosis [71]. Carotid ultrasound played a pivotal role in this trial since it was used to select potential candidates for enrollment. Doppler velocity measurements were used to identify individuals with a stenosis of 60% diameter or greater. Carotid Doppler ultrasound was used as a screening test but the intention was to insure that all individuals who underwent carotid arteriography and surgery had a carotid artery stenosis of at least 60%. For this reason, the selected Doppler velocity threshold was set to a value high enough to detect at least 95% individuals with carotid stenosis of 60% or more. In ACAS, the measured specificity of carotid ultrasound was above 97% [72]. Carotid ultrasound was, however, used according to a very strict protocol and quality control. In order to qualify carotid stenosis, participating centers had to show evidence of a strong correlation between Doppler measurements and the results of carotid arteriography for 50 carotid arteries. Early results showed marked variations between centers [72], with some centers having diagnostic performance worse than would be expected through random measurements. The diagnostic performance of carotid Doppler ultrasound improved with better instrumentation and compliance with the imaging protocol [73]. These results are very different than those reported for the centers participating in the NASCET study [74]. The sensitivity and specificity of carotid ultrasound in NASCET were 68 and 67%, respectively, when compared retrospectively with central angiographic readings for carotid stenosis of 70% or more. This result, although it applies to a-one-for-all-devices PSV (peak systolic velocity) threshold for symptomatic individuals enrolled in the NASCET study, is not an acceptable performance for a screening test. The results of the carotid Doppler ultrasound studies performed without validation in the NASCET study generated some controversy. Certain methodological issues played a role in the poor diagnostic performance of Doppler ultrasound in NASCET. Because of the absence of any quality assurance program, variations in patient selection, imaging devices and performance and differences in the imaging protocols [74,76,77] likely contributed to the poor results reported for Doppler ultrasound. The obvious remedies would have included the use of a standard imaging protocol, a certification program for qualifying both sonographers and laboratories, the implementation of a quality assurance/improvement by a central coordinating/training center and adoption of locally validated screening criteria.

In both ACAS and NASCET, the use of carotid ultrasound in the assessment of the degree of carotid stenosis had a variable effect on the final results. In the ACAS Trial, carotid artery Doppler velocity measurements for grading carotid artery stenosis severity failed to show a dose–response effect, as opposed to the results of the NASCET using angiography. In NASCET, the greater the degree of stenosis on angiography, the greater was the benefit of surgery. In NASCET, the degree of carotid stenosis measured by Doppler velocity estimates did not, however, relate to the benefit of surgery [74]. In ACAS, carotid ultrasound measurements did not show an association with the risk of a future stroke, despite the implementation of a standard imaging protocol. However, it is possible that this may represent a selection bias in the way in which these asymptomatic individuals were selected for the ACAS study, since arteriographic estimates of carotid stenosis also did not show a dose–response effect in this trial. The asymptomatic patients had very few events in the ACAS Trial (1–2% of stroke risk per year in surgical and medical arms) and the benefits of surgery were not related to the severity of stenosis as measured on the arteriogram [71].

It is difficult to reconcile these reports from large multi-center studies with the reports, coming mostly from single academic centers, that show carotid Doppler velocity measurements to have high sensitivity and specificity. A meta-analysis of studies comparing carotid ultrasound with carotid angiography demonstrated that for the diagnosis of carotid stenosis of 70–99% versus less than 70%, carotid ultrasound had a pooled sensitivity (the probability of a positive test if a condition exists) of 86% and a pooled specificity (the probability of a negative test if a condition does not exist) of 87% [78]. For detection of carotid occlusion, carotid ultrasound had a sensitivity of 96% and a specificity of 100%. Most Doppler studies do not agree on the cut-off velocity values for the degree of carotid stenosis, despite efforts to standardize these criteria [79]. Currently, the NASCET method is considered the preferred standard in reporting the degree of carotid stenosis in clinical routine. The National Quality Forum in the US introduced a performance measure that imaging methods should refer to NASCET stenosis in interpretation of carotid studies (see also Chapter 6).

Carotid ultrasound criteria for detection of carotid stenosis

Because of Doppler velocity measurement variability, there are discrepant criteria for Doppler parameters of carotid stenosis that are being used in numerous clinical ultrasound laboratories and medical practices. Each carotid ultrasound laboratory must, therefore, develop and validate its own criteria to grade carotid stenosis. These parameters must be validated with other imaging modalities and surgical findings and an ongoing quality control program must be implemented. All of these are assured in the laboratories that are certified by the Intersocietal Commission for Accreditation of Vascular Laboratories (ICVL) or other accredited ultrasound associations. The sensitivity and specificity of duplex ultrasound for the detection of high-grade carotid stenosis should be as high as 85% as in certified ultrasound laboratories that keep a rigorous quality control and assurance of ultrasound measurements and performance of sonologists. In clinical practice, however, the sensitivity and specificity of duplex ultrasound for detecting carotid stenosis are more likely to be about 70%.

The most important ultrasound parameters for the assessment of the degree of carotid stenosis include a peak systolic velocity (PSV), end-diastolic velocity (EDV) and systolic velocity ICA/CCA ratio. These parameters must be evaluated in the pre-stenotic, stenotic and post-stenotic regions of the investigated carotid artery. The degree of stenosis can also be assessed visually from gray-scale ultrasound images (B-mode) and cross-checked with color Doppler imaging. Color Doppler imaging can guide Doppler velocity determination in order to select the most critical site of stenosis for Doppler velocity measurements. The examples of carotid ultrasound criteria for the degree of carotid stenosis are widely available (Table 8.2, Figure 8.5) and can be used as a template to validate individual laboratory criteria for the estimation of carotid stenosis [75,80].

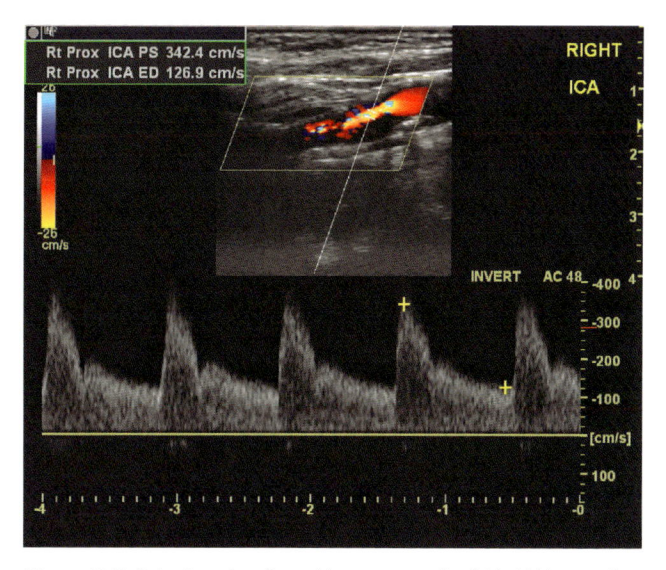

Figure 8.5 Color Doppler of carotid artery stenosis of 80–99% according to the Northern Manhattan Study diagnostic ultrasound criteria (Table 8.2; peak systolic velocity = 342.4 cm s^{-1}, diastolic velocity = 126.9 cm s^{-1}).

Carotid stenosis in multi-center clinical trials

Differences in imaging devices, imaging protocols and skills of sonographers likely have an effect on diagnostic performance of Doppler ultrasound in various multi-center studies [77,81,82]. The additional variability exists at the level of individual ultrasound laboratories. Despite these multiple sources of the variability, Doppler ultrasound can be implemented at more that one center with proper quality assurance protocols. The multi-center clinical trials with carotid ultrasound assessment of the degree of carotid stenosis need to implement strategies to reduced variability of the ultrasound results across the centers. These include appropriate implementation of a central coordinating, training and reading center, a standard imaging protocol, a certification program for qualifying both sonographers and laboratories, a quality assurance program and adoption of locally validated screening criteria. All of these strategies were adopted in an ongoing Carotid Revascularization Endarterectomy versus Stent Trial (CREST) [83]. In addition, CREST required that all participating ultrasound laboratories were certified

Table 8.2 Carotid diagnostic ultrasound criteria for the degree of carotid artery stenosis[a] in the Northern Manhattan Study [80]

Carotid stenosis (%)	Peak systolic velocity (cm s^{-1})	Peak diastolic velocity (cm s^{-1})	Systolic velocity ICA/CCA ratio	Diastolic velocity ICA/CCA ratio
0	<120	<40	<1.8	<2.4
1–39	<120	<40	<1.8	<2.4
40–59	<170	<40	<1.8	<2.4
60–79	>170	>40	>1.8	>2.4
80–99	>250	>100	>3.7	<5.5
100% occlusion	N/A	N/A	N/A	N/A

[a]Gray-scale imaging and color Doppler flow imaging (CDFI) are included in the diagnostic criteria. Gray-scale imaging provides anatomic information about the location and orientation of vessels as well as size, location, surface characteristics and composition of atherosclerotic plaques. Plaques are classified as homogeneous (uniform echo pattern) or heterogeneous (complex echo pattern with mixed densities, sonolucent areas). CDFI diagnostic criteria of the classification of carotid stenosis include three sources of information: (1) the Doppler frequency spectrum, (2) measurement of the residual vessel lumen and (3) characteristic color flow patterns. Asymmetric blood flow patterns must be considered. [Editor's comment: the ICA/CCA diastolic velocity ratio is not recommended by the Society of Radiologists in Ultrasound Multidisciplinary Criteria for grading carotid stenosis (79)].

by the ICVAL or other professional accreditation associations. The purpose of CREST is to compare the performance of carotid artery stenting and carotid endarterectomy in preventing stroke, and also the effect of these procedures on subsequent MI or mortality rates in both asymptomatic and symptomatic patients with carotid stenosis of 70% or more on ultrasound (or >60% by angiography in asymptomatic and >50% ipsilateral stenosis in symptomatic patients). At completion, CREST may be able to provide the evidence for implementation of carotid ultrasound as a screening tool for the assessment of the risk of future stroke in patients with carotid stenosis across multiple centers and ultrasound laboratories.

Carotid ultrasound in epidemiological studies and quality assurance

There have been several large epidemiologic studies of carotid artery stenosis and its natural history (Table 8.3).

In the Cardiovascular Health Study [8], a large multicenter study of individuals aged 65 years or more in four communities in the US, an increased risk of having a stroke or TIA was associated with the degree of stenosis measured by Doppler ultrasound. The risk of stroke was much greater in subjects with velocities above 250 cm s^{-1} (75% stenosis) than for individuals with stenosis of 50–75% (Doppler velocities between 150 and 225 cm s^{-1}) [8]. In addition, Doppler velocity measurements made in asymptomatic individuals were directly associated with the risk of a future stroke [84]. A dose–response association was seen between Doppler velocities and incident stroke: the higher the measured Doppler velocity, the greater was the chance of experiencing a subsequent stroke during a 5-year follow-up. However, the prevalence of individuals with blood flow velocities above 150 cm s^{-1}, i.e. the equivalent of a 50% diameter stenosis, was less than 5% in individuals who had no evidence of cerebrovascular symptoms when they were evaluated with Doppler ultrasound. These results were similar to those of the other studies that reported the prevalence of carotid artery stenosis over 50% on ultrasound of 2–8%. Furthermore, a very strict protocol and quality assurance program was used in CHS. The CHS study was conducted in four very distinct geographic regions of the US. All sonographers used the same imaging device, were trained in the same imaging protocol and were given feedback as to their technique during review of their images at a central reading center.

Gray-scale (B-mode) imaging of the atherosclerotic plaque

Much attention has been focused on the measurement of atherosclerotic plaque when determining whether a lesion is significant from the perspective of surgical interventions. However, stenotic lesions causing a 50% or more carotid luminal narrowing have a prevalence of less than 10% in the general population whereas most lesions, if present, cause less than 50% narrowing of arterial diameter [80]. Therefore, the emphasis should be shifted towards a more global evaluation of the extent of carotid artery disease and possible associations with cardiovascular risk factors.

Gray-scale imaging alone, without the use of duplex or color Doppler ultrasound, has been shown to have a low sensitivity and specificity for grading the severity of carotid disease as compared with arteriography and pathology [75]. While Doppler velocity evaluations circumvent this problem in diagnostic accuracy, the gray-scale information on the carotid ultrasound imaging is important in order to evaluate

Table 8.3 Prevalence of a symptomatic carotid stenosis of 50% or greater on duplex ultrasound in the general population

Study	Setting	No.	Age (years)	Carotid stenosis (%)
Josse [2]	General population screening	526	45–84	2.4–6.1
Salonen [3]	Population-based, Finland	412	42–60	2.3–4.8
Colgan [4]	Health fair	348	24–94	4
Fowl [5]	Veterans volunteers	153	>50	6.5
Jungquist [6]	Population-based, Sweden	478	68	5
O'Leary [7]	Framingham Study	1189	66–93	8
O'Leary [8]	Cardiovascular Health Study	5201	>65	6.2
Prati [9]	Population-based, Italy	1348	18–99	2.1
Pujia [10]	Retirement homes	239	65–94	5
Willeit [11]	Population-based, Italy	909	40–79	5.8
Mannami [12]	Japanese population	1694	50–79	4.4
Rundek [61]	Population-based, Northern Manhattan Study (NOMAS)	2189	>40	4 (stenosis 40–60%) <1 (stenosis >60%)

the severity of carotid artery disease for lesions of less than 50% diameter reduction (where Doppler velocities are less than 150 cm s^{-1}). Plaques of low echodensity (hypoechoic or echolucent) in a combination with color Doppler imaging can be measured accurately [80,84]. In CHS, the degree of atherosclerotic plaque was subjectively quantified as absent (0%), 1–24% diameter narrowing or 25–49% diameter narrowing if the Doppler velocity was less than 150 cm s^{-1}. For velocities above 150 cm s^{-1} but less than 250 cm s^{-1}, the lesion was graded as 50–74% diameter stenosis narrowing. For velocities above 250 cm s^{-1}, the stenosis was graded as 75–99% stenosis [8,84]. Totally occluded carotid arteries with no detectable Doppler flow signals were distinguished from sub-totally occluded arteries with the low-amplitude blood flow signals with the aid of color Doppler imaging [75]. This semi-quantitative scale showed an association with cardiovascular risk factors: the higher the category of plaque formation, the more an individual has cardiovascular risk factors in CHS and also in the Framingham Heart Study [7,8].

Cardiovascular risk factors and subclinical carotid artery disease

Where did the expression "cardiovascular risk factors" come from? After the end of World War II, Public Health scientists were mostly focused on infectious diseases. In the late 1940s, a well-focused effort was directed towards understanding the factors responsible for the apparent epidemic of cardiovascular diseases in the US population. The ground-breaking Framingham Study was an example of a well-coordinated effort to measure various health parameters in a large suburban population [7]. The defined cohort, made up of volunteers, was then followed in time. With the development of cardiovascular events such as myocardial infarction and strokes, a database relating these events to certain parameters such as blood pressure and cholesterol levels was established. With time, these data generated enough events to indicate that the major culprits for incident cardiovascular events included diabetes, smoking, high blood pressure and elevated cholesterol levels. These measures became recognized as risk factors for cardiovascular disease and stroke.

Cardiovascular risk factors include age, gender, diabetes, history of cigarette smoking, hypertension, increased LDL cholesterol and decreased HDL cholesterol are also risk factors for subclinical carotid disease. These risk factors can be further refined to include cigarette pack-years smoked, increased blood pressure and further lipoprotein sub-fractions such as Lp(a) and apolipoprotein B, or a combination of selected risk factors such as in the metabolic syndrome [86–88]. Several hundred risk factors for vascular disease have been identified and their treatment or control is crucial in order to reduce substantially the public health burden of vascular disease [89]. Potential novel treatments, such as the "polypill," and the detection of subclinical vascular disease as a risk assessment tool and as surrogate outcome are important new strategies in the reduction of the burden of vascular disease. Prevention of cardiovascular disease and stroke has moved beyond secondary prevention to the early identification and treatment of individuals thought to be at risk [90].

Global vascular risk assessment is now recommended as standard practice in vascular disease prevention and therapeutic strategies ranging from individuals at high risk (aggressive risk factor management) to those at low risk (periodic monitoring). Global risk stratification appears to carry its greatest benefit for the large segment of the population comprising individuals who are asymptomatic and have "intermediate" vascular risk on the basis of current risk measures. Non-invasive techniques such as ultrasound for assessing vascular wall status or cardiovascular function are useful tools in these individuals because they provide a more accurate assessment of vascular risk and possibly reclassify low-risk individuals to a high risk category [91]. Vascular risk determination by ultrasonographic measures of subclinical vascular disease may lead to more aggressive treatments and more effective prevention.

The presence of carotid arterial wall changes such as increased carotid artery IMT [91] and small non-stenotic carotid plaques [61] have served as markers of pre- or subclinical atherosclerotic burden and early detectable vascular disease and as surrogate endpoints for the evaluation of the effects of preventive therapies in clinical trials [92,93]. Ultrasound is an important and reliable tool to measure these quantitative (carotid IMT, plaque thickness, plaque area, volume) or semi-quantitative (plaque echodensity) changes and lesions. They can serve as a powerful non-invasive tool for determining the effects of risk factor exposure and risk of future vascular disease.

Plaque characterization

Early surgical series showed that the appearance of endarterectomy specimens correlated with the appearance on B-mode ultrasound, with hypoechoic areas representing areas of hemorrhage [94–96]. These early studies on carotid plaque characteristics were biased to patients with high degrees of stenosis and, therefore, fairly large plaques. The main focus of the ultrasound examination was to confirm whether or not a plaque was "dangerous," i.e. at high risk for causing a stroke. Ultrasound studies also focused on the plaque surface irregularity and the capacity for detecting ulcerations (Figure 8.6) [96,97].

The accuracy of ultrasound in detecting ulceration has been marginal in symptomatic patients with carotid stenosis, as the severity of carotid stenosis is still the most important factor associated with the risk of recurrent stroke.

The concept of a vulnerable plaque in the coronary artery system has, over the years, come to be recognized as a major cause of acute myocardial infarction. According to

PART IV Ultrasound in Stroke Prevention and Treatment

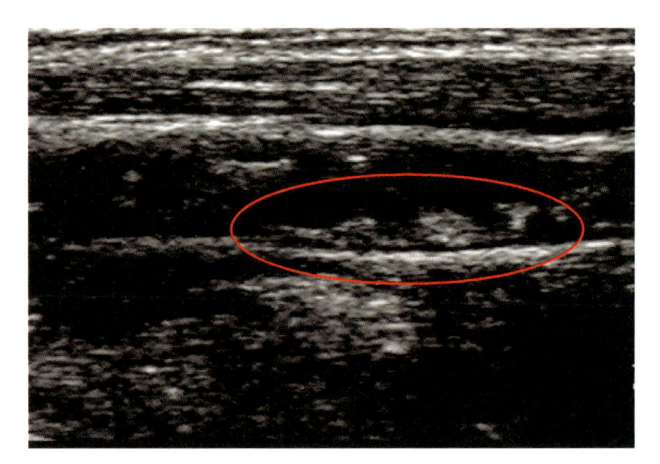

Figure 8.6 Irregular plaque surface with possible ulceration on the B-mode carotid ultrasound.

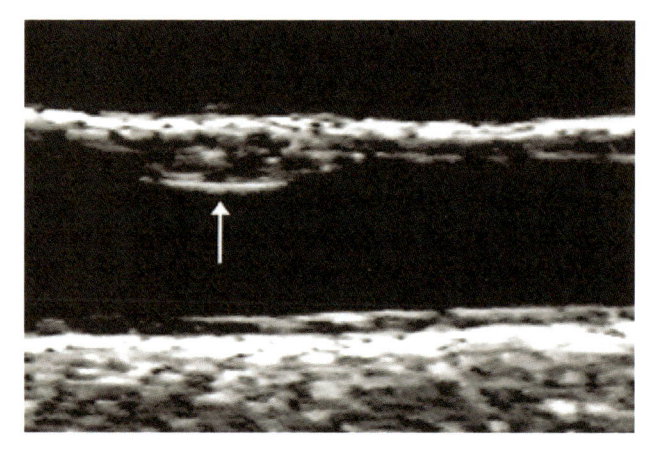

Figure 8.7 Hypoechoic, or dark, echolucent plaque on B-mode imaging (note that the plaque content under a bright cap is as dark as the medium).

this theory, a complex mechanism of cholesterol deposition, inflammation and cap thinning will cause an "active" plaque to rupture abruptly into the artery lumen, thus exposing its thrombogenic core. Therefore, rupture of high-risk, vulnerable plaques is responsible for coronary thrombosis, the main cause of unstable angina, acute myocardial infarction and sudden cardiac death [98]. In addition, half of the plaques likely to rupture and cause thrombosis of the coronary arteries cause less than 50% diameter narrowing. Until they cause the first ischemic cardiac event, these lesions are asymptomatic. Analogous to the acute coronary artery syndrome wherein perfusion failure is not the primary mechanism, "rupture-prone" or "unstable" plaques may be important in the pathophysiology of embolic stroke [99], which may account for 15–70% of all ischemic strokes [100]. While the degree of carotid stenosis is still the most powerful predictor of ischemic stroke among those individuals with severe stenosis, plaque characteristics, such as plaque surface irregularity and echo-morphology, aid in the identification of "unstable" plaques and stroke risk stratification among individuals without carotid stenosis and among those with carotid stenosis beyond the degree of stenosis [101,102]. Hence patients in the NASCET and ECST trials with less than 70% stenosis are not risk free and the challenge is to identify those patients with less severe plaques who are at particular risk of athero-thrombotic events due to plaque instability.

The exact mechanisms linking echolucent plaques, irregular plaque surface morphology and ischemic stroke are unclear. A strong correlation between carotid plaque surface irregularity and microscopic plaque rupture and hemorrhage has been observed in a correlative study of angiography with histology [103]. Plaques prone to rupture have reduced cap thickness, a large necrotic-lipid core and a severe inflammatory infiltrate on histology. Recently, intraplaque hemorrhage secondary to rupture of the intraplaque vasa vasorum has been advocated as a mechanism for carotid plaque vulnerability [80]. Plaque rupture with ulceration is most likely the dominant mechanism leading to thrombus formation, subsequent cerebral embolization and cerebral ischemia.

Definition of plaque echogenicity or echodensity

Plaque echogenicity is defined as hypoechoic or echolucent (dark on ultrasound) and hyperechoic or echodense (bright on ultrasound) in comparison with the echodensity of surrounding media as the reference, such as blood (dark on ultrasound, lowest reflection of the ultrasound beam), vessel wall (lighter than blood), soft tissue (lighter than blood) and bone (the brightest on ultrasound, the highest reflection of the ultrasound beam) [104].

Plaque characterization may be performed using a qualitative scoring system:
- *Type 1:* hypoechoic or echolucent, plaque that contains a homogeneous distribution of echoes (with the exception of an echogenic rim thought to represent a fibrous cap) (Figure 8.7).
- *Type 2:* hypoechoic or echolucent, plaque that contains a heterogeneous distribution of echoes (50% or more of the plaque has hypoechoic elements) (Figure 8.8).

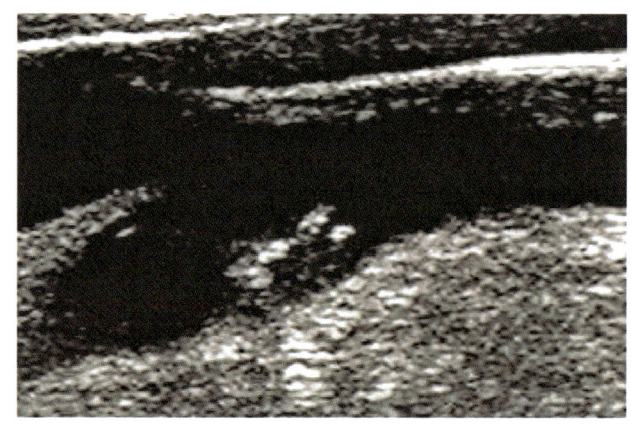

Figure 8.8 Hypoechoic, or echolucent, plaque that contains a heterogeneous distribution of echoes (50% or more of the plaque has hypoechoic elements) on B-mode imaging.

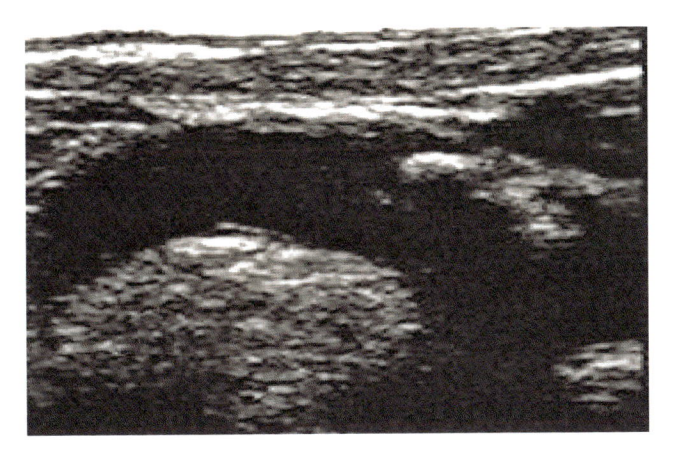

CHAPTER 8 Cardiovascular Risk Factors and Carotid Ultrasound

Figure 8.9 Hypoechoic, or echolucent, plaque that contains a heterogeneous distribution of echoes (50% or more of the plaque has hyperechoic elements) on B-mode imaging.

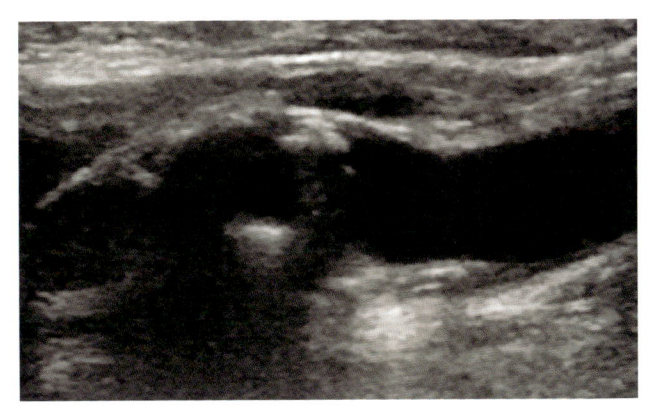

Figure 8.11 Hyperechoic, or echodense, calcified plaque that contains extensive acoustic shadowing to preclude evaluation of the plaque characteristics.

- *Type 3:* hyperechoic or echodense, plaque that contains a heterogeneous distribution of echoes (50% or more of the plaque has hyperechoic elements) (Figure 8.9).
- *Type 4:* hyperechoic or echodense, plaque that contains a homogeneous distribution of echoes (the plaque is made up completely of hyperechoic elements) (Figure 8.10).
- *Type 5:* hyperechoic or echodense, calcified plaque that contains acoustic shadowing extensive to preclude evaluation of the plaque characteristics (Figure 8.11).

These metrics of carotid artery plaque are qualitative or semi-quantitative. Recently, quantitative measures of plaque echogenicity have been developed using computer-assisted methods.

The gray-scale median: a computer-assisted index of plaque echogenicity

The gray-scale median (GSM) index can be obtained from the standard B-mode images of the vessel walls and plaque. Images are captured and analyzed on a computerized platform using a specific algorithm. The GSM index is generated after the color Doppler effect has been subtracted and echo frequencies analyzed in individual pixels determining differences in echogenicity (Figure 8.12).

Several studies have consistently correlated low GSM index (hypoechoic plaques) with lipid-rich and necrotic material and also intraplaque hemorrhage [105]. In addition, selected areas of the plaque can be further analyzed by normalized image analyses to increase the precision of the plaque echogenicity index [106]. GSM analysis of the plaque echolucency may be a useful tool in the assessment of carotid plaque embolic potential in clinical practice. However, the clinical relevance of the GSM index has yet to be proven. Although a relatively large number of studies have reported a good reliability of ultrasound evaluation of plaque echogenicity and a high correlation with pathological specimens, criticism remains as to whether the results have been fully consistent and whether some common technical guidelines can be followed. A recent critical review of major studies on the correlation between ultrasonographic plaque

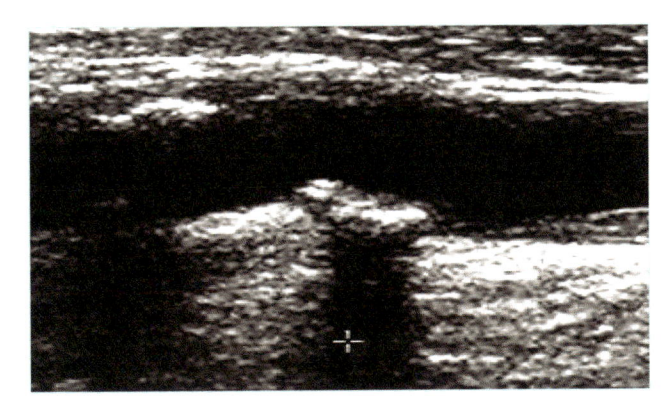

Figure 8.10 Hyperechoic, or echodense, plaque that contains a homogeneous distribution of echoes (the plaque is made up completely of hyperechoic elements).

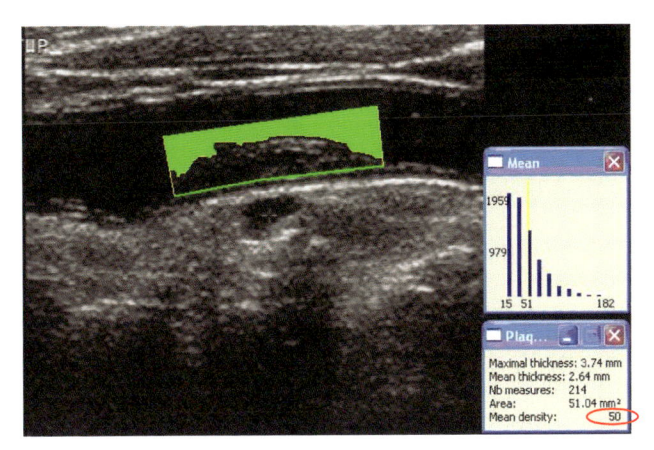

Figure 8.12 The gray-scale median (GSM) index measured on the B-mode image of the carotid plaque (GMS is expressed as a mean density of 50).

167

features and histological characteristics has emphasized a poor consistency among different studies [107]. Further technological development of the ultrasound imaging, use of contrast agents and molecular imaging will soon allow for a better characterization of plaque morphology.

Echolucent (hypoechoic) plaque and risk of stroke

The presence of hypoechoic carotid plaques has been related to abnormalities on computed tomograms of the brain [108]. Large longitudinal prospective studies have shown that hypoechoic lesions are associated with the likelihood of future stroke and MI in individuals who are asymptomatic at the time of their ultrasound examination [109,110]. In the Cardiovascular Health Study among asymptomatic individuals who were followed up for a mean of 3 years, echolucent carotid plaques were associated with a twofold increased risk of stroke and with a 2.3-fold increased risk of stroke among those who had echolucent plaques in combination with carotid stenosis >50% [109]. In the Tromsø study among asymptomatic individuals with carotid stenosis, echolucent plaques were associated with a five times greater risk of stroke. This increased risk was independent of the degree of stenosis and cardiovascular risk factors [110]. Conversely, several smaller studies have reported an association between echolucent plaques and increased risk of stroke only among patients who already had had a stroke [111]. Small sample sizes, hospital-based study designs and patient characteristics mostly likely accounted for the difference.

In addition to increased risk of stroke, echolucent plaque may be a major contributing factor for higher complication rates after carotid stenting than expected. In the Imaging in Carotid Angioplasty and Risk of Stroke (ICAROS) study [112], patients with echolucent carotid plaques, as measured by the ultrasound gray-scale median (GSM) index, had a greater 30-day risk of stroke (7%) after carotid stenting in comparison with those with less echolucent plaques (1.5%). This indicates that patient selection for carotid revascularization may need to be redefined to account for the ultrasonographic characteristics of carotid plaque in addition to the degree of carotid stenosis. Darker and softer plaques may be more vulnerable to mechanical intravascular manipulation and even deployment of the protection device prior to stenting may dislodge some of its material causing embolization.

Echodense (hyperechoic, calcified) plaque and risk of stroke

Deposition of calcium in carotid plaques has been associated with plaque stability as these lesions are often seen in long-standing asymptomatic plaques. The mechanism by which the "protective" effects of plaque calcification may explain plaque stability may be that such calcification is the last "healing" event in the process of plaque activity. These plaques become less 'active' by being less prone to rupture, sub-intimal dissection and hemorrhage and therefore become stable. Supportive evidence for a stable course and lower risk of stroke for patients with carotid plaques with higher calcium content came from a computed tomography (CT) study [113]. Although B-mode ultrasound may be less technically accurate in the detection of plaque calcification, there is histopathological evidence that echodense plaques represent a higher calcium-to-lipid ratio content, with the highest calcium content in homogeneously echodense plaques [80].

Calcified plaques are considered a good prognostic feature based on the lower rates of stroke [114,115]. However, several recent studies have shown opposite results. Echodense carotid plaques have been associated with an increased risk of stroke [116,117]. A similar observation was reported for the coronary calcium score, which was significantly associated with an increased risk of vascular events [118]. The paradoxical effect of plaque calcification on the risk of stroke may be explained by its association with a presence of echolucent (active) plaques in different vascular beds, which may be associated with an increased risk of vascular events. Calcified plaque is therefore a marker rather than a causative lesion for stroke. A patient with evidence of echodense or calcified "non-vulnerable" carotid plaque still may be considered a "vulnerable patient."

Carotid artery intima-media thickness

In 1986, a group of investigators reported to a strong association between the presence of atherosclerosis and an ultrasonographic measurement of the thickness of the aortic wall. This measurement was also performed for the carotid artery wall and was shown to correlate with the presence of cardiovascular risk factors [119–121]. In addition, carotid IMT has been shown to be significantly associated with traditional vascular risk factors in young adults (<35 years) [122,123].

The measurement consists of determining the distance between the leading edge of the lumen to wall interface of the artery and the interface between the media and adventitia on the artery wall (Figure 8.13). The combined width of this anatomic region is defined as the carotid intima-media thickness (IMT). Ultrasonic measurement of carotid IMT correlates well with histology and is a reliable measure of subclinical atherosclerosis *in vivo* [119].

Carotid IMT is being increasingly used for risk stratification in individuals and as an endpoint in intervention studies [124]. Several panels, including the American Society of Echocardiography and Vascular Medicine, have recently supported the use of carotid IMT in vascular risk stratification in mild to moderate risk individuals and outlined the recommendations for the IMT protocols [125–127].

Since its first evaluation *in vitro*, measurements of intima-media thickness have also been applied to large population

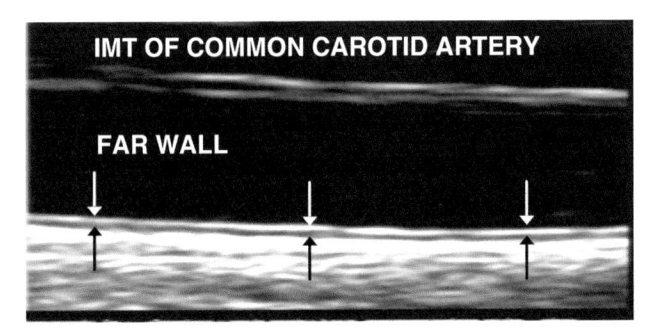

Figure 8.13 IMT of the far wall of the common carotid artery. The measurements consist of determining the distance between the leading edge of the lumen to wall interface of the artery and the interface between the medium and adventitia on the artery wall.

groups. The first two studies to look at this in a systematic way were the Atherosclerosis Risk in Communities (ARIC) [128] and Kuopio heart studies [129]. Both studies showed clear associations between carotid IMT and risk of clinical vascular events. A number of longitudinal studies have examined the relationship between IMT and future events, most frequently the incidence of cardiac events [myocardial infarction (MI), angina pectoris, coronary intervention] and cerebrovascular events (stroke or transient ischemic attack) [130–137]. Recently, carotid IMT was approved by the FDA for use in clinical trials of human subjects as a valid marker of atherosclerosis and a surrogate secondary endpoint of vascular outcomes.

Carotid IMT and prediction of incident vascular events

Since 1997, there have been at least 12 large longitudinal studies, including ARIC, CHS, Rotterdam and MESA, that have assessed the predictive power of carotid IMT for incident vascular events [130–138]. In all of them, IMT was a significant predictor of events independent of the traditional vascular risk factors, with relative risks that ranged from 1.3 to 8.5. For instance, in the ARIC study, every 0.19 mm increment in the mean IMT was associated with a significant adjusted 38% increase for women and 17% increase for men in the risk of a coronary event [128]. In the CHS, a 1 SD increment in carotid IMT (0.20 mm CCA) resulted in a 36% increased risk of stroke or MI after adjustment for age, sex and other risk factors. This effect was more powerful than a 5.5 year increment in age or a 21.5 mmHg increase in systolic blood pressure [139]. There was a clear dose–response relationship. Carotid IMT has also shown to predict future vascular events in patients with diabetes [140] and end-stage renal disease requiring hemodialysis [141].

Carotid IMT in clinical trials

Carotid IMT measurements have been substantially used in randomized controlled trials (RCTs) to evaluate the efficacy of various interventions [124]. In these trials, IMT is used as an alternative endpoint (surrogate) for cardiovascular morbidity and mortality on the premise that change in carotid IMT reflects change in vascular risk. The main advantage of using carotid IMT in a trial as an outcome variable over morbidity and mortality is the considerable reduction in sample size and follow-up time.

Carotid IMT as a surrogate outcome marker was evaluated in numerous randomized clinical trials of statins, ACE inhibitors, beta-blockers, calcium channel blockers and glitazones [142–154]. Rates of change in carotid IMT, as observed in the control groups of these trials, differ considerably across studies, mostly because of different populations and intervention studied. The overall weighed rate of change in mean common carotid IMT based on data from 13 studies was 0.0147 mm per year (95% CI 0.0122 to 0.0173), with a median SD of 0.053 mm. Carotid IMT progression has acceptable longitudinal repeatability and significant correlation with other markers of atherosclerosis. However, data on the longitudinal relationship of carotid IMT change with change in the risks of vascular events are still limited and under intense investigation.

What is carotid IMT measurement?

Carotid IMT is a continuous measure and is, therefore, measurable in all individuals. Since it is a continuous measure, mean values or increasing increments of IMT are typically used to determine the magnitude of associations with vascular risk factors or incident vascular events. Alternatively, definitions and prevalence of an "abnormal" carotid IMT can be based on a relative scale. That is, compared with those with a carotid IMT below a given threshold or cut-point, individuals with IMT above this level may be classified as abnormal based on increased risk for higher levels of vascular risk factors or incident vascular disease [125]. In this way, comparisons can be made for different age groups across a wide age range.

Longitudinal studies have used different IMT measurement methods in different populations [93]. The technical requirements needed to perform IMT measurements are demanding and therefore technical performance of IMT protocol is one of the possible sources of the heterogeneity between the studies. The other sources of heterogeneity between the studies include the details of the ultrasound protocol, namely the precise definitions of the carotid segments investigated (a various combination of IMT measured in the common and internal carotid artery and carotid bulb), the use of mean or maximum IMT at each carotid segment, the measurement of near- and far-wall or only far-wall IMT and whether IMT is measured on only one or on both sides of the neck.

The reproducibility of IMT has improved considerably over recent decades. Interestingly, none of the study population characteristics except for the duration of follow-up

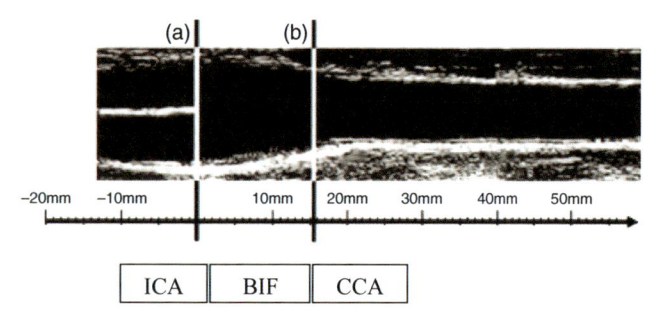

PART IV Ultrasound in Stroke Prevention and Treatment

Figure 8.14 IMT measurements in different carotid segments. Anatomic landmarks may be used as reference points, such as (A) the tip of the flow divider and (B) the beginning of the bulb widening. IMT in the common carotid artery (CCA) can be defined as 10–0 mm before the bulb widening, IMT in bifurcation (BIF) can be defined as the segment between the beginning of the bulb widening and the tip of the flow divider and IMT in the internal carotid artery (ICA) can be defined as 0–10 mm distal from the tip of the flow divider [93].

significantly explained the heterogeneity between the studies in the meta-analysis [93]. Despite the limited statistical power of the meta-analysis, the parameters such as the position of the carotid segment (Figure 8.14) do not significantly influence the hazard estimates for vascular events.

There are pros and cons of each carotid IMT measurement protocol. Nevertheless, the use of a standardized protocol in a laboratory is strongly recommended for future studies in a recent consensus document [127]. In addition, it is recommended that IMT measurements are performed in plaque-free areas. Most of the ultrasound protocols used in the epidemiological studies do not state explicitly how to deal with plaques, but, given that all of them use clear anatomic landmarks, it is likely that plaque thickness measurements are incorporated in the IMT measurements. In general population-based studies with a low prevalence of plaque, this is unlikely to be a major confounding factor. However, plaque may not be a rare finding as its prevalence in the general population can be as high as 60% among those over the age of 40 years and almost 100% among those over the age of 70 years [155]. The prevalence of carotid plaque should not be underestimated in studies of preclinical atherosclerotic burden as the presence of plaque may be an important confounder in the predictive models of IMT. Separate characterization of plaque and IMT is therefore prudent to derive better information on the risk of vascular diseases.

Carotid IMT measurement protocol

To ensure clinically relevant results, adoption of the ultrasound protocol of one of the large studies such as ARIC, CHS or MESA is suggested, preferably the one with a population similar to that of the intended study. If a single protocol is established in an individual ultrasound laboratory in the future, it should show good reproducibility and a solid database that demonstrates the clinical relevance of IMT measured by this specific protocol. Only following this recommendation may the comparisons of the vascular risks according to the levels of carotid IMT be compared between the studies.

A standardized carotid IMT protocol uses internal landmarks (e.g. the tip of the flow divider between the internal and external carotid arteries and the jugular vein) to allow evaluation of the carotid arteries in a systematic and reproducible fashion and the use of fixed and optimal angles of interrogation (Figure 8.14). The carotid IMT may be derived from the common carotid, carotid bifurcation and internal carotid artery segments and also from both the near and far carotid artery walls.

The technical properties of the ultrasound device and the expertise of the sonographer are important factors for obtaining precise IMT measurements. A comparison of the CHS results with ARIC shows site-specific acquisition of data in more than 97% of instances for the CHS protocol [139]. For the ARIC study, data completeness for the common carotid artery was 79%, dropping to 41% in the proximal internal carotid artery [156]. The number of missing IMT in various carotid sites has dropped significantly in most recent studies due to new advances in high-resolution and high-definition ultrasound and training and teaching programs that have improved the sonographers' performance and assured quality of data acquisition.

IMT image analysis

Carotid IMT measurements are usually performed off-line from digital images on a specifically designed reading station or platform. Some of the novel ultrasound equipment may already have an IMT package installed on their commercially available systems. The use of single calipers to measure IMT is not recommended due to a large error of measurement. Sampling of a large number of points along the artery wall is preferable and is easy to obtain by the automated computer-assisted edge detection systems that use more sophisticated imaging algorithms (Figure 8.15) [127,157].

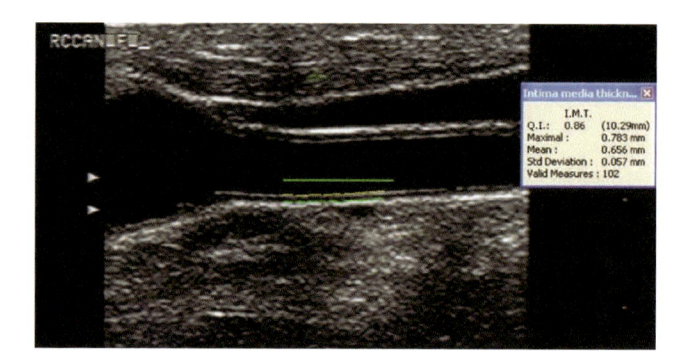

Figure 8.15 IMT measurements performed in the far wall of the common carotid artery by the automated computer assisted edge detection software.

High-precision IMT measurements with edge detectors have found application in the serial measurement of wall thickness changes over time. Measurements using sophisticated edge detectors can track the progression or regression of atherosclerotic disease and have been substantially tested in clinical trials of the various lipid-, blood pressure- and glucose-lowering clinical trials [124].

Most large epidemiological studies and clinical trials used specialized algorithms to measure IMT [93,158,159]. This approach decreases the variability and increases the precision of IMT measurements. This translates into an increase in statistical power for detecting associations with risk factors in smaller groups of subjects. With sufficient precision, the IMT measurement may be perfected enough to be used as a screening variable at the level of the individual patient.

Carotid IMT measurements are one of the most powerful measurement techniques for subclinical cardiovascular disease. With improvements in technology and improved edge detection algorithms, a precise estimate of the atherosclerotic burden by ultrasound measurement of carotid IMT in individual patients is likely to be an important screening tool in preventive vascular medicine.

Summary

The role of carotid ultrasound is expanding beyond that of a diagnostic test that is used efficiently in symptomatic patients or even one where carotid Doppler ultrasound can be used to identify the asymptomatic patient with a high-grade carotid artery stenosis. Gray-scale imaging of early plaque deposition and carotid artery wall thickness is applicable to the majority of individuals with subclinical atherosclerosis who are at the mild to moderate risk of cardiovascular disease and stroke. Using IMT measurements, individuals who have suffered changes related to exposure to cardiovascular risk factors can now be identified. These individuals may profit from early presymptomatic drug interventions and lifestyle modification at a stage sufficiently early that atherosclerotic changes can at least stabilize and possibly regress. The major limitations to the generalized application of this technology are the need for quality assurance protocols and measurement technologies that go beyond the scope of most diagnostic vascular laboratories. The implementation of quality imaging training programs and harmonization of ultrasound protocols will soon allow for the wide use of these technologies in preventive vascular medicine.

References

1 Wardlaw JM, Chappell FM, Best JJ, et al. NHS Research and Development Health Technology Assessment Carotid Stenosis Imaging Group. Non-invasive imaging compared with intra-arterial angiography in the diagnosis of symptomatic carotid stenosis: a meta-analysis. Lancet 2006;**367**(9521): 1503–12.

2 Josse MO, Touboul PJ, Mas JL, et al. Prevalence of asymptomatic internal carotid artery stenosis. Neuroepidemiology 1987;**6**(3):150–2.

3 Salonen R, Seppanen K, Rauramaa R, et al. Prevalence of carotid atherosclerosis and serum cholesterol levels in eastern Finland. Arteriosclerosis 1988;**8**:788–792.

4 Colgan MP, Strode GR, Sommer JD, et al. Prevalence of asymptomatic carotid disease: results of duplex scanning in 348 unselected volunteers. J Vasc Surg 1988;**8**(6):674–8.

5 Fowl RJ, Marsch JG, Love M, et al. Prevalence of hemodynamically significant stenosis of the carotid artery in an asymptomatic veteran population. Surg Gynecol Obstet 1991;**172**(1):1316.

6 Jungquist G, Hanson BS, Isacsson SO, et al. Risk factors for carotid artery stenosis: an epidemiological study of men aged 69 years. J Clin Epidemiol 1991;**44**(4–5):347–53.

7 O'Leary DH, Anderson KM, Wolf PA, et al. Cholesterol and carotid atherosclerosis in older persons: the Framingham Study. Ann Epidemiol 1992;**2**(1–2):147–53.

8 O'Leary DH, Polak JF, Kronmal RA, et al., on behalf of the CHS Collaborative Research Group. Distribution and correlates of sonographically detected carotid artery disease in the Cardiovascular Health Study. Stroke 1992;**23**:1752–60.

9 Prati P, Vanuzzo D, Casaroli M, et al. Prevalence and determinants of carotid atherosclerosis in a general population. Stroke 1992;**23**:1705–11.

10 Pujia A, Rubba P, Spencer MP. Prevalence of extracranial carotid artery disease detectable by echo-Doppler in an elderly population. Stroke 1992;**3**:818–22.

11 Willeit J, Kiechl S. Prevalence and risk factors of asymptomatic extracranial carotid artery atherosclerosis: a population-based study. Arterioscler Thromb 1993;**13**:661–8.

12 Mannami T, Konishi M, Baba S, et al. Prevalence of asymptomatic carotid atherosclerotic lesions detected by high-resolution ultrasonography and its relation to cardiovascular risk factors in the general population of a Japanese city: the Suita study. Stroke 1997;**28**:518–25.

13 Chen WH, Ho DS, Ho SL, et al. Prevalence of extracranial carotid and vertebral artery disease in Chinese patients with coronary artery disease. Stroke 1998;**29**:631–4.

14 Kallikazaros I, Tsioufis C, Sideris S, et al. Carotid artery disease as a marker for the presence of severe coronary artery disease in patients evaluated for chest pain. Stroke 1999;**30**: 1002–7.

15 Zimarino M, Cappelletti L, Venarucci V, et al. Age-dependence of risk factors for carotid stenosis: an observational study among candidates for coronary arteriography. Atherosclerosis 2001;**159**:165–73.

16 Ambrosetti M, Carotid stenosisorati P, Salerno M, et al. Newly diagnosed carotid atherosclerosis in patients with coronary artery disease admitted for cardiac rehabilitation. Ital Heart J 2004;**5**(11):840–3.

17 Komorovsky R, Desideri A, Coscarelli S, et al. Impact of carotid arterial narrowing on outcomes of patients with acute coronary syndromes. Am J Cardiol 2004;**93**:1552–5.

18 Tanimoto S, Ikari Y, Tanabe K, et al. Prevalence of carotid artery stenosis in patients with coronary artery disease in Japanese population. *Stroke* 2005;**36**:2094–8.

19 Barnes RW, Nix ML, Sansonetti D, et al. Late outcome of untreated asymptomatic carotid disease following cardiovascular operations. *J Vasc Surg* 1985;**2**(6):843–9.

20 Faggioli GL, Curl GR, Ricotta JJ. The role of carotid screening before coronary artery bypass. *J Vasc Surg* 1990;**12**(6):724–9.

21 Vigneswaran WT, Sapsford RN, Stanbridge RD. Disease of the left main coronary artery: early surgical results and their association with carotid artery stenosis. *Br Heart J* 1993;**70**(4):342–5.

22 D'Agostino RS, Svensson LG, Neumann DJ, et al. Screening carotid ultrasonography and risk factors for stroke in coronary artery surgery patients. *Ann Thorac Surg* 1996;**62**:1714–23.

23 Birincioglu L, Arda K, Bardakci H, et al. Carotid disease in patients scheduled for coronary artery bypass: analysis of 678 patients. *Angiology* 1999;**50**(1):9–19.

24 Rath PC, Agarwala MK, Dhar PK, et al. Carotid artery involvement in patients of atherosclerotic coronary artery disease undergoing coronary artery bypass grafting. *Indian Heart J* 2001;**53**(6):761–5.

25 Kawarada O, Yokoi Y, Morioka N, et al. Carotid stenosis and peripheral artery disease in Japanese patients with coronary artery disease undergoing coronary artery bypass grafting. *Circ J* 2003;**67**:1003–6.

26 Simons PCG, Algra A, van der Graaf Y, et al., for the SMART Study Group. Carotid artery stenosis in patients with peripheral arterial disease: the SMART study. *J Vasc Surg* 1999;**30**:519–25.

27 Ballotta E, Da Giau G, Renon L, et al. Symptomatic and asymptomatic carotid artery lesions in peripheral vascular disease: a prospective study. *Int J Surg Invest* 1999;**1**(4):357–63.

28 Pilcher JM, Danaher J, Khaw KT. The prevalence of asymptomatic carotid artery disease in patients with peripheral vascular disease. *Clin Radiol* 2000;**55**:56–61.

29 Cina CS, Safar HA, Maggisano R, et al. Prevalence and progression of internal carotid artery stenosis in patients with peripheral arterial occlusive disease. *J Vasc Surg* 2002;**36**:75–82.

30 Louie J, Isaacson JA, Zierler RE, et al. Prevalence of carotid and lower extremity arterial disease in patients with renal artery stenosis. *Am J Hypertens* 1994;**7**(5):436–9.

31 Missouris CG, Papavassiliou MB, Khaw K, et al. High prevalence of carotid artery disease in patients with atheromatous renal artery stenosis. *Nephrol Dial Transplant* 1998;**13**:945–8.

32 Polak JF, O'Leary DH, Kronmal RA, et al. Sonographic evaluation of carotid artery atherosclerosis in the elderly: relationship of disease severity to stroke and transient ischemic attack. *Radiology* 1993;**188**:363–70.

33 Longstreth WT Jr, Shemanski L, Lefkowitz D, et al. Asymptomatic internal carotid artery stenosis defined by ultrasound and the risk of subsequent stroke in the elderly. The Cardiovascular Health Study. *Stroke* 1998;**29**:2371–6.

34 Comerota AJ, Cranley JJ, Cook SE. Real-time B-mode carotid imaging in diagnosis of cerebrovascular disease. *Surgery* 1981;**89**:718–29.

35 Leary DH, Anderson KM, Wolf PA, et al. Cholesterol and carotid atherosclerosis in older persons: the Framingham Study. *Ann Epidemiol* 1992;**2**:147–53.

36 Leary DH, Polak JF, Kronmal RA, et al. Distribution and correlates of sonographically detected carotid artery disease in the Cardiovascular Health Study. The CHS Collaborative Research Group. *Stroke* 1992;**23**:1752–60.

37 Dawber TR. *The Framingham Study. The Epidemiology of Atherosclerotic Disease. A Commenwealth Fund Book.* Cambridge, MA: Harvard University Press, 1980.

38 Selhub J, Jacques PF, Bostom AG, et al. Association between plasma homocysteine concentrations and extracranial carotid-artery stenosis. *N Engl J Med* 1995;**332**:286–91.

39 De Angelis M, Scrucca L, Leandri M, et al. Prevalence of carotid stenosis in type 2 diabetic patients asymptomatic for cerebrovascular disease. *Diabetes Nutr Metab* 2003;**16**(1):48–55.

40 Bonora E, Kiechlk S, Willeit J, et al. Carotid atherosclerosis and coronary heart disease in the metabolic syndrome. Prospective data from the Bruneck Study. *Diabetes Care* 2003;**26**:1251–7.

41 Tell GS, Polak JF, Ward BJ, et al. Relation of smoking with carotid artery wall thickness and stenosis in older adults. The Cardiovascular Health Study. The Cardiovascular Health Study (CHS) Collaborative Research Group. *Circulation* 1994;**90**(6):2905–8.

42 Whisnant J, Homer D, Ingall T, et al. Duration of cigarette smoking is the strongest predictor of severe extracranial carotid artery atherosclerosis. *Stroke* 1990;**21**:707–14.

43 Risley P, Jerrard-Dunne P, Sitzer M, et al. Carotid Atherosclerosis Progression Study. Promoter polymorphism in the endotoxin receptor (CD14) is associated with increased carotid atherosclerosis only in smokers: the Carotid Atherosclerosis Progression Study (CAPS). *Stroke* 2003;**34**(3):600–4.

44 Manolio TA, Kronmal RA, Burke GL, et al., for the CHS Collaborative Research Group. Short-term predictors of incident stroke in older adults. The Cardiovascular Health Study. *Stroke* 1996;**27**:1479–86.

45 Hollander M, Bots ML, Iglesias del Sol A, et al. Carotid plaques increase the risk of stroke and subtypes of cerebral infarction in asymptomatic elderly. The Rotterdam Study. *Circulation* 2002;**105**:2872–7.

46 Sacco RL, Benjamin EJ, Broderick JP, et al. American Heart Association Prevention Conference. IV. Prevention and Rehabilitation of Stroke. Risk factors. *Stroke* 1997;**28**:1507–17.

47 Chambers BR, Norris JW. Outcome in patients with asymptomatic neck bruits. *N Engl J Med* 1986;**315**:860–5.

48 Mackey AE, Abrahamowicz M, Langlois Y, et al. Outcome of asymptomatic patients with carotid disease. *Neurology* 1997;**48**:896–903.

49 Bock RW, Gray-Weale AC, Mock PA, et al. The natural history of asymptomatic carotid artery disease. *J Vasc Surg* 1993;**17**(1):160–9.

50 Halliday A, Mansfield A, Marro J, et al.; MRC Asymptomatic Carotid Surgery Trial (ACST) Collaborative Group. Prevention of disabling and fatal strokes by successful carotid endarterectomy in patients without recent neurological symptoms: randomized controlled trial. *Lancet* 2004;**363**(9420):1491–502.

51 Norris JW, Zhu CZ, Bornstein NM, et al. Vascular risks of asymptomatic carotid stenosis. *Stroke* 1991;**22**(12):1485–90.

52 Nicolaides AN, Kakkos SK, Griffin M, et al.; Asymptomatic Carotid Stenosis and Risk of Stroke (ACSRS) Study Group.

Severity of asymptomatic carotid stenosis and risk of ipsilateral hemispheric ischaemic events: results from the ACSRS study. *Eur J Vasc Endovasc Surg* 2005;**30**:275–84.

53 Norris JW, Zhu CZ, Bornstein NM, et al. Vascular risks of asymptomatic carotid stenosis. *Stroke* 1991;**22**:1485–90.

54 Hedblad B, Janzon L, Jungquist G, et al. Factors modifying the prognosis in men with asymptomatic carotid artery disease. *J Intern Med* 1998;**243**(1):57–64.

55 Love BB, Grover-McKay M, Biller J, et al. Coronary artery disease and cardiac events with asymptomatic and symptomatic-cerebrovascular disease. *Stroke* 1992;**23**; 939–45.

56 Mackey AE, Abrahamowicz M, Langlois Y, et al. Outcome of asymptomatic patients with carotid disease. *Neurology* 1997;**48**:896–903.

57 Chimowitz MI, Weiss DG, Cohen SL, et al. Cardiac prognosis of patients with carotid stenosis and no history of coronary artery disease. Veterans Affairs Cooperative Study Group 167. *Stroke* 1994;**25**(4):759–65.

58 Joakimsen O, Bonaa KH, Mathiesen EB, et al. Prediction of mortality by ultrasound screening of a general population for carotid stenosis: the Tromso Study. *Stroke* 2000;**31**:1871–6.

59 Lewis RF, Abrahamowicz M, Cote R, et al. Predictive power of duplex ultrasonography in asymptomatic carotid disease. *Ann Intern Med* 1997;**127**:13–20.

60 Roederer GO, Langlois YE, Jager KA, et al. The natural history of carotid arterial disease in asymptomatic patients with cervical bruits. *Stroke* 1984;**15**:605–13.

61 Rundek T, Arif H, Boden-Albala B, et al. Carotid plaque, a subclinical precursor of vascular events: the Northern Manhattan Study. *Neurology* 2008;**70**(14):1200–7.

62 Polak JF, Shemanski L, O'Leary DH, et al. Hypoechoic plaque at US of the carotid artery: an independent risk factor for incident stroke in adults aged 65 years or older. Cardiovascular Health Study. *Radiology* 1998;**208**(3):649–54.

63 Hunt KJ, Evans GW, Folsom AR, et al. Acoustic shadowing on B-mode ultrasound of the carotid artery predicts ischemic stroke: the Atherosclerosis Risk in Communities (ARIC) study. *Stroke* 2001;**32**(5):1120–1126.

64 Hollander M, Bots ML, Iglesias del Sol A, et al. Carotid plaques increase the risk of stroke and subtypes of cerebral infarction in asymptomatic elderly: the Rotterdam Study. *Circulation* 2002;**105**:2872–7.

65 Spence JD, Eliasziw M, DiCicco M. Carotid plaque area. A tool for targeting and evaluating vascular preventive therapy. *Stroke* 2002;**33**:2916–22.

66 Carra G, Visona A, Bonanome A, et al. Carotid plaque morphology and cerebrovascular events. *Int Angiol* 2003;**22**: 284–9.

67 Spence JD. Technology Insight: ultrasound measurement of carotid plaque-patient management, genetic research and therapy evaluation. *Nat Clin Pract Neurol* 2006;**2**(11):611–9.

68 Brook RD, Bard RL, Patel S, et al. A negative carotid plaque area test is superior to other noninvasive atherosclerosis studies for reducing the likelihood of having underlying significant coronary artery disease. *Arterioscler Thromb Vasc Biol* 2006;**26**(3):656–62.

69 Johnsen SH, Mathiesen EB, Joakimsen O, et al. Carotid atherosclerosis is a stronger predictor of myocardial infarction in women than in men: a 6-year follow-up study of 6226 persons: the Tromsø Study. *Stroke* 2007;**38**(11):2873–80.

70 Barnett PA, Spence JD, Manuck SB, et al. Psychological stress and the progression of carotid atherosclerosis. *J Hypertens* 1997;**15**:49–55.

71 Executive Committee for the Asymptomatic Carotid Atherosclerosis Study. Endarterectomy for asymptomatic carotid artery stenosis. *JAMA* 1995;**273**:1421–8.

72 Howard G, Baker WH, Chambless LE, et al. An approach for the use of Doppler ultrasound as a screening tool for hemodynamically significant stenosis (despite heterogeneity of Doppler performance). A multi-center experience. Asymptomatic Carotid Atherosclerosis Study Investigators. *Stroke* 1996;**27**:1951–7.

73 Schwartz SW, Chambless LE, Baker WH, et al. Consistency of Doppler parameters in predicting arteriographically confirmed carotid stenosis. Asymptomatic Carotid Atherosclerosis Study Investigators. *Stroke* 1997;**28**:343–7.

74 Eliasziw M, Rankin RN, Fox AJ, et al. Accuracy and prognostic consequences of ultrasonography in identifying severe carotid artery stenosis. *Stroke* 1995;**26**:1747–52.

75 Zwiebel WJ. Duplex sonography of the cerebral arteries: efficacy, limitations and indications. *Am J Radiol* 1992;**158**:29–36.

76 Hunink MGM, Polak JF, Barlan MM, et al. Detection and quantification of carotid artery stenosis: efficacy of various Doppler velocity parameters. *AJR Am J Roentgenol* 1993;**160**:619–25.

77 Kuntz KM, Polak JF, Whittemore AD, et al. Duplex ultrasound criteria for the identification of carotid stenosis should be laboratory specific. *Stroke* 1997;**28**:597–602.

78 Nederkoorn PJ, van der Graaf Y, Hunink MG. Duplex ultrasound and magnetic resonance angiography compared with digital subtraction angiography in a carotid artery stenosis: a systematic review. *Stroke* 2003;**34**:1324–32.

79 Grant EG, Benson CB, Moneta GL, et al. Carotid artery stenosis: gray-scale and Doppler US diagnosis – Society of Radiologists in Ultrasound Consensus Conference. *Radiology* 2003;**229**:340–6.

80 Moussa I, Rundek T, Mohr JP, eds. *Risk Stratification and Management of Patients with Asymptomatic Carotid Artery Disease*. New York: Taylor & Francis, 2007.

81 Criswell BK, Langsfeld M, Tullis MJ, et al. Evaluating institutional variability of duplex scanning in the detection of carotid artery stenosis. *Am J Surg* 1998;**176**:591–7.

82 Ranke C, Creutzig A, Becker H, et al. Standardization of carotid ultrasound: a hemodynamic method to normalize for interindividual and interequipment variability. *Stroke* 1999;**30**: 402–6.

83 Hobson RW II, Howard VJ, Roubin GS, et al.; CREST. Credentialing of surgeons as interventionalists for carotid artery stenting: experience from the lead-in phase of CREST. *J Vasc Surg* 2004;**40**(5):952–7.

84 Leary DH, Polak JF, Wolfson SK Jr, et al. Use of sonography to evaluate carotid atherosclerosis in the elderly. The Cardiovascular Health Study. CHS Collaborative Research Group. *Stroke* 1991;**22**:1155–63.

85 Gronholdt ML, Nordestgaard BG, Nielsen TG, et al. Echolucent carotid artery plaques are associated with elevated levels of fasting and postprandial triglyceride-rich lipoproteins. *Stroke* 1996;**27**:2166–72.

86 Rundek T, White H, Boden-Albala B, et al. The metabolic syndrome and subclinical carotid atherosclerosis: the Northern Manhattan Study. *J Cardiometab Syndr* 2007;**2**(1):24–9.

87 Jeng JS, Sacco RL, Kargman DE, et al. Apolipoproteins and carotid artery atherosclerosis in an elderly multiethnic population: the Northern Manhattan stroke study. *Atherosclerosis* 2002;**165**(2):317–25.

88 Paultre F, Tuck CH, Boden-Albala B, et al. Relation of Apo(a) size to carotid atherosclerosis in an elderly multiethnic population. *Arterioscler Thromb Vasc Biol* 2002;**22**(1):141–6.

89 Radziszewska B, Hart RG, Wolf PA, et al. Clinical research in primary stroke prevention: needs, opportunities and challenges. *Neuroepidemiology* 2005;**25**(2):91–104.

90 Goldstein LB, Adams R, Alberts MJ, et al. Primary prevention of ischemic stroke: a guideline from the American Heart Association/American Stroke Association Stroke Council. *Stroke* 2006;**37**:1583–633.

91 Stein JH, Fraizer MC, Aeschlimann SE, et al. Vascular age: integrating carotid intima-media thickness measurements with global coronary risk assessment. *Clin Cardiol* 2004;**27**(7):388–92.

92 Wilson PW, Hoeg JM, D'Agostino RB, et al. Cumulative effects of high cholesterol levels, high blood pressure and cigarette smoking on carotid stenosis. *N Engl J Med* 1997;**337**:516–22.

93 Lorenz MW, Markus HS, Bots ML, et al. Prediction of clinical cardiovascular events with carotid intima-media thickness: a systematic review and meta-analysis. *Circulation* 2007;**115**(4):459–67.

94 Lusby RJ, Ferrell LD, Ehrenfeld WK, et al. Carotid plaque hemorrhage. Its role in production of cerebral ischemia. *Arch Surg* 1982;**117**:1479–88.

95 Gray-Weale AC, Graham JC, Burnett JR, et al. Carotid artery atheroma: comparison of preoperative B-mode ultrasound appearance with carotid endarterectomy specimen pathology. *J Cardiovasc Surg* 1988;**29**:676–81.

96 Bluth EI, Kay D, Merritt CR, et al. Sonographic characterization of carotid plaque: detection of hemorrhage. *AJR Am J Roentgenol* 1986;**146**:1061–5.

97 Donnell TF, Erdoes L, Mackey WC, et al. Correlation of B-mode ultrasound imaging and arteriography with pathologic findings at carotid endarterectomy. *Arch Surg* 1985;**120**:443–9.

98 Fuster V, Moreno PR, Fayad ZA, et al. Atherothrombosis and high-risk plaque. Part I: evolving concepts. *J Am Coll Cardiol* 2005;**46**(6):937–54.

99 Rundek T. Beyond percent stenosis: carotid plaque surface irregularity and risk of stroke. *Int J Stroke* 2007;**2**(3):169–71.

100 Foulkes MA, Wolf PA, Price TR, et al. The Stroke Data Bank: design, methods and baseline characteristics. *Stroke* 1998;**19**:547–54.

101 Prabhakaran S, Rundek T, Ramas R, et al. Carotid plaque surface irregularity predicts ischemic stroke: the Northern Manhattan Study. *Stroke* 2006;**37**(11):2696–701.

102 Mathiesen EB, Bonaa KH, Joakimsen O. Echolucent plaques are associated with high risk of ischemic cerebrovascular events in carotid stenosis: the Tromsø study. *Circulation* 2001;**103**:2171–5.

103 Lovett JK, Gallagher PJ, Hands LJ, et al. Histological correlates of carotid plaque surface morphology on lumen contrast imaging. *Circulation* 2004;**110**:2190–7.

104 De Bray JM, Baud JM, Dauzat M. Consensus concerning the morphology and the risk of carotid plaques. *Cerebrovasc Dis* 1996;**7**:289–96.

105 Tegos TJ, Sohail M, Sabetai MM, et al. Echomorphologic and histopathologic characteristics of unstable carotid plaques. *AJNR Am J Neuroradiol* 2000;**21**:1937–44.

106 Denzel C, Balzer K, Muller KM, et al. Relative value of normalized sonographic in vitro analysis of arteriosclerotic plaques of internal carotid artery. *Stroke* 2003;**34**:1901–6.

107 Lovett JK, Redgrave JN, Rothwell PM. A critical appraisal of the performance, reporting and interpretation of studies comparing carotid plaque imaging with histology. *Stroke* 2005;**36**:1091–7.

108 Geroulakos G, Hobson RW, Nicolaides A. Ultrasonographic carotid plaque morphology in predicting stroke risk. *Br J Surg* 1996;**83**:582–7.

109 Polak JF, Shemanski L, O'Leary DH, et al. Hypoechoic plaque at US of the carotid artery: an independent risk factor for incident stroke in adults aged 65 years or older. Cardiovascular Health Study. *Radiology* 1998;**208**:649–54.

110 Johnsen SH, Mathiesen EB, Joakimsen O, et al. Carotid atherosclerosis is a stronger predictor of myocardial infarction in women than in men: a 6-year follow-up study of 6226 persons: the Tromsø Study. *Stroke* 2007;**38**(11):2873–80.

111 Gronholdt ML, Nordestgaard BG, Schroeder TV, et al. Ultrasonic echolucent carotid plaques predict future strokes. *Circulation* 2001;**104**:68–73.

112 Biasi GM, Froio A, Dietrich EB, et al. Carotid plaque echolucency increases the risk of stroke in carotid stenting. The Imaging in Carotid Angioplasty and Risk of Stroke (ICAROS) Study. *Circulation* 2004;**110**:756–62.

113 Shaalan WE, Cheng H, Gewertz B, et al. Degree of carotid plaque calcification in relation to symptomatic outcome and plaque inflammation. *J Vasc Surg* 2004;**40**:262–9.

114 European Carotid Plaque Study Group. Carotid artery plaque composition and relationship to clinical presentation and ultrasound B-mode imaging. *Eur J Vasc Surg* 1995;**10**:23–30.

115 Reilly LM, Lusby RJ, Hugues L, et al. Carotid plaque histology using real-time ultrasonography: clinical and therapeutic implications. *Am J Surg* 1997;**113**:1352–8.

116 Prabhakaran S, Singh R, Zhou X, et al. Presence of calcified carotid plaque predicts vascular events: the Northern Manhattan Study. *Atherosclerosis* 2007;**195**(1):e197–201.

117 Fanning NF, Walters TD, Fox AJ, et al. Association between calcification of the cervical carotid artery bifurcation and white matter ischemia. *AJNR Am J Neuroradiol* 2006;**27**(2):378–83.

118 Greenland P, LaBree L, Azen SP, et al. Coronary artery calcium score combined with Framingham score for risk prediction in asymptomatic individuals. *JAMA* 2004;**291**:210–5.

119 Pignoli P, Tremoli E, Poli A, et al. Intimal plus medial thickness of the arterial wall: a direct measurement with ultrasound imaging. *Circulation* 1986;**74**:1399–406.

120 Poli A, Tremoli E, Colombo A, et al. Ultrasonographic measurement of the common carotid artery wall thickness in hypercholesterolemic patients. A new model for the quantitation and follow-up of preclinical atherosclerosis in living human subjects. *Atherosclerosis* 1988;**70**:253–61.

121 Lorenz MW, von Kegler S, Steinmetz H, et al. Carotid intima-media thickening indicates a higher vascular risk

across a wide age range: prospective data from the Carotid Atherosclerosis Progression Study (CAPS). *Stroke* 2006;**37**: 87–92.
122 Davis PH, Dawson JD, Riley WA, et al. Carotid intimal-medial thickness is related to cardiovascular risk factors measured from childhood through middle age: the Muscatine Study. *Circulation* 2001;**104**(23):2815–9.
123 Freedman DS, Dietz WH, Tang R, et al. The relation of obesity throughout life to carotid intima-media thickness in adulthood: the Bogalusa Heart Study. *Int J Obes Relat Metab Disord* 2004;**28**(1):159–66.
124 Bots ML, Evans GW, Riley WA, et al. Carotid intima-media thickness measurements in intervention studies: design options, progression rates and sample size considerations: a point of view. *Stroke* 2003;**34**(12):2985–94.
125 Stein JH, Korcarz CE, Hurst RT, et al.; American Society of Echocardiography Carotid Intima-Media Thickness Task Force. Use of carotid ultrasound to identify subclinical vascular disease and evaluate cardiovascular disease risk: a consensus statement from the American Society of Echocardiography Carotid Intima-Media Thickness Task Force. Endorsed by the Society for Vascular Medicine. *J Am Soc Echocardiogr* 2008;**21**(2):93–111.
126 Roman MJ, Naqvi TZ, Gardin JM, et al.; American Society of Echocardiography; Society for Vascular Medicine and Biology. American Society of Echocardiography Report. Clinical application of noninvasive vascular ultrasound in cardiovascular risk stratification: a report from the American Society of Echocardiography and the Society for Vascular Medicine and Biology. *Vasc Med* 2006;**11**(3):201–11.
127 Touboul PJ, Hennerici MG, Meairs S, et al. Mannheim carotid intima-media thickness consensus (2004–2006). An update on behalf of the Advisory Board of the 3rd and 4th Watching the Risk Symposium, 13th and 15th European Stroke Conferences, Mannheim, Germany, 2004 and Brussels, Belgium, 2006. *Cerebrovasc Dis* 2007;**23**(1):75–80.
128 Heiss G, Sharrett AR, Barnes R, et al. Carotid atherosclerosis measured by B-mode ultrasound in populations: associations with cardiovascular risk factors in the ARIC study. *Am J Epidemiol* 1991;**134**:250–6.
129 Salonen R, Salonen J. Determinants of carotid intima-media thickness: a population-based ultrasonography study. *J Intern Med.* 1991;**229**:225–31.
130 Bots ML, Hoes AW, Koudstaal PJ, et al. Common carotid intima-media thickness and risk of stroke and myocardial infarction: the Rotterdam Study. *Circulation* 1997;**96**:1432–7.
131 Chambless LE, Heiss G, Folsom AR, et al. Carotid-artery intima and media thickness as a risk factor for myocardial infarction and stroke in older adults. Cardiovascular Health Study Collaborative Research Group. *N Engl J Med* 1999;**340**:14–22.
132 Chambless LE, Folsom AR, Clegg LX, et al. Carotid wall thickness is predictive of incident clinical stroke: the Atherosclerosis Risk in Communities (ARIC) Study. *Am J Epidemiol* 2000;**151**:478–87.
133 Iglesias del Sol A, Bots ML, Grobbee DE, et al. Carotid intima-media thickness at different sites: relation to incident myocardial infarction; the Rotterdam Study. *Eur Heart J* 2002;**23**:934–40.
134 Hollander M, Hak AE, Koudstaal PJ, et al. Comparison between measures of atherosclerosis and risk of stroke: the Rotterdam Study. *Stroke* 2003;**34**:2367–72.
135 Kitamura A, Iso H, Imano H, et al. Carotid intima-media thickness and plaque characteristics as a risk factor for stroke in Japanese elderly men. *Stroke* 2004;**35**:2788–94.
136 Rosvall M, Janzon L, Berglund G, et al. Incident coronary events and case fatality in relation to common carotid intima-media thickness. *J Intern Med* 2005;**257**:430–7.
137 Rosvall M, Janzon L, Berglund G, et al. Incidence of stroke is related to carotid IMT even in the absence of plaque. *Atherosclerosis* 2005;**179**:325–31.
138 Fernandes VR, Polak JF, Edvardsen T, et al. Subclinical atherosclerosis and incipient regional myocardial dysfunction in asymptomatic individuals: the Multi-Ethnic Study of Atherosclerosis (MESA). *J Am Coll Cardiol* 2006;**47**(12):2420–8.
139 O Leary DH, Polak JF, Kronmal RA, et al. Thickening of the carotid wall. A marker for atherosclerosis in the elderly? Cardiovascular Health Study Collaborative Research Group. *Stroke* 1996;**27**:224–31.
140 Matsumoto K, Sera Y, Nakamura H, et al. Correlation between common carotid arterial wall thickness and ischemic stroke in patients with type 2 diabetes mellitus. *Metabolism* 2002;**51**(2): 244–7.
141 Nishizawa Y, Shoji T, Maekawa K, et al. Intima-media thickness of carotid artery predicts cardiovascular mortality in hemodialysis patients. *Am J Kidney Dis* 2003;**41**(S3):S76–9.
142 Lonn EM, Yusuf S, Dzavik V, et al., for the SECURE Investigators. Effects of ramipril and vitamin E on atherosclerosis. The study to evaluate carotid ultrasound changes in patients treated with ramipril and vitamin E (SECURE). *Circulation* 2001;**103**: 919–25.
143 Blankenhorn DH, Johnson RL, Nessim SA, et al. The Cholesterol Lowering Atherosclerosis Study (CLAS): design, methods and baseline results. *Control Clin Trials* 1987;**8**:356–87.
144 Furberg CD, Adams HP, Applegate WB, et al., for the Asymptomatic Carotid Artery Progression Study (ACAPS) Research Group. Effect of lovastatin on early carotid atherosclerosis and cardiovascular events. *Circulation* 1994;**90**:1679–87.
145 Crouse JR, Byington RP, Bond MA, et al. Pravastatin, Lipids and Atherosclerosis in the Carotid Arteries (PLAC-II). *Am J Cardiol* 1995;**75**:455–9.
146 Smilde TJ, van Wissen S, Wollersheim H, et al. Effect of aggressive versus conventional lipid lowering on atherosclerosis progression in familial hypercholesterolaemia (ASAP): a prospective, randomised, double-blind trial. *Lancet* 2001;**357**: 577–81.
147 Taylor AJ, Kent SM, Flaherty PJ, et al. ARBITER: Arterial Biology for the Investigation of the Treatment Effects of Reducing cholesterol. A randomized trial comparing the effects of atorvastatin and pravastatin on carotid intima medial thickness. *Circulation* 2002;**106**:2055–60.
148 Crouse JR, Grobbee DE, O'Leary DH, et al. Measuring effects on intima media thickness: an evaluation of rosuvastatin – the METEOR study. *Atheroscler Suppl* 2002;**3**:94, Abstract 136.
149 Mack WJ, Selzer RH, Hodis HN, et al. One-year reduction and longitudinal analysis of carotid intima-media thickness associated with colestipol/niacin therapy. *Stroke* 1993, **24**:1779–83.

150 Kastelein JJ, Akdim F, Stroes ES, *et al.*; ENHANCE Investigators. Simvastatin with or without ezetimibe in familial hypercholesterolemia. *N Engl J Med* 2008;**358**(14):1431–43.

151 Bots ML, Visseren FL, Evans GW, *et al.*; RADIANCE 2 Investigators. Torcetrapib and carotid intima-media thickness in mixed dyslipidaemia (RADIANCE 2 study): a randomised, double-blind trial. *Lancet* 2007;**370**(9582):153–60.

152 Brown MJ, Palmer CR, Castaigne A, *et al.* Morbidity and mortality in patients randomized to double-blind treatment with a long-acting calcium-channel blocker or diuretic in the International Nifedipine GITS study: Intervention as a Goal in Hypertension Treatment (INSIGHT). *Lancet* 2000;**356**:366–72.

153 Ubels FL, Terpstra WF, Smit AJ. Carotid intima-media thickness: influence of drug treatment and clinical implications. *Neth J Med* 1999;**55**:188–95.

154 Sidhu JS, Kaposzta Z, Markus HS, *et al.* Effect of rosiglitazone on common carotid intima-media thickness progression in coronary artery disease patients without diabetes mellitus. *Arterioscler Thromb Vasc Biol* 2004;**24**:930–4.

155 Rundek T, Brook RD, Spence JD. Letter by Rundek *et al.* regarding article, "Prediction of clinical cardiovascular events with carotid intima-media thickness: a systematic review and meta-analysis." *Circulation* 2007;**116**(9):e317.

156 Howard G, Burke GL, Evans GW, *et al.* Relations of intimal-medial thickness among sites within the carotid artery as evaluated by B-mode ultrasound. ARIC Investigators. Atherosclerosis Risk in Communities. *Stroke* 1994;**25**:1581–7.

157 Baldassarre D, Tremoli E, Amato M, *et al.* Reproducibility validation study comparing analog and digital imaging technologies for the measurement of intima-media thickness. *Stroke* 2000;**31**:1104–1110.

158 Bond MG, Wilmoth SK, Enevold GL, *et al.* Detection and monitoring of asymptomatic atherosclerosis in clinical trials. *Am J Med* 1989;**86**:33–6.

159 Bots M, Mulder P, Hofman A, *et al.* Reproducibility of carotid vessel wall thickness measurements. The Rotterdam Study. *J Clin Epidemiol* 1994;**47**:921–30.

9 Applications of Functional Transcranial Doppler (fTCD)

Konstantinos Vadikolias[1] & Georgios Tsivgoulis[2]
[1]Democritus University of Thrace, Alexandroupolis, Greece
[2]University of Alabama Hospital, Birmingham, AL, USA and Democritus University of Thrace, Alexandroupolis, Greece

Introduction

Neuroimaging modalities with high spatial resolution including positron emission tomography (PET), single photon emission computed tomography (SPECT), xenon-clearance technique and functional magnetic resonance imaging (fMRI) are currently used to assess regional cerebral blood flow (rCBF) changes during cognitive functions [1–9]. However, most rCBF techniques are invasive, time consuming and expensive. Additionally, the low temporal resolution of these techniques limits the real-time representation of the dynamic or cognitive task effect in the cerebral blood flow [10,11]. Another potentially attractive alternative is the real-time monitoring of changes in blood flow velocity (FV) during cognitive functions using functional transcranial Doppler (fTCD), which is a term used to characterize TCD measurements during the simultaneous performance of cognitive tasks. Interestingly, Aaslid [12] had demonstrated increased blood flow velocities (FVs) in the posterior cerebral arteries in response to visual stimulation using TCD 5 years before the first fMRI study was published [13]. The advantages of fTCD are related to the excellent temporal resolution and the real-time assessment of changes in flow parameters in intracranial circulation. Consequently, fTCD may be considered as a promising tool for the evaluation of cerebral autoregulation and vasomotor reactivity during dynamic tests but also for the assessment of blood flow changes during cognitive tasks. This chapter summarizes the applications of fTCD, potential advantages and disadvantages and technical considerations related to the limitations of this neuroimaging modality.

Physiological background

A specific cognitive function results in increased local neural activity. The regional increase in neuronal activity leads to a local vasodilation, either directly or indirectly via an increase in local energy consumption. This mechanism is characterized as "metabolic coupling" [14,15]. More specifically, the "neurovascular coupling" adapts local cerebral blood flow in accordance with the metabolic needs and activity of the underlying cortex [16]. The exact way in which rCBF and synaptic activity are connected is subject to investigation [14]. Experimental data suggest that nitric oxide participates in the increase in rCBF by augmenting regional glucose metabolism [17–19].

In contrast with the dilatation of the small cerebral arterioles, the diameter of the large cerebral arteries can be regarded as constant. Angiographic measurements showed that cerebral arteries with a cross-section larger than 2.5 mm do not change their diameter during hypercapnia or after administration of vasopressin [20,21]. This condition is most probably fulfilled according to the findings of more recent studies [22,23]. The changes of the diameter of the small arterioles and the constancy of the diameter of the basal cerebral arteries lead to FV changes. In other words, changes in FVs in the large basal arteries are not a result of their own vasomotor activity but reflect changes in the blood demand in their perfusion areas and changes in local neuronal activity [24]. Therefore, CBF modifications are nearly proportional to velocity modifications in the basal cerebral arteries. fTCD relies on FV changes in the supplying basal cerebral arteries, which correspond to alterations in rCBF [25]. The proportionality between FV and CBF in the supplying arteries can be deduced mathematically, under the assumption that several flow and vessel characteristics, such as stable vessel diameter, laminar flow and constancy of blood viscosity, are present [14,25]. Although these prerequisites cannot be assumed in practice, a close relationship between rCBF changes due to local neural activity and corresponding FV alterations has been demonstrated [26].

Cerebrovascular Ultrasound in Stroke Prevention and Treatment, 2nd edition. Edited by Andrei V. Alexandrov. © 2011 Blackwell Publishing Ltd.

PART IV Ultrasound in Stroke Prevention and Treatment

Therefore, the monitoring of FV alterations in the supplying basal cerebral arteries by fTCD reflects the rCBF changes during the specific cognitive task.

How to perform a fTCD investigation: technical considerations and practical recommendations

Devices, hardware and software

A standard depth and the lowest possible sample volume (3 mm) are preferable. The probes are attached and fixed with a rubber ribbon in order to obtain the maximum signal intensity at the predetermined insonation depth. Different probe holder fixation systems (e.g. adhesive fixation, elastic headbands with a base support on two earplugs and on the nasal ridge, screw-topped probe fixation systems) that allow optional adjustments over a large range in temporal windows are commercially available.

Software specifications such as automatic artifact rejection and the extension of storage capacity which allows the offline analysis of data offer additional capabilities. Other characteristics, such as the automatic estimation of mean values in a defined time interval, are available. Specific programs for automated analysis of event-related changes in FV and for artifact detection and rejection have been developed. In many studies, the program AVERAGE developed by Deppe et al. [27] has been used. This program provides several steps of data preprocessing, i.e. data normalization, artifact management, noise reduction and heart beat analysis. A more complete analysis using Fourier analysis of mean flow velocity (MFV) time series, called functional transcranial Doppler spectroscopy (fTCDS), has recently been described [28].

Examination technique – cognitive tasks

Patients with extra- or intra-cranial steno-occlusive arterial disease or lesions that could influence the normal pattern of blood flow are regularly excluded from fTCD assessments. A sitting position in front of a computer screen in a quiet room with dimmed light is usually selected. It is preferable to perform a trial period of recording prior to the examination in order to ensure the stability of the probes and the comfortable seating of the subjects. It is also crucial to avoid movements and speaking (depending on the function tested). A clear explanation of each task and command before the beginning is recommended to avoid the need for any verbal instruction or auditory stimulation during the study. In order to control for compliance, a subsequent task could be used after the end of each test or at the end of the entire examination. Alternatively, verbalizing in a low voice is suggested in order to minimize the risk of signal artifacts [25].

After recording the baseline values, the investigator starts addressing commands of the different specific tasks, usually

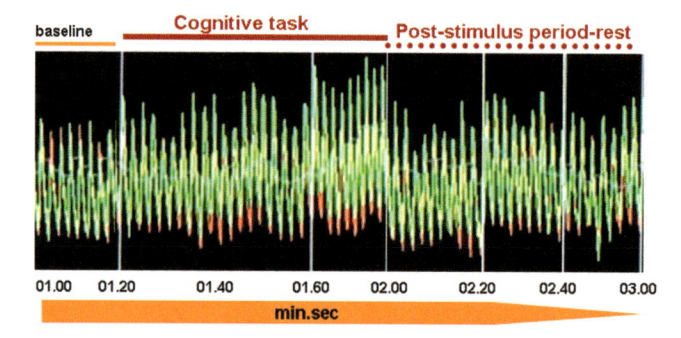

Figure 9.1 Offline-mode analysis. The software allows time windows to be defined corresponding to a specific cognitive task as well as the pre- and post-stimulus periods. The green–red recording presents the simultaneous fluctuations of mean FV values for the defined interval bilaterally.

separated in different epochs. Most common is the presentation of the stimuli (on-cycle) followed by an off-period of 15–30 s (off-cycle). The "on" and "off" cycles are repeated but should not be extended to more than 20 trials because of response habituation [10,29]. During the performance of a specific task an increase in FVs is recorded. During the offline analysis, the intervals corresponding to the performance of each task for the rest and baseline periods are defined in the recorded diagram on the basis of time measurements and the cues marking the start and end of each task. According to the software used, the mean values for each interval can be calculated (Figure 9.1). The comparison of event-related blood flow velocity changes within the territories of two cerebral arteries can serve to evaluate the most activated area. As a measure of quantification of the differences of the left and the right recordings, the lateralization indices (LI) are used based on the percentage change of blood FV from baseline.

In the study of Rihs et al. [30], an overall fTDC language lateralization index (LI) was defined as follows:

$$LI = \mathrm{mean}\,V\mathrm{shift}_{\mathrm{language\ tasks}} - \mathrm{mean}\,V\mathrm{shift}_{\mathrm{visuospatial\ tasks}}$$

where V shift is the change in left MCA blood flow velocity divided by right MCA blood flow velocity during activity compared with rest.

For the calculation of LI for a specific task, a simplified equation in which positive value means left-hemispheric dominance and a negative value right-hemispheric dominance is

$$LI\text{-}N = \Delta V_L - \Delta V_R = \frac{V_{LE} - V_{LH}}{V_{LH}} - \frac{V_{RE} - V_{RH}}{V_{RH}}$$

where L = left, R = right, $LI\text{-}N$ = lateralization index based on mean values of mean velocities during the performance of a specific task (N), ΔV = percentage difference of mean FV during a cognitive task/baseline, V_{LE}, V_{RE} = mean average value of mean FV during the task and V_{LH}, V_{RH} = mean average value of mean baseline FV value.

A more detailed and precise equation is used with the AVERAGE program [27,31,32]. The LI is calculated as the maximum difference of the FV curves in two arteries according to

$$LI_{fTCD} = \frac{1}{t_{int} \int_{t_{max}-0.5t_{int}}^{t_{max}+0.5t_{int}} \Delta V(t) dt}$$

where $\Delta V(t) = dV(t)$ left $- dV(t)$ right is the difference between the relative velocity changes of the left and right MCAs, t_{max} represents the latency of the absolute maximum of $\Delta V(t)$ during a defined interval and t_{int} represents the chosen integration time period. In other words, to make this measure less sensitive to spikes, the LI is calculated as mean FV difference of a 2 s interval (t_{int}) enclosing the maximum difference.

Special attention should be paid to the choice of the period that will be used as the baseline reference value. Usually the task performance follows the alternating rest–activation strategy [33]. Many studies use the last pre-test interval of each rest phase as baseline measurement for the subsequent cognitive task [31,34–37]. Other investigators estimate the mean baseline value as the average of mean values of all the rest phases [29,38,39]. This issue becomes more complex if we take into account that according to previous observations there is a short phase of increase in FV at the end of the stimulus [40] and also a post-stimulus "undershooting reaction" [11,40,41] (Figure 9.2). During the post-stimulus period FVs have been shown to decrease below the level of the pre-stimulus period. In a recent study [41], this post-stimulus "undershooting reaction" was quantified and it was indicated that the blood flow in the more activated dominant hemisphere was more "stable" and with lesser FV fluctuations than the non-dominant one during successive alternative periods of activation and rest. According to these reports, it is preferable to schedule adequate rest periods between the epochs and to avoid including the post-stimulus periods in the calculation of mean pre-test baseline values.

The selection of cognitive tasks is dependent on the specific function that will be examined. For example, checkerboard stimulus or viewing pictures with increasing complexity (structure, color and depth) has been used as visual stimuli [40]. The word generation task showed the greater activation pattern of the dominant hemisphere in studies of language lateralization [41–46]. Attention tasks have been used in order to investigate attention deficits [37]. Known standardized tests and scales such as the Wisconsin Card Sorting Test (WCST) and the Tower of Hanoi puzzle (TOH) were transferred into computer programs and were used in fTCD studies [47–50]. Special tasks suitable for children have been proposed [51,52].

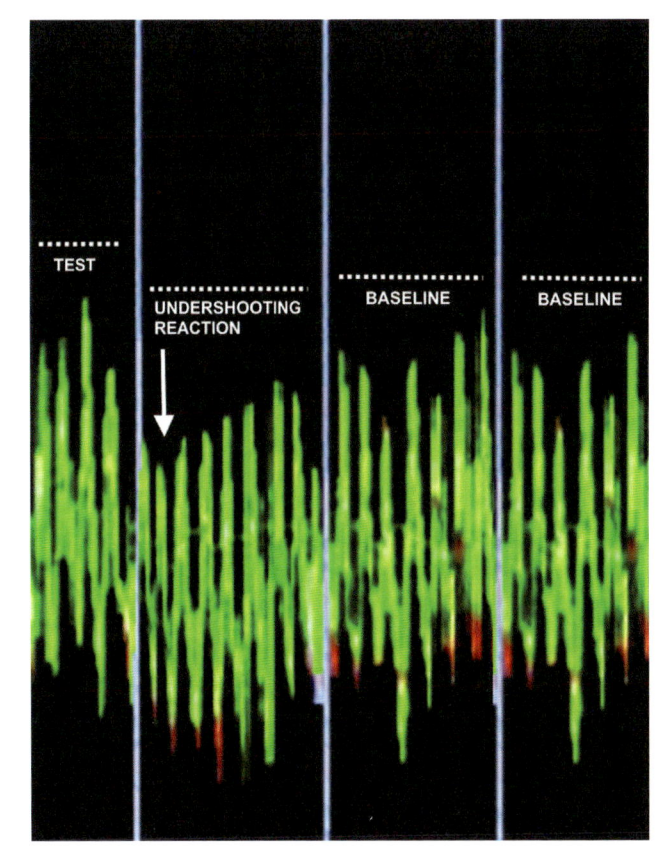

Figure 9.2 Undershooting reaction. During the post-stimulus period FVs have been shown to decrease below the level of the pre-stimulus period (arrow). Mean value including this sort period could be lower than the baseline value (Multidop T2s TCD device, DWL Elektronische Systeme, Sipplingen, Germany; Aristotle University 2nd Department of Neurology, Neurosonology Laboratory, Director Prof. N. Artemis).

Validation studies

In several validation studies, the technique of fTCD was directly compared with other methods [30,31,45,53–58]. The intracarotid amobarbital procedure, otherwise known as the Wada test [53], is considered as the gold standard method for the determination of language dominance. In the comparative study of Knecht *et al.* [31], fTCD results were concordant with the results of the Wada test in every case. Although the fact that the methods of fMRI and fTCD record different phenomena (the oxyhemoglobin/deoxyhemoglobin ratio and the FVs in the basal arteries, respectively), their results were concordant [54] and the evoked FV changes as expressed by lateralization indices (LI) showed a strong linear relation [55]. In a study on spatial attention, fMRI results in three out of 15 subjects (20%) were different to fTCD results [56]. However, after a more detailed analysis of their activation pattern, the final results were concordant in these cases also.

A highly significant correlation between the Wada test and fTCD has been reported not only in healthy individuals, but also in patients [30]. Moreover, in another comparative study, fTCD and the Wada test were in good agreement regarding hemispheric language lateralization in all patients, even children, in patients with low IQ and in non-native speakers [45]. Significant correlations were also found between neuropsychologic task performance, TCD changes and PET blood flow changes in comparative fTCD and PET studies [57,58].

The evaluation of the statistical parameters of reliability (i.e. retest reliability coefficients, consistency, signal-to-noise ratios) is crucial when monitoring possible shifts in FVs bilaterally. There are not a great number of fTCD studies explicitly dealing with this issue (Table 9.1). The introduction of interhemispheric indices improves significantly the inter- and intra-observer reproducibility [59]. A satisfactory inter-observer reproducibility in measurements repeated within hours was found ($r = 0.92$) and also a good intra-observer reproducibility was estimated in measurements repeated with a 2-month interval (correlation coefficient $r = 0.80$) in the study of Bay-Hansen et al. [59]. In the study of Knecht et al. [43], LIs obtained from repeated examinations in 10 subjects showed a high test–retest reproducibility ($r = 0.95$, $P < 0.0001$) and identical results were found on 10 repeated assessments of LI in the same subject. Over repeated examinations during a line bisection task, the index of lateralization of 20 healthy subjects showed a high test–retest reproducibility ($r = 0.9$, $P < 0.01$ in the study of Flöel et al. [60].

Limitations

The main limitation of fTCD is related to the fact that 5–10% of the healthy Caucasian population exhibits an insufficient temporal ultrasound window. Moreover, the absolute FVs cannot be measured precisely by TCD, since the difference between the emitted and received frequencies is influenced by the angle between the ultrasonic beam and the flow direction of the blood stream. However, in the examination of MCAs, the angle between the ultrasonic beam and the vessel is usually so small that the deviation resulting from it

Table 9.1 Summary of studies on reliability of fTCD measurements

Participants	Cognitive task	Parameters examined	Results	Study (Ref.)
11 (1 with epilepsy)	Word generation task (language lateralization)	1 Test–retest reproducibility 2 10 repeated assessments of LI in the same subject	1 High correlation coefficient ($r = 0.95$, $p < 0.0001$) 2 No statistically significant variation ($p = 0.8$)	43
30 healthy	Rest	1 Inter-observer reproducibility 2 Intra-observer reproducibility	1 $r = 0.92$ 2 $r = 0.8$	59
20 healthy	Line bisectioning task	1 Test–retest reproducibility 2 10 repeated assessments of LI in the same subject	1 $r = 0.9$, $p < 0.01$ 2 Overlapped confidence intervals	60
20 healthy	13 verbal and visuospatial tasks	Test–retest repeatability	8/13 tasks $r = 0.52$-0.83	61
20 healthy	Language lateralization: 6 tests	Repeatability coefficient	95–100%	62
16 children aged 2–9 years	Picture-description language task	1 LIs test–retest reliability 2 10 times task repetition in a single subject 3 Accuracy (SE_{LI})[a] 4 Signal-to-noise ratio (CV) over time	1 High ($r_{tt} = 0.87$, $p > 0.01$) 2 No trend indicating any practice or habituation effects 3 No changes ($p = 0.87$) 4 No changes over time ($p = 0.37$)	52
10 healthy participants	A series of cognitive tasks – language lateralization	1 Average difference between first and second measurements 2 Repeatability coefficient – BSI[b] limits of agreement	1 $p > 0.05$ 2 Good repeatability, 90–100% of the LI values for each task were within the limits of agreement	41

[a]SE_{LI} = standard error first examination and second examination.
[b]British Standards Institution.

can almost be neglected [63]. Prior to the beginning of the recordings, the probes are fixed in the headband in a stable position in order to obtain the maximum signal intensity at the predetermined insonation depth. Furthermore, the use of the relative FV changes can give more accurate results independent of the insonation angle not only for the MCAs but also for the others cerebral arteries [24,27].

The real-time TCD recordings can be responsible for certain technical limitations. In fact, FV modulations due to a defined stimulus are small in contrast to spontaneous fluctuations of the blood flow velocity resulting from processes such as arousal, respiration or ventricular contractions [26]. These non-specific modulations can exceed the stimulus-related response in FV up to 10-fold [64]. As a consequence, it is important to avoid movements of the subjects or the examiners during the entire duration of the examination. It is also recommended to mark involuntary movements (e.g. coughing) in order to take them into account during the offline data analysis. The use of averaging stimulus-related FV modulations or the use of indices for the estimation of the related changes minimizes probable errors.

Another potential methodological shortcoming is the impact of pathological conditions of the vessel on flow characteristics. For example, in the vicinity of stenotic vessels, there is a risk of a non-laminar (turbulent) flow pattern depending on the degree of the stenosis and the perfusion pressure. If fTCD is applied in these vessel segments with turbulent flow, proportionality of CBFV and rCBF is not assured [26]. For this reason, an overall evaluation of extracranial and intracerebral circulation prior to the performance of fTCD study is recommended.

Applications of fTCD

The method of fTCD is currently used with a wide variety of cognitive tasks in order to examine different functions. The most frequently insonated arteries are the MCAs, mainly in studies concerning cognitive functions and language lateralization. ACAs are insonated in studies which use arithmetic problems or complex cognitive tasks and PCAs mainly in studies concerning visual and color perception. Cognitive tasks have shown comparable FV changes in young and old subjects [65,66], suggesting that the hemodynamic response to neuronal activation is unaffected by aging alone. The most prominent fTCD applications are outlined below (Table 9.2).

Vision and visual perception
Visual perception was among the first issue of interest. Aaslid [12] compared FV changes in the PCA and MCA under simple light stimulation. The increase in FV measured in the PCA was significantly greater than that in the MCA. Conrad and Klingelhofer [40] observed differences in the activation pattern of FVs during dynamic checkerboard-pattern stimulation and white screen stimulation. FV changes have been studied in relation to the frequency [67] and the intensity [68] of intermittent light stimulation. Dominance for color perception in the right hemisphere in right-handers has been reported in another fTCD study [69]. A right-hemispheric specialization for visuospatial processing was found after the use of visual imagination tasks [70].

Auditory perception
In an elegant study by Klingelhofer *et al.* [71], "white noise" resulted in significant but relatively small bilateral changes in FV, in contrast to speech that led to more pronounced reactions, especially of left hemisphere in right-handed subjects. The study of music perception is also an interesting issue. FV increases without significant lateralization have been found during passive music perception, but a greater increase in FV was recorded in the right MCA during the effort to identify a known melody between others [72]. In a study with professional (right-handed) musicians, no lateralization during passively listening to music was found, but there was a greater increase in FVs in the right MCA during the task of identification of the melodies [73]. Musicians and non-musicians seem to show differences in lateralization of musical stimuli with a right hemisphere lateralization during harmony perception in non-musicians and an attentive mode of listening contributing to a left hemisphere lateralization in musicians [74].

Language and motor activation
The hemispheric dominance for language has been examined widely using different tests such as word generation task [41–47,75], word association task [76], word fluency tasks [41,70,77], assignment of words to semantic categories, word meaning and synonyms [77–79], syntax and logical completion of sentences [36,42,77,79] and reading aloud [41,42,77,79].

Simple finger movements showed a greater increase in FV in the MCA contralateral to the side of movement [71], and the same was reported for opening and closing of the fist [80].

Executive functions
FV changes in ACAs have been studied during a simple subtraction task (seven serial subtractions, starting with the number 1000), and a slight but significant bilateral FV increase was reported [81]. FV reactions have also been recorded during addition, subtraction and multiplication tasks [82]. Changes in ACAs and MCAs bilaterally were also recorded during the performance of computer versions of the Wisconsin Card Sorting Test (WCST) [49,50].

Anticipation of somatosensoric stimuli was examined in fTCD studies [83,36,84]. Visuospatial tasks, referred to as "faces" and "designs," were used for the activation of the

Table 9.2 Assessment of cognitive functions using different cognitive tasks

Artery – insonation depth	Cognitive tasks (examples)	Function	Summary of studies (Ref.)
MCA (46–55 mm)	• Word generation task • Verbal fluency • Synonyms – comparison of words • Syntax – sentence construction • Picture-description language task • Reading task • Semantic decision task • Reading aloud	Language	29,30,31,41–47,52,55,66,70,77–79
MCA	• Comparison of faces • Comparison of designs.	Right-hemispheric activation	29,30,36,79
MCA	• Visual-imaging task	Visuospatial attention	56,70,71,
MCA	• Finger movements	Motor function	71,80
PCA	• Dark and color stimulation	Color perception	69
PCA-P2	• White screen stimulation • Checkerboard pattern • Picture viewing • Reading test • Repetitive light stimulation at different frequencies	Occipital lobe function	40,67,68,97
ACA A1, MCA A1	• Wisconsin Card Sorting Test	Frontal lobe function	48,49
MCA	• Cube perspective test	Spatial orientation	47
MCA	• Phonological memory task • Verbal working memory task	Working memory	35
MCA M1, ACA, PCA-P2	• Subtraction		81,82
MCA	• Music pieces (language – rhythm –melody)	Music perception	38, 72–74
MCA	• Tonic alertness • Phasic alertness • Go/NoGo • Divided attention	Attention	37
MCA	• Line bisection task	Spatial attention	60,87
MCA	• Cued tactile stimuli • Non-cued tactile stimuli	Anticipation of somatosensoric stimuli	36,84,85
MCA	• Watching movie scenes • Picture sequences of emotion-related content	Emotional processes	88,89

right hemisphere [79]. In order to examine spatial processing, more complex tests are used such as recognizing certain symbols only by touching them [71,85], visual discrimination and perceptual speed of identical pictures [36], three-dimensional puzzle, computer game, visual search task, comparison of pairs of complex geometric figures, mental rotation [79], "line bisectioning" [87,60], visuospatial and verbal working memory tasks [35]. In these cases, the results are more complex since in many instances a bilateral activation is reported.

Furthermore, FV changes have been examined during the performance of video games [82], watching movie scenes of different emotional content [88] and presentation of images with emotional content [89]. The findings support the assumption of a greater activation of the right hemisphere during emotional processes. FV changes in MCAs have also been studied during the execution of memory tasks. Different attention tasks have been used in order to estimate attention deficits [37].

fTCD studies in patients with neurological disorders

The great majority of fTCD studies have included normal subjects. There are several reasons for this. First, the performance of cognitive tasks demands good cooperation and a full comprehension of the entire procedure. Second, TCD recordings require normal baseline values and laminar blood flow. Despite these technical limitations, fTCD has also been used in patients with neurological diseases. An important attempt is the evaluation of language dominance in epileptic patients. This issue is of great interest in the presurgical evaluation of patients with medically intractable focal epilepsies because fTCD could be an alternative to the Wada test method, which is an invasive technique carrying certain risks.

fTCD has also been used in autistic children [90], in patients with dementia [91] and schizophrenia [50,92], in stroke patients with normal large extracranial and intracranial vessels [93], in aphasic patients [94], in patients during generalized spike-wave activity [95], in migraine [96], in smoking young adults [97] and in patients with tumors [30]. Efforts have been made to detect potential shifts of lateralization with stroke patients during the course of their recovery. Moreover, the activation of areas in the infarcted hemisphere, soon after stroke onset, seemed to be a predictor of recovery from aphasia [93,98].

Conclusions

fTCD offers a wide range of applications in studying brain functions in normal subjects and neurological patients. From a practical point of view, non-invasiveness is one of its most important advantages. No medications or contrast injections need to be administered. There are no limitations concerning patient selection such as phobias, obesity, compatibility with pacemakers or surgical materials that result in exclusion of a substantial number of patients from fMRI. fTCD seems to be an ideal instrument for the investigation of brain functions in all ages, in large cohorts and in longitudinal studies. This research area may constitute a challenge for future investigation especially under the auspices of a well-organized blind study with a standardized methodology in order to estimate better the potential ability to complement neuroimaging techniques and the Wada test in the presurgical evaluation of patients. Other interesting areas could be the investigation of executive brain functions and brain plasticity on the basis of defined criteria and a complete description of laboratory settings.

References

1. Phelps ME, Mazziota JC, Huang SC. Study of cerebral function with positron computed tomography. *J Cereb Blood Flow Metab* 1982;**2**:113–62.
2. Squire LR, Ojemann JG, Miezin FM, et al. Activation of the hippocampus in normal humans: a functional anatomical study of memory. *Proc Natl Acad Sci USA* 1992;**89**(5):1837–41.
3. Borbély K, Nagy D, Tóth M, et al. Speech activation SPECT and plasticity of language networks. *J Neuroradiol* 2005;**32**(5):345–7.
4. Binder JR, Swanson SJ, Hammeke TA, et al. Determination of language dominance using functional MRI: a comparison with the Wada test. *Neurology* 1996;**46**(4):978–84.
5. Pujol J, Deus J, Losilla JM, et al. Cerebral lateralization of language in normal left-handed people studied by functional MRI. *Neurology* 1999;**52**(5):1038–43.
6. Desmond JE, Sum JM, Wagner AD, et al. Functional MRI measurement of language lateralization in Wada- tested patients. *Brain* 1995;**118**(6):1411–9.
7. Gaillard WD, Pugliese M, Grandin CB, et al. Cortical localization of reading in normal children: an fMRI language study. *Neurology* 2001;**57**:47–54.
8. Lehéricy S, Cohen L, Bazin B, et al. Functional MR evaluation of temporal and frontal language dominance compared with the Wada test. *Neurology* 2000;**54**:1625–33.
9. Jansen A, Sehlmeyer C, Pfleiderer B, et al. Assessment of verbal memory by fMRI: lateralization and functional neuroanatomy. *Clin Neurol Neurosurg* 2009;**111**(1):57–62.
10. Daffertshofer M. Functional Doppler testing. In: Hennerici M, Meairs S, eds. *Cerebrovascular Ultrasound*. Cambridge: Cambridge University Press, 2001: 341–59.
11. Klingerhofer J, Sander D. Transcranial Doppler ultrasonography monitoring during cognitive testing. In: Tegeler CH, Babikian VL, Gomez CR, eds. *Neurosonology*. St. Louis, MO: Mosby, 1996: 200–13.
12. Aaslid R. Visually evoked dynamic blood flow response of the human cerebral circulation. *Stroke* 1987;**18**:771–7.
13. Kwong KK, Belliveau JW, Chesler DA, et al. Dynamic magnetic resonance imaging of human brain activity during primary sensory stimulation. *Proc Natl Acad Sci USA* 1992;**89**(12):5675–9.
14. Deppe M, Ringelstein EB, Knecht S. The investigation of functional brain lateralization by transcranial Doppler sonography. *NeuroImage* 2004;**21**:1124–46.
15. Jueptner M, Weiller C,. Review: does measurement of regional cerebral blood flow reflect synaptic activity? Implications for PET and fMRI. *NeuroImage* 1995;**2**:148–56.
16. Logothetis N, Pauls J, Augath M, et al. Neurophysiological investigation of the basis of the fMRI signal. *Nature* 2001;**412**:150–7.
17. Iadecola C. Regulation of the cerebral microcirculation during neural activity: is nitric oxide the missing link? *Trends Neurosci* 1993;**16**:206–14.
18. Brian JEJ, Faraci FM, Heistad DD. Recent insights into the regulation of cerebral circulation. *Clin Exp Pharmacol Physiol* 1996;**23**(6–7):449–57.
19. Faraci FM, Brian JE. Nitric oxide and the cerebral circulation. *Stroke* 1994;**25**(3):692–703.
20. Huber P, Handa J. Effect of contrast material, hypercapnia, hyperventilation, hypertonic glucose and papaverine on the diameter of the cerebral arteries. Angiographic determination in man. *Invest Radiol* 1967;**2**(1):17–32.
21. Krapf R, Markwalder TM, Linder HR. Failure to demonstrate a vasoconstrictive effect of vasopressin on the internal carotid and middle cerebral arteries: a transcranial ultrasound Doppler study. *Ultrasound Med Biol* 1987;**13**(3):131–4.

22 Giller CA, Bowman G, Dyer H, et al. Cerebral arterial diameters during changes in blood pressure and carbon dioxide during craniotomy. *Neurosurgery* 1993;**32**:737–47.

23 Serrador JM, Picot PA, Rutt BK, et al. MRI measures of middle cerebral artery diameter in conscious humans during simulated orthostasis. *Stroke* 2000;**31**:1672–8.

24 Dushek S, Schandry R. Functional transcranial Doppler sonography as a tool in psychophysiological research. *Psychophysiology* 2003;**40**:436–54.

25 Lohmann H, Ringelstein E, Knecht S. Functional transcranial Doppler sonography. In: Baumgartner RW, ed. *Handbook on Neurovascular Ultrasound. Frontiers of Neurology and Neuroscience*, Vol. 21. Basel: Karger, 2006: 251–60.

26 Clark JM, Skolnick BE, Gelfand R, et al. Relationship of 133Xe cerebral blood flow to middle cerebral arterial flow velocity in men at rest. *J Cereb Blood Flow Metab* 1996;**16**:1255–62.

27 Deppe M, Knecht S, Henningsen H, et al. AVERAGE: a Windows program for automated analysis of event related cerebral blood flow. *J Neurosci Methods* 1997;**75**:147–54.

28 Njemanze PC. Cerebral lateralisation for facial processing: gender-related cognitive styles determined using Fourier analysis of mean cerebral blood flow velocity in the middle cerebral arteries. *Laterality* 2007;**12**(1):31–49.

29 Droste DW, Harders AG, Rastogi E. A transcranial Doppler study of blood flow velocity in the middle cerebral arteries performed at rest and during mental activities. *Stroke* 1989;**20**: 1005–11.

30 Rihs F, Sturzenegger M, Gutbrod K, et al. Determination of language dominance: Wada test confirms functional transcranial Doppler sonography. *Neurology* 1999;**52**:1591–6.

31 Knecht S, Deppe M, Ebner A, et al. Noninvasive determination of language lateralization by functional transcranial Doppler sonography: a comparison with the Wada test. *Stroke* 1998;**29**:82–86.

32 Deppe M, Knecht S, Lohmann H, et al. A method for the automated assessment of temporal characteristics of functional hemispheric lateralization by transcranial Doppler sonography. *J Neuroimaging* 2004;**14**:226–30.

33 Stroobant N, Vingerhoets G. Transcranial Doppler ultrasonography monitoring of cerebral hemodynamics during performance of cognitive tasks: a review. *Neuropsychol Rev* 2000;**10**(4): 213–31.

34 Bulla-Hellwig M, Vollmer J, Gotzen A, et al. Hemispheric asymmetry of arterial blood flow velocity changes during verbal and visuospatial tasks. *Neuropsychologia* 1996;**34**:987–91.

35 Cupini LM, Matteis M, Troisi E, et al. Bilateral simultaneous transcranial Doppler monitoring of flow velocity changes during visuospatial and verbal working memory tasks. *Brain* 1996;**119**:1249–53.

36 Knecht S, Deppe M, Backer M, et al. Regional cerebral blood flow increases during preparation for and processing of sensory stimuli. *Exp Brain Res* 1997;**116**:309–14.

37 Matteis M, Bivona U, Catani S, et al. Functional transcranial Doppler assessment of cerebral blood flow velocities changes during attention tasks. *J Neurol* 2009;**16**:81–7.

38 Droste DW, Harders AG, Rastogi E. Two transcranial Doppler studies on blood flow velocity in both middle cerebral arteries during rest and the performance of cognitive tasks. *Neuropsychologia* 1989;**27**:1221–30.

39 Harders AG, Laborde G, Droste DW, et al. Brain activity and blood flow velocity changes: a transcranial Doppler study. *Int J Neurosci* 1989;**47**:91–102.

40 Conrad B, Klingelhofer J. Dynamics of regional cerebral blood flow for various visual stimuli. *Exp Brain Res* 1989;**77**:437–41.

41 Vadikolias K, Artemis N, Mitsias PD, et al. Evaluation of the stability of blood flow over time in the dominant hemisphere: a functional transcranial Doppler study. *J Cereb Blood Flow Metab* 2007;**27**(11):1870–7.

42 Stroobant N, Buijs D, Vingerhoets G. Variation in brain lateralization during various language tasks: a functional transcranial Doppler study. *Behav Brain Res* 2009;**199**:190–6.

43 Knecht S, Deppe M, Ringelstein EB, et al. Reproducibility of functional transcranial Doppler-sonography in determining hemispheric language lateralization. *Stroke* 1998;**29**:1155–9.

44 Knecht S, Deppe M, Drager B, et al. Language lateralization in healthy right-handers. *Brain* 2000;**123**:74–81.

45 Knake S, Haag A, Hamer HM, et al. Language lateralization in patients with temporal lobe epilepsy: a comparison of functional transcranial Doppler sonography and the Wada test. *NeuroImage* 2003;**19**(3):1228–32.

46 Knecht S, Henningsen H, Deppe M, et al. Successive activation of both cerebral hemispheres during cued word generation. *Neuroreport* 1996;**29**;7(3):820–4.

47 Dorst J, Haag A, Knake S, et al. Functional transcranial Doppler sonography and a spatial orientation paradigm identify the non-dominant hemisphere. *Brain Cogn* 2008;**68**:53–8.

48 Schuepbach D, Merlo MCG, Goenner F, et al. Cerebral hemodynamic response induced by the Tower of Hanoi puzzle and Wisconsin Card Sorting Test. *Neuropsychologia* 2002;**40**:39–53.

49 Schuepbach D, Hell D, Baumgartner RW. Lateralization of cerebral hemodynamics during Wisconsin Card Sorting Test: a functional transcranial Doppler sonography study. *Clin Neurophysiol* 2005;**116**:1041–8.

50 Feldmann D, Schuepbach D, von Rickenbach B, et al. Association between two distinct executive tasks in schizophrenia: a functional transcranial Doppler sonography study. *BMC Psychiatry* 2006;**6**:25.

51 Bishop DVM, Watt H, Papadatou-Pastou M. An efficient and reliable method for measuring cerebral lateralization during speech with functional transcranial Doppler ultrasound. *Neuropsychologia* 2009;**47**:587–90.

52 Lohmann H, Drager B, Muller-Ehrenberg B et al. Language lateralization in young children assessed by functional transcranial Doppler sonography. *NeuroImage* 2005;**24**:780–90.

53 Wada J, Rasmussen T. Intracarotid injection of sodium amytal for the lateralization of cerebral speech dominance. *J Neurosurg* 1960;**17**:266–82.

54 Schmidt P, Krings T, Willmes K, et al. Determination of cognitive hemispheric lateralization by "functional" transcranial Doppler cross-validated by functional MRI. *Stroke* 1999;**30**:939–45.

55 Deppe M, Knecht S, Papke K, et al. Assessment of hemispheric language lateralization: a comparison between fMRI and fTCD. *J Cereb Blood Flow Metab* 2000;**20**:263–8.

56 Jansen A, Floel A, Deppe M, et al. Determining the hemispheric dominance of spatial attention: a comparison between fTCD and fMRI. *Hum Brain Mapp* 2004;**23**:168–80.

57 Uzuner N, Ak I, Gücüyener D, et al. Cerebral hemodynamic patterns with technetium Tc-99m exametazime single

photon emission computed tomography and transcranial Doppler sonography: a validation study using visual stimulation. *J Ultrasound Med* 2002;**21**(9):955–9.
58. Sabri O, Owega A, Schreckenberger M, et al. A truly simultaneous combination of functional transcranial Doppler sonography and H$_2$^{15}O PET adds fundamental new information on differences in cognitive activation between schizophrenics and healthy control subjects. *J Nucl Med* 2003;**44**(5):671–81.
59. Bay-Hansen J, Ravn T, Knudsen GM. Application of interhemispheric index for transcranial Doppler sonography velocity measurements and evaluation of recording time. *Stroke* 1997;**28**:1009–14.
60. Flöel A, Lohmann H, Breitenstein C, et al. Reproducibility of hemispheric blood flow increases during line bisectioning. *Clin Neurophysiol* 2002;**113**(6):917–24.
61. Stroobant N, Vingerhoets G. Test–retest reliability of functional transcranial Doppler ultrasonography. *Ultrasound Med Biol* 2001;**27**(4):509–14.
62. Vadikolias K, Artemis N, Tripsianis G, et al. Functional transcranial Doppler (fTCD): test–retest reliability of the method in determining hemispheric lateralization. *J Neurol* 2004;**251**(S3):160–1.
63. Widder, B. *Doppler- und Duplexsonographie der hirnversorgenden Arterien*, 5th edn. Berlin: Springer, 1999.
64. Diehl RR, Diehl B, Sitzer M, et al. Spontaneous oscillations in cerebral blood flow velocity in normal humans and in patients with carotid artery disease. *Neurosci Lett* 1991;**127**:5–8.
65. Groschel K, Terborg C, Schnaudigel S, et al. Effects of physiological aging and cerebrovascular risk factors on the hemodynamic response to brain activation: a functional transcranial Doppler study. *Eur J Neurol* 2007;**14**:125–31.
66. Knake S, Haag A, Pilgramm G, et al. Language dominance in mesial temporal lobe epilepsy: a functional transcranial Doppler sonography study of brain plasticity. *Epilepsy Behav* 2006;**9**:345–8.
67. Gomez SM, Gomez CR, Hall IS. Transcranial Doppler ultrasonographic assessment of intermittent light stimulation at different frequencies. *Stroke* 1990;**21**:1746–8.
68. Sturzenegger M, Newell DW, Aaslid R. Visually evoked blood flow response assessed by simultaneous two-channel transcranial Doppler using flow velocity averaging. *Stroke* 1996;**27**:2256–61.
69. Njemanze PC, Gomez CR, Horenstein S. Cerebral lateralization and color perception: a transcranial Doppler study. *Cortex* 1992;**28**:69–75.
70. Silvestrini M, Cupini LM, Matteis M, et al. Bilateral simultaneous assessment of cerebral flow velocity during mental activity. *J Cereb Blood Flow Metab* 1994;**14**, 643–8.
71. Klingelhofer J, Matzander G, Sander D, et al. Assessment of functional hemispheric asymmetry by bilateral simultaneous cerebral blood flow velocity monitoring. *J Cereb Blood Flow Metab* 1997;**17**:577–85.
72. Matteis M, Silvestrini M, Troisi E, et al. Transcranial Doppler assessment of cerebral flow velocity. Transcranial Doppler sonography in psychophysiological research during perception and recognition of melodies. *J Neurol Sci* 1997;**149**: 57–61.
73. Vollmer-Haase J, Finke K, Hartje W, et al. Hemispheric dominance in the processing of J.S. Bach fugues: a transcranial Doppler sonography (TCD) study with musicians. *Neuropsychologia* 1998;**36**:857–67.
74. Evers S, Dannert J, Rodding D, et al. The cerebral haemodynamics of music perception. A transcranial Doppler sonography study. *Brain* 1999;**122**(1):75–85.
75. Varnadore AE, Roberts AE, McKinney WM. Modulations in cerebral hemodynamics under three response requirements while solving language-based problems: a transcranial Doppler study. *Neuropsychologia* 1997;**35**:1209–14.
76. Markus HS, Boland M. Cognitive activity monitored by noninvasive measurement of cerebral blood flow velocity and its application to the investigation of cerebral dominance. *Cortex* 1992;**28**:575–81.
77. Vingerhoets G, Stroobant N. Lateralization of cerebral blood flow velocity changes during cognitive tasks. A simultaneous bilateral transcranial Doppler study. *Stroke* 1999;**30**: 2152–8.
78. Hartje W, Ringelstein EB, Kistinger B, et al. Transcranial Doppler ultrasonic assessment of middle cerebral artery blood flow velocity changes during verbal and visuospatial cognitive tasks. *Neuropsychologia* 1994;**32**:1443–52.
79. Rihs F, Gutbrod K, Gutbrod B, et al. Determination of cognitive hemispheric dominance by "stereo" transcranial Doppler sonography. *Stroke* 1995;**26**:70–3.
80. Orlandi G, Murri, L. Transcranial Doppler assessment of cerebral flow velocity at rest and during voluntary movements in young and elderly healthy subjects. *Int J Neurosci* 1996;**84**:45–53.
81. Kelley RE, Chang JY, Scheinman NJ, et al. Transcranial Doppler assessment of cerebral flow velocity during cognitive tasks. *Stroke* 1992;**23**:9–14.
82. Thomas C, Harer C. Simultaneous bihemispherical assessment of cerebral blood flow velocity changes during a mental arithmetic task. *Stroke* 1993;**24**:614–5.
83. Backer M, Deppe M, Zunker P, et al. Tuning to somatosensory stimuli during focal attention. *Cerebrovasc Dis* 1994;**4**(Suppl 3):3.
84. Backer M, Knecht S, Deppe M, et al. Cortical tuning: a function of anticipated stimulus intensity. *Neuroreport* 1999;**10**: 293–6.
85. Kelley RE, Chang JY, Suzuki S, et al. Selective increase in the right hemisphere transcranial Doppler velocity during a spatial task. *Cortex* 1993;**29**:45–52.
86. Droste D, Harders A, Liberti, G. Bilateral simultaneous transcranial Doppler monitoring during the performance of a verbal fluency task and a face recognition task. *J Psychophysiol* 1996;**10**:303–9.
87. Floel A, Knecht S, Lohmann H, et al. Language and spatial attention can lateralize to the same hemisphere in healthy humans. *Neurology* 2001;**57**:1018–24.
88. Stoll M, Hamann GF, Mangold, R, et al. Emotionally evoked changes in cerebral hemodynamics measured by transcranial Doppler sonography. *J Neurol* 1999;**246**:127–33.
89. Troisi, E, Silvestrini M, Matteis M, et al. Emotion-related cerebral asymmetry: hemodynamics measured by functional ultrasound. *J Neurol* 1999;**246**:1172–6.
90. Bruneau N, Dourneau MC, Garreau B, et al. Blood flow response to auditory stimulations in normal, mentally retarded and autistic children: a preliminary transcranial Doppler ultrasonographic study of the middle cerebral arteries. *Biol Psychiatry* 1992;**32**:691–9.

91 Asil T, Uzuner N. Differentiation of vascular dementia and Alzheimer disease: a functional transcranial Doppler ultrasonographic study. *J Ultrasound Med* 2005;**24**(8):1065–70.

92 Owega A, Klingelhofer J, Sabri O, et al. Cerebral blood flow velocity in acute schizophrenic patients: a transcranial Doppler ultrasonography study. *Stroke* 1998;**29**:1149–54.

93 Silvestrini M, Caltagirone C, Cupini LM, et al. Activation of healthy hemisphere in poststroke recovery. A transcranial Doppler study. *Stroke* 1993;**24**:1673–7.

94 Silvestrini M, Troisi E, Matteis M, et al. Involvement of the healthy hemisphere in recovery from aphasia and motor deficit in patients with cortical ischemic infarction: a transcranial Doppler study. *Neurology* 1995;**45**(10):1815–20.

95 Diehl B, Knecht S, Deppe M, et al. Cerebral hemodynamic response to generalized spike-wave discharges. *Epilepsia* 1998;**39**:1284–9.

96 Backer M, Sander D, Hammes MG, et al. Altered cerebrovascular response pattern in interictal migraine during visual stimulation. *Cephalalgia* 2001;**21**(5):611–6.

97 Oláh L, Raiter Y, Candale C, et al. Visually evoked cerebral vasomotor response in smoking and nonsmoking young adults, investigated by functional transcranial Doppler. *Nicotine Tob Res* 2008;**10**(2):353–8.

98 Silvestrini M, Troisi E, Matteis M, et al. Correlations of flow velocity changes during mental activity and recovery from aphasia in ischemic stroke. *Neurology* 1998;**50**:191–5.

10 Transcranial Doppler in the Detection and Quantitation of Patent Foramen Ovale and Other Right-to-Left Circulatory Shunts

Annabelle Lao[1], Cindy J. Fuller[2] & Jill T. Jesurum[2]
[1]Santo Thomas University, Manila, Philippines
[2]Swedish Heart & Vascular Institute, Seattle, WA, USA

Introduction

Patent foramen ovale (PFO) is a relatively common source of right-to-left circulatory shunt (RLS), occurring in approximately 25% of the population [1]. Large-diameter PFOs, which predispose patients to intermittent paradoxical emboli through RLS, have been implicated in cryptogenic stroke, transient ischemic attack (TIA), platypnea–orthodeoxia syndrome, decompression illness in scuba divers, cerebral fat embolism syndrome and transient global amnesia [2,3]. Transcranial Doppler can be used to detect and quantify the magnitude of RLS and to assess the presence of residual RLS after transcatheter PFO closure. This chapter presents clinical applications of TCD in the detection and quantitation of RLS.

Prevalence of PFO

The foramen ovale is an opening in the interatrial septum resulting from incomplete coverage of the ostium secundum – an opening within the septum primum – by the septum secundum. The foramen ovale serves as a one-way valve for physiologic right-to-left shunting of oxygenated blood *in utero*. Blood from the placenta enters the right atrium through the inferior vena cava and crosses the foramen ovale into the systemic circulation. Postnatal lung expansion and initiation of the pulmonary circulation reverse the atrial pressure gradient, causing functional closure of the foramen ovale. Fibrosis follows closure, and complete fusion of the interatrial septae occurs by 2 years of age in most individuals [4]. Lack of septal fusion results in a PFO, a potential hole that can be opened by reversal of the interatrial pressure gradient or by an intracardiac catheter (Figure 10.1).

Cerebrovascular Ultrasound in Stroke Prevention and Treatment, 2nd edition. Edited by Andrei V. Alexandrov. © 2011 Blackwell Publishing Ltd.

Familial PFO prevalence is consistent with autosomal dominant inheritance [5]. Female siblings of stroke patients with PFO are more likely to have PFO than siblings of stroke patients without PFO [odds ratio (OR) 9.8, $p < 0.01$] [6]. Interestingly, this finding was not seen in male siblings of stroke patients with PFO. Autopsy studies showed the presence of PFO in 17–29% of the general population [1,7,8]. Non-invasive population-based studies showed similar prevalence of PFO in the general population, ranging from 17% by transthoracic echocardiography (TTE) [9] to 25.6% by transesophageal echocardiography (TEE) [5]. There was no sex difference seen in either study. The prevalence of PFO declined with age, from 30% among persons aged <30 years to 20% among persons aged >80 years; however, PFO size increased with age [10].

PFO and ischemic stroke

Over 40% of ischemic strokes that occur in young people (aged <55 years) are cryptogenic [11]. The prevalence of PFO is higher in patients with cryptogenic stroke than in those with known stroke etiology (61% versus 19%) [12]. PFO may serve as a conduit for paradoxical cerebral embolism that could be the mechanism for some cryptogenic strokes. A 13–56% prevalence of PFO among young ischemic stroke patients has been reported [13–18]. The risk of stroke in young patients (patients aged <55 years) with a PFO was greater than age-matched controls without PFO [OR 3.10, 95% confidence interval (CI) 2.29 to 4.21] [19]. A recent study showed an association of PFO with cryptogenic stroke among older patients (aged >55 years) (OR 2.92, 95% CI 1.70 to 5.01, $p < 0.001$) [20]. The risk of stroke recurrence in 3 years among patients with PFO was 7.2% and increased to 16.3% among patients with cryptogenic stroke [21]. Risk of stroke is also increased by large PFO diameter (>2 mm) [22,23] and large magnitude of RLS measured by TEE or TCD [21,24,25].

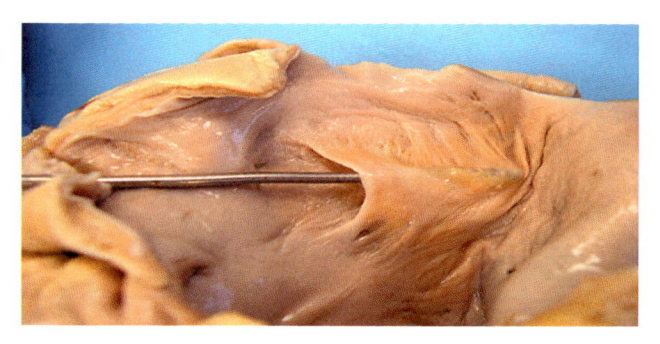

Figure 10.1 Autopsy specimen of patent foramen ovale, as seen from the left atrium. Reproduced from Desai et al. [10], with permission from Nature Publishing Group.

Patent foramen ovale may be associated with other risk factors for stroke. Atrial septal aneurysm (ASA) is defined as a hypermobile septum primum with ≥10 mm excursion into either atrium. Although the presence of isolated ASA is <1% in the general population [26], the prevalence in patients with cryptogenic stroke is 4–25% [13]. The coexistence of ASA with PFO increased the OR for stroke to 15.59 (95% CI 2.83 to 85.87) [19]. The presence of both PFO and ASA is a significant predictor for recurrent stroke [hazard ratio (HR) 4.17, 95% CI 1.47 to 11.84] [21,27]. Inherited prothrombotic disorders have been associated with PFO in patients with cryptogenic stroke, particularly the prothrombin gene G20210 mutation [28–30].

The source of paradoxical cerebral emboli in patients with PFO is unknown; however, Cramer et al. [12] reported that the incidence of pelvic deep vein thrombosis was higher in patients with cryptogenic stroke (20%) and patients with cryptogenic stroke and PFO (22%) than in patients with stroke of determined origin (4%; $p < 0.025$). Patients with cryptogenic stroke were significantly younger and had fewer risk factors for atherosclerosis than were those with stroke of known cause. The prevalence of PFO was 61% in the cryptogenic stroke group and 19% in those with a determined origin of stroke. The finding that most patients with cryptogenic stroke and pelvic deep vein thrombosis also had a PFO supports paradoxical embolism as the stroke mechanism.

As many patients with PFO are asymptomatic [1,31], there is no currently recommended treatment for primary prevention of stroke or TIA. The current standard secondary prevention strategy is warfarin or antiplatelet drugs such as aspirin or clopidogrel [32]. Surgical closure of PFO has been abandoned for transcatheter closure, which involves percutaneous implantation of a device that occludes the PFO tunnel and is endothelialized within 2–4 months [33,34]. Several single-center trials performed since 2002 have reported recurrent stroke rates of 0–6% following closure [35–39]. The reported clinical studies of PFO closure for prevention of recurrent stroke are shown in Table 10.1. Older patients (aged >55 years) were more likely to have recurrent stroke following PFO closure than younger patients (6.6% versus 1.4%, $p = 0.03$) [38], which may have been due to increased prevalence of hypertension and hyperlipidemia in the older patients. In another series of patients who underwent PFO closure, older patients (aged >55 years) were more likely to experience new onset atrial fibrillation post-procedure than younger patients (14/40 versus 2/47, respectively, $p < 0.025$) [40].

The US Food and Drug Administration (FDA) approved two PFO closure devices under a Humanitarian Device Exemption, which was withdrawn in 2006 when it was ascertained that the population that could be treated with these devices was >4000 patients per year [32]. Randomized trials of transcatheter PFO closure versus medical therapy (warfarin, aspirin, clopidogrel) to prevent recurrent stroke have not been completed; however, Khairy et al. [41] reviewed data from 10 PFO closure studies and six medical therapy studies and reported a 1-year recurrence rate of 3.8–12.0% for medical therapy compared with 0–4.9% for surgical or transcatheter PFO closure.

PFO and migraine

Migraine headache affects 8–13% of the population [42,43]. An association between migraine headache and PFO has

Table 10.1 Summary of major studies ($N > 100$ patients) since 2002 of transcatheter PFO closure and stroke recurrence[a]

Study	No. of patients (% female)	Mean follow-up (range) (years)	Stroke recurrence after closure (%)	No. with residual RLS (%)
Onorato et al. (2003) [39]*	256 (41)	1.6 (0.1–2.8)	0	NA (2)
Windecker et al. (2004) [36]	150 (47)	2.3 (0.6–4.0)	1	26 (17)
Schuchlenz et al. (2005) [37]	167 (46)	2.8	0.6	NA
Harms et al. (2007) [38]*	237 (52)	1.6	3.4	72 (34)
Slavin et al. (2007) [35]	131 (50)	2.5 (0.3–5.4)	0	11 (8)

[a]Asterisks refer to studies in which RLS prior to and after PFO closure was assessed by TCD. NA, data not available.

Table 10.2 Major studies of transcatheter PFO closure for migraine prevention[a]

Study	No. (% female)	Mean age (SD) (years)	No. (%) with MA+	Mean follow-up	Migraines resolved	Reduced severity or frequency	Unchanged
Wilmshurst et al. (2000) [53]	21 (48)	NA	16 (76)	1.5–32 mo (range)	48% (44% MA+, 60% MA−)	38% (50% MA+, 0% MA−)	14% (6% MA+, 40% MA−)
Schwerzmann et al. (2004) [54]	48 (65)	49 (11) MA+, 42 (12) MA−	37 (77)	1.7 yr	NA	54% MA+, 62% MA−	3 MA+ and large residual shunt
Azarbal et al. (2005) [58]	37 (66)	NA	20 (54)	12 mo	75% MA+, 40% MA−	5% MA+, 40% MA−	NA
Reisman et al. (2005) [56]	57 (67)	47 (12)	39 (68)	37 wk	56% (54% MA+, 62% MA−)	14% (14% MA+, 15% MA−)	30% (32% MA+, 23% MA−)
Anzola et al. (2006) [55]	50 (82)	NA	40 (80)	12 mo	36%	52%	8%
Slavin et al. (2007) [35]	50 (75)	46 (12)	40 (80)	30 mo	64% (68% MA+, 50% MA−)	21% (13% MA+, 40% MA−)	NA
Dubiel et al. (2008) [59]	46 (76)	44 (14)	24 (52)	38 mo	24% (33% MA+, 14% MA−)	63% (58% MA+, 68% MA−)	NA

[a]Abbreviations: NA, data not available; MA+, migraine with aura; MA−, migraine without aura; yr, years; mo, months; wk, weeks.

been recognized, although the mechanisms are still debated and poorly understood [44]. The prevalence of PFO may be 47–67% in migraine with aura patients, 23–47% in those without aura and 17–25% among controls [45–48]. It has been postulated that large RLS was causally related to migraine and increased the risk of stroke among migraineurs [49,50]. More patients who had migraine with aura and stroke were found to have RLS (84%) than migraineurs with aura but without stroke (38.1%, $p < 0.001$) and population controls (12.2%, $p < 0.001$) [51]. The odds ratio of having migraine in the presence of PFO with moderate or large RLS was 7.78 (95% CI 2.53 to 29.3, $p < 0.001$) [47], suggesting that interatrial communication may be associated with migraine pathogenesis. These data have led to the theory that interatrial transit of microemboli or vasoactive compounds through the PFO evade pulmonary filtration and affect cerebral vasoreactivity leading to migrainous symptoms, ischemic stroke or both [47]. Gori et al. [52], however, reported that the extent of RLS did not correlate with the severity of migraine with aura.

Transcatheter closure of PFO caused complete resolution or marked reduction in migraine frequency in several non-randomized studies [35,53–56] (Table 10.2). Reisman et al. [56] reported complete migraine resolution in 56% of patients and 14% of patients reported a significant (>50%) reduction in migraine frequency. In the same study, patients reported an 80% reduction in the mean number of migraine episodes per month after PFO closure (6.8 ± 9.6 before closure versus 1.4 ± 3.4 after closure, $p < 0.001$). Migraine Intervention with STARFlex Technology (MIST) is the only randomized, double-blind trial of PFO closure and migraine treatment completed to date. The trial failed to meet the primary endpoint of complete migraine resolution. Three subjects (4.3%) experienced total cessation of migraines after PFO closure; 42% had a >50% reduction in headache days relative to 23% of patients in the sham closure group ($p = 0.038$) [57]. Other randomized trials of PFO closure and migraine are still in progress. At this time, the FDA has not approved transcatheter PFO closure for migraine outside ongoing randomized trials.

PFO and decompression sickness

Patent foramen ovale is a risk factor for decompression sickness (DCS) in deep-sea divers [60]. The prevalence of PFO among divers who suffered from DCS was 59.5% compared with 36.1% in normal controls ($p = 0.06$); when the numbers of divers with large RLS were compared, 51.3% had DCS compared with 25% of controls ($p = 0.03$) [61]. Divers with PFO and DCS were more likely to have mobility of the interatrial septum than divers with PFO but without DCS ($p = 0.02$) [62]. Divers are more likely to have brain abnormalities on MRI than non-divers, regardless of history of DCS [63]. The presence of PFO resulted in a 4.5-fold increase in DCS events and two times more ischemic brain lesions on MRI than divers without PFO [64]. The prevalence of multiple brain lesions in divers with large PFO was 23% compared with 0% in other divers ($p = 0.004$) [65]. Closure of

Table 10.3 Diagnostic parameters of single-gated TCD when compared with TEE[a]

Study	N	Sensitivity (%)	Specificity (%)	PPV (%)	NPV (%)	Accuracy (%)
Di Tullio et al. (1993) [69]	27	68	100	100	83	87
Klotzsch et al. (1994) [73]	111	91.3	93.8	91.3	91.3	92.8
Job et al. (1994) [74]	137	89	92			
Devuyst et al. (1997) [75]	37	100	55	83	100	81
Kwiecinski et al. (1994) [76]	61	85	85	87	82	85

[a] Abbreviations: PPV, positive predictive value; NPV, negative predictive value

PFO resulted in complete cessation of DCS in 100% of divers in one study [66].

Methods of PFO detection

The current gold standard for detection of PFO is TEE with contrast injection (c-TEE), which allows quantitative assessment of the degree of intra-cardiac shunting and visualization of the cardiac anatomy [67]. When compared with autopsy, c-TEE showed sensitivity and specificity of 89% and 100%, respectively; for color Doppler TEE, both sensitivity and specificity were equal to 100% [68]. The sensitivity of c-TEE in detecting a PFO may be increased most effectively by the Valsalva maneuver (VM); however, there may be inadequate Valsalva in TEE since sedation is required and patients may not be able to comply with instructions.

Transthoracic echocardiography is also used in PFO detection, but sensitivity and specificity are compromised because of inadequate heart visualization [69]. Several studies using TTE showed low sensitivity (47–75%), with a specificity of 92–100% compared with TEE [69–71]. A newer transthoracic method, transmitral Doppler (TMD), promises to increase sensitivity in detecting RLS to 94% due to increased bubble detection for patients with suboptimal two-dimensional windows [71].

Transcranial Doppler is comparable to c-TEE for detecting PFO-related RLS (type A, class II evidence) [72]. When compared with c-TEE, TCD sensitivity ranges from 68 to 100% and specificity from 55 to 100% [69,73–76] (Table 10.3). Contrast TCD (c-TCD) does not require sedation of the patient, thus ensuring better collaboration during VM. However, it does not provide any information concerning the morphology of the interatrial septum or the size of PFO. Detection of RLS with c-TCD does not imply the presence of PFO, as RLS through a ventricular septal defect or extracardiac shunt through a pulmonary arteriovenous malformation may also be present. Contrast-enhanced TEE is the most sensitive to detect PFO, followed by c-TCD and c-TTE [69]. However, when clinically significant RLS detection is concerned, c-TCD can reliably detect cerebral embolic conduction [69].

TCD has been augmented by power M-mode (PMD), a technology allowing power display with Doppler velocity and frequency signals over selectable depth ranges along the transducer beam [77]. Power M-mode TCD enhances sensitivity over single-gated TCD examination by detecting more microembolic signals (MES) following revised criteria [78,79] (Table 10.4). Spencer et al. [78] reported 98%

Table 10.4 Criteria for quantitation of microembolic signals (MES) with single-gated TCD versus power M-mode TCD (PMD) [79][a]

Single-gated TCD	PMD
Transient, lasting <300 ms At least 3 dB higher signal intensity than that of the highest blood flow signal	MES visible at least 3 dB higher than the highest spontaneous PMD display if background flow signal MES reflects motion in one direction at a minimum spatial extent of 7.5 mm and a minimum temporal extent of 30 ms. An MCA MES moves toward the probe with a positively sloped track. An ACA MES moves away from the probe with negatively sloped track
Unidirectional Snap, chirp audible sound	The MES must traverse a specific depth determined by the highest intensity of the insonated artery to avoid repeated counting of the same embolus

[a] Abbreviations: MCA, middle cerebral artery; ACA, anterior cerebral artery.

Table 10.5 Patent foramen ovale diagnosis contingency tables of three ultrasound modalities compared with PFO catheter probing [78][a]

Ultrasound modality	PPV (%)	NPV (%)	Sensitivity (%)	Specificity (%)	Accuracy (%)
TTE (N = 30)	95	0.09	64	50	63
TEE (N = 56)	96	17	91	33	88
PMD (N = 100)	96	50	98	33	94

[a]Abbreviations: PPV, positive predictive value; NPV, negative predictive value; TTE, transthoracic echocardiography; TEE, transesophageal echocardiography; PMD, power M-mode transcranial Doppler.

sensitivity and 94% accuracy when detecting PFO with PMD compared with a probe patent PFO, which compared favorably with other ultrasound modalities (Table 10.5).

Contrast-enhanced TCD detection of right-to-left shunts

An early International Consensus Meeting [80] recommended a standard examination procedure for the detection of RLS using contrast TCD. Intravenous access should be obtained with an 18-gauge needle inserted into the antecubital vein and the patient should be in the supine position. At least one middle cerebral artery (MCA) is insonated. The contrast agent is prepared using 9 ml of isotonic saline solution and 1 ml of air mixed with a three-way stopcock by exchange of saline–air mixture between the syringes at least 10 times and injected as a bolus during normal respiration (rest). The examination is repeated using the VM. Contrast agent is injected 5 s before the start of the VM; the overall VM duration should be 10 s. The time when the first MES appears at the MCA level will be noted.

Several methodological improvements have been proposed to increase the sensitivity of TCD. Recommendations were:

1 performing the procedure twice in a supine position;
2 using 10 ml of contrast agent, either saline or galactose base medium;
3 a 25–40 s time window to exclude other sources of shunting;
4 use of bilateral recording; and
5 performing VM for 5 s at 5–10 s after contrast injection [80–84].

Galactose-based contrast agent was shown to yield more MES than agitated saline contrast agent [85,86]; however, galactose contrast is unapproved for use in the US. A Doppler probe placed over the left sternum border can be used to detect the arrival of the contrast bolus in the right atrium and serve as a signal for the patient to initiate Valsalva strain [78]. Introduction of contrast via the inferior vena cava from femoral vein injection is preferentially directed towards the fossa ovalis and crosses the PFO more readily than an injection from an antecubital vein (100% versus 75% during VM; $p < 0.01$), thus allowing for increased detection of RLS [87]; however, this is not practical for outpatient assessments.

An expanded TCD protocol was developed to evaluate whether additional injections of agitated saline in different positions would improve RLS detection [88]. The four positions tested were supine, right lateral decubitus, upright sitting and sitting with right lateral leaning. If the initial supine testing was negative, all of the other positions will also be negative. If the supine position was positive for RLS, change in body position increased the MES count by up to 42%, thereby increasing the shunt grade. The highest MES count was obtained in the sitting position [88].

Shunt grading/quantitation

There are two grading systems available for detection and quantitation of RLS by TCD. The International Consensus Criteria (ICC) [80] present a four-level categorization according to the MES count:

1 0 MES (negative result);
2 (2) 1–10 MES;
3 >10 MES or shower ("shower" is >25 MES); and
4 curtain (MES too numerous for a single MES to be identified [31]).

The results should be documented for resting (normal respiration) and VM testing separately.

Spencer's Logarithmic Scale (SLS) [78], on the other hand, uses a six-point logarithmic scale:

- negative test (no MES),
- grade I (1–10 MES);
- grade II (11–30 MES);
- grade III (31–100 MES);
- grade IV (101–300 MES); and
- grade V (>300 MES; shower or curtain pattern).

PART IV Ultrasound in Stroke Prevention and Treatment

Table 10.6 Accuracy parameters for the International Consensus Criteria and Spencer Logarithmic Scale to detect large PFO, as determined by TEE [89]

Criteria	Sensitivity (%)	Specificity (%)	PPV (%)	NPV (%)	Accuracy (%)
International Consensus (any positive MES count)	100	72.4	32.1	100	64.1
Spencer Logarithmic Scale grade III+ (>30 MES)	100	91.3	60	100	85.5

[a]Abbreviations: PPV, positive predictive value; NPV, negative predictive value.

The minimum MES count suggestive of clinically relevant RLS is controversial. A comparison of the ICC and SLS grading systems in the detection and quantification of large and functional RLS showed that SLS grade ≥III can predict large RLS and decrease the likelihood of false-positive TCD diagnosis when compared with TEE [89] (Table 10.6). This study is in concordance with a study done by Serena et al. [31], where only showers and curtain patterns were associated with increased risk of stroke. In addition, Anzola et al. [25] reported that the presence of large RLS assessed by TCD was the only independent predictor of recurrent stroke.

Clinical applications of TCD in RLS detection and quantitation

The ICC [80] recommends insonation of at least one MCA for RLS diagnosis and frequently adequate bilateral temporal bone windows cannot be found. Increasing age, sex and ethnicity have been associated with inadequacy of the window [90,91]. However, the ability to obtain reliable measurement of MES from a single temporal bone window may be compromised by asymmetry between left and right cerebral circulations, as can occur with carotid artery disease [92,93]. A retrospective study was performed to determine if unilateral detection of MES with PMD yielded similar results to bilateral detection for assessment of RLS [94]. Recorded data from 87 patients with confirmed PFO were re-analyzed. At rest, significantly more MES were detected with bilateral versus unilateral detection ($p = 0.01$), but not following Valsalva ($p = 0.13$). Unilateral and bilateral detection were equally able to detect large RLS (grades IV or V) following VM ($p = 1.00$). For patients aged ≥55 years ($N = 41$), the right side yielded greater MES than the left side (mean difference 9% ± 37; 95% CI −3 to 21%) at rest ($p = 0.01$), but not following VM (mean difference 1% ± 25; 95% CI −7 to 9%, $p = 0.10$) [94].

Another potential method to assess RLS in the presence of inadequate temporal bone windows is by insonation of the vertebrobasilar circulation (VBC) via the transoccipital window. When compared with right MCA detection, VBC detection showed 57% sensitivity and 100% specificity at rest and 84% sensitivity and 100% specificity after VM [95]. There were positive correlations between MES detected by MCA and VBC insonation both at rest (κ = 0.91, $p < 0.01$) and following VM (κ = 0.93, $p < 0.01$). The sensitivity and specificity of detecting medium and large RLS following VM reached 100% [95].

As mentioned earlier, TCD cannot rule out other sources of RLS. Jesurum et al. [96] assessed the ability of PMD to detect secondary sources of RLS while the PFO tunnel was occluded with a sizing balloon prior to transcatheter PFO closure in 88 patients. Patients who had significant RLS during balloon occlusion had a higher proportion of residual RLS following deployment of the septal occluder device than those who did not have RLS during balloon occlusion ($N = 83$; 94% versus 57%, respectively; $p = 0.004$). At routine final follow-up evaluation (162 days ± 122, $n = 65$), 12 (92%) patients who had significant secondary RLS during PFO balloon occlusion had residual RLS; 10 of these (83%) had large RLS (>100 MES). In contrast, patients who did not have secondary RLS during balloon occlusion were less likely to have residual RLS at follow-up (chi-square, $p = 0.004$ versus baseline secondary RLS-positive patients) [96].

TCD has been used to determine the potential impact of RLS on migraine. Migraineurs with and without aura had larger RLS than non-migraineurs; however, there was no difference in the magnitude of RLS between migraineurs with and without aura ($p = 0.06$). Migraineurs with a history of stroke had larger RLS than migraineurs without stroke history ($p = 0.04$), stroke patients without migraine ($p = 0.007$) and non-migraineurs without a history of stroke ($p < 0.0001$) [49]. In contrast, in a cohort of patients with PFO who all had a history of cerebrovascular events [97], migraineurs had a higher proportion of large RLS at both rest and following VM than non-migraineurs ($p = 0.04$ and 0.01, respectively). These differences were despite similarities in atrial septal anatomy assessed by intracardiac echocardiography. When migraineurs were compared based on the presence or absence of aura, migraineurs without aura had larger RLS than migraineurs with aura at rest ($p = 0.02$) but not following VM ($p = 0.2$). All of these patients underwent

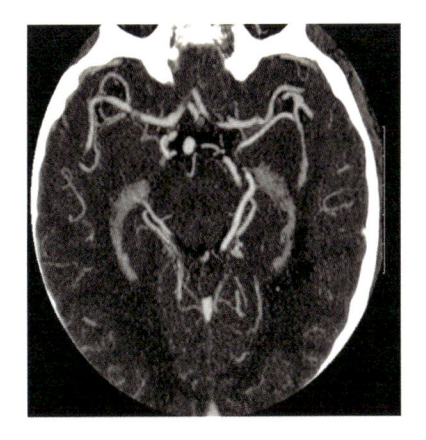

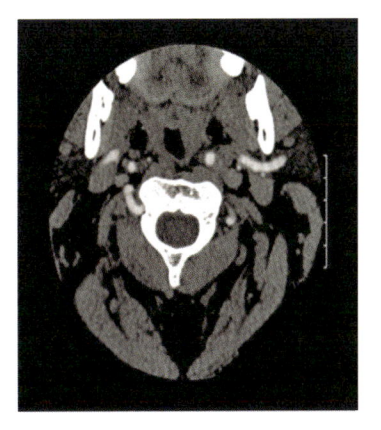

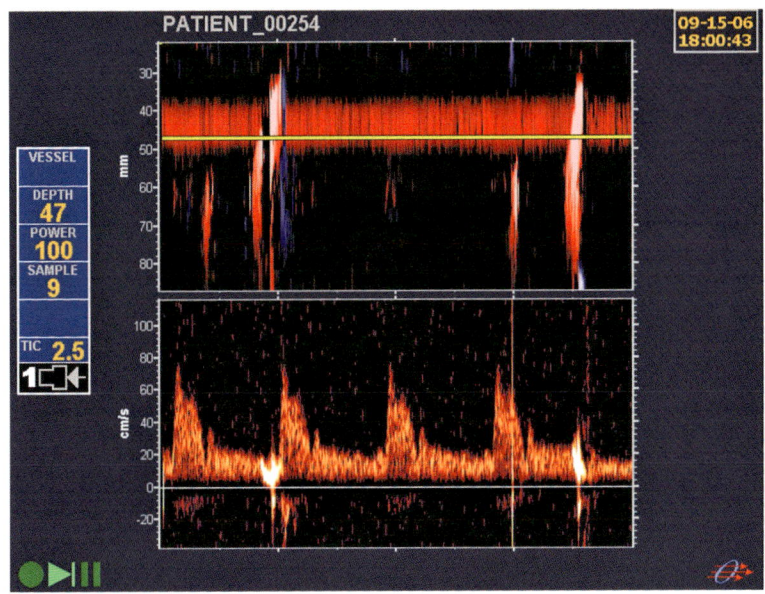

CHAPTER 10 Transcranial Doppler in the Detection and Quantitation PFO

Figure 10.2 Impact of TCD findings on patient management.

PFO closure for prevention of recurrent stroke and 92% of the cohort had large RLS (SLS grades IV–V) following VM, so the results are difficult to generalize [97].

Although migraine relief is a common outcome after PFO closure, the effect of residual RLS on headache frequency is unknown. In a small single-center analysis ($N = 67$) [98], migraine relief ($\geq$50% reduction in frequency) was independent of closure status [77% complete closure (SLS grades 0–II) versus 83% incomplete closure (SLS grades $\geq$III); $p = 0.76$] at late follow-up (540 days; 95% CI 537 to 711). Following PFO closure, patients experienced significantly reduced migraine frequency (4.4 ± 6.3 to 1.7 ± 4.5 events per month, $p < 0.001$). Thirty-six (54%) migraineurs experienced complete migraine relief and 17 (25%) experienced substantial relief. Migraineurs with aura were 4.5 times more likely to experience migraine relief than migraineurs without aura (6.4 and 1.4, respectively, $p = 0.02$), despite a similar degree of complete closure (68% migraineurs with aura versus 59% migraineurs without aura, $p = 0.56$) [98]. Transcatheter PFO closure may reduce RLS below a threshold where microemboli or vasoactive chemicals may trigger migraine.

Summary

TCD is a sensitive, non-invasive method for the detection of RLS due to PFO. Standardized protocols have been established for proper diagnosis. Unilateral or bilateral MCA or transoccipital approaches may be used. In conjunction with intracardiac echocardiography, TCD can be used to assess the presence of secondary RLS in patients undergoing PFO closure. Finally, TCD can be used as a tool to assess outcomes in patients after intervention to close PFO.

Case illustrations

Case 1

A 43-year-old man, a non-smoker without history of hypertension, diabetes or alcohol abuse, suddenly developed weakness of the right arm and leg after lifting weights. On examination he is alert, with non-fluent aphasia and plegia in the right extremities. His total NIHSS score is 10 points. Brain CT scan showed an acute infarct in the left parietal lobe while CTA and carotid examination were unremarkable. TEE showed a >4 mm septal defect with right-to-left shunting following agitated saline injection. TCD showed <30 MB in supine position, which increased to curtain appearance when done in sitting position (on both rest and Valsalva maneuver).

Case 2

An 83-year-old man with end-stage renal disease suddenly developed acute loss of consciousness, seizures and left hemiparesis after his central hemodialysis access catheter was manipulated. CTA showed air in the cavernous sinus. TCD (Figure 10.2) showed circulating emboli.

First, in cases of cryptogenic stroke we use TCD even after negative cardiac echo studies to double-check if the shunt was missed due to inability to perform Valsalva well (TTE) or suboptimal imaging of heart chambers (TEE) or if shunt is extra-cardiac (i.e. possible pulmonary AVM). If RLS is found, it prompts further investigations for deep venous thrombosis or pro-coagulable state so that shunt may not be a mere bystander but a conduit for thrombi leading to paradoxical embolization. This may prompt clinicians to consider more than aspirin (i.e. antiplatelet therapy) for secondary stroke prevention, particularly in the immediate phase to 1 year following stroke or TIA.

Second, information from TCD can be obtained during the first encounter with the patient, i.e. in the emergency room, stroke unit, outpatient clinic and prior to cardiac imaging. Positive TCD RLS test should alert cardiologists to be more diligent in ascertaining the shunt.

Finally, the presence of a shunt may explain pathogenesis of stroke in patients when one would suspect paradoximal embolism last as in the elderly patient above (unless one clearly documented catheter manipulation prior to stroke) or in cases of fat embolism after bone fracture or platypnea–orthodeoxia symptoms (that could be found in professional-level athletes with PFO). Young patients with stroke, particularly women taking birth control pills who smoke, should be carefully tested for RLS [98].

References

1 Hagen PT, Scholz DG, Edwards WD. Incidence and size of patent foramen ovale during the first 10 decades of life: an autopsy study of 965 normal hearts. *Mayo Clin Proc* 1984;**59**:17–20.

2 Meier B, Lock JE. Contemporary management of patent foramen ovale. *Circulation* 2003;**107**:5–9.

3 Klotzsch C, Sliwka U, Berlit P, et al. An increased frequency of patent foramen ovale in patients with transient global amnesia. Analysis of 53 consecutive patients. *Arch Neurol* 1996;**53**:504–8.

4 Kerut EK, Norfleet WT, Plotnick GD, et al. Patent foramen ovale: a review of associated conditions and the impact of physiological size. *J Am Coll Cardiol* 2001;**38**:613–23.

5 Meissner I, Whisnant JP, Khandheria BK, et al. Prevalence of potential risk factors for stroke assessed by transesophageal echocardiography and carotid ultrasonography: the SPARC study. Stroke Prevention: Assessment of Risk in a Community. *Mayo Clin Proc* 1999;**74**:862–9.

6 Arquizan C, Coste J, Touboul PJ, et al. Is patent foramen ovale a family trait? A transcranial Doppler sonographic study. *Stroke* 2001;**32**:1563–6.

7 Seib G. Incidence of the patent foramen ovale cordis in adult American whites and American negroes. *Am J Anat* 1934;**55**:511–25.

8 Thompson T, Evans V. Paradoxical embolism. *Q J Med* 1930;**23**:135–52.

9 Di Tullio MR, Sacco RL, Sciacca RR, et al. Patent foramen ovale and the risk of ischemic stroke in a multiethnic population. *J Am Coll Cardiol* 2007;**49**:797–802.

10 Desai AJ, Fuller CJ, Jesurum JT, et al. Patent foramen ovale and cerebrovascular diseases. *Nat Clin Pract Cardiovasc Med* 2006;**3**:446–55.

11 Sacco RL, Ellenberg JH, Mohr JP, et al. Infarcts of undetermined cause: the NINCDS Stroke Data Bank. *Ann Neurol* 1989;**25**:382–90.

12 Cramer SC, Rordorf G, Maki JH, et al. Increased pelvic vein thrombi in cryptogenic stroke: results of the Paradoxical Emboli from Large Veins in Ischemic Stroke (PELVIS) study. *Stroke* 2004;**35**:46–50.

13 Lechat P, Mas JL, Lascault G, et al. Prevalence of patent foramen ovale in patients with stroke. *N Engl J Med* 1988;**318**:1148–52.

14 Webster MW, Chancellor AM, Smith HJ, et al. Patent foramen ovale in young stroke patients. *Lancet* 1988;**ii**:11–2.

15 Cabanes L, Mas JL, Cohen A, et al. Atrial septal aneurysm and patent foramen ovale as risk factors for cryptogenic stroke in patients less than 55 years of age. A study using transesophageal echocardiography. *Stroke* 1993;**24**:1865–73.

16 de Belder MA, Tourikis L, Leech G, et al. Risk of patent foramen ovale for thromboembolic events in all age groups. *Am J Cardiol* 1992;**69**:1316–20.

17 Di Tullio M, Sacco RL, Gopal A, et al. Patent foramen ovale as a risk factor for cryptogenic stroke. *Ann Intern Med* 1992;**117**:461–5.

18 Hausmann D, Mugge A, Becht I, et al. Diagnosis of patent foramen ovale by transesophageal echocardiography and association with cerebral and peripheral embolic events. *Am J Cardiol* 1992;**70**:668–72.

19 Overell JR, Bone I, Lees KR. Interatrial septal abnormalities and stroke: a meta-analysis of case-control studies. *Neurology* 2000;**55**:1172–9.

20 Handke M, Harloff A, Olschewski M, et al. Patent foramen ovale and cryptogenic stroke in older patients. *N Engl J Med* 2007;**357**:2262–8.

21 De Castro S, Cartoni D, Fiorelli M, et al. Morphological and functional characteristics of patent foramen ovale and their embolic implications. *Stroke* 2000;**31**:2407–13.

22 Steiner MM, Di Tullio MR, Rundek T, et al. Patent foramen ovale size and embolic brain imaging findings among patients with ischemic stroke. *Stroke* 1998;**29**:944–8.

23 Homma S, Sacco RL, Di Tullio MR, et al. Effect of medical treatment in stroke patients with Patent Foramen Ovale: Patent Foramen Ovale in Cryptogenic Stroke Study. *Circulation* 2002;**105**:2625–31.

24 Stone DA, Godard J, Corretti MC, et al. Patent foramen ovale: association between the degree of shunt by contrast transesophageal echocardiography and the risk of future ischemic neurologic events. *Am Heart J* 1996;**131**:158–61.

25 Anzola GP, Zavarize P, Morandi E, et al. Transcranial Doppler and risk of recurrence in patients with stroke and patent foramen ovale. *Eur J Neurol* 2003;**10**:129–35.

26 Hanley PC, Tajik AJ, Hynes JK, et al. Diagnosis and classification of atrial septal aneurysm by two-dimensional echocardiography: report of 80 consecutive cases. *J Am Coll Cardiol* 1985;**6**:1370–82.

27 Mas JL, Arquizan C, Lamy C, et al. Recurrent cerebrovascular events associated with patent foramen ovale, atrial septal aneurysm or both. *N Engl J Med* 2001;**345**:1740–6.

28 Karttunen V, Hiltunen L, Rasi V, et al. Factor V Leiden and prothrombin gene mutation may predispose to paradoxical embolism in subjects with patent foramen ovale. *Blood Coagul Fibrinol* 2003;**14**:261–8.

29 Lichy C, Reuner KH, Buggle F, et al. Prothrombin G20210A mutation, but not factor V Leiden, is a risk factor in patients with persistent foramen ovale and otherwise unexplained cerebral ischemia. *Cerebrovasc Dis* 2003;**16**:83–7.

30 Pezzini A, Del Zotto E, Magoni M, et al. Inherited thrombophilic disorders in young adults with ischemic stroke and patent foramen ovale. *Stroke* 2003;**34**:28–33.

31 Serena J, Segura T, Perez-Ayuso MJ, et al. The need to quantify right-to-left shunt in acute ischemic stroke: a case–control study. *Stroke* 1998;**29**:1322–8.

32 Slottow TL, Steinberg DH, Waksman R. Overview of the 2007 Food and Drug Administration Circulatory System Devices Panel meeting on patent foramen ovale closure devices. *Circulation* 2007;**116**:677–82.

33 Bailey CE, Allaqaband S, Bajwa TK. Current management of patients with patent foramen ovale and cryptogenic stroke: our experience and review of the literature. *WMJ* 2004;**103**:32–6.

34 Jux C, Wohlsein P, Bruegmann M, et al. A new biological matrix for septal occlusion. *J Interv Cardiol* 2003;**16**:149–52.

35 Slavin L, Tobis JM, Rangarajan K, et al. Five-year experience with percutaneous closure of patent foramen ovale. *Am J Cardiol* 2007;**99**:1316–20.

36 Windecker S, Wahl A, Nedeltchev K, et al. Comparison of medical treatment with percutaneous closure of patent foramen ovale in patients with cryptogenic stroke. *J Am Coll Cardiol* 2004;**44**:750–8.

37 Schuchlenz HW, Weihs W, Berghold A, et al. Secondary prevention after cryptogenic cerebrovascular events in patients with patent foramen ovale. *Int J Cardiol* 2005;**101**:77–82.

38 Harms V, Reisman M, Fuller CJ, et al. Outcomes after transcatheter closure of patent foramen ovale in patients with paradoxical embolism. *Am J Cardiol* 2007;**99**:1312–5.

39 Onorato E, Melzi G, Casilli F, et al. Patent foramen ovale with paradoxical embolism: mid-term results of transcatheter closure in 256 patients. *J Interv Cardiol* 2003;**16**:43–50.

40 Kiblawi FM, Sommer RJ, Levchuck SG. Transcatheter closure of patent foramen ovale in older adults. *Catheter Cardiovasc Interv* 2006;**68**:136–42; discussion 143–4.

41 Khairy P, O'Donnell CP, Landzberg MJ. Transcatheter closure versus medical therapy of patent foramen ovale and presumed paradoxical thromboemboli: a systematic review. *Ann Intern Med* 2003;**139**:753–60.

42 Schwerzmann M, Nedeltchev K, Meier B. Patent foramen ovale closure: a new therapy for migraine. *Catheter Cardiovasc Interv* 2007;**69**:277–84.

43 Lipton RB, Bigal ME, Diamond M, et al. Migraine prevalence, disease burden and the need for preventive therapy. *Neurology* 2007;**68**:343–9.

44 Wilmshurst P, Nightingale S. Relationship between migraine and cardiac and pulmonary right-to-left shunts. *Clin Sci (Lond)* 2001;**100**:215–20.

45 Anzola GP, Magoni M, Guindani M, et al. Potential source of cerebral embolism in migraine with aura: a transcranial Doppler study. *Neurology* 1999;**52**:1622–5.

46 Domitrz I, Mieszkowski J, Kwiecinski H. The prevalence of patent foramen ovale in patients with migraine (in Polish). *Neurol Neurochir Pol* 2004;**38**:89–92.

47 Schwerzmann M, Nedeltchev K, Lagger F, et al. Prevalence and size of directly detected patent foramen ovale in migraine with aura. *Neurology* 2005;**65**:1415–8.

48 Demirtas Tatlidede A, Oflazoglu B, Erten Celik S, et al. Prevalence of patent foramen ovale in patients with migraine. *Agri* 2007;**19**:39–42.

49 Anzola GP, Morandi E, Casilli F, et al. Different degrees of right-to-left shunting predict migraine and stroke: data from 420 patients. *Neurology* 2006;**66**:765–7.

50 Giardini A, Donti A, Formigari R, et al. Spontaneous large right-to-left shunt and migraine headache with aura are risk factors for recurrent stroke in patients with a patent foramen ovale. *Int J Cardiol* 2007;**120**:357–62.

51 Wilmshurst P, Nightingale S, Pearson M, et al. Relation of atrial shunts to migraine in patients with ischemic stroke and peripheral emboli. *Am J Cardiol* 2006;**98**:831–3.

52 Gori S, Morelli N, Fanucchi S, et al. The extent of right-to-left shunt fails to correlate with severity of clinical picture in migraine with aura. *Neurol Sci* 2006;**27**:14–7.

53 Wilmshurst PT, Nightingale S, Walsh KP, et al. Effect on migraine of closure of cardiac right-to-left shunts to prevent recurrence of decompression illness or stroke or for haemodynamic reasons. *Lancet* 2000;**356**:1648–51.

54 Schwerzmann M, Wiher S, Nedeltchev K, et al. Percutaneous closure of patent foramen ovale reduces the frequency of migraine attacks. Neurology 2004;**62**:1399–401.

55 Anzola GP, Frisoni GB, Morandi E, et al. Shunt-associated migraine responds favorably to atrial septal repair. A case-control study. Stroke 2006;**37**:430–4.

56 Reisman M, Christofferson RD, Jesurum J, et al. Migraine headache relief after transcatheter closure of patent foramen ovale. J Am Coll Cardiol 2005;**45**:493–5.

57 Dowson A, Mullen MJ, Peatfield R, et al. Migraine Intervention with STARFlex Technology (MIST) Trial: A prospective, multicenter, double-blind, sham-controlled trial to evaluate the effectiveness of patent foramen ovale closure with STARFlex septal repair implant to resolve refractory migraine headache. Circulation 2008;**117**:1397–404.

58 Azarbal B, Tobis J, Suh W, et al. Association of interatrial shunts and migraine headaches: impact of transcatheter closure. J Am Coll Cardiol 2005;**45**:489–92.

59 Dubiel M, Bruch L, Schmehl I, et al. Migraine headache relief after percutaneous transcatheter closure of interatrial communications. J Interv Cardiol 2008;**21**:32–7.

60 Moon RE, Camporesi EM, Kisslo JA. Patent foramen ovale and decompression sickness in divers. Lancet 1989;**i**:513–4.

61 Germonpre P, Dendale P, Unger P, et al. Patent foramen ovale and decompression sickness in sports divers. J Appl Physiol 1998;**84**:1622–6.

62 Cartoni D, De Castro S, Valente G, et al. Identification of professional scuba divers with patent foramen ovale at risk for decompression illness. Am J Cardiol 2004;**94**:270–3.

63 Koch AE, Kampen J, Tetzlaff K, et al. Incidence of abnormal cerebral findings in the MRI of clinically healthy divers: role of a patent foramen ovale. Undersea Hyperb Med 2004;**31**:261–8.

64 Schwerzmann M, Seiler C, Lipp E, et al. Relation between directly detected patent foramen ovale and ischemic brain lesions in sport divers. Ann Intern Med 2001;**134**:21–4.

65 Knauth M, Ries S, Pohimann S, et al. Cohort study of multiple brain lesions in sport divers: role of a patent foramen ovale. BMJ 1997;**314**:701–5.

66 Wilmshurst PT, Nightingale S, Walsh KP, et al. Effect on migraine of closure of cardiac right-to-left shunts to prevent recurrence of decompression illness or stroke or for haemodynamic reasons. Lancet 2000;**356**:1648–51.

67 Pearson AC, Labovitz AJ, Tatineni S, et al. Superiority of transesophageal echocardiography in detecting cardiac source of embolism in patients with cerebral ischemia of uncertain etiology. J Am Coll Cardiol 1991;**17**:66–72.

68 Schneider B, Zienkiewicz T, Jansen V, et al. Diagnosis of patent foramen ovale by transesophageal echocardiography and correlation with autopsy findings. Am J Cardiol 1996;**77**:1202–9.

69 Di Tullio M, Sacco RL, Venketasubramanian N, et al. Comparison of diagnostic techniques for the detection of a patent foramen ovale in stroke patients. Stroke 1993;**24**:1020–4.

70 Belkin RN, Pollack BD, Ruggiero ML, et al. Comparison of transesophageal and transthoracic echocardiography with contrast and color flow Doppler in the detection of patent foramen ovale. Am Heart J 1994;**128**:520–5.

71 Kerr AJ, Buck T, Chia K, et al. Transmitral Doppler: a new transthoracic contrast method for patent foramen ovale detection and quantification. J Am Coll Cardiol 2000;**36**:1959–66.

72 Sloan MA, Alexandrov AV, Tegeler CH, et al. Assessment: transcranial Doppler ultrasonography: report of the Therapeutics and Technology Assessment Subcommittee of the American Academy of Neurology. Neurology 2004;**62**:1468–81.

73 Klotzsch C, Janssen G, Berlit P. Transesophageal echocardiography and contrast-TCD in the detection of a patent foramen ovale: experiences with 111 patients. Neurology 1994;**44**:1603–6.

74 Job FP, Ringelstein EB, Grafen Y, et al. Comparison of transcranial contrast Doppler sonography and transesophageal contrast echocardiography for the detection of patent foramen ovale in young stroke patients. Am J Cardiol 1994;**74**:381–4.

75 Devuyst G, Despland PA, Bogousslavsky J, et al. Complementarity of contrast transcranial Doppler and contrast transesophageal echocardiography for the detection of patent foramen ovale in stroke patients. Eur Neurol 1997;**38**:21–5.

76 Kwiecinski H, Mieszkowski J, Torbicki A, et al. Detection of patent foramen ovale by transcranial Doppler ultrasonography (in Polish). Neurol Neurochir Pol 1994;**28**:29–34.

77 Moehring MA, Spencer MP. Power M-mode Doppler (PMD) for observing cerebral blood flow and tracking emboli. Ultrasound Med Biol 2002;**28**:49–57.

78 Spencer MP, Moehring MA, Jesurum J, et al. Power M-mode transcranial Doppler for diagnosis of patent foramen ovale and assessing transcatheter closure. J Neuroimaging 2004;**14**:342–9.

79 Saqqur M, Dean N, Schebel M, et al. Improved detection of microbubble signals using power M-mode Doppler. Stroke 2004;**35**:e14–7.

80 Jauss M, Zanette E. Detection of right-to-left shunt with ultrasound contrast agent and transcranial Doppler sonography. Cerebrovasc Dis 2000;**10**:490–6.

81 Droste DW, Lakemeier S, Wichter T, et al. Optimizing the technique of contrast transcranial Doppler ultrasound in the detection of right-to-left shunts. Stroke 2002;**33**:2211–6.

82 Droste DW, Kriete JU, Stypmann J, et al. Contrast transcranial Doppler ultrasound in the detection of right-to-left shunts: comparison of different procedures and different contrast agents. Stroke 1999;**30**:1827–32.

83 Schwarze JJ, Sander D, Kukla C, et al. Methodological parameters influence the detection of right-to-left shunts by contrast transcranial Doppler ultrasonography. Stroke 1999;**30**:1234–9.

84 Droste DW, Silling K, Stypmann J, et al. Contrast transcranial Doppler ultrasound in the detection of right-to-left shunts: time window and threshold in microbubble numbers. Stroke 2000;**31**:1640–5.

85 Droste DW, Reisener M, Kemeny V, et al. Contrast transcranial Doppler ultrasound in the detection of right-to-left shunts. Reproducibility, comparison of 2 agents and distribution of microemboli. Stroke 1999;**30**:1014–8.

86 Uzuner N, Horner S, Pichler G, et al. Right-to-left shunt assessed by contrast transcranial Doppler sonography: new insights. J Ultrasound Med 2004;**23**:1475–82.

87 Hamann GF, Schatzer-Klotz D, Frohlig G, et al. Femoral injection of echo contrast medium may increase the sensitivity of testing for a patent foramen ovale. Neurology 1998;**50**:1423–8.

88. Lao AY, Sharma VK, Tsivgoulis G, et al. Effect of body positioning during transcranial Doppler detection of right-to-left shunts. Eur J Neurol 2007;**14**:1035–9.
89. Lao AY, Sharma VK, Tsivgoulis G, et al. Detection of right-to-left shunt: comparison between the International Consensus and Spencer Logarithmic Scale criteria. J Neuroimaging 2008;**18**:402–6.
90. Grolimund P, Seiler RW, Aaslid R, et al. Evaluation of cerebrovascular disease by combined extracranial and transcranial Doppler sonography. Experience in 1,039 patients. Stroke 1987;**18**:1018–24.
91. Halsey JH. Effect of emitted power on waveform intensity in transcranial Doppler. Stroke 1990;**21**:1573–8.
92. Tsutsui JM, Xie F, Cano M, et al. Detection of retained microbubbles in carotid arteries with real-time low mechanical index imaging in the setting of endothelial dysfunction. J Am Coll Cardiol 2004;**44**:1036–46.
93. Kim DW, Min JH, Lee YS. Transcranial Doppler in asymptomatic carotid stenosis representing hemodynamic impairment: correlation study with magnetic resonance imaging. J Neuroimaging 2004;**14**:331–5.
94. Jesurum JT, Fuller CJ, Moehring MA, et al. Unilateral versus bilateral middle cerebral artery detection of right-to-left shunt by power m-mode transcranial Doppler. J Neuroimaging 2009;**19**:235–41.
95. Del Sette M, Dinia L, Rizzi D, et al. Diagnosis of right-to-left shunt with transcranial doppler and vertebrobasilar recording. Stroke 2007;**38**:2254–6.
96. Jesurum JT, Fuller CJ, Renz J, et al. Diagnosis of secondary source of right-to-left shunt with balloon occlusion of patent foramen ovale and power M-mode transcranial Doppler. JACC Cardiovasc Intv 2009;**2**:561–7.
97. Jesurum JT, Fuller CJ, Velez CA, et al. Migraineurs with patent foramen ovale have larger right-to-left shunt despite similar atrial septal features. J Headache Pain 2007;**8**:209–16.
98. Jesurum JT, Fuller CJ, Kim CJ, et al. Migraine relief occurs following patent foramen ovale closure despite residual right-to-left shunt in late follow-up. Am J Cardiol 2008;**102**:916–20.

11 Ultrasound in Neurocritical Care

Andrew D. Barreto MD & James C. Grotta MD
University of Texas–Houston Medical School, Houston, TX, USA

Introduction

The subspecialty of neurocritical care is a relatively new, but rapidly advancing, field of medicine. Before the advent of intracranial pressure monitoring in the 1980s, neurologic critical care consisted predominantly of neurosurgical postoperative patients. Monitoring of these patients' neurological status comprised serial physical examinations. Due to the complexity of damage and depressed mental status of these patients, these crude "neuro-checks" often revealed only irreversible injury.

In the twenty-first century, sophisticated monitors and sensors have largely replaced (but not eliminated) the bedside clinical examination. Although clinical changes are still very important, the concept of advanced neuromonitoring has evolved to provide ultra-early warning that permanent injury may be imminent. The ideal neuromonitor should be non-invasive, continuous, real-time and have a high sensitivity and specificity for predicting both intracranial alterations, therapy success or need for modifications, in addition to long-term clinical outcomes. Along with pressure monitoring, brain oxygen tension, continuous electroencephalography and metabolism, transcranial Doppler (TCD) ultrasound can allow the prediction of long-term outcome in patients suffering from neurological diseases.

This chapter provides an overview of the current applications of ultrasound in the intensive care unit (ICU). Specifically, the use of TCD ultrasound in cerebral perfusion and intracranial pressure prediction is reviewed. Additional important ICU applications of ultrasound, such as predicting malignant middle cerebral infarction, intracranial hemorrhage detection and brain death determination, are discussed.

Assessment of vasospasm

TCD monitoring in the setting of post-subarachnoid vasospasm is probably the most widely known role for ultrasound in the neurocritical care unit. TCD has multiple advantages in monitoring patients at risk for vasospasm including its non-invasiveness, portability, low cost and ease of repeatability. Evidence for TCD monitoring in the clinical setting of vasospasm associated with subarachnoid hemorrhage will not be discussed as it is covered in greater detail in other chapters.

TCD for assessment of cerebral hemodynamics

TCD and cerebral perfusion pressure

Measurement of cerebral perfusion pressure (CPP) is critical in many neurologic diseases, including traumatic brain injury (TBI), malignant infarction and intracerebral hemorrhage. CPP measurement through ICP monitoring has been recommended as standard of care in all cases of severe, but salvageable, TBI [1]. CPP is calculated by subtracting the ICP from mean arterial pressure (MAP). The rate of mortality has been shown to be greater in those having mean ICPs greater than 20 mmHg and in patients with consistently low CPP (<55 mmHg) [2]. Therefore, the Brain Trauma Foundation's guidelines recommend a CPP of at least 60 mmHg [3].

CPP measurement depends on accurate ICP monitoring, which usually involves the placement of invasive parenchymal or intraventricular devices. Although these pressure monitors provide valuable information, they are not without risk. Risk of infection, hemorrhage, poor positioning or malfunction can all complicate device utilization [4]. Therefore, techniques or technologies aimed at non-invasive CPP estimation in order to guide treatment strategies have been sought. Several methods of estimating CPP using TCD have been described.

In the mid-1980s, Aaslid et al. introduced the first measurement of estimated CPP, which was based on Fourier analysis of TCD flow velocity and the arterial pressure [5]. The formula related the first harmonic component of the arterial pressure to the spectral pulsatility index. Although this method was sensitive to detect changes in CPP over time, it proved to have a limited absolute accuracy (the 95% prediction error was as wide as ±27 mmHg). Czosnyka et al. compared invasively measured CPP with both

Cerebrovascular Ultrasound in Stroke Prevention and Treatment, 2nd edition.
Edited by Andrei V. Alexandrov. © 2011 Blackwell Publishing Ltd.

Aaslid *et al.*'s estimation of CPP and their own estimation formula in 96 patients with head injury [6]. Their formula used time-averaged mean, systolic and diastolic values of TCD from the middle cerebral artery. Estimation of CPP was associated with better 95% confidence limits compared with Aaslid *et al.*'s estimation (±21 versus ±29 mmHg). The estimated CPP was less than 10 mmHg in 71% of the actual CPP measurements. Although this work was promising, the degree of error was still too great to consider replacing invasive means of monitoring. Therefore, a subsequent validation of this method was performed in another cohort of 25 head injury patients. The authors found 50% smaller 95% confidence intervals than with previous methods [7]. In this small series, 80% of the absolute differences between measured and estimated CPP were less than 10 mmHg and 90% of cases less than 13 mmHg.

TCD and ICP estimation

Rather than estimating CPP directly, others have attempted to use TCD to estimate ICP non-invasively. Schmidt *et al.* developed a non-invasive assessment of "simulated" ICP which was correlated with invasive-ICP measurements obtained from parenchymal monitors [8]. In 11 intensive care patients (eight with TBI), they collected TCD flow velocities, arterial blood pressure (ABP) and developed a mathematical formula used to generate ICP simulation. Using the waveforms from the ICP measurements, 2 MHz TCD waveforms and APB (measured by radial arterial line), a computer program fit the best model between APB and TCD which approximated the ICP waveform and pressure (Figure 11.1). Importantly, at the time of recording, no patients had cerebral vasospasm or intracranial stenosis. The mean absolute difference between computed and measured ICP was 4.0 ± 1.8 mmHg. The authors concluded that, considering 5 mmHg as a crucial threshold for the mean absolute difference, eight of the 11 patients could have been precisely treated for ICP abnormalities using the simulated ICP measurements. Furthermore, the authors felt that even less precise simulations of the absolute values still accurately predicted ICP changes and trends.

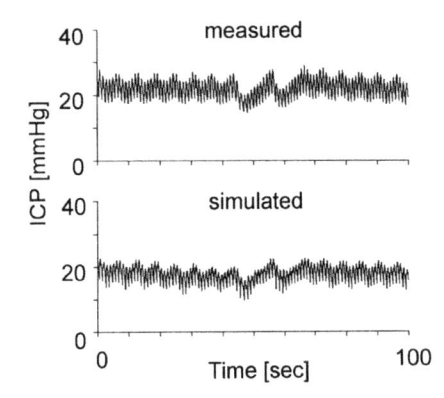

Figure 11.1 Measured and simulated ICP in one patient. Respiratory modulations can also be observed. Reproduced from Schmidt *et al.* [8] with permission from Wolters Kluwer.

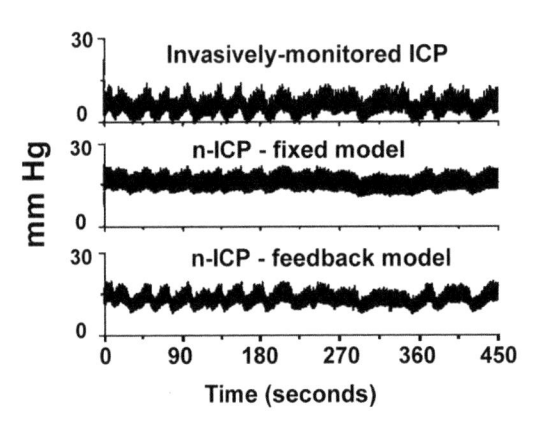

Figure 11.2 Curves of measured ICP compared with a non-invasive ICP measure (n-ICP). The feedback model showed similar ICP dynamics which remained blunted in the fixed model of ICP calculation. Adapted from Schmidt *et al.* [9] with permission from Wolters Kluwer.

The same group later improved the accuracy for ICP estimation by using an adaptive model [9]. They incorporated a corrective factor for the current state of the patient's cerebral autoregulation (SCA) to enhance the predictive model. Again, the estimated ICPs were calculated using 167 recordings of blood pressure and TCD velocity waveforms from a larger patient sample size ($n = 145$). The SCA feedback-controlled, non-invasive ICP assessment showed higher accuracy than the original corresponding (fixed) constant procedure described above and predicted ICP dynamics more accurately and with less dampening (Figure 11.2). The mean error of estimated ICP was 7.6 mmHg in the fixed model and 6.9 mmHg in the adaptive model ($p < 0.005$). Although the model was improved using the adaptive design, the observed degree of accuracy was probably still too high for routine clinical design-making. However, since not every neurological patient will receive invasive ICP-monitoring (e.g. stroke patients), some may have unrecognized elevated ICP and be missed. The authors pointed out that non-invasive ICP assessment using TCD ultrasound measurements could be a helpful tool in early intracranial hypertension diagnosis. This is especially true in patients without decompression and in centers where neurosurgical expertise is not immediately available.

Pulsatility index and ICP

The pulsatility index (PI) is a calculated ratio which provides information about impedance to flow. Notably, in contrast to TCD velocity measurements, PI is a ratio that is not subject to problems of insonation angle. Originally described in 1974 by Gosling and King [10], the PI can be used to describe the compliance of the brain. In the setting of increased intracranial pressure in TBI, cerebral edema increases distal vascular resistance which results

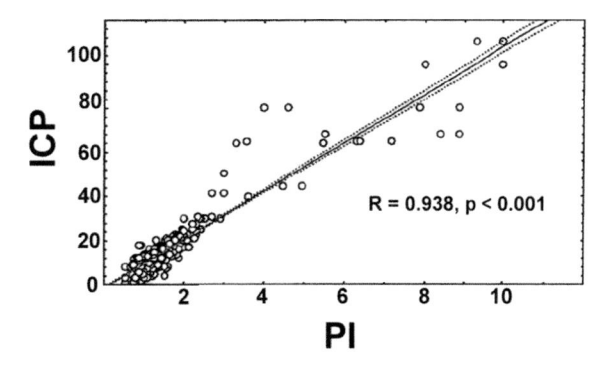

Figure 11.3 Graph demonstrating significant correlation between ICP and PI. Dotted lines are 95% confidence interval. Adapted from Bellner et al. [12] with permission from Elsevier.

in an increase in PI that can be assessed by TCD. When high ICPs are managed either medically or surgically, the PI values decrease. In one study, PI values were shown to decrease significantly by an average of 33% postoperatively in series of 19 TBI patients who underwent decompressive hemicraniectomy [11]. Interestingly, greater reductions in PI were noted in the decompressed hemisphere, indicating reduction in cerebrovascular resistance.

Correlation between increased ICP and high PI has been described in TBI patients [12–19]. Homburg et al. investigated 10 head-injured patients and demonstrated a positive correlation between PI and epidural pressure ($r = 0.82$) [14]. Similarly, Moreno et al. performed TCD measurements of 125 consecutive severe TBI (GCS < 9) patients within 24 h of admission [16]. They also reported a significant correlation between invasively measured ICP and PI ($r^2 = 0.69$, $p < 0.0001$). In another study, by Bellner et al., of 81 neurosurgical patients (21 with TBI), 658 TCD measurements were compared to invasive ICP readings [12]. The authors demonstrated excellent correlation between ICP and PI (Figure 11.3). The regression line was ICP = 11.1 × PI − 1.43. In patients with ICPs between 10 and 40, the sensitivity and specificity to detect an ICP > 20 mmHg was 89 and 92%, respectively. The authors concluded that the TCD-measured PI can provide guidance in managing intracranial hypertension in the critical care setting.

TCD PI has also been shown to correlate well with cerebral perfusion pressure in patients with TBI. In one study of 41 severe TBI patients, Chan et al. found that when CPP decreased below a critical value of 70 mmHg, a progressive increase in TCD PI was observed ($r = -0.942$, $p < 0.0001$) [20]. This decline was also accompanied by a significant fall in SjO_2, which indicates an increase in oxygen extraction by the brain to maintain its metabolic needs when CBF falls due to a reduction in cerebral blood flow. It was concluded that when there is no ICP monitor in place or there is suspicion of an inaccurate ICP measurement, TCD PI may be useful in detecting low CPP. Of note, PI can also be affected by systemic hemodynamics and carbon dioxide concentrations in blood and should be interpreted with much caution.

TCD and cerebral autoregulation

Cerebral autoregulation (CA) represents the brain's ability to maintain a stable environment in the presence of changes in either systemic blood pressure or cerebral perfusion pressure. For example, if CA is intact, a decrease in mean arterial pressure (MAP) will provoke a compensatory vasodilation, an increase in cerebral blood volume, resulting in an increase in ICP. Thus, with intact CA, MAP and ICP will be divergent. Conversely, if CA fails, a decrease in blood pressure will not result in compensatory dilation and, therefore, the ICP will fall. In this case, the MAP and ICP changes take place in the same direction. After cerebral insults such as TBI, an intact CA system protects against secondary damage such as delayed ischemic insults or harmful brain edema.

Cerebral autoregulatory disturbances can precede autoregulatory failure. TCD monitoring has been suggested as a potential non-invasive, real-time tool for monitoring the status of CA. In the setting of malignant MCA infarction, TCD velocities of the ipsi- and contralateral MCA have been shown to have different degrees of autoregulation in response to changes in head position and hypertensive challenges [21,22]. For instance, in one study, when norepinephrine increased the mean arterial pressure by 10 mmHg, the ipsilateral MCA velocity rose to 36% higher than pre-blood pressure augmentation whereas the contralateral increased by only 18%. This finding supports earlier reports that clinically important ICP gradients can be compartmentalized [23].

Disturbances in cerebral autoregulation have been described using TCD-based measurements that correlate with poor outcome. Some have suggested that using these measurements to guide treatment decisions may provide additional information regarding prognosis. For instance, Czosnyka et al. described six head-injury patients with normal CPP (>70 mmHg) but disturbed autoregulation (as measured by TCD), all of whom experienced a poor outcome [24]. Software packages and algorithms for CA estimation are available with certain TCD units; however, their practical utility and significance for therapeutic decision making require further studies.

Clinical outcome prediction and TCD

Traumatic brain injury

In addition to providing non-invasive measurements of ICP in TBI patients, TCD has been used to predict clinical outcomes. In one series, a TCD admission flow velocity of less than 28 cm s^{-1} correctly predicted early death in 80% of all deaths [25]. Patients who made a good recovery or had only moderate disability at 6 months showed a significant increase in mean velocity from 36.2 cm s^{-1} at admission to 47.8 cm s^{-1} at discharge, in contrast to those who were severely disabled, in whom velocity generally remained low. In another study, Lang et al. used TCD to study the predictive capabilities of cerebral autoregulation (CA) in 37 TBI patients [26]. They were able to demonstrate impaired CA in the first 5 days after TBI. The presence of impaired CA was significantly correlated with poor clinical outcome as measured by the Glasgow Outcome Scale (GOS).

As described above, Moreno et al. [16] correlated PI with ICP in a large group of TBI patients. Six months after injury, patients who experienced a good outcome (complete recovery or moderate disability) had a mean PI of 1.0, whereas patients with a poor outcome (death, severe disability or vegetative state) had a mean PI of 1.6 ($p < 0.0001$). The authors concluded that if performed within the first 24 h of severe head injury, TCD is valid in predicting long-term clinical outcome. These findings were corroborated by van Santbrink et al., who also found that low MCA velocities and high PI within 24 h of severe TBI were significantly associated with poor outcome [27].

Intracerebral hemorrhage

Non-traumatic, spontaneous intracerebral hemorrhage (ICH) is a devastating disease with 30-day mortality rates greater than 30% [28]. Mortality in the first few hours or days after ICH is attributable to increased ICP and tissue shifts, which can lead to brain herniation and death. Since ICP has been correlated with pulsatility index (PI), TCD has been investigated as a potential tool to predict neurologic worsening and clinical outcome in the setting of ICH.

Mayer et al. studied 30 supratentorial hemorrhages with bilateral 2 MHz TCD ultrasound monitoring [29]. The MCA was insonated continuously at a depth of 45–60 mm. The ipsilateral-to-contralateral pulsatility ratio was found to be significantly higher in patients with large versus small ICH (1.29 versus 1.06, $p = 0.001$). In a multivariable logistic regression analysis, the contralateral PI was highly correlated with IVH volume ($r = 0.76$, $r^2 = 0.58$, $p < 0.001$). In addition, the ratio of ipsilateral-to-contralateral PI ($r = 0.65$, $r^2 = 0.42$, $p = 0.0002$) correlated primarily with ICH and surrounding edema volume. The authors pointed out that the ratio of ipsilateral-to-contralateral pulsatility may provide a clinically useful, non-invasive measure of compartmentalized mass effect in patients with acute ICH. Notably, since localized mechanical damage and even transtentorial herniation can be seen in the absence of a global increase in intracranial pressure, TCD monitoring offers additional important data which have the advantage of being both non-invasive and non-irradiating [30,31]. However, further study was still needed to clarify the time course and prognostic significance of TCD waveform asymmetries in patients with large ICH.

To address the issue of prognostic significance, Marti-Fabregas et al. performed bilateral MCA TCD measurements within 12 of symptom onset in 48 patients with supratentorial non-traumatic ICH [32]. The first TCD was performed at a mean of 5.6 ± 3.6 h from symptom onset. Logistic regression revealed only Glasgow Coma Scale score and contralateral MCA PI as independent predictors of 30-day mortality. A cutoff of 1.75 for the unaffected hemisphere PI predicted death with a sensitivity of 80%, specificity of 94%, positive predictive value of 86% and negative predictive value of 91%. The authors concluded that TCD PI values of >1.75 can be used in patients with ICH to predict poor survival probability.

Although estimation of ICP using non-invasive techniques is attractive in theory, widespread adoption has not gained popularity. Several factors may explain this phenomenon. First, the lack of acoustic windows represents an inherent limitation of TCD-based ICP estimates. It is well known that approximately 10–15% of patients lack temporal windows [33]. Second, performance of TCD still requires specialized training and operator expertise which is not widely available. Third, direct and reliable calculation of absolute ICP values from TCD spectra remains an elusive goal. Lastly, well-designed, controlled trials providing evidence that non-invasive measures of CPP or ICP are non-inferior to invasive measures in terms of directing treatment and improving clinical outcome are lacking.

Duplex ultrasound imaging

Two-dimensional imaging of intracranial structures can be achieved using transcranial color-coded duplex sonography (TCCS). Brain parenchyma, ventricles and intracranial vessels have all been visualized using this technology [34–40]. Importantly, since cranial CT scans usually require transportation of critically ill patients, ultrasound imaging can provide valuable bedside data to enhance clinical decision-making.

Intracranial parenchymal assessment

Cranial computed tomography (CT) and magnetic resonance imaging (MRI) remain the standard methods for radiological diagnosis in suspected stroke. However, duplex ultrasound has been investigated to determine how it compares with CT. Maurer et al. judged TCCS against cranial CT scan in a group of 151 acute stroke patients. A total of 67 of the patients were infarctions, 60 were ICH and 24 had no focal lesions [41]. After excluding 12% of patients due to insufficient acoustic bone windows, 95% of the diagnoses were in agreement with CT. Despite two hemorrhages missed because of lack of temporal windows, the sensitivity of ultrasound in the detection of ICH was 94% and the specificity was 95%. The authors concluded that if CT is not readily available, TCCS may complement the clinical examination in patients with acute stroke. Caution has to be exercised since duplex ultrasound provides limited views of brain parenchyma and small bleedings or lacunar lesions may be below duplex resolution.

Mass effect after stroke

The mass effect which results from space-occupying cytotoxic edema causes horizontal displacement of the brainstem, which alters the level of consciousness. Midline shift in the brainstem of ≥4 mm has been demonstrated to correlate with low 14-day probability of survival [42], while mortality of malignant middle cerebral artery infarction reaches 80% [43]. A meta-analysis of hemicraniectomy for malignant MCA patients demonstrated a 50% reduction in mortality [44], which resulted in a number-needed-to-treat of 2 in order to prevent one death [44]. Although follow-up cranial CTs are performed to detect these changes, duplex ultrasound can be used to follow midline shift. Recommendations from the combined analysis of hemicraniectomy trials [44] point to individualized decision-making on when to intervene, and this provides an opportunity for duplex technology to be investigated in management of these patients. Bertram et al. prospectively performed TCCS and cranial CT in consecutive space-occupying ischemic (seven patients with MCA infarction) and hemorrhagic lesions (10 patients with large basal ganglia hemorrhage) [45]. Measurements of midline shift were based upon depth of the third ventricle. Linear regression analysis revealed a high correlation between transcranial duplex sonography and CT (Figure 11.4). Similar findings were reported by other groups who found a high correlation between these two techniques in 18 ($r = 0.87$) [35] and 62 ($r = 0.93$) [46] consecutive stroke patients.

In comparison with neuroimaging, even invasive intracranial pressure monitoring may not detect early midline shift, uncal herniation or neurological deterioration. Since intracranial pressure can remain normal in patients with midline shift and clinical herniation [47], duplex technology may represent a novel way to predict clinical worsening before irreversible deficits occur.

Until the recent advances in portable CT units, which are still only available in larger hospitals, serial CT scans required at least 1 h of nursing attention. Critically ill patients must be transported to the scanner room and placed in a flat position. The supine position is unfavorable for patients with raised intracranial pressures as it further increases ICP and may increase morbidity [48]. In addition, radiation exposure from repeated CT scans is not without risk. It is estimated that 1–2% of all cancers in the US may be attributable to CT studies [49]. TCCS offers a safe, non-invasive method to monitor space-occupying effects of strokes and complement traditional CT studies.

Hemorrhagic transformation

TCCS has been investigated for the detection of hemorrhagic transformation (HT) in the early phase of cerebral infarction. Seidel et al. performed repetitive studies in 32 patients with acute ischemic stroke in the middle cerebral artery territory beginning at 12 h and extending to 5 days from symptom onset [50]. HT was identified as hyperechogenicity in the MCA territory. Size and localization of infarction were determined by cranial CT. In 10 of 11 patients, TCCS detected HT as confirmed by CT (sensitivity 91%, specificity 95%). The authors concluded that duplex transcranial ultrasound is a promising tool for depicting HT in patients with acute hemispheric stroke and might be suitable for monitoring purposes. Note, however, the above-mentioned limitations for parenchymal imaging.

Localization during ICU procedures

Duplex ultrasound imaging has proven beneficial for bedside guidance of invasive procedures including percutaneous drainage, paracentesis, thoracentesis, inferior vena cava filter placement and venous access (Figure 11.5). Traditional methods of central venous access have relied on anatomical landmarks which serve as guidelines for procedural protocols. These landmarks do not take into account variability of anatomy and presence of thrombosis, which lead to both unsuccessful procedures and increased rates of complications. Complication rates related to central line placement have been reported to range

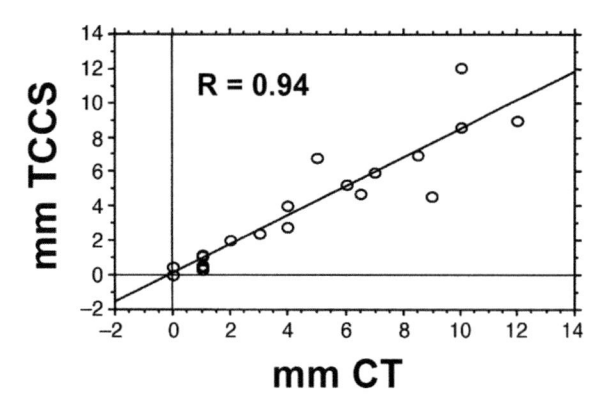

Figure 11.4 Linear regression plot of transcranial duplex sonography versus CT scan; mm = milimeters of shift. Adapted from Bertram et al. [45].

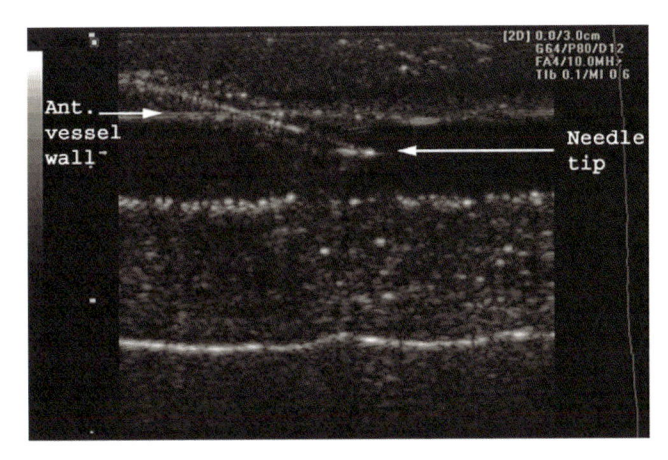

Figure 11.5 Ultrasound-guided central venous cannulation. Images demonstrates the needle advancing through the vessel wall. Reproduced from Abboud and Kendall [67] with permission from Elsevier.

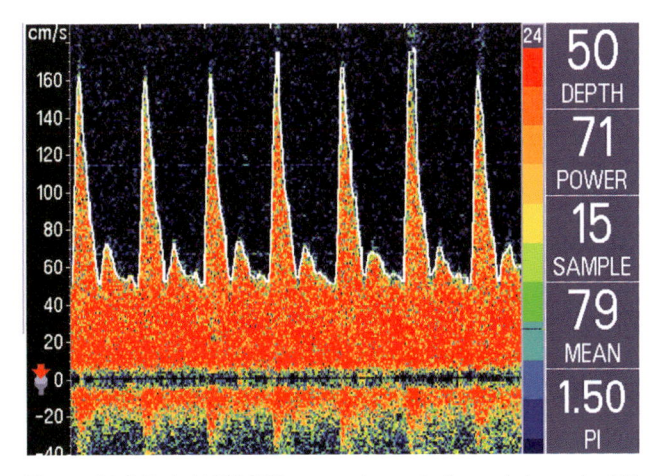

Figure 11.6 Typical MCA TCD pattern demonstrating early increasing ICP.

from 0.3 to 19%, depending on insertion site and the definition of the complication [51–53].

A meta-analysis which included 18 randomized controlled studies compared anatomical- with ultrasound-guided central venous cannulation [54]. Briefly, the study concluded that 2D ultrasound guidance was more effective than the landmark method for all outcomes for central access in adults. The relative risks of failed attempts, complications and failed first attempts were reduced by 86, 57 and 41%, respectively. Significantly fewer attempts were required for success and the duration of the procedure was decreased when using ultrasound. Further, ultrasound guidance has been shown to be cost-effective when compared with anatomical guidance [55].

Decompression of obstructive hydrocephalus involves the placement of ventriculostomy catheters which are also guided by anatomical landmarks. Despite the frequency of the procedure, data are scant regarding the accuracy of free-hand ventriculostomy. Obbens *et al.* reported a 2% failure rate in Ommaya reservoir implantation [56]. Ultrasound-guided stereotaxis has been shown to be precise in a canine model [57], but human data are less extensive. In one study, duplex ultrasound-guided ventriculostomy placement was assessed through a burr hole in 46 patients [58]. An average of 1.1 punctures was necessary to reach the ventricular system. Exact placement of all catheters except one was achieved when the ventricle could be visualized by ultrasound. However, it is still not clear if the systematic application of ultrasound guidance would result in a significant reduction in failure rates or reduced complications.

Brain death

Laws in many countries require confirmation of loss of cerebral function before brain death can be confirmed. Confirmatory tests include electroencephalography and/or cerebral blood flow. Angiography has been considered the gold standard historically, but is laborious and difficult to perform because patients must be transferred from the intensive care unit to the angiography suite.

In contrast, transcranial Doppler ultrasound has emerged as an accepted form of confirming the clinical diagnosis of brain death. The details of TCD criteria in determining brain death are described elsewhere in this book, but will be briefly outlined here with clinical examples.

To begin, since approximately 10% of patients lack an acoustic window for insonation, it is desirable to establish the windows and demonstrate cerebral perfusion prior to the onset of brain death. As the intracranial pressures elevate, the TCD waveforms exhibit a characteristic high-resistant profile. The pulsatility index increases as the diastolic velocities reduce in amplitude (Figure 11.6). As the cerebral perfusion pressure approaches zero, TCD waveforms progress into systolic spikes. Later, diastolic waveforms eventually reverse direction, resulting in a reverberating pattern. (Figure 11.7) illustrates the technetium-99 hexamethylpropylenamine oxime (HMPAO) scan of an individual who had suffered a massive brainstem hemorrhage and later developed reverberating flow on TCD. In comparison, (Figure 11.8) illustrates a radionucleotide CBF scan in a patient with absent cerebral function, but diastolic flow was still present (i.e. the patient had not reached a reverberating pattern).

The sensitivity of brain death detection using TCD criteria is not 100%. False negatives do occur, especially if a time has elapsed between brain death and the ultrasound scan [59]. Nevertheless, due to its reported specificity of 97–100% [60–63], TCD is included in Germany's brain death guidelines [64] and received Class A, level II evidence for the determination of cerebral circulatory arrest/brain death by the American Academy of Neurology [65]. Hospitals may have their own protocols for determination of brain death

PART IV Ultrasound in Stroke Prevention and Treatment

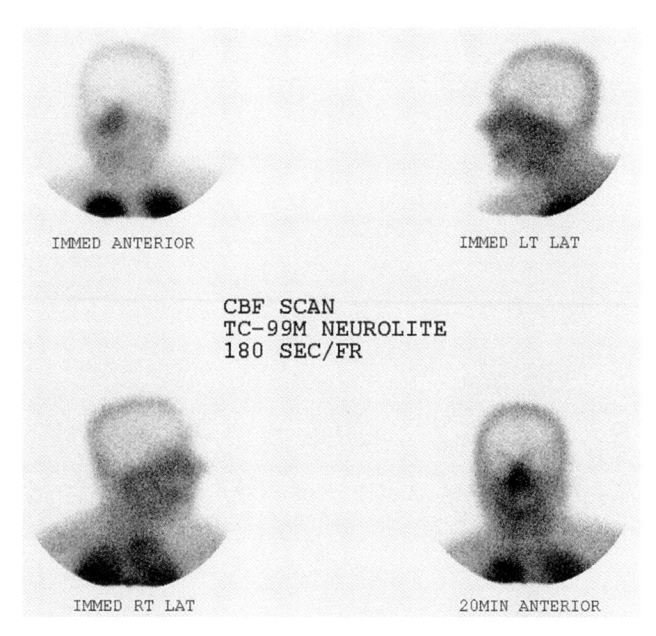

Figure 11.7 Cerebral blood flow scan: immediately (IMMED) after injection and 20 min later demonstrating no intracranial perfusion ("hollow-skull phenomenon").

and it is important to reconcile practice of TCD in this setting with specific rules established at a given hospital. A clinician who performs neurological evaluation of potentially brain-dead patient may use TCD as an extension of this examination or a screening test. Findings of positive end-diastolic flow may rule out a complete cerebral circulatory arrest at the time of examination and postpone more definitive brain perfusion scanning. Alternatively, if a reverberating (or oscillating) pattern is found, this information can be used to explain to the patient's family what is happening and in itself this can help in decision-making and offer humanitarian value.

Summary

Neurocritical care is rapidly becoming a sought-after subspecialty. In the US, the United Council for Neurologic Subspecialties (UCNS) approved the neurological subspecialty area of neuro-intensive care for membership by the UCNS Board in October 2005 and offers a yearly certification examination. Currently, trainees are expected to receive 24 months of experience, which includes 12 months of ICU time. Recommended elective rotations include Doppler laboratory experience, but this is not mandatory [66]. As discussed in this chapter, ultrasound can provide valuable information to help supplement clinical decision-making and improve diagnostic and prognostic accuracy. Therefore, future trainees in neurocritical care fellowship programs would benefit from receiving ultrasound instruction as it has become increasingly more ubiquitous.

Ultrasound in the neurological intensive care unit offers a safe, repeatable, non-invasive, rapid and inexpensive modality for important diagnostic and treatment strategies. As worries over radiation exposure and gadolinium-associated complications have intensified, ultrasound technology remains an important tool for use in critically ill patients.

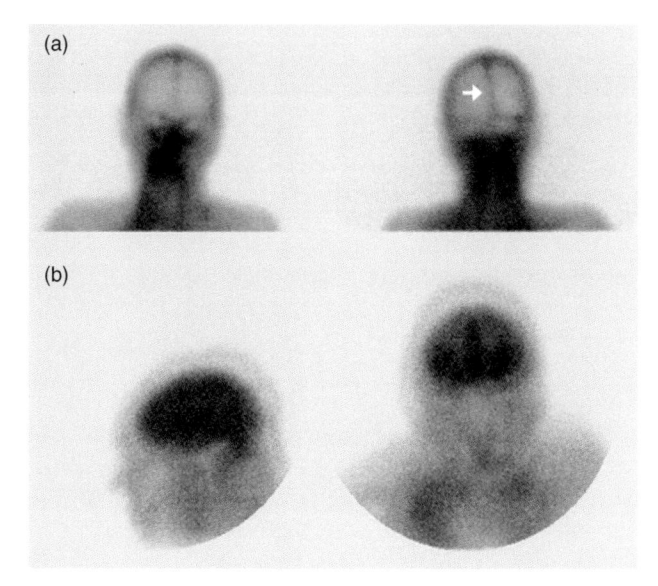

Figure 11.8 Tc-99 HMPAO CBF scans. (A) Partial intracranial perfusion. White arrow = venous sinus perfusion. (B) Normal, full perfusion for reference.

References

1 Bratton SL, Chestnut RM, Ghajar J, *et al*. Guidelines for the management of severe traumatic brain injury. VI. Indications for intracranial pressure monitoring. *J Neurotrauma* 2007;**24** Suppl 1:S37–44.

2 Balestreri M, Czosnyka M, Hutchinson P, *et al*. Impact of intracranial pressure and cerebral perfusion pressure on severe disability and mortality after head injury. *Neurocrit Care* 2006;**4**: 8–13.

3 Brain Trauma Foundation, American Association of Neurological Surgeons, Joint Section on Neurotrauma and Critical Care. Intracranial pressure treatment threshold. *J Neurotrauma* 2000;**17**: 493–5.

4 Guyot LL, Dowling C, Diaz FG, *et al*. Cerebral monitoring devices: analysis of complications. *Acta Neurochir Suppl* 1998;**71**:47–9.

5 Aaslid R, Lundar T, Lindegaard K-F, *et al*. Estimation of cerebral perfusion pressure from arterial blood pressure and transcranial Doppler recordings. In: Miller JD, Teasdale GM, Rowan JO, *et al*., eds. *Intracranial Pressure VI*. Berlin: Springer, 1986: 226–9.

6. Czosnyka M, Matta BF, Smielewski P, et al. Cerebral perfusion pressure in head-injured patients: a noninvasive assessment using transcranial Doppler ultrasonography. *J Neurosurg* 1998;**88**:802–8.
7. Schmidt EA, Czosnyka M, Matta BF, et al. Non-invasive cerebral perfusion pressure (nCPP): evaluation of the monitoring methodology in head injured patients. *Acta Neurochir Suppl* 2000;**76**:451–2.
8. Schmidt B, Klingelhofer J, Schwarze JJ, et al. Noninvasive prediction of intracranial pressure curves using transcranial Doppler ultrasonography and blood pressure curves. *Stroke* 1997;**28**:2465–72.
9. Schmidt B, Czosnyka M, Raabe A, et al. Adaptive noninvasive assessment of intracranial pressure and cerebral autoregulation. *Stroke* 2003;**34**:84–9.
10. Gosling RG, King DH. Arterial assessment by Doppler-shift ultrasound. *Proc R Soc Med* 1974;**67**:447–9.
11. Bor-Seng-Shu E, Hirsch R, Teixeira MJ, et al. Cerebral hemodynamic changes gauged by transcranial Doppler ultrasonography in patients with posttraumatic brain swelling treated by surgical decompression. *J Neurosurg* 2006;**104**:93–100.
12. Bellner J, Romner B, Reinstrup P, et al. Transcranial Doppler sonography pulsatility index (PI) reflects intracranial pressure (ICP). *Surg Neurol* 2004;**62**:45–51; discussion 51.
13. Boishardy N, Granry JC, Jacob JP, et al. Value of transcranial Doppler ultrasonography in the management of severe head injuries (in French). *Ann Fr Anesth Reanim* 1994;**13**:172–6.
14. Homburg AM, Jakobsen M, Enevoldsen E. Transcranial Doppler recordings in raised intracranial pressure. *Acta Neurol Scand* 1993;**87**:488–93.
15. McQuire JC, Sutcliffe JC, Coats TJ. Early changes in middle cerebral artery blood flow velocity after head injury. *J Neurosurg* 1998;**89**:526–32.
16. Moreno JA, Mesalles E, Gener J, et al. Evaluating the outcome of severe head injury with transcranial Doppler ultrasonography. *Neurosurg Focus* 2000;**8**:e8.
17. Rath SA, Richter HP. Transcranial Doppler sonography as a reliable diagnostic tool in craniocerebral trauma (in German). *Unfallchirurg* 1993;**96**:569–75.
18. Shiogai T, Nagayama K, Damrinjap G, et al. Morphological and hemodynamic evaluations by means of transcranial power Doppler imaging in patients with severe head injury. *Acta Neurochir Supp.* 1998;**71**:94–100.
19. Splavski B, Radanovic B, Vrankovic D, et al. Transcranial Doppler ultrasonography as an early outcome forecaster following severe brain injury. *Br J Neurosurg* 2006;**20**:386–90.
20. Chan KH, Miller JD, Dearden NM, et al. The effect of changes in cerebral perfusion pressure upon middle cerebral artery blood flow velocity and jugular bulb venous oxygen saturation after severe brain injury. *J Neurosurg* 1992;**77**:55–61.
21. Schwarz S, Georgiadis D, Aschoff A, et al. Effects of induced hypertension on intracranial pressure and flow velocities of the middle cerebral arteries in patients with large hemispheric stroke. *Stroke* 2002;**33**:998–1004.
22. Schwarz S, Georgiadis D, Aschoff A, et al. Effects of body position on intracranial pressure and cerebral perfusion in patients with large hemispheric stroke. *Stroke* 2002;**33**:497–501.
23. Sahuquillo J, Poca MA, Arribas M, et al. Interhemispheric supratentorial intracranial pressure gradients in head-injured patients: are they clinically important? *J Neurosurg* 1999;**90**:16–26.
24. Czosnyka M, Smielewski P, Kirkpatrick P, et al. Monitoring of cerebral autoregulation in head-injured patients. *Stroke* 1996;**27**:1829–34.
25. Chan KH, Miller JD, Dearden NM. Intracranial blood flow velocity after head injury: relationship to severity of injury, time, neurological status and outcome. *J Neurol Neurosurg Psychiatry* 1992;**55**:787–91.
26. Lang EW, Lagopoulos J, Griffith J, et al. Noninvasive cerebrovascular autoregulation assessment in traumatic brain injury: validation and utility. *J Neurotrauma* 2003;**20**:69–75.
27. van Santbrink H, Schouten JW, Steyerberg EW, et al. Serial transcranial Doppler measurements in traumatic brain injury with special focus on the early posttraumatic period. *Acta Neurochir (Wien)* 2002;**144**:1141–9.
28. Broderick JP, Adams HP Jr, Barsan W, et al. Guidelines for the management of spontaneous intracerebral hemorrhage: a statement for healthcare professionals from a special writing group of the Stroke Council, American Heart Association. *Stroke* 1999;**30**:905–15.
29. Mayer SA, Thomas CE, Diamond BE. Asymmetry of intracranial hemodynamics as an indicator of mass effect in acute intracerebral hemorrhage. A transcranial Doppler study. *Stroke* 1996;**27**:1788–92.
30. Janny P, Papo I, Chazal J, et al. Intracranial hypertension and prognosis of spontaneous intracerebral haematomas. A correlative study of 60 patients. *Acta Neurochir (Wien)* 1982;**61**:181–6.
31. Papo I, Janny P, Caruselli G, et al. Intracranial pressure time course in primary intracerebral hemorrhage. *Neurosurgery* 1979;**4**:504–11.
32. Marti-Fabregas J, Belvis R, Guardia E, et al. Prognostic value of pulsatility index in acute intracerebral hemorrhage. *Neurology* 2003;**61**:1051–6.
33. Rajamani K, Gorman M. Transcranial Doppler in stroke. *Biomed Pharmacother* 2001;**55**:247–57.
34. Behnke S, Becker G. Sonographic imaging of the brain parenchyma. *Eur J Ultrasound* 2002;**16**:73–80.
35. Seidel G, Gerriets T, Kaps M, et al. Dislocation of the third ventricle due to space-occupying stroke evaluated by transcranial duplex sonography. *J Neuroimaging* 1996;**6**:227–30.
36. Seidel G, Kaps M, Dorndorf W. Transcranial color-coded duplex sonography of intracerebral hematomas in adults. *Stroke* 1993;**24**:1519–27.
37. Seidel G, Kaps M, Gerriets T. Potential and limitations of transcranial color-coded sonography in stroke patients. *Stroke* 1995;**26**:2061–6.
38. Seidel G, Kaps M, Gerriets T, et al. Evaluation of the ventricular system in adults by transcranial duplex sonography. *J Neuroimaging* 1995;**5**:105–8.
39. Becker G, Bogdahn U, Strassburg HM, et al. Identification of ventricular enlargement and estimation of intracranial pressure by transcranial color-coded real-time sonography. *J Neuroimaging* 1994;**4**:17–22.
40. Bogdahn U, Becker G, Winkler J, et al. Transcranial color-coded real-time sonography in adults. *Stroke* 1990;**21**:1680–8.
41. Maurer M, Shambal S, Berg D, et al. Differentiation between intracerebral hemorrhage and ischemic stroke by transcranial color-coded duplex-sonography. *Stroke* 1998;**29**:2563–7.

42 Pullicino PM, Alexandrov AV, Shelton JA, et al. Mass effect and death from severe acute stroke. *Neurology* 1997;**49**:1090–5.

43 Hacke W, Schwab S, Horn M, et al. "Malignant" middle cerebral artery territory infarction: clinical course and prognostic signs. *Arch Neurol* 1996;**53**:309–15.

44 Vahedi K, Hofmeijer J, Juettler E, et al. Early decompressive surgery in malignant infarction of the middle cerebral artery: a pooled analysis of three randomised controlled trials. *Lancet Neurol* 2007;**6**:215–22.

45 Bertram M, Khoja W, Ringleb P, et al. Transcranial colour-coded sonography for the bedside evaluation of mass effect after stroke. *Eur J Neurol* 2000;**7**:639–46.

46 Stolz E, Gerriets T, Fiss I, et al. Comparison of transcranial color-coded duplex sonography and cranial ct measurements for determining third ventricle midline shift in space-occupying stroke. *AJNR Am J Neuroradiol* 1999;**20**:1567–71.

47 Schwab S, Aschoff A, Spranger M, et al. The value of intracranial pressure monitoring in acute hemispheric stroke. *Neurology* 1996;**47**:393–8.

48 Feldman Z, Kanter MJ, Robertson CS, et al. Effect of head elevation on intracranial pressure, cerebral perfusion pressure and cerebral blood flow in head-injured patients. *J Neurosurg* 1992;**76**:207–11.

49 Brenner DJ, Hall EJ. Computed tomography – an increasing source of radiation exposure. *N Engl J Med* 2007;**357**: 2277–84.

50 Seidel G, Cangur H, Albers T, et al. Transcranial sonographic monitoring of hemorrhagic transformation in patients with acute middle cerebral artery infarction. *J Neuroimaging* 2005;**15**:326–30.

51 Sznajder JI, Zveibil FR, Bitterman H, et al. Central vein catheterization. Failure and complication rates by three percutaneous approaches. *Arch Intern Med* 1986;**146**:259–61.

52 Mansfield PF, Hohn DC, Fornage BD, et al. Complications and failures of subclavian-vein catheterization. *N Engl J Med* 1994;**331**:1735–8.

53 Merrer J, De Jonghe B, Golliot F, et al. Complications of femoral and subclavian venous catheterization in critically ill patients: a randomized controlled trial. *JAMA* 2001;**286**:700–7.

54 Hind D, Calvert N, McWilliams R, et al. Ultrasonic locating devices for central venous cannulation: meta-analysis. *BMJ* 2003;**327**:361.

55 Calvert N, Hind D, McWilliams R, et al. Ultrasound for central venous cannulation: economic evaluation of cost-effectiveness. *Anaesthesia* 2004;**59**:1116–20.

56 Obbens EA, Leavens ME, Beal JW, et al. Ommaya reservoirs in 387 cancer patients: a 15-year experience. *Neurology* 1985;**35**: 1274–8.

57 Brown FD, Rachlin JR, Rubin JM, et al. Ultrasound-guided periventricular stereotaxis. *Neurosurgery* 1984;**15**:162–4.

58 Strowitzki M, Moringlane JR, Steudel W. Ultrasound-based navigation during intracranial burr hole procedures: experience in a series of 100 cases. *Surg Neurol* 2000;**54**:134–44.

59 Kuo JR, Chen CF, Chio CC, et al. Time dependent validity in the diagnosis of brain death using transcranial Doppler sonography. *J Neurol Neurosurg Psychiatry* 2006;**77**:646–9.

60 Hassler W, Steinmetz H, Gawlowski J. Transcranial Doppler ultrasonography in raised intracranial pressure and in intracranial circulatory arrest. *J Neurosurg* 1988;**68**:745–51.

61 Hassler W, Steinmetz H, Pirschel J. Transcranial Doppler study of intracranial circulatory arrest. *J Neurosurg* 1989;**71**:195–201.

62 Petty GW, Wiebers DO, Meissner I. Transcranial Doppler ultrasonography: clinical applications in cerebrovascular disease. *Mayo Clin Proc* 1990;**65**:1350–64.

63 Zurynski Y, Dorsch N, Pearson I, et al. Transcranial Doppler ultrasound in brain death: experience in 140 patients. *Neurol Res* 1991;**13**:248–52.

64 Haupt WF, Rudolf J. European brain death codes: a comparison of national guidelines. *J Neurol* 1999;**246**:432–7.

65 Sloan MA, Alexandrov AV, Tegeler CH, et al. Assessment: transcranial Doppler ultrasonography: report of the Therapeutics and Technology Assessment Subcommittee of the American Academy of Neurology. *Neurology* 2004;**62**:1468–81.

66 United Council for Neurologic Subspecialties. *Neurocritical Care Fellowship Program Requirements*, http://www.ucns.org/globals/axon/assets/3675.pdf (accessed 30 June 2010).

67 Abboud PA, Kendall JL. Ultrasound guidance for vascular access. *Emerg Med Clin North Am* 2004;**22**:749–73.

12 Cerebral Vasospasm after Subarachnoid Hemorrhage

Mark R. Harrigan[1], David W. Newell[2] & Andrei V. Alexandrov[1]
[1]University of Alabama Hospital, Birmingham, AL, USA
[2]University of Washington, Seattle, WA, USA

Introduction

Cerebral vasospasm is a delayed sustained contraction of the cerebral arteries, which can be induced by blood products that remain in contact with the cerebral vessel wall following subarachnoid hemorrhage [1,2]. Vasospasm is a common complication of subarachnoid hemorrhage (SAH) which is often responsible for delayed ischemic neurological deficits (DINDS) in these patients [1–4]. The most common cause of spontaneous SAH is from the rupture of cerebral aneurysms [5–7]. However, subarachnoid hemorrhage can also occur from other causes, such as head injury and following neurosurgical operations for other lesions, and these hemorrhages can also lead to vasospasm. A more in-depth understanding of cerebral vasospasm has been possible through the development of non-invasive diagnostic techniques such as transcranial Doppler (TCD) [8,9] and techniques to measure cerebral blood flow [10–12], and also from experimental models of vasospasm [13–15]. The pathophysiology of vasospasm and the role of TCD and blood flow studies in the diagnosis and management of patients with cerebral vasospasm is discussed in this chapter.

Biologic and physiological aspects of vasospasm

Hemoglobin and other products from the breakdown of blood around the outside of the cerebral vessels can enter the vessel walls and induce biochemical changes leading to sustained muscular contraction and also structural changes of the vessel characterized by collagen deposition [2]. Contractile and structural changes result in severe narrowing of the cerebral arteries that in turn can produce increased vascular resistance in the conducting vessels and secondary decreases in cerebral blood flow. Vasospasm most frequently occurs in the basal cerebral vessels as they course through the basal cisterns, which parallels the typical deposition of blood following rupture of aneurysms [4]. Occasionally, vasospasm can be found in the more distally located cerebral vessels, depending on the location of aneurysmal subarachnoid hemorrhage and the location of the blood deposited around the vessels. The location and extent of the subarachnoid bleeding is determined by a non-contrast CT scan of the (Figure 12.1). CT scans can be graded for the presence of blood using the Fischer Grades [16] described in Table 12.1. The location and the thickness of the blood clots deposited in the subarachnoid space have predictive value of the risk of vasospasm and subsequent development of delayed ischemic deficits [4,16].

Vasospasm following SAH will occur and cause some degree of vessel narrowing in most patients [1,2,4,17,18]. Clinical severity of SAH measured with Hunt–Hess Grades [19] (Table 12.2) or the Glasgow Coma Scale [20, 21], clot burden and hydrocephalus on CT [22] and velocity changes on transcranial Doppler [23] are generally predictive of vasospasm development and progression to delayed neurological deficits.

The majority of these patients, however, do not develop vessel narrowing to the point of reducing blood flow to ischemic levels. Most patients will therefore only sustain transient mild or moderate narrowing of the cerebral vessels and undergo spontaneous resolution without development of DIND. Severe vasospasm will cause greater vessel narrowing with reduction of blood flow to ischemic thresholds and development of delayed ischemic neurologic deficits [24]. The onset of DIND indicates that compensatory mechanisms, including recruitment of collateral circulation, autoregulation of the cerebral blood flow and increases in oxygen extraction fraction, are no longer adequate to provide sufficient blood flow.

Cerebrovascular Ultrasound in Stroke Prevention and Treatment, 2nd edition.
Edited by Andrei V. Alexandrov. © 2011 Blackwell Publishing Ltd.

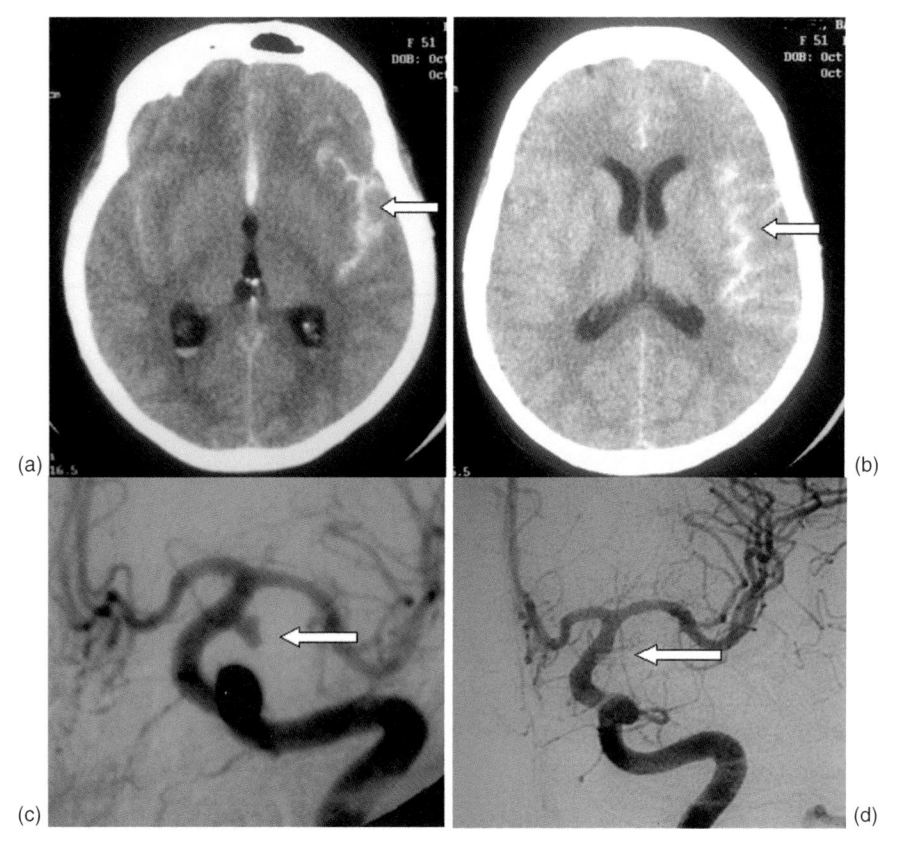

PART IV Ultrasound in Stroke Prevention and Treatment

Figure 12.1 CT appearance of SAH and aneurysm location. Illustration of a CT scan of the head [(a) and (b)] in a patient following a recent subarachnoid hemorrhage illustrating thick vertical layers of blood (arrows) in the intra-hemispheric and left Sylvian fissure, placing the patient at risk for vasospasm in these locations. Angiogram in the came patient [(c) and (d)] showing a posterior communicating artery aneurysm before [(b), arrow)] and after [(n) clipping].

Clinical and diagnostic features of DIND and vasospasm

The diagnosis of delayed ischemic neurological deficit is generally made on clinical grounds, when a patient develops a new neurologic deficit that is not explained by other causes. Delayed neurologic deterioration in patients with SAH can occur from causes other than vasospasm, including hydrocephalus, edema, hemorrhage, sepsis, electrolyte disturbance or seizures. Clinical suspicion of DINDs due to vasospasm is usually triggered by either a decreased level of consciousness or focal neurologic signs, including speech deficits or weakness. Vasospasm causing frontal lobe ischemia may present as confusion, agitation, apathy or electrolyte disturbances. A so-called cerebral salt-wasting syndrome or unexplained increase in urinary output after subarachnoid hemorrhage [25,26] may precede the onset of neurologic deficits. Ischemic symptoms in the posterior circulation may be associated with a decreased level of consciousness and breathing abnormalities or can be subtle and can include diplopia and other brain stem signs such as decreased gag reflex.

Ancillary diagnostic studies including CT scanning, TCD and blood flow measurements have a role in supporting the diagnosis of DIND since there is uncertainty in some cases whether the degree of vasospasm present in a patient is responsible for the clinical symptoms. The CT scan can

Table 12.1 Fisher Grades of SAH on CT scans

Grade	CT demonstration of SAH
1	No blood detected
2	Diffuse or vertical layers <1 mm thick
3	Localized subarachnoid clot or layers ≥1 mm thick
4	Intracerebral or intraventricular clot with diffuse or no SAH

Table 12.2 Hunt–Hess Classification of SAH

Grade	Description
I	Asymptomatic or mild headache with mild nuchal rigidity
II	Moderate or severe headache, nuchal rigidity, no neurological deficit other than nerve palsy
III	Mild focal deficit, drowsiness or confusion
IV	Stupor, moderate to severe hemiparesis, possible early decerebrate rigidity and vegetative disturbances
V	Deep coma, decerebrate rigidity, moribund appearance

CHAPTER 12 Cerebral Vasospasm after Subarachnoid Hemorrhage

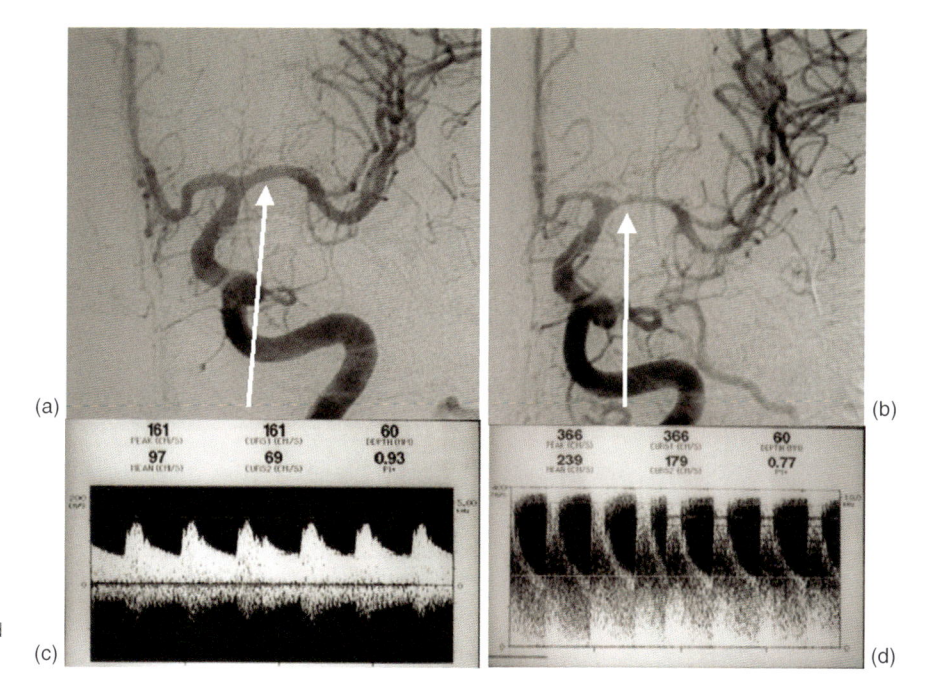

Figure 12.2 The proximal middle cerebral artery vasospasm. A left internal carotid angiogram [(a) and (b)] showed the middle cerebral arteries before (a) and after (b) the onset of vasospasm. Transcranial Doppler recordings [(c) and (d)] of the corresponding left middle cerebral blood flow velocities at baseline (c) before the onset of vasospasm and after development of severe spasm (d).

rule out hydrocephalus, edema or hemorrhage as a cause of new neurologic deficits. It is also useful to ascertain whether a new infarct is present, using CT, before proceeding to endovascular therapy such as angioplasty [27], since the presence of significant infarction has been associated with increased complications following angioplasty with or without papaverine [28–31].

Post-traumatic vasospasm, or vasospasm following head injury, is now increasingly recognized as a clinical entity with potentially significant consequences [32–34]. Following trauma, bleeding in the subarachnoid space can leave blood deposited around the basal cerebral arteries and can lead to delayed cerebral vessel narrowing and ischemia. Martin *et al.* suggested that patients with significant post-traumatic subarachnoid hemorrhage be examined frequently by TCD for the presence of vasospasm and also hypo- or hyperperfusion states after brain injury [35].

Use of transcranial Doppler and cerebral blood flow studies for vasospasm

TCD had one of the first applications in the identification of cerebral vasospasm after SAH [8,9]. TCD can be used to detect vasospasm and the amount of blood on the CT scan correlated with the degree of subsequent velocity elevations [23]. Although TCD does not allow one to measure cerebral blood flow [36,37], numerous studies showed that TCD can be useful in detecting and monitoring the degree of vasospasm following subarachnoid hemorrhage, following the time course of spasm, and also to evaluate the effects of treatment for vasospasm used alone or in conjunction with CBF studies [38–42].

The degree of vasospasm in the basal vessels is inferred from the amount of acceleration of blood flow velocity through the vessels as they become narrowed [38] (Figure 12.2, Table 12.3). As a practical matter it is always important to obtain baseline TCD measurements in patients with subarachnoid hemorrhage and to frequently (daily or every other day) repeat examinations throughout the hospital stay. Lindegaard *et al.* [38] showed that vasospastic middle cerebral arteries usually demonstrate velocities greater than 120 cm s^{-1}, with velocity being inversely related to arterial diameter, and velocities greater than 200 cm s^{-1} are predictive of a 1 mm residual MCA lumen diameter or less. Note that a normal MCA diameter is approximately 3 mm.

Table 12.3 Stages of vasospasm[a]

Stage	Vessel narrowing	TCD velocity	CBF	DIND
I	↑	↑	⇔	No
II	↑↑	↑↑	⇔	No
III	↑↑↑	↑↑↑	↓↓	No
IV	↑↑↑↑	↑↑↑↑ or ↑↑↑	↓↓↓	Yes

[a]This table shows relative changes in vessel narrowing, TCD velocities, CBF and delayed neurologic deficits according to the progressive stages of vasospasm. ↑ = mild, ↑↑ = moderate, ↑↑↑ = severe, ↑↑↑↑ = very severe, ⇔ = no change. Abbreviations: TCD = transcranial Doppler, CBF = cerebral blood flow, DIND = delayed ischemic neurologic deficit.

Single-photon emission computed tomography (SPECT) is one of several methods that can be used to evaluate regional cerebral blood flow in patients with vasospasm following SAH [41]. Other methods to evaluate blood flow include xenon computed tomography (Xe-CT) [37], radioactive xenon-133 with external detectors, positron emission tomography (PET) and either thermodilution or laser Doppler cortical flow probes. The information gained from CBF methods can be complementary to information provided by TCD and the neurologic examination and can be helpful in deciding on different treatment regimens in patients following subarachnoid hemorrhage [42]. However, TCD mean flow velocity measurements do not allow the calculation of cerebral blood flow volume and should not substitute CBF measurements [36,37,43,44]. TCD velocity information is helpful in predicting the degree of vessel narrowing, spasm progression or regression and compensatory vasodilation.

The changes in velocity on TCD have been correlated with vessel narrowing measured using angiography and the best correlations are in the middle cerebral artery [38,39]. Sloan et al. evaluated the sensitivity and specificity of TCD for vasospasm in the middle cerebral artery and the vertebrobasilar system [45,46]. It is recommended that the extracranial internal carotid artery velocity be recorded also when assessing anterior circulation vasospasm because increased or decreased velocities can also be caused by blood flow changes, i.e. hyperdynamic state with hypertension–hypervolemia. By recording velocity in the MCA and ICA, a Lindegaard ratio [47,48] between the mean flow velocities (MCA/ICA) can be calculated which may help in differentiating spasm severity and the relative contribution of hyperemia (see also Chapter 6).

Vasospasm can be limited to distal vascular distributions in a relatively small percentage of cases and can be missed by TCD [49]. Although TCD is insensitive for detecting far distal vasospasm (i.e. M3 or distal M2 MCA), distal spasm affecting proximal M2 segments of the MCA can be detected (Figure 12.3). Far distal spasm can often be predicted by the distribution of blood in more distal locations on the initial CT scan following subarachnoid hemorrhage. Newell et al. reported that isolated distal vessel spasm causing significant neurologic deficit is unusual after subarachnoid hemorrhage, but does exist [49]. Cerebral blood flow methods such as Xe-CT or SPECT are useful for confirming this diagnosis.

We employ TCD to perform daily monitoring in patients with subarachnoid hemorrhage preoperatively and in the postoperative period. The routine use of blood flow studies may also be helpful in guiding therapy for vasospasm. Yonas et al. utilized CBF measurements with Xe-CT and documented decreased cerebral blood flow specific to territories supplied by vasospastic vessels [43]. When combined with routine TCD detection of vasospasm, Xe-CT CBF or SPECT evaluation may prove valuable in determining which

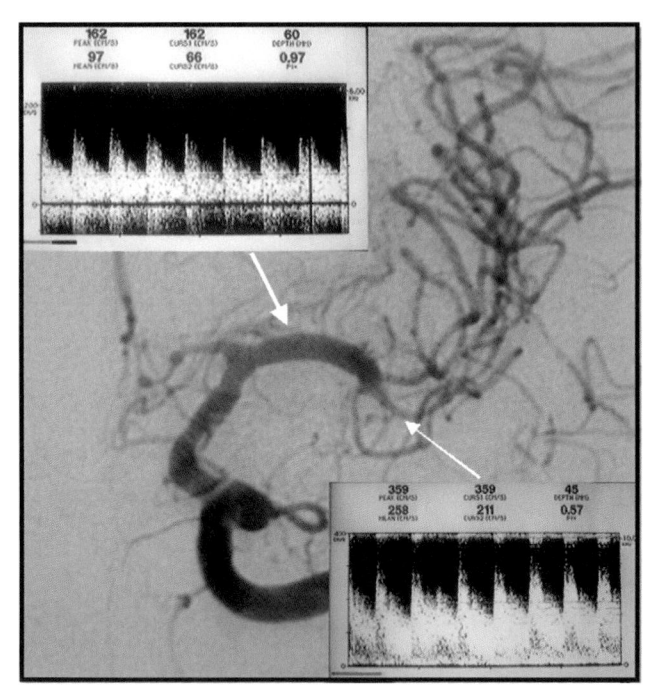

Figure 12.3 M2 MCA vasospasm. A left internal carotid angiogram showed improvement in vessel diameter after balloon angioplasty for a severe proximal M1 MCA vasospasm (see Figures 12.1 and 12.2). TCD showed mean flow velocities of 97 cm s^{-1} in the M1 MCA after angioplasty (upper waveform) and the M2 MCA mean flow velocities of 258 cm s^{-1} (lower waveform), indicating development of spasm in more distal branches.

patients will ultimately benefit from angioplasty and may also be useful to predict when earlier intervention during the asymptomatic period might be beneficial. Moreover, CBF imaging techniques such as Xe-CT and SPECT assess tissue perfusion, which complements the assessment of vessel diameter provided by TCD.

Options for treatment of vasospasm

Various medications have been evaluated in human clinical studies for their effect on reducing ischemic complications from vasospasm [3,30,31, 0]. Calcium channel blockers, which are cerebral-selective, have been shown to be effective in improving outcome after subarachnoid hemorrhage and are now used routinely [51,52].

Another therapy which is routinely employed for the prevention and treatment of ischemic deficits following subarachnoid hemorrhage is triple-H therapy, which denotes induced hypertension, hypervolemia and hemodilution [50]. The triple-H therapy utilizes crystalloid and colloid solutions and also vasopressors to increase blood pressure. Therapies including triple-H therapy and calcium channel blockers are often not completely effective in eliminating delayed ischemic neurological deficits (DINDS) from cerebral vasospasm. Endovascular therapy using angioplasty and/or papaverine offers an additional modality for treatment in patients with vasospasm.

Zubkov *et al.* first reported the use of endovascular techniques to dilate vasospastic cerebral arteries mechanically in a series of patients [27]. These encouraging results established that mechanical dilation of cerebral arteries affected by vasospasm can result in a sustained treatment effect and thereby may benefit patients who are affected by cerebral ischemia from vasospasm. Subsequent reports from the US verified the findings of Zubkov *et al.* and led to further development of balloon angioplasty for the treatment of vasospasm [28,29].

Treatment of vasospasm with papaverine has also been employed recently with renewed interest in the treatment of distal spasm that cannot be directly reached by balloon-carrying catheters. Currently, papaverine and balloon angioplasty are the most common endovascular therapies being employed in the treatment of cerebral vasospasm [30,31]. Papaverine infusion is accomplished using small repeated injections with a super-selective catheter positioned just proximal to the affected area of a vessel using an infusion of 300 mg per side or 600 mg total dose. Balloon angioplasty is performed also using transfemoral catheterization with a road mapping imaging technique available for accurate balloon placement. A soft silicone micro-balloon catheter is used and is introduced just proximal to the spastic segments. Papaverine can also be used as an adjunct to facilitate dilation of vessel segments prior to the introduction of the balloon catheter. The balloon is inflated under low pressure multiple times while advancing it into the spastic segments. Careful attention is paid not to pass the catheter into a branch or a small vessel and not to over-inflate the artery past the original diameter, which will minimize the risk of vessel rupture.

Angioplasty in the anterior circulation can be performed in the supraclinoid carotid arteries and proximal middle cerebral arteries, including the M2 branches. Angioplasty can also be performed in both vertebral arteries, the basilar artery, proximal posterior cerebral arteries and, occasionally, the proximal superior cerebellar arteries. The anterior cerebral artery system has not previously been accessible for balloon angioplasty, but recent advances in catheters make it possible to dilate the A1 segments in some patients.

Elliott *et al.* observed relative improvements in CBF, using SPECT at 24 h following treatment of vasospasm, with balloon angioplasty significantly more often than with papaverine infusion [53]: 71% of vessel segment territories demonstrated improved CBF at 24 h following balloon angioplasty whereas only 31% of vessel segment territories showed improvement within 24 h following papaverine infusion. These results are consistent with TCD observations that balloon angioplasty is superior to papaverine infusion when used alone for the treatment of proximal vasospasm. TCD can be used to monitor flow velocities at the site of angioplasty to document the sustained effect of the interventional procedure.

Other studies have also shown that TCD and other variables can monitor triple-H therapy and predict outcomes after subarachnoid hemorrhage [54,55].

Conclusions

The occurrence of stroke and permanent ischemic brain damage from cerebral vasospasm continues to be a clinical problem in patients following SAH and is a potentially preventable or reversible condition. Prompt recognition and treatment of this condition depends in part on accurate diagnosis that can be facilitated using TCD and cerebral blood flow studies. Although asymptomatic patient selection for early angioplasty to prevent the onset of DIND remains controversial, TCD can be used to:
1 detect asymptomatic vasospasm onset;
2 follow spasm progression and facilitate triple-H-therapy;
3 identify patients with severe vasospasm;
4 monitor the effect of therapies and interventions; and
5 detect spasm resolution.

References

1 Weir B, Grace M, Hansen J, *et al.* Time course of vasospasm in man. *J Neurosurg* 1978;**48**:173–8.
2 Sloan MA. Cerebral vasoconstriction: physiology, pathophysiology and occurrence in selected cerebrovascular disorders. In: Caplan LR, ed. *Brain Ischemia: Basic Concepts and Their Clinical Relevance*. Berlin: Springer, 1994.
3 Fleischer AS, Raggio JF, Tindall GT. Aminophylline and isoproterenol in the treatment of cerebral vasospasm. *Surg Neurol* 1977;**8**:117–21.
4 Kistler JP, Crowell RM, Davis KR, *et al.* The relation of cerebral vasospasm to the extent and location of subarachnoid blood visualized by CT scan: a prospective study. *Neurology* 1983;**33**:424–36.
5 Oldenkott P, Stolz C. Subarachnoid hemorrhage. The diagnostic guiding symptom: the blood containing liquor. Cause, clinical aspects, treatment problems and prognosis (in German). *Med Welt* 1969;**23**:1326–31.
6 Niizuma H, Kwak R, Otabe K, *et al.* Angiography study of cerebral vasospasm following the rupture of intracranial aneurysms: Part II. Relation between the site of aneurysm and the occurrence of the vasospasm. *Surg Neurol* 1979;**11**:263–7.
7 Reynolds AF, Shaw CM. Bleeding patterns from ruptured intracranial aneurysms: an autopsy series of 205 patients. *Surg Neurol* 1981;**15**:232–5.
8 Aaslid R, Markwalder TM, Nornes H. Noninvasive transcranial Doppler ultrasound recording of flow velocity in basal cerebral arteries. *J Neurosurg* 1982;**57**:769–74.

9 Lindegaard KF, Nornes H, Bakke SJ, et al. Cerebral vasospasm after subarachnoid haemorrhage investigated by means of transcranial Doppler ultrasound. *Acta Neurochir (Wien)* 1988;**42** Suppl:P81–4.

10 Bohm E, Aronson G, Hugosson R, et al. Cerebral circulatory conditions in patients with ruptured aneurysms measured by an intravenous radioactive-indicator technique. *Acta Neurol Scand* 1968;**44**:33–42.

11 Grubb RL Jr, Raichle ME, Eichling JO, et al. Effects of subarachnoid hemorrhage on cerebral blood volume, blood flow and oxygen utilization in humans. *J Neurosurg* 1977;**46**: 446–53.

12 Meyer CH, Lowe D, Meyer M, et al. Progressive change in cerebral blood flow during the first three weeks after subarachnoid hemorrhage. *Neurosurgery* 1983;**12**:58–76.

13 Barry KJ, Gogjian MA, Stein BM. Small animal model for investigation of subarachnoid hemorrhage and cerebral vasospasm. *Stroke* 1979;**10**:538–41.

14 Rothberg CS, Weir B, Overton TR. Treatment of subarachnoid hemorrhage with sodium nitroprusside and phenylephrine: an experimental study. *Neurosurgery* 1979;**5**:588–95.

15 Megyesi JF, Vollrath B, Cook DA, et al. In vivo animal models of cerebral vasospasm: a review. *Neurosurgery* 2000;**46**: 448–60.

16 Fischer CM, Kistler JP, Davis JM. Relation of cerebral vasospasm to subarachnoid hemorrhage visualized by computed tomographic scanning. *Neurosurgery* 1980;**6**:1–9.

17 Heros RC, Zervas NT, Varsos V. Cerebral vasospasm after subarachnoid hemorrhage: an update. *Ann Neurol* 1983;**14**: 599–608.

18 Mayberg MR: Cerebral vasospasm. *Neurosurg Clin North Am* 1998;**9**:615–27.

19 Hunt WE, Hess RM. Surgical risk as related to time of intervention in the repair of intracranial aneurysms. *J Neurosurg* 1968;**28**:14–20.

20 Teasdale G, Jennett B. Assessment of coma and impaired consciousness – a practical guide. *Lancet* 1974;**ii**(7872):81–4.

21 Teasdale GM, Murray L. Revisiting the Glasgow Coma Scale and Coma Score. *Intensive Care Med* 2000;**26**:153–4.

22 Black PM. Hydrocephalus and vasospasm after subarachnoid hemorrhage from ruptured intracranial aneurysms. *Neurosurgery* 1986;**18**:12–6.

23 Seiler RW, Grolimund P, Aaslid R, et al. Cerebral vasospasm evaluated by transcranial ultrasound correlated with clinical grade and CT-visualized subarachnoid hemorrhage. *J Neurosurg* 1986;**64**:594–600.

24 Yamakami I, Isobe K, Yamaura A, et al. Vasospasm and regional cerebral blood flow (rCBF) in patients with ruptured intracranial aneurysm: serial rCBF studies with the xenon-133 inhalation method. *Neurosurgery* 1983;**13**:394–401.

25 Berendes E, Scherer R, Schuricht G, et al. Massive natriuresis and polyuria after triple craniocervical subarachnoid hemorrhage: cerebral salt wasting syndrome? *(in German) Anasthesiol Intensivmed Notfallmed Schmerzther* 1992;**27**:445–8.

26 Harrigan MR. Cerebral salt wasting syndrome. *Crit Care Clin* 2001;**17**:125–38.

27 Zubkov YN, Nikiforov BM, Shustin VA. Balloon catheter technique for dilatation of constricted cerebral arteries after aneurysmal subarachnoid hemorrhage. *Acta Neurochir (Wien)* 1984;**70**:65–79.

28 Higashida RT, Halbach VV, Cahan LD, et al. Transluminal angioplasty for treatment of intracranial arterial vasospasm. *J Neurosurg* 1989;**71**:648–53.

29 LeRoux PD, Newell DW, Eskridge J, et al. Severe symptomatic vasospasm: the role of immediate postoperative angioplasty. *J Neurosurg* 1994;**80**:224–9.

30 Kaku Y, Yonekawa Y, Tsukahara T, et al. Superselective intra-arterial infusion of papaverine for the treatment of cerebral vasospasm after subarachnoid hemorrhage. *J Neurosurg* 1992;**77**:842–7.

31 Kassell NF, Helm G, Simmons N, et al. Treatment of cerebral vasospasm with intra-arterial papaverine. *J Neurosurg* 1992;**77**:848–52.

32 Lee JH, Martin NA, Alsina G, et al. Hemodynamically significant cerebral vasospasm and outcome after head injury: a prospective study. *J Neurosurg* 1997;**87**:221–33.

33 Zubkov AY, Pilkington AS, Bernanke DH, et al. Posttraumatic cerebral vasospasm: clinical and morphological presentations. *J Neurotrauma* 1999;**16**:763–70.

34 Zubkov AY, Lewis AI, Raila FA, et al. Risk factors for the development of post-traumatic cerebral vasospasm. *Surg Neurol* 2000;**53**:126–30.

35 Martin NA, Patwardhan RV, Alexander MJ, et al. Characterization of cerebral hemodynamic phases following severe head trauma: hypoperfusion, hyperemia and vasospasm. *J Neurosurg* 1997;**87**:9–19.

36 Romner B, Brandt L, Berntman L, et al. Simultaneous transcranial Doppler sonography and cerebral blood flow measurements of cerebrovascular CO2-reactivity in patients with aneurysmal subarachnoid haemorrhage. *Br J Neurosurg* 1991;**5**:31–7.

37 Clyde BL, Resnick DK, Yonas H, et al. The relationship of blood velocity as measured by transcranial Doppler ultrasonography to cerebral blood flow as determined by stable xenon computed tomographic studies after aneurysmal subarachnoid hemorrhage. *Neurosurgery* 1996;**38**:896–904.

38 Lindegaard KF, Nornes H, Bakke SJ, et al. Cerebral vasospasm after subarachnoid haemorrhage investigated by means of transcranial Doppler ultrasound. *Acta Neurochir Suppl (Wien)* 1988;**42**:81–4.

39 Sloan MA. Transcranial Doppler monitoring of vasospasm after subarachnoid hemorrhage. In: Tegeler CH, Babikian VL, Gomez CR, eds. *Neurosonology*. St. Louis, MO: Mosby, 1996: 156–71.

40 Giller CA, Purdy P, Giller A, et al. Elevated transcranial Doppler ultrasound velocities following therapeutic arterial dilation. *Stroke* 1995;**26**:123–7.

41 Lewis DH, Eskridge JM, Newell DW, et al. Brain SPECT and the effect of cerebral angioplasty in delayed ischemia due to vasospasm. *J Nucl Med* 1992;**33**:1789–96.

42 Rajendran JG, Lewis DH, Newell DW, et al. Brain SPECT used to evaluate vasospasm after subarachnoid hemorrhage: correlation with angiography and transcranial Doppler. *Clin Nucl Med* 2001;**26**:125–30.

43 Yonas H, Sekhar L, Johnson SW, et al. Determination of irreversible ischemia by xenon-enhanced computed tomographic monitoring of cerebral blood flow in patients with symptomatic vasospasm. *Neurosurgery* 1989;**24**:368–72.

44 Kontos HA. Validity of cerebral arterial blood flow calculations from velocity measurements. *Stroke* 1989;**20**: 1–3.
45 Sloan MA, Haley EC, Kassell NF, *et al*. Sensitivity and specificity of transcranial Doppler ultrasonography in the diagnosis of vasospasm following subarachnoid hemorrhage. *Neurology* 1989;**39**:1514–8.
46 Sloan MA, Burch CM, Wozniak MA, *et al*. Transcranial Doppler detection of vertebrobasilar vasospasm following subarachnoid hemorrhage. *Stroke* 1994;**25**:2187–97.
47 Lindegaard KF, Nornes H, Bakke SJ, *et al*. Cerebral vasospasm diagnosis by means of angiography and blood velocity measurements. *Acta Neurochir (Wien)* 1989;**100**:12–24.
48 Lindegaard KF. The role of transcranial Doppler in the management of patients with subarachnoid haemorrhage: a review. *Acta Neurochir (Suppl)* 1999;**72**:59–71.
49 Newell DW, Grady MS, Eskridge JM, *et al*. Distribution of angiographic vasospasm after subarachnoid hemorrhage: implications for diagnosis by transcranial Doppler ultrasonography. *Neurosurgery* 1990;**27**:574–7.
50 Awad IA, Carter LP, Spetzler RF, *et al*. Clinical vasospasm after subarachnoid hemorrhage: response to hypervolemic hemodilution and arterial hypertension. *Stroke* 1987;**18**:365–72.
51 Barker FG, Ogilvy CS. Efficacy of prophylactic nimodipine for delayed ischemic deficit after subarachnoid hemorrhage: a metaanalysis. *J Neurosurg* 1996;**84**:405–14.
52 Feigin VL, Rinkel GJ, Algra A, *et al*. Calcium antagonists in patients with aneurysmal subarachnoid hemorrhage: a systematic review. *Neurology* 1998;**50**:844–66.
53 Elliott JP, Newell DW, Lam DJ, *et al*. Comparison of balloon angioplasty and papaverine infusion for the treatment of vasospasm following aneurysmal subarachnoid hemorrhage. *J Neurosurg* 1998;**88**:277–84.
54 Quereshi AI, Suarez JI, Bhardwaj A, *et al*. Early predictors of outcome in patients receiving hypervolemic and hypertensive therapy for symptomatic vasospasm after subarachnoid hemorrhage. *Crit Care Med* 2000;**28**:824–9.
55 Qureshi AI, Sung GY, Razumovsky AY, *et al*. Early identification of patients at risk for symptomatic vasospasm after aneurismal subarachnoid hemorrhage. *Crit Care Med* 2000;**28**:984–90.

13 Intra-Operative TCD Monitoring

Zsolt Garami & Alan B. Lumsden
The Methodist Hospital, Houston, TX, USA

Monitoring carotid endarterectomy

Introduction
Carotid endarterectomy (CEA) was introduced by Eastcott *et al.* [1] and its efficacy and durability were established in two large randomized trials for symptomatic patients with carotid stenosis [2,3]. The number-needed-to-treat to prevent one stroke is 8:1 for symptomatic patients with ≥70 carotid stenosis and 15:1 for those with 50–69% stenosis [4]. In asymptomatic patients, the overall risk of stroke is low, i.e. 2% per year, and CEA offers a small protection by reducing it to 1% per year if complication rate from angiography and surgery is ≤2% [5]. Peri-operative complications from CEA in symptomatic patients amounted to 6.5% in the NASCET trial [6] and are even higher in general practice [7].

Non-invasive monitoring of CEA can identify patients developing ischemia during surgery. Cerebral blood flow measurements [8,9], electroencephalography (EEG) [9–14], evoked potentials [15–16], cerebral oximetry [17,18], direct stump pressure measurements [19,20] and ultrasound [21–25] can be used for this purpose. If CEA is performed under local anesthesia, patient status also can be checked with repeat clinical examinations [26]. EEG and cerebral oximetry are very sensitive to the development of cerebral ischemia even before clinical changes become apparent [9–18]; however, these methods can miss ischemia, particularly with general anesthesia [27,28], and are limited in ability to determine the mechanism by which ischemia develops. Ultrasound can provide sensitivity equal to EEG to detect cerebral ischemia [28] and demonstrates in real time the mechanism by which ischemia has developed, i.e. embolism, hypo-perfusion, thrombosis or hyper-perfusion [29]. Although multi-center randomized trials of monitoring techniques targeted to reduce peri-operative stroke or TIA are lacking, several prospective studies showed very low complication rates with monitoring compared with historic controls [29–32], and a single-center randomized trial investigated reduction of microemboli after CEA as a surrogate marker for the risk of peri-operative stroke [33,34].

Cerebrovascular Ultrasound in Stroke Prevention and Treatment, 2nd edition. Edited by Andrei V. Alexandrov. © 2011 Blackwell Publishing Ltd.

A theoretical case (Figure 13.1) presented below demonstrates a variety of previously reported typical TCD findings during CEA [21–25,28–32], their on-line interpretation and responses to prevent possible complications.

Case presentation
A 68-year-old man with past history of hypertension, smoking and leg claudication had a sudden onset of slurred speech and right arm weakness lasting for 10 min with complete resolution. On examination, he has no neurological symptoms. Carotid ultrasound showed an 80% left ICA stenosis and a 30% right ICA stenosis. MRI showed no DWI/FLAIR abnormalities and MRA showed a flow gap in the left ICA bulb.

Diagnostic considerations
Clinical examination and vascular imaging studies are consistent with a severe carotid stenosis in a patient with recent TIA. The motor symptoms and possible speech impairment point to the left hemispheric TIA. This patient appears an appropriate candidate for the left carotid endarterectomy and CEA under general anesthesia is scheduled.

Ultrasound findings pre-clamp
The left MCA flow signals were identified with TCD at the depth of 55 mm and a 2 MHz transducer was fixed for continuous monitoring using Marc series headframe (Spencer Technologies, Seattle, WA, USA). Ultrasound findings are summarized in a graph (Figure 13.1) where solid black lines identify waveforms detected during uncomplicated course of the CEA and red lines indicate flow changes that necessitate correction. Interpretation of TCD findings provided below, differential diagnosis and possible corrective measures were derived from previous publications [21–25, 28–33].

During wound preparation and left carotid exposure, TCD monitoring showed a blunted left MCA flow signal and numerous embolic signals of short duration and variable velocities.

Interpretation, differential diagnosis and management
TCD showed a delayed systolic flow acceleration in the MCA ipsi-lateral to a severe carotid stenosis since this is a

CHAPTER 13 Intra-Operative TCD Monitoring

TCD Monitoring During Carotid Endarterectomy

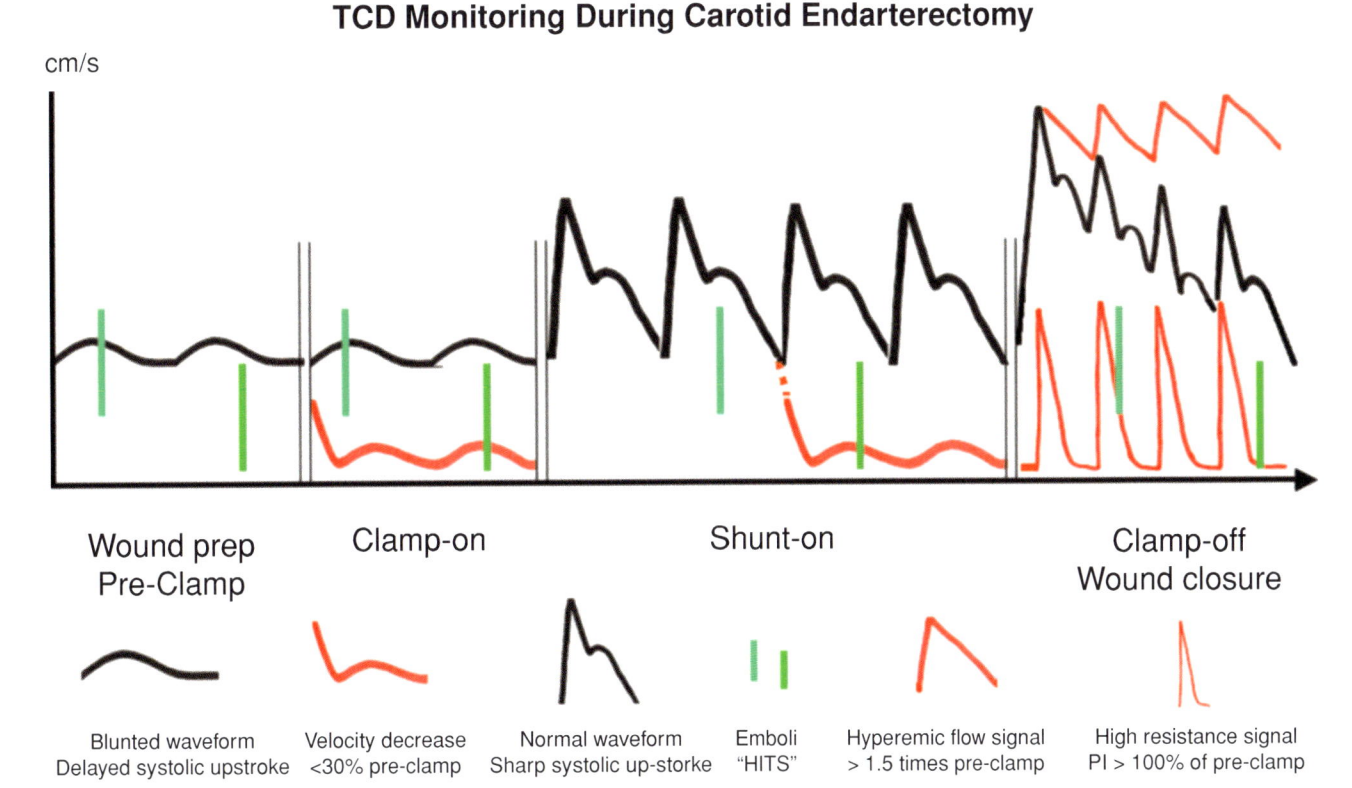

Figure 13.1 Summary of TCD monitoring findings during carotid endarterectomy.

flow-limiting lesion and the MCA is dilated in an attempt to attract collateral flow.

The differential diagnosis includes:

1 Vessel identification, i.e. terminal ICA, PCA versus MCA flow detection if the sample volume is 10 mm or greater and transducer angulation is not slightly upwards and anterior.
2 ICA stenosis progression if a pre-surgical TCD showed normal systolic flow acceleration in the MCA. If a blunted flow signal was present on baseline TCD and a reduction in the MCA flow velocities was noted, this finding could be attributable to the changes in the angle of insonation and cerebral blood flow reduction due to general anesthesia.
3 Waveform/velocity changes due to lowering of BP and decrease in cardiac output/brain metabolic demand with general anesthesia.

TCD also showed numerous embolic signals before surgical dissection of the carotids. The differential diagnosis includes:

1 Spontaneous embolization from the active carotid plaque since patients with symptomatic carotid stenosis TCD can detect on average four embolic signals per hour in the MCA unilateral to a severe symptomatic ICA stenosis [35].
2 Spontaneous embolization from a proximal source, i.e. artificial heart valves, heart chambers or aortic arch atheroma. In this situation, an assessment of the contralateral MCA flow signals may reveal similar or higher rates of embolic signals [36,37] unrelated to the carotid stenosis or surgical maneuvers.
3 Embolic signals that appear in relation to surgical maneuvers. For example, skin preparation, surgical skin dissection and carotid exposure may cause mechanical compression of very soft plaques and dislodge micro-particles from the plaque surface or pre-exposed core [29]. In this case, a nurse and surgeon may consider more gentle skin and wound preparation and modification of carotid exposure techniques. This observation may be particularly useful for surgical residents in training.

Ultrasound findings with carotid clamping

The left MCA flow waveform and velocity did not change after carotid cross-clamping and several embolic signals were detected at and in a few seconds after cross-clamping.

Interpretation, differential diagnosis and management

No change in the flow velocities after cross-clamping can be expected if the MCA unilateral to the severe carotid stenosis is not dependent on the residual flow through the lesion and collateralization of flow occurs through the communicating arteries. However, the differential diagnosis should include erroneous vessel identification, i.e. PCA that will not show significant changes with carotid clamping.

The appearance of several embolic signals can also be expected since clamping may dislodge micro-particles due to mechanical stress to the vessel wall. The worrisome explanation may be that the clamp was not advanced distal enough to compress the vessel beyond the edge of carotid plaque. Nevertheless, these embolic signals represent microscopic particles that probably do not cause any detectable damage unless they are too numerous and are associated with a significant velocity decrease.

TCD can also detect a significant drop in the unilateral MCA velocity (red line). This flow phenomenon can be expected in patients who still have their MCA flow being dependent on the residual flow through the proximal carotid stenosis, particularly if an "isolated MCA" is present. These flow findings can be expected if pre-surgical angiography showed the absence of intracranial collaterals with incomplete circle of Willis ("trapped" MCA). The differential diagnosis includes:

1 Blood pressure drop. Arterial BP reading or assessment of the contralateral MCA waveform can help to identify this reason.
2 Transducer displacement. Therefore, the use of a firm and reliable fixation device is of paramount importance.

Flow velocity decrease on TCD can be transient, therefore requiring no immediate corrective action. Although it usually takes just a few seconds, it may take up to 2 min for the MCA flow velocity to recover after cross-clamping due to recruitment of additional collaterals [38].

The TCD velocity decrease is considered significant if it falls below 30% of the pre-clamp values [29]. To trust the numeric output of a TCD unit, the flow signal should be optimized and the online readings should be taken at the end of the sweep. If flow signals are weak, the sonographer should know how to measure the velocity manually, calculate the mean flow velocity values and quickly estimate the velocity change. Experienced observers can estimate the velocity change by visual inspection of the real-time display and some surgeons would prefer to see the display or to have this information available for them as soon as possible.

A TCD velocity decrease below 30% of the pre-clamp value may be dangerous for the patient if it persists for longer than 2 min. This velocity drop indicates:
1 Lack of collateral recruitment [29, 38].
2 A significant decrease in cerebral blood flow since the angle of insonation remained constant [29,39,40].

This information can be helpful to identify potential candidates for selective shunting.

Although studies showed that placement of shunts during every surgery may result in lower complication rates, data are yet insufficient to determine if selective or routine shunting result in improved outcomes [41]. In this case, the information presented below can help to identify problems with shunt function during CEA.

Ultrasound findings after shunt placement

Shunt insertion resulted in left MCA flow velocity increase and improved systolic flow acceleration. A few embolic signals were also detected.

Interpretation, differential diagnosis and management

TCD showed improvement in the early systolic flow acceleration since the shunt delivers blood flow using unilateral carotid artery and the hemisphere becomes less dependent on the collateral flow.

TCD findings of increased flow velocities are likely associated with a higher flow rate through the MCA since the angle of insonation remained unchanged.

TCD also showed several embolic signals during and after shunt placement. The differential diagnosis includes:
1 Most likely harmless air microbubbles since shunt placement introduces miniscule amounts of air into the arterial tree and these bubbles are so small in size that they can pass through the brain circulation into the venous collectors without causing detectable brain damage (hence further studies of cognitive impairment post-carotid revascularization may point to the opposite).
2 Particulate embolization with plaque fragments or microthrombi that may originate or form at the shunt edges during its preparation and insertion. Shunt placement may also cause a small mechanical stress to the vessel wall or to the plaque edges if present at the site of insertion.
3 Spontaneous embolization from a proximal source that could have been present before surgery.

Since embolic signals were not associated with a significant velocity decrease, their size was likely to be too small to cause any significant obstruction to flow and no immediate action is required. However, persistence of multiple emboli without any proximal source includes the following differential algorithm:
1 Shunt placement still allows air entrance into the circulation. Tightening of vessel wall incision around shunt insertion sites may be considered.
2 Distal shunt edge may be dislodging plaque components is a distal plaque formation is present. The distal ICA inspection may be performed.
3 Distal shunt position may cause turbulence with microcavitation bubble formation. Shunt alignment with the vessel and its position may be revised.
4 Shunt placement re-introduces a greater flow volume into the distal ICA and this flow may be dislodging microparticles, particularly if the distal or intracranial ICA disease is present.

During shunting, TCD can show a sudden velocity drop below pre-clamp values (red line). The differential diagnosis for this finding includes:
1 Transducer displacement. The sonographer should pay attention to changes in patient head position and surgical

manipulations to make sure that these flow findings are not due to an artifact.

2 Blood pressure drop. Use the arterial blood pressure reading to identify this mechanism (if deployed, bilateral TCD monitoring can demonstrate the influence of central hemodynamics).

3 Kink of the shunt. A surgeon may have re-positioned the shunt and this may cause the shunt lumen to embed into the vessel wall. A simple shunt re-orientation over the surgical field may restore the flow.

4 Shunt thrombosis. Despite its rare occurrence, this possibility should be considered since the motionless blood in the shunt cannot be distinguished from the moving blood with a simple visual inspection. If shunt thrombosis is present, its patency should be quickly restored to avoid distal hypoperfusion and/or embolization.

After carotid clamp placement, if the MFV drops below 50% of baseline (delta% <50%) then this suggests that the cerebral hemisphere cannot recruit adequate collaterals (Figure 13.2). The distal arterial tree will become maximally dilated so that the PI may also decrease. This indicates the need for shunting. However, after monitoring CEA with TCD, the experienced TCD sonographer realizes that routine shunt placement in CEA exposes patients to embolization during both shunt insertion and removal. Nevertheless, there is no consensus in the literature regarding selective versus routine shunting. Several normal flow velocity and waveform changes are expected during CEA. Post-stenotic waveforms are seen at baseline at start of the procedure (Figure 13.2A). The dampened waveforms are seen on the spectral display of the ipsilateral MCA and depend on the severity of the carotid stenosis. As stated previously, usually only the MCA and ACA are monitored during the procedure but there are uncommon circumstances where a brief insonation of the ophthalmic artery can be helpful.

Prior to skin incision, baseline values are established. The delta% is set at 100% and the automatic MES detection

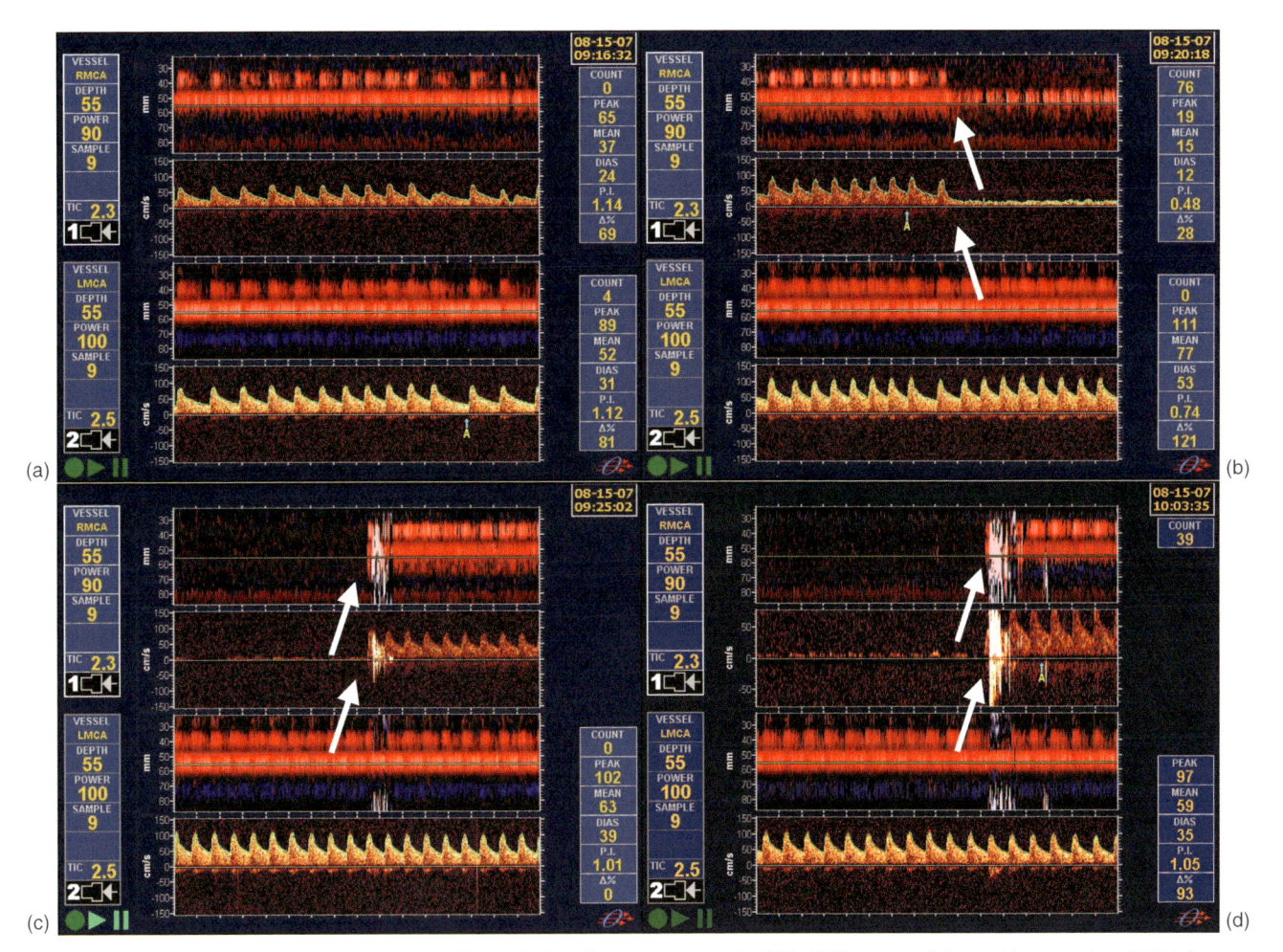

Figure 13.2 Bilateral MCA monitoring during CEA with application of shunt. (A) Manipulation of the carotid bulb during dissection causing cardiac rhythm disturbance and microemboli. (B) Clamp applied to the carotid artery (white arrows) with marked reduction of MCA flow (>50% decrease in MFV). (C) Placement of shunt with restoration of MCA flow and associated embolic shower (white arrows). (D) Removal of shunt and arterial clamp with embolic shower (white arrows).

is activated. Manipulating the carotid bulb during skin preparation and dissection can affect the cardiac rhythm (Figure 13.2A). It is helpful to insonate bilateral MCAs so that cardiac rhythm, waveform changes and microembolic signatures can be compared with the contralateral side. In addition, in some patients, MES may be seen during skin preparation, dissection and handling of the carotid artery.

Once the ICA is clamped, an abrupt change in flow is seen (Figure 13.2B). Additional vasodilation can occur and the existing collaterals are augmented by recruitment of new sources. In patients with an intact circle of Willis, collateral pathways consist of blood flow derived from the contralateral ICA or vertebral arteries: anterior cross-filling via the anterior communicating artery, and posterior cross-filling via the posterior communicating artery. Recruitment of these collateral pathways requires an intact circle of Willis and often leads to only minor decreases in the PI and MFV.

When the circle of Willis is incomplete and there are insufficient collateral pathways to maintain adequate MCA flow, a significant MFV drop is seen and can be accompanied by dramatic decrease in PI (Figure 13.2B). In the example in (Figure 13.2), the MFV decreased from 37 to 15 cm s^{-1}. Application of a shunt is usually accompanied by a small embolic shower and restoration of waveform amplitude (Figure 13.2C). Again, because of the extra time and the risk of embolization, our practice is to place shunts selectively in patients meeting TCD criteria (>50% decrease in MFV) as discussed previously. Once the shunt is in place, improved MCA flow is noted almost immediately (Figure 13.2C).

Repair of the stenotic carotid lesion can be appreciated after the shunt is removed and the artery unclamped (Figure 13.2D). Note that small embolic showers are detected both during shunt placement/removal and in removing the arterial clamp. Repair of the carotid stenosis often results in improved waveforms and PI value normalization. Care should be taken that the TCD display scale has not been altered when comparing baseline (Figure 13.2A) and post-repair waveforms and velocities (Figure 13.2D) in the spectral display.

In cases where sufficient collaterals exist, CEA without shunting can be performed. After the arterial clamp is applied to the carotid artery, a drop in MFV is seen (Figure 13.2B). If MFV remains <50% of baseline, than shunt placement can be safely avoided. In the example in Figure 13.3, a drop in MFV is seen but, as collateral pathways are recruited, the spectral waveform flow velocities improve within 30 s (Figure 13.3C). After the clamp is removed, MFV and waveforms normalize. Note the elevated PI and sharp systolic upstroke in the spectral waveform in this patient with chronic hypertension (Figure 13.3A and D).

Ultrasound findings after shunt and cross-clamp removal

The left MCA flow velocity immediately increased to above pre-clamp and on-shunt values. Over the next minute, the flow velocities gradually decreased by approximately 50% and stabilized at values within a 30% difference with the contralateral side (data not shown).

The waveform showed vertical systolic upstroke, i.e. normal flow acceleration. Several embolic signals were detected within the first 2 min of cross-clamp release.

Interpretation, differential diagnosis and management

TCD showed a transient hyperemic response after normal flow was re-established in the carotid artery. Usually there is a short phase of decreased flow velocities associated with shunt removal and a transient velocity increase can be expected after clamp removal.

If the velocity increase is ≥1.5 times the pre-clamp values, it may indicate hyper-perfusion [29]. If this velocity increase persists for longer than 2 min without a trend towards velocity decrease, the differential diagnosis includes:
1 A benign finding, if overall mean flow velocity does not exceed 80 cm s^{-1} or 130% of the contralateral side.
2 The velocity increase with blood pressure increase due to passive autoregulation.
3 Potential development of the hyper-perfusion syndrome, if the velocity increase ×1.5 persists for longer than 2 min.

Potential measures that can be used to prevent hyper-perfusion early after cross-clamp release include:
1 Hyperventilation or increased oxygenation.
2 Pharmacological blood pressure decrease.
3 Partial ICA cross-clamp and slow release.
The last measure can be used to limit the incoming flow temporarily, slowly increase its amount over time, and thus to "remind" the brain to autoregulate the incoming flow.

TCD often detects emboli early after cross-clamp release. The presence of embolic signals may be attributable to the following sources:
1 Air microbubbles, trapped or introduced by manipulations with shunt and cross-clamp removal.
2 Spontaneous emboli from a proximal source.
3 Particulate emboli, originating at the incompletely removed plaque edges or thrombus in the ICA.

It can be expected that several emboli (usually microbubbles) can be detected upon cross-clamp release. After spontaneous embolization from a cardiac or aortic source has been excluded, the persistence of frequent emboli is worrisome. If the continuing presence of emboli is associated with re-establishment of a blunted MCA waveform or a significant velocity decrease, surgical revision is warranted. If these TCD findings were obtained after wound closure, i.e. in

CHAPTER 13 Intra-Operative TCD Monitoring

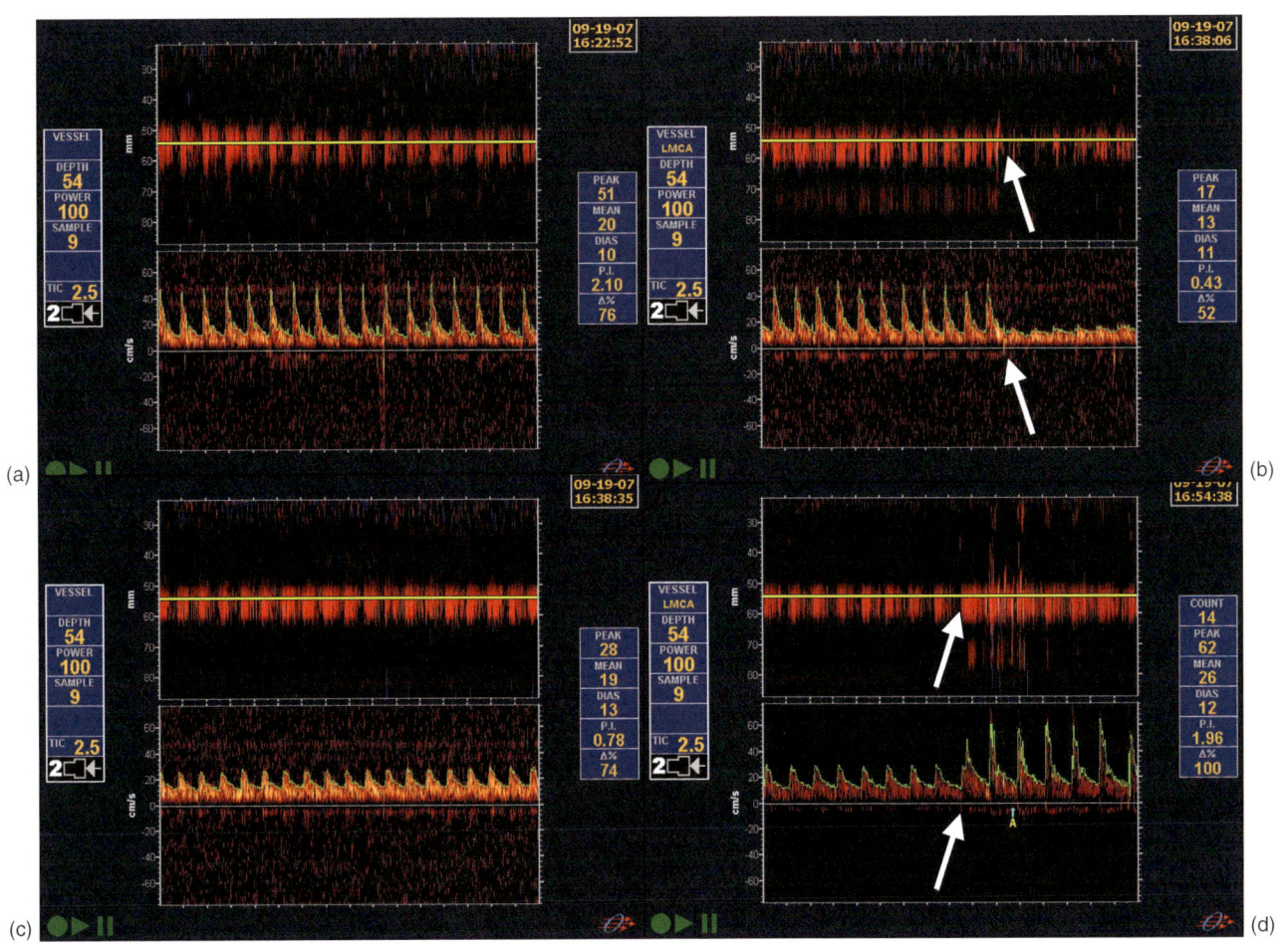

Figure 13.3 Unilateral MCA monitoring of CEA showing adequate MCA flow after arterial clamping. (A) Baseline MCA insonation prior to start of the procedure showing an elevated pulsatility index in this patient with chronic hypertension. (B) Application of carotid artery clamp (white arrow) with drop in MFV from 20 to 13. (C) Restoration of flow velocities within 30 s demonstrating the adequacy of collaterals. No shunt was used. (D) Release of arterial clamp without emboli shower (white arrow).

the recovery room, a duplex ultrasound examination of the extracranial carotids can be performed to detect the presence of a fresh thrombus in the ICA.

Shortly after cross-clamp release, TCD can show a spiky high-resistance signal in the MCA (Figure 13.1, red line) [31]. This is an abnormal waveform that indicates high resistance to flow at the site or just distal to insonation depth. The abrupt appearance of this flow signal is rare and indicates thrombo-embolism in the MCA. In this situation, an urgent angiography may be performed to visualize the site and extent of occlusion and this patient may be a candidate for an experimental intra-arterial intervention, i.e. thrombolysis, mechanical clot disruption or removal.

Chronic carotid stenosis with long-standing cerebral hypoperfusion causes arterial autoregulatory dysfunction. The distal cerebral arterial tree becomes chronically dilated and is unable to regulate flow by constriction after correction of the stenosis. The increased blood flow exceeds the metabolic demands of the tissue and causes tissue hyperemia. Persistent severe headache, seizures and intracranial hemorrhage (ICH) are uncommon but serious complications of hyperperfusion. The incidence of ICH with hyperperfusion is estimated at 2% [23]. Contralateral carotid disease, high-grade ipsilateral stenosis and poor collateral pathways are associated with an increased risk of hyperemia. Use of an intraoperative shunt during CEA can be associated with TCD defined hyperperfusion syndrome [29].

Cerebral hyperperfusion by TCD criteria is defined as a >150% increase in MFV from the pre-clamp MFV during CAS or CEA [29] (Figure 13.4). Several investigators and our own experience suggest that strict interpretation of the TCD hyperperfusion criteria will overestimate its incidence. Immediate MCA MFV measurements after ballooning or clamp release often show a transient hyperperfusion that normalizes before the end of the procedure. This probably reflects previous perturbation of the autoregulatory

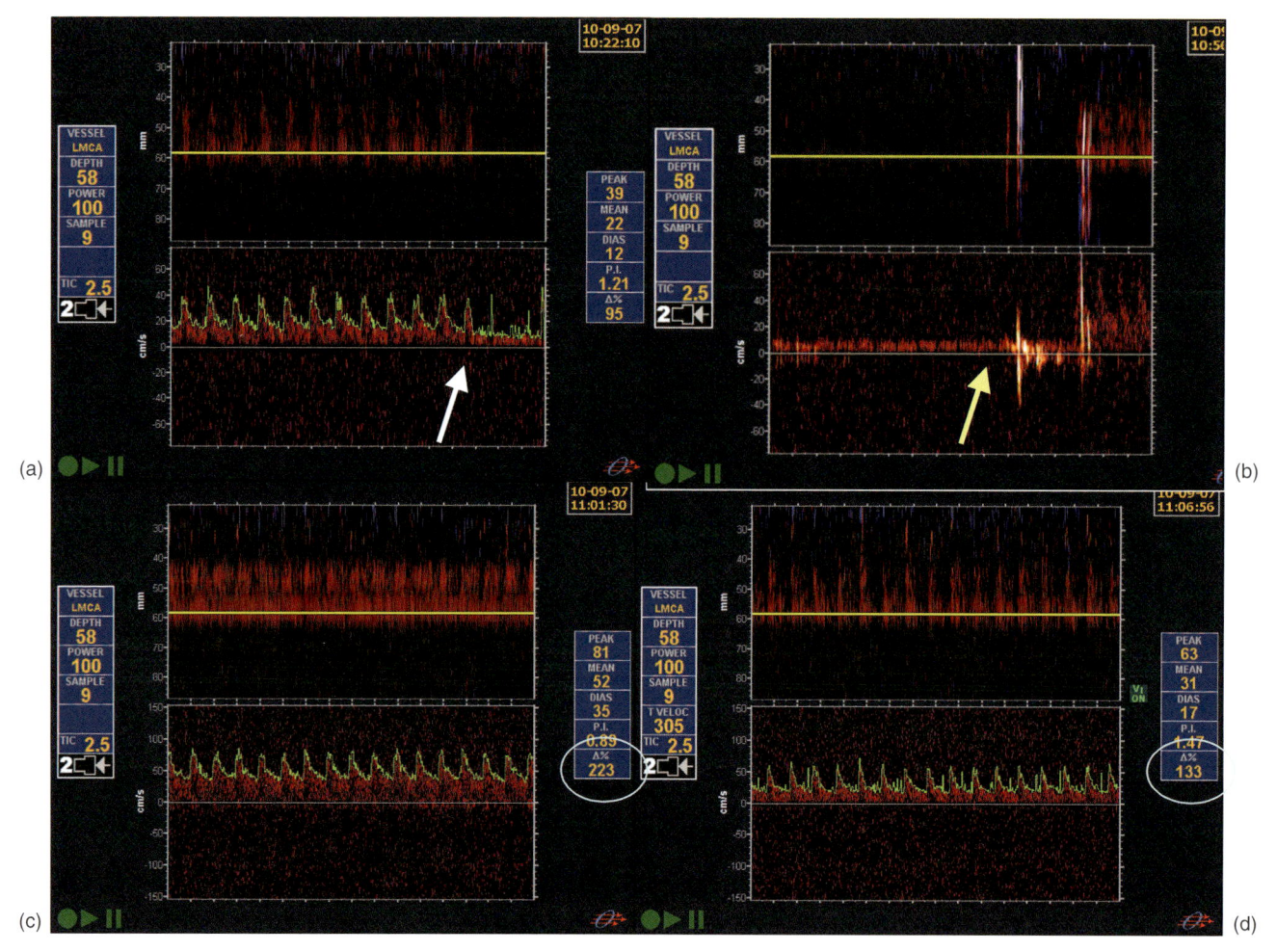

PART IV Ultrasound in Stroke Prevention and Treatment

Figure 13.4 Left MCA TCD showing hyperperfusion after carotid artery unclamping during CEA. (A) Clamp applied to carotid artery (thin white arrow). (B) Clamp release (thin yellow arrow). (C) Hyperperfusion phenomenon: >150% increase in MFV (curved white arrow) from pre-clamp value (22 → 52 = 236% increase). The MFV increase persisted past 2 min and corrective measures were taken. (D) After hyperventilation for several minutes, the MFV is reduced.

system that corrects over several minutes. Our technique is to make sure that arterial hypertension is avoided after cross-clamp release and wait 2 minutes after correction of stenosis to allow for restoration of the autoregulatory system. After 2 minutes, if signs of hyperemia still persist, we make the diagnosis of hyperperfusion and initiate appropriate treatment, i.e., further blood pressure management, hyperventilation and possibly re-clamping the ICA followed by a slow clamp release.

Follow-up

This patient (Figure 13.1) underwent successful and uneventful left carotid endarterectomy. Repeat carotid duplex 2 weeks after surgery showed no residual stenosis in the left ICA and a mild (approximately 30%) right ICA stenosis. Repeat duplex examinations were scheduled at 1 and 6 months after surgery. The patient receives aspirin 350 mg [42] and clopidogrel 75 mg daily [43] and remains asymptomatic during follow-up. However, the safety of combining aspirin and clopidogrel long-term has come into question with results of the clinical trials [44,45]. Given his history of symptomatic peripheral arterial disease, this patient will continue on plavix monotherapy after 1 month of dual antiplatelets. Flow findings/criteria presented in the schematic Figure 13.1 could also be applied to monitoring of the carotid stenting procedures with a few nuances described in the section below.

Carotid artery stenting (CAS)

Since carotid artery stenting (CAS) was approved for clinical use, it has become an alternative to carotid endarterectomy (CEA) in selected patients. Strokes related to CAS also are usually due to perioperative hypoperfusion, hyperperfusion or, most commonly, thromboembolism. Published stroke rates range between 2 and 10% [46]. In addition to symptomatic thromboembolic events, silent subclinical brain embolism occurs at an even higher rate. Monitoring for such events is critical to prevent, diagnose and treat procedure-related embolism.

With the increasing incidence of carotid stenting procedures, there is less histopathologic information usually attained during endarterectomy available to link clinical events to brain embolism. Carotid stents are sometimes deployed without any neurophysiological or real-time neurovascular monitoring, which severely limits the clinician's ability to intervene when complications arise. TCD is the only examination able to monitor intracranial blood flow in real time, thus detecting both asymptomatic and symptomatic cerebrovascular events as they actually happen.

TCD shows the blood flow direction and velocity in the intracranial vessels, adding physiologic information to the anatomical images obtained with other imaging modalities. TCD can also detect potential collateral flow signals in the ophthalmic, anterior communicating and posterior communicating arteries caused by hemodynamically significant carotid stenosis. Understanding the collateral flow patterns can affect the intervention, e.g. CEA versus CAS, whether or not to place a shunt during CEA and deciding which embolic protection method to use during CAS based on the patient's intracranial flow patterns. Unlike CEA, sudden flow velocity and waveform changes are not generally seen in CAS except a severe lesion crossing with the wire and briefly during balloon angioplasty/stent deployment. Since no arterial clamping is needed, flow is expected to remain antegrade in the cerebral circulation. Contralateral ICA occlusion may be one of the indications to perform CAS over CEA. Acute hypoperfusion is less of a concern since there is no arterial clamping; however, CAS is generally associated with a higher rate of microembolic signals and even brief periods of delayed washout may be of concern. Hyperperfusion and, especially, thromboembolism are the major complications associated with CAS.

Wires and catheters can dislodge atherosclerotic debris and thrombus in a diseased aortic arch and cause embolization to both cerebral hemispheres. In recent studies, performing an aortic arch angiogram was one of the worst embolic offenders. The incidence of TCD-detected MCA microemboli increased with the frequency of wire and catheter manipulation within the aortic arch. In addition to atherosclerotic emboli, contrast injections in the aortic arch and the carotid artery allow air bubbles to embolize to the brain and are detected as MES by TCD. It is unclear how these air microbubbles affect the intracranial circulation and if they contribute to cerebral ischemia or cognitive dysfunction.

There are currently several techniques to reduce embolization during CAS. The most prominent contenders are the distal filter deployment and reversal of carotid artery flow. Both techniques show MES when a wire is passed in the aortic arch, the carotid artery and in crossing the lesion. Injection of contrast into the carotid system appears on TCD as a bright reflection associated with MES. Even when using a distal filter wire, stent deployment is still associated with distal embolic showers.

The interest in using covered stents to contain atheromatous debris waned due to higher in-stent re-stenosis rates compared with bare metal stents. Nevertheless, fewer MES were detected by TCD with the use of covered stents. Flow reversal techniques are being developed to reduce stent deployment embolization further. Early reports show significant reductions in MES during stent deployment with flow reversal techniques [47]. Depending on the exact flow reversal technique, flow reversal is commonly seen in the ACA and terminal ICA on peri-procedural TCD monitoring.

There is also increasing evidence that embolic phenomena persist after CAS even without intravascular manipulation. Rapp *et al* performed diffusion-weighted magnetic resonance imaging at 1 and 48 h after CAS [48]. The majority of new lesions were detected 48 h after CAS, indicating that thromboembolism continues after the procedure when protection devices have been removed. Post-procedure TCD can detect these post-procedure emboli in real time, whereas MRI remains the tool to show only the end result of the damage.

Problematic TCD findings during carotid interventions, depending on the interpretation, dictate what remedial action is needed to correct the situation. For example, hypoperfusion indicates the need for shunting during CEA (Figure 13.2). Conversely, hyperperfusion indicates hyperemia after clamp removal and would prompt corrective hyperventilation and blood pressure management (Figure 13.5). In other examples, dampened waveforms and low velocities may indicate the presence of thrombus, prompting further investigation, possibly urgent thrombectomy. Distal embolic showers without artery manipulation may indicate the presence of proximal thrombus or dissection.

MCA insonation during CAS is valuable in the detection of proximal ICA dissection occurring during angioplasty, clamping or endarterectomy. Typically these lesions produce multiple MES in the ipsilateral MCA even without arterial manipulation. If suspected, ICA dissection can be visualized with B-mode ultrasound. Two lumens can be seen with an intimal flap present. The true and false lumens will have different waveform morphologies, velocity and pulsatility indices. However, TCD suggestion of ICA dissection should be confirmed by alternative means, e.g. angiography or surgical re-exploration [49,50].

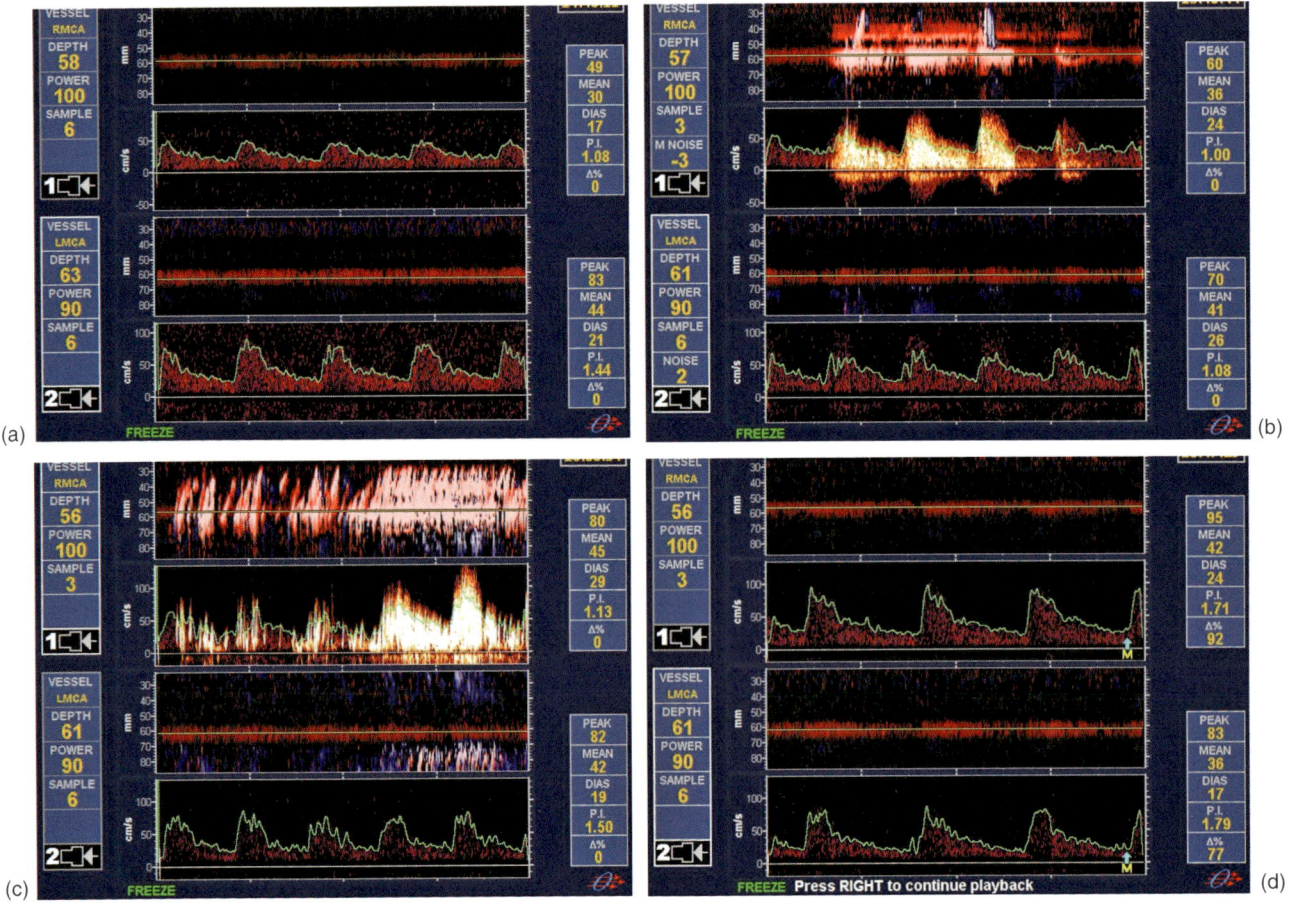

PART IV Ultrasound in Stroke Prevention and Treatment

Figure 13.5 Bilateral MCA monitoring during right CAS. (A) Baseline insonation before the start of the procedure. The right MCA is shown at the top and the left MCA is at the bottom of each TCD screen. (B) Injection of contrast into right common carotid artery (only channel showing bright contrast signals). (C) Embolic shower during carotid stent deployment. The MCA spectral waveform shows minimal disturbance (green outline). (D) Post-stent result. There is improvement in the right MCA spectral waveform and MFV.

Cardiac surgery monitoring

Retrograde cerebral perfusion

Three primary mechanisms cause injury to brain tissues after cardiac and aortic operations: "mechanical" injury from cerebral embolism, blood flow alterations leading to reperfusion injury and environmental, pharmacological and patient-related factors influencing postoperative state [51].

In addition to other methods that extend safe circulatory arrest, i.e. cerebroplegia, antegrade perfusion via the innominate artery and hypothermia, retrograde cerebral perfusion (RCP) via superior vena cava cannulation was initially suggested to reverse massive air embolism [52] and later developed to maintain cerebral blood flow during surgical repairs involving the aortic arch [53]. A transvenous brain retro-perfusion procedure has also been applied in acute ischemic stroke in an attempt to reverse ischemic damage [54].

At surgery, RCP is performed during profound hypothermic circulatory arrest that by itself offers neuroprotection [55]. When added to profound hypothermic circulatory arrest, RCP significantly reduced neurological dysfunction, providing superior brain protection [56–58].

To deliver blood to the brain in a retrograde fashion, the superior vena cava is cannulated and connected to a cardiopulmonary bypass machine. In a few seconds on bypass, a trickle blood flow appears from the brachio-cephalic arteries descending to the aorta. It has been a matter of controversy whether this blood reaches the brain tissue or is being shunted from venous collectors to large intracranial arteries. Without ultrasound monitoring, it is not clear how the bypass pressure and flow volume settings should be adjusted to achieve blood flow delivery to the brain since electroencephalography shows no cerebral electrical activity due to hypothermia. It has also been a matter of controversy whether the capillary bed is perfused during RCP [59,60].

CHAPTER 13 Intra-Operative TCD Monitoring

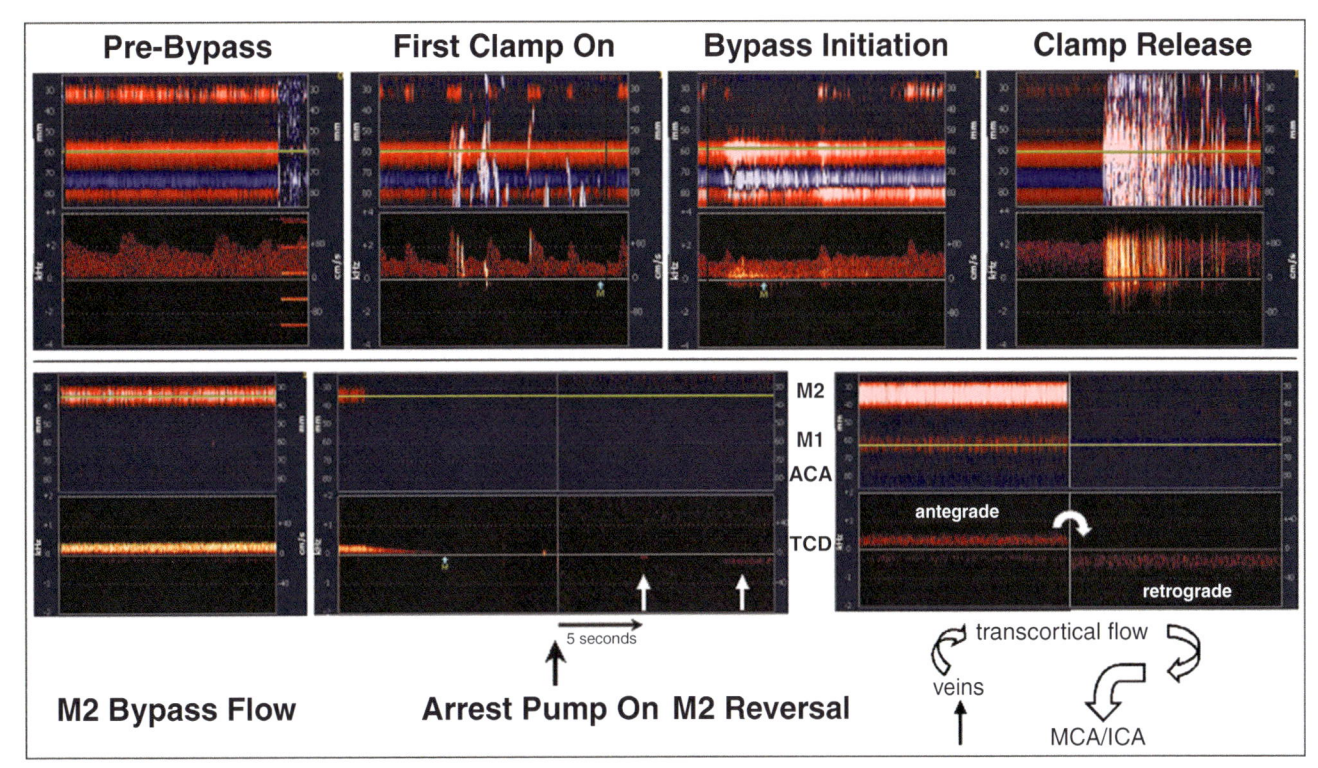

Figure 13.6 The Pre-Bypass flow has a low-resistance signature on the M-mode TCD that also shows antegrade M2, M1 MCA flows as well as the A1 ACA flow. The artifact at the end of the sweep is caused by electrical cautery. The First Clamp On image displays multiple embolic signals in both MCA and ACAs. Note that M-mode provides tracks of emboli in time and space. Emboli can be mapped to the arterial branches that they pass by depth and direction and also time delays along the horizontal axis. The M-mode display yields more emboli than a single-gate spectral TCD. The Bypass Initiation image shows changes in systolic acceleration towards non-pulsatile perfusion and also changes in flow signal intensity due to introduction of a new pool of blood with different impedance. The Clamp Release image shows a shower of emboli (mostly air microbubbles) passing towards the brain. The M2 Bypass Flow is a non-pulsatile antegrade flow at 30–40 mm depths with transtemporal insonation. During induction of a complete arrest of cerebral circulation, M2 flow signals disappear on the M-mode display first since at any given depth M-mode is less sensitive than a single-gate spectral TCD display. The flow signals on spectral TCD disappear last, indicating complete arrest of cerebral circulation with the bypass pump being turned off. After the pump has been turned on (arrow), flow signals appear in the M2 MCA approximately 5 s later. The flow direction is reversed, implying that this flow has reached the MCA by retrograde filling of its branches from the venous circulation. The 5 s delay may be caused by the time necessary to fill up the veins since these vessels have the greatest intracranial compartmental capacity to accommodate flow volume. The reversed flow signals are much weaker in intensity and have lower velocities since these parameters are indirectly proportional to the flow volume, which is reduced during retro-perfusion. Finally, a low-intensity retrograde flow establishes through the M1 MCA (bottom right image) and the diagram illustrates the passage of blood from venous collectors to the proximal intracranial arteries of the circle of Willis.

Although TCD cannot directly access parenchymal perfusion of the brain, it can detect typical flow reversal in the proximal MCA in animal models of RCP [61]. In humans, the TCD beam can be steadily focused on the M2 or M1 MCA and the direction of flow in these segments can change with effective retro-perfusion [62–65]. However, failure to reverse flow on TCD occurred in up to 40% of patients undergoing RCP in previous studies. Perhaps this lack of flow reversal on TCD should be used to change or optimize perfusion settings to achieve flow reversal in basal cerebral arteries.

We routinely monitor aortic surgeries with TCD and detect flow reversal in the M2–M1 MCA segments during RCP. We were able to achieve 100% detection of flow reversal in MCAs in the presence of temporal windows and in other arteries if these windows were absent [66]. If no reversal was achieved with initial low volume RCP, the volume was raised up to 600 cm^3 until flow reversal was detected by TCD. The following case illustrates intraoperative flow findings.

Ultrasound findings

TCD showed a low-resistance flow towards the transducer in the MCA before bypass initiation (Figure 13.6, upper left image). The first aortic cross-clamp produced a cluster of embolic signals (Figure 13.6). Note that more signals are seen on M-mode display than on a single-channel TCD since M-mode simultaneously displays several vessels and shows

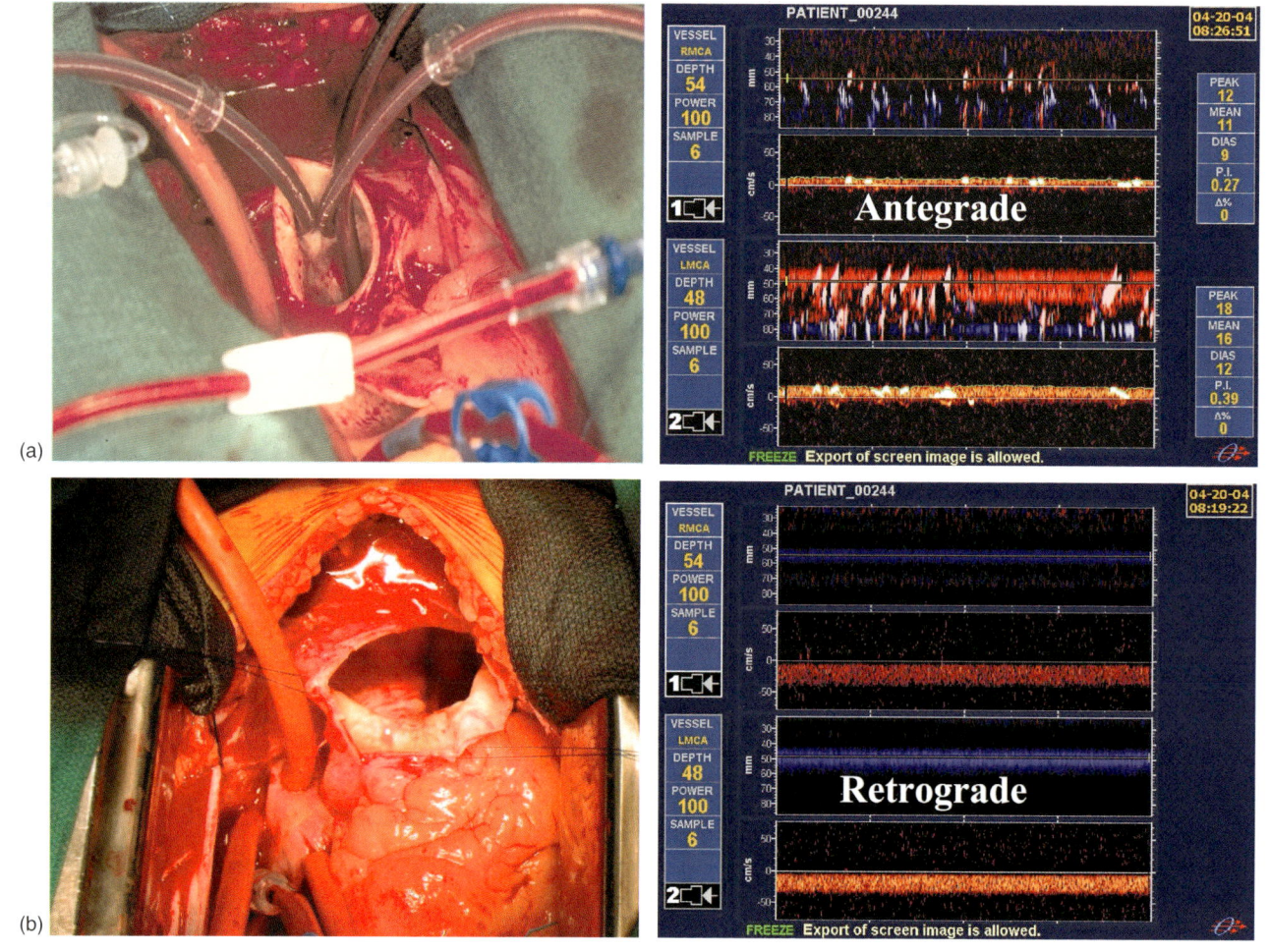

PART IV Ultrasound in Stroke Prevention and Treatment

Figure 13.7 Cannulation with antegrade cerebral perfusion (A) and retrograde cerebral perfusion via venous cannulas (B).

the emboli course in both time and space. The MCA flow signal intensity increases during bypass initiation (Figure 13.6) since a new pool of blood with different impedance is being introduced into circulation. The aortic clamp release produced a shower of embolic signals that likely represent air microbubbles (Figure 13.6, upper right image).

The bottom row of images (Figure 13.6) shows M2 MCA flow on normal bypass, during hypothermia and cessation of antegrade perfusion (arrest) followed by initiation of brain retro-perfusion and subsequent reversal in flow direction. Note that reversed flow appears 5–10 s after the retroperfusion pump was turned on and this flow has decreased signal intensity compared with antegrade pre-arrest flow.

TCD detection of multiple embolic signals during bypass surgery has been studied extensively [67–70]. The cannula and bypass blood may contain numerous air microbubbles detectable by TCD. Their appearance correlates with surgical manipulations and quality of filtering systems. The size of these bubbles was shown to be small enough to pass through brain vasculature without causing harm. However, a cumulative number of these embolic signatures may be related to neuro-psychological deficits after bypass surgery. Also, brain embolization with lipid aggregates may be responsible for small capillary-arteriolar dilations (SCADs), and these microcirculatory lesions may be the patho-morphological substrate of neurological dysfunction after bypass surgery [68,69]. Since TCD cannot yet differentiate gaseous from solid, particularly lipid emboli, the value of just emboli counting remains uncertain.

Antegrade cerebral perfusion (ACP) is a cardiopulmonary bypass technique that was used first with special cannulation procedures to perfuse the brain during neonatal and infant aortic arch reconstruction. It is used in lieu of deep hypothermic circulatory arrest (DHCA) and therefore has the theoretical advantage of protecting the brain from hypoxic ischemic injury [64]. During antegrade cannulation of innominate artery or operative field becomes occupied by cannulas and by alternative axcilliary artery cannulation could free up the operating field.

During ACP, the brain is not protected from direct arterial embolization (Figure 13.7), and during RCP that could provide essential benefit during extended prolonged circulatory arrest surgeries [71,72].

Prior to undertaking intraoperative TCD monitoring, sufficient clinical and practical experience must be obtained. A suboptimal interrogation window through the skull is also a limiting factor for TCD monitoring.

Thromboembolism, hypoperfusion and hyperperfusion are the primary causes of stroke in the operating room. TCD monitoring of the MCA is a valuable tool that quickly alerts clinicians to these complications. Because TCD monitors in real time, the clinician can make procedural changes sooner than with other monitoring modalities. However, for intraoperative TCD to be effective, it requires a team that is able to interpret and act on the TCD findings.

References

1 Eastcott HHG, Pickering GW, Rob CG. Reconstruction of internal carotid artery in a patient with intermittent attacks of hemiplegia. *Lancet* 1954;**ii**:954.
2 North American Symptomatic Carotid Endarterectomy Trial Collaborators. Beneficial effect of carotid endarterectomy in symptomatic patients with high-grade carotid stenosis. *N Engl J Med* 1991;**325**:445–53.
3 European Carotid Surgery Trialists' Collaborative Group. Randomised trial of endarterectomy for recently symptomatic carotid stenosis: final results of the MRC European Carotid Surgery Trial (ECST). *Lancet* 1998;**351**:1379–87.
4 Barnett HJ, Taylor DW, Eliasziw M, et al. Benefit of carotid endarterectomy in patients with symptomatic moderate or severe stenosis. North American Symptomatic Carotid Endarterectomy Trial Collaborators. *N Engl J Med* 1998;**339**:1415–25.
5 Executive Committee of the Asymptomatic Carotid Atherosclerosis Study. Endarterctomy for asymptomatic carotid artery stenosis. *JAMA* 1995;**273**:1421–8.
6 Ferguson GG, Eliasziw M, Barr HW, et al. The North American Symptomatic Carotid Endarterectomy Trial: surgical results in 1415 patients. *Stroke* 1999;**30**:1751–8.
7 Chaturvedi S, Aggarwal R, Murugappan A. Results of carotid endarterectomy with prospective neurologist follow-up. *Neurology* 2000;**26**:55:769–72.
8 Sundt TM. The ischemic tolerance of neural tissue and the need for monitoring and selective shunting during carotid endarterectomy. *Stroke* 1983;**14**:93–8.
9 Sharbrough FM, Messik JM, Sundt TM. Correlation of continuous electroencephalograms with cerebral blood flow measurements during carotid endarterectomy. *Stroke* 1973;**4**:674–83.
10 Blackshear WM, Di Carlo V, Seifert KB, et al. Advantages of continuous electroencephalographic monitoring during carotid surgery. *J Cardiovasc Surg* 1986;**27**:146–53.
11 Cho I, Smullens SN, Streletz LJ, et al. The value of intraoperative EEG monitoring during carotid endarterectomy. *Ann Neurol* 1986;**20**:508–12.
12 Blume WT, Ferguson GG, McNeil DK. Significance of EEG changes at carotid endarterectomy. *Stroke* 1986;**17**:891–7.
13 McCarthy WJ, Park AE, Koushanpour E, et al. Carotid endarterectomy. Lessons from intraoprative monitoring – a decade of experience. *Ann Surg* 1996;**224**:291–307.
14 Balotta E, Daigau G, Saladini M, et al. Results of electroencephalographic monitoring during 369 consecutive carotid artery revascularizations. *Eur Neurol* 1997;**37**:43–7.
15 Kearse LA, Brown EN, McPeck K. Somatosensory evoked potential sensitivity relative to electroencephalography for cerebral ischemia during carotid endarterectomy. *Stroke* 1992;**23**:498–505.
16 Haupt WF, Horsch S. Evoked potential monitoring in carotid surgery: a review of 994 cases. *Neurology* 1992;**42**:835–8.
17 Duncan LA, Ruckley CV, Wildsmith JAW. Cerebral oximetry: a useful monitor during carotid artery surgery. *Anesthesiology* 1995;**50**:1041–5.
18 Samra SK, Dorje P, Zelenock GB, et al. Cerebral oximetry in patients undergoing carotid endarterectomy under regional anesthesia. *Stroke* 1996;**27**:49–55.
19 Cherry KJ, Roland CF, Hallett JW, et al. Stump pressure, the contralateral carotid artery and electroencephalographic changes. *Am J Surg* 1991;**162**:185–9.
20 Harada RN, Comerota AJ, Good GM, et al. Stump pressure, electroencephalographic changes and the contralateral carotid artery: another look at selective shunting. *Am J Surg* 1995;**170**:148–53.
21 Padayachee TS, Bishop CCR, Gosling RG, et al. Monitoring middle cerebral artery blood flow velocity during carotid endarterectomy. *Br J Surg* 1986;**73**:98–100.
22 Steiger HJ, Schaffler L, Boll J, et al. Results of microsurgical carotid endarterectomy: a prospective study with transcranial Doppler and EEG monitoring and selective shunting. *Acta Neurochir (Wien)* 1989;**100**:31–8.
23 Spencer MP, Thomas GI, Nicholls SC, et al. Detection of middle cerebral artery emboli during carotid endarterectomy using transcranial Doppler ultrasonography. *Stroke* 1990;**21**:415–23.
24 Ackerstaff RGA, Janes C, Moll FL, et al. The significance of emboli detection by means of transcranial Doppler ultrasonography monitoring in carotid endarterectomy. *J Vasc Surg* 1995;**21**:415–23.
25 Canthelmo NL, Babikian VL, Samaraweera RN, et al. Cerebral microembolism and ischemic changes associated with carotid endarterectomy. *J Vasc Surg* 1998;**27**:1024–31.
26 Benjamin ME, Silva MB, Watt C, et al. Awake patient monitoring to determine the need for shunting during carotid endarterectomy. *Surgery* 1993;**114**:673–81.
27 Haupt WF, Erasmi-Korber H, et al. Intraoperative recording of parietal SEP can miss hemodynamic infarction during carotid endarterectomy: a case study. *Electroencephalogr Clin Neurophysiol* 1994;**92**:86–8.
28 Arnold M, Sturzenegger M, Schaffler L, et al. Continuous intraoperative monitoring of middle cerebral artery flow velocities and electroencephalography during carotid endarterectomy. *Stroke* 1997;**28**:1345–50.
29 Spencer MP. Transcranial Doppler monitoring and causes of stroke from carotid endarterectomy. *Stroke* 1997;**28**:685–91.

30 Jansen C, Ramos LM, van Heesewijk JP, et al. Impact of microembolism and hemodynamic changes in the brain during carotid endarterectomy. *Stroke* 1994;**25**:992–7.

31 Ackerstaff RG, Moons KG, van de Vlasakker CJ, et al. Association of intraoperative transcranial Doppler monitoring variables with stroke from carotid endarterectomy. *Stroke* 2000;**31**:1817–23.

32 Babikian VL, Canthelmo NL. Cerebrovascular monitoring during carotid endarterectomy. *Stroke* 2000;**31**:1799–801.

33 Levy CR, O'Malley HM, Fell G, et al. Transcranial Doppler detected cerebral mircoembolism following carotid endarterectomy. High intensity signal loads predict postoperative cerebral ischemia. *Brain* 1997;**120**:621–9.

34 Kaposzta Z, Baskerville PA, Madge D, et al. L-Arginine and S-nitrosoglutathione reduce embolization in humans. *Circulation* 2001;**103**:2371–5.

35 Siebler M, Kleinschmidt A, Sitzer M, et al. Cerebral microembolism in symptomatic and asymptomatic high-grade internal carotid artery stenosis. *Neurology* 1994;**44**:615–8.

36 Georgiadis D, Grosset DG, Kelman A, et al. Prevalence and characteristics of intracranial mircoembolic signals in patients with different types of prosthetic cardiac valves. *Stroke* 1994;**25**;587–92.

37 Sliwka U, Ulrich J, Wissuma D, et al. Occurrence of transcranial Doppler high-intensity transient signals in patients with potential cardiac sources of embolism: a prospective study. *Stroke* 1995;**26**:2067–70.

38 Babikian VL, Canthelmo NL, Wijman CAC. Neurovascular monitoring during carotid endarterectomy. In: Babikian VL, Wechsler LR, eds. *Transcranial Doppler Ultrasonography*, 2nd edn. Boston: Butterworth-Heinemann, 1999: 233.

39 Kontos HA. Validity of cerebral arterial blood flow calculations from velocity measurements. *Stroke* 1989;**20**:1–3.

40 Aaslid R, Lindegaard KF, Sorteberg W, et al. Cerebral autoregulation dynamics in humans. *Stroke* 1989;**20**:45.

41 Counsell C, Salinas R, Naylor R, et al. Routine or selective carotid artery shunting for carotid endarterectomy (and different methods of monitoring in selective shunting). *Cochrane Database Syst Rev* 2000;(2):CD000190.

42 Taylor DW, Barnett HJ, Haynes RB, et al. Low-dose and high-dose acetylsalicylic acid for patients undergoing carotid endarterectomy: a randomized controlled trial. ASA and Carotid Endarcetectomy (ACE) Trial Collaborators. *Lancet* 1999;**353**:2179–84.

43 CAPRIE Steering Committee. A randomized, blinded trial of clopidogrel versus aspirin in patients at risk of ischaemic events. *Lancet* 1996;**348**:1329–32.

44 Yusuf S, Zhao F, Mehta SR, et al.; Clopidogrel in Unstable Angina to Prevent Recurrent Events Trial Investigators. Effects of clopidogrel in addition to aspirin in patients with acute coronary syndromes without ST-segment elevation. *N Engl J Med* 2001;**345**:494–502.

45 Albers GW, Amarenco P. Combination therapy with clopidogrel and aspirin: can the CURE results be extrapolated to cerebrovascular patients? *Stroke* 2001;**32**:2948.

46 Chen CI, Iguchi Y, Garami Z, et al. Analysis of emboli during carotid stenting with distal protection device. *Cerebrovasc Dis* 2006;**21**(4):223–8.

47 Garami Z, Charlton-Ouw KM, Broadbent KC, et al. A practical guide to transcranial Doppler monitoring during carotid interventions, Part 1: basics and blood flow changes. *Vasc Ultrasound Today* 2008;**13**(1), 1–24.

48 Rapp JH, Wakil L, Sawhney R, et al. Subclinical embolization after carotid artery stenting: new lesions on diffusion-weighted magnetic resonance imaging occur postprocedure. *J Vasc Surg*. 2007;**45**(5):867–72; discussion 872–4.

49 Garami Z, Charlton-Ouw KM, Broadbent KC, et al. A practical guide to transcranial Doppler monitoring during carotid interventions, Part 2: protocol and interpretation. *Vasc Ultrasound Today* 2008;**13**(2), 25–52.

50 Garami ZF, Bismuth J, Charlton-Ouw KM, et al. Simultaneous pre- and post-filter transcranial Doppler monitoring during carotid artery stenting. *J Vasc Surg* 2009;**49**(2):340–4.

51 Swain JA. Cardiac surgery and the brain. *N Engl J Med* 1993;**329**:1119–20.

52 Mills NL, Ochsner JL. Massive air embolism during cardiopulmonary bypass. Causes, prevention and management. *J Thorac Cardiovasc Surg* 1980;**80**:708–17.

53 Ueda Y, Miki S, Kusuhara K, et al. Deep hypothermic systemic circulatory arrest and contiuous retrograde cerebral perfusion for surgery of aortic arch aneurysm. *Eur J Cardiothorac Surg* 1992;**6**:36–41.

54 Frazee JG, Luo X, Luan G, et al. Retrograde transvenous neuroperfusion: a back door treatment for stroke. *Stroke* 1998;**29**:1912–6.

55 Gillinov AM, Redmond JM, Zehr KJ, et al. Superior cerebral protection with profound hypothermia during circulatory arrest. *Ann Thorac Surg* 1993;**55**:1432–9.

56 Safi HJ, Iliopoulos DC, Gopinath SP, et al. Retrograde cerebral perfusion during profound hypothermia and circulatory arrest in pigs. *Ann Thorac Surg* 1995;**59**:1107–12.

57 Safi HJ, Brien HW, Winter JN, et al. Brain protection via cerebral retrograde perfusion during aortic arch aneurysm repair. *Ann Thorac Surg* 1993;**56**:270–6.

58 Safi HJ, Letsou GV, Iliopoulos DC, et al. Impact of retrograde cerebral perfusion on ascending aortic and arch aneurysm repair. *Ann Thorac Surg* 1997;**63**:1601–7.

59 Ehrlich MP, Hagl C, McCullough JN, et al. Retrograde cerebral perfusion provides negligible flow through brain capillaries in the pig. *J Thorac Cardiovasc Surg* 2001;**122**:331–8.

60 Pagano D, Boivin CM, Faroqui MH, et al. Surgery of thoracic aorta with hypothermic circulatory arrest: experience with retrograde perfusion via superior vena cava and demonstration of perfusion. *Eur J Cardiothorac Surg* 1996;**10**:833–8.

61 Razumovsky AY, Tseng EE, Hanley DF, et al. Cerebral hemodynamic changes during retrograde brain perfusion in dogs. *J Neuroimaging* 2001;**11**:171–8.

62 Sakahashi H, Hashimoto A, Aomi S, et al. Transcranial Doppler measurement of middle cerebral artery blood flow during continuous retrograde cerebral perfusion (in Japanese). *Nippon Kyobu Geka Gakkai Zasshi* 1994;**42**:1851–7.

63 Quigley RL, Fuller BC, Sampson LN, et al. Passive retrograde cerebral perfusion during routine cardiac valve surgery reverses middle cerebral artery blood flow and reduces risk of stroke. *J Heart Valve Dis* 1997;**6**:288–91.

64 Tanoe Y, Tominaga R, Ochiai Y, *et al*. Comparative study of retrograde and selective cerebral perfusion with transcranial Doppler. *Ann Thorac Surg* 1999;**67**:672–5.

65 Wong C, Bonser RS. Retrograde perfusion and true reverse brain blood flow in humans. *Eur J Cardiothorac Surg* 2000;**17**:597–601.

66 Garami Z, Estrera A, Scheinbaum R, *et al*. Monitoring of cerebral blood flow with power mode Doppler TCD during retrograde cerebral perfusion. *Cerebrovasc Dis* 2002;**13**(Suppl 4):38.

67 Clark RE, Brillman J, Davis DA, *et al*. Microemboli during coronary artery bypass grafting. Genesis and effect on outcome. *J Thorac Cardiovasc Surg* 1995;**109**(2):249–57.

68 Stump DA, Kon NA, Rogers AT, *et al*. Emboli and neuropsychological outcome following cardiopulmonary bypass. *Echocardiography* 1996;**13**:555–8.

69 Brown WR, Moody DM, Challa VR, *et al*. Histologic studies of brain microemboli in humans and dogs after cardiopulmonary bypass. *Echocardiography* 1996;**13**:559–6.

70 Brown WR, Moody DM, Challa VR, *et al*. Longer duration of cardiopulmonary bypass is associated with greater numbers of cerebral microemboli. *Stroke* 2000;**31**:707–13.

71 Estrera AL, Garami Z, Miller CC III, *et al*. Cerebral monitoring with transcranial Doppler ultrasonography improves neurologic outcome during repairs of acute type A aortic dissection. *J Thorac Cardiovasc Surg* 2005;**129**(2):277–85.

72 Estrera AL, Garami Z, Miller CC, *et al*. Acute type A aortic dissection complicated by stroke: can immediate repair be performed safely? *J Thorac Cardiovasc Surg* 2006;**132**(6):1404–8.

14 Intracranial Stenosis

Vijay K. Sharma[1] & K.S. Lawrence Wong[2]
[1]Division of Neurology, National University Hospital, Singapore
[2]Department of Medicine and Therapeutics, Chinese University of Hong Kong, Prince of Wales Hospital, Hong Kong, China

Introduction

Intracranial atherosclerosis leads to cerebrovascular events that account for at least 10% of all ischemic strokes in North America, but it is one of the most common causes of stroke worldwide, especially among stroke patients of Asian, African or Hispanic ancestry [1–6]. The presence of intracranial atherosclerosis is associated with an increased risk of recurrent stroke ranging from 10 to 50% per year [3–8].

The diagnosis of intracranial large artery stenosis requires vascular imaging of the craniocervical circulation. For decades, conventional digital subtraction angiography (DSA) had been the only method to visualize the intracranial circulation in clinical practice. However, the invasive nature of conventional angiography and the risk of periprocedural complications [9] hindered its widespread use in the evaluation of intracranial vascular lesions in stroke patients.

Computed tomographic angiography (CTA) has recently been introduced as a new sensitive and specific tool for the assessment of cerebral vasculature [10,11]. CTA is preferable to magnetic resonance angiography (MRA) since the depiction of the anatomy of the circle of Willis by the former is more reliable [12]. CTA has an excellent yield in the diagnosis of intracranial steno-occlusive disease when compared with digital subtraction angiography (DSA) [10,13]. However, MRA has the advantages of not requiring intravenous contrast injection (especially problematic in patients with diabetes or renal disease) and many other added information such as atherosclerotic plaque morphology.

Transcranial Doppler (TCD) ultrasound permits the study of large numbers of patients safely and reliably in clinical practice.[14,15]. Intracranial arterial steno-occlusive lesions cause characteristic alterations in the Doppler signals, including focal increases in velocity, local spectral turbulence, prestenotic and/or post-stenotic changes and various collateral flow patterns. Stenosis and/or occlusion of the ICA siphon, proximal (M1) segment of middle cerebral artery, intracranial vertebral artery, proximal basilar artery and proximal (P1) segment of posterior cerebral artery can be reliably detected by TCD. Sensitivity, specificity, positive predictive values and negative predictive values of TCD are generally higher in anterior circulation than the vertebrobasilar circulation owing to less tortuosity of the former and the technical problems in studying the latter [14,15].

In a recent study, we validated TCD with CTA in patients with acute cerebral ischemia, performed within 2 h of each other, by experienced neurosonologists. We found that bedside TCD examination yields satisfactory agreement with urgent brain CTA in the evaluation of patients with acute cerebral ischemia. TCD can provide real-time flow findings that are complementary to information provided by CTA [16]. Intracranial arterial stenotic lesions in the internal carotid distribution are dynamic and can evolve over time, and the progression may be associated with new ipsilateral stroke or TIA or major vascular events [17]. Existing data suggest an association between the degree of stenosis and recurrent stroke, with higher degrees of stenosis and the number of vessels affected predicting worse prognosis [17–19].

One of the important limitations of TCD is an insufficient temporal acoustic window, and this can be a limiting factor in a significant number of cases, depending upon the population studied [20,21]. The yield of TCD in cases with suboptimal acoustic windows can be enhanced with the help of various contrast agents. Furthermore, the ability to assess the intracranial arteries by TCD remains as much an art as it is science and remains "operator dependent." However, when TCD is performed and interpreted by experienced neurosonologists, it provides a higher yield with results comparable to those of contrast angiography, especially if these two investigations are performed closer in time to each other [16].

Focal intracranial disease

One of the basic aims of TCD in patients with cerebrovascular ischemia is to diagnose a moderate to severe (≥50%)

Cerebrovascular Ultrasound in Stroke Prevention and Treatment, 2nd edition.
Edited by Andrei V. Alexandrov. © 2011 Blackwell Publishing Ltd.

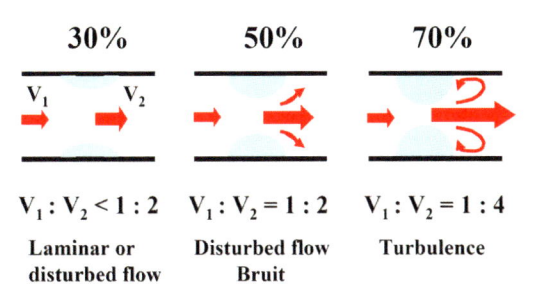

CHAPTER 14 Intracranial Stenosis

Stenosis and Flow Velocity

Figure 14.1 Relationship between pre- and post-stenotic velocities in a vessel with straight walls and no bifurcations.

stenosis in the relevant intracranial arterial segment. The relationship among the mean flow velocities (MFV) obtained from various intracranial arteries usually follows the normal hierarchy: MCA ≥ ACA ≥ siphon ≥ PCA ≥ BA ≥ VA. Velocity values can be equal between these arterial segments or sometimes exceed by 5–10 cm s^{-1}, i.e. ACA > MCA or BA > ICA. likely due to the angle of insonation or common anatomic variations.

As a rule, for a vessel with straight walls, a 50% diameter reduction doubles the velocity and a 70% stenosis triples the velocity at the exit of stenosis compared with a prestenotic segment or with the contralateral side (Figure 14.1). Warfarin–Aspirin Stroke in Intracranial Disease (WASID) trial identified a significant higher stroke risk in patients with intracranial stenosis at 50% diameter reduction or greater on contrast angiography [8,22]. (Figure 14.2) However, this may not always correlate well with TCD findings. Such an example is shown in Figure 14.2 (DSA estimation) and 3 (TCD estimation).

Various diagnostic criteria have been used to diagnose a ≥50% stenosis in different intracranial arteries. These criteria are by no means absolute and each neurovascular laboratory should validate their results against contrast angiography (CTA or DSA).

Middle cerebral artery (MCA) stenosis

Primary findings for a ≥50% MCA stenosis include a focal mean flow velocity increase (MFV ≥ 100 cm s^{-1}), and/or peak systolic velocity increase (PSV ≥ 140 cm s^{-1}), and/or inter-hemispheric MFV difference of ≥30% in adults free of abnormal circulatory conditions [17,23,24–35]. In a recent meta-analysis, we demonstrated a spectral MFV of >100 cm s^{-1} to be the most balanced and accurate parameter regarding a diagnostic velocity threshold [36]. However, MFV is heart-rate dependent, so it is important to record the heart rate during examination. To improve the predictive value of 100 cm s^{-1} threshold, we use the ratio with a homologous or a proximal MCA segment of ≥2 [33]. A ≥70% MCA stenosis will produce a stenotic:prestenotic ratio of 3:1 or greater (Figure 14.3).

If velocities are affected by anemia, congestive heart failure and other circulatory conditions, then a focal MFV difference of ≥30% between neighboring or homologous arterial segments should be applied. Adult patients with anemia or hyperthyroidism often have MCA mean flow velocities in the range 60–110 cm s^{-1}. In children with sickle cell disease, an MCA MFV up to 170 cm s^{-1} is considered normal [37,38].

A stenosis in the MCA may also be suspected if indirect flow disturbances are detected by TCD. These important additional findings may include:
1 Bruit or disturbed flow distal to the stenosis suggesting turbulence (Figure 14.4).
2 An increased unilateral anterior cerebral artery (ACA) MFV indicating compensatory flow diversion [39,40] (Figure 14.4). This finding may also indicate A1 ACA or an ICA bifurcation stenosis with a side-to-side ACA MFV ratio ≥1.2.
3 A low-frequency noise produced by non-harmonic co-vibrations of the vessel wall and musical murmurs due to harmonic co-vibrations producing pure tones.

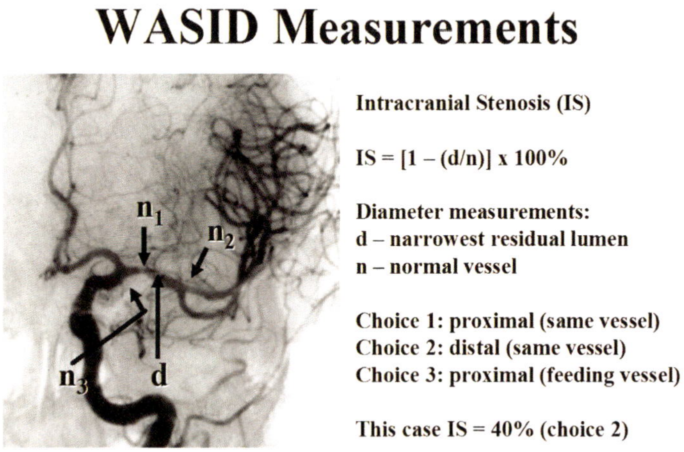

WASID Measurements

Intracranial Stenosis (IS)

IS = [1 − (d/n)] × 100%

Diameter measurements:
d – narrowest residual lumen
n – normal vessel

Choice 1: proximal (same vessel)
Choice 2: distal (same vessel)
Choice 3: proximal (feeding vessel)

This case IS = 40% (choice 2)

Figure 14.2 Method used for estimating a stenosis in the intracranial arteries by Warfarin–Aspirin Symptomatic Intracranial Disease (WASID) trial criteria.

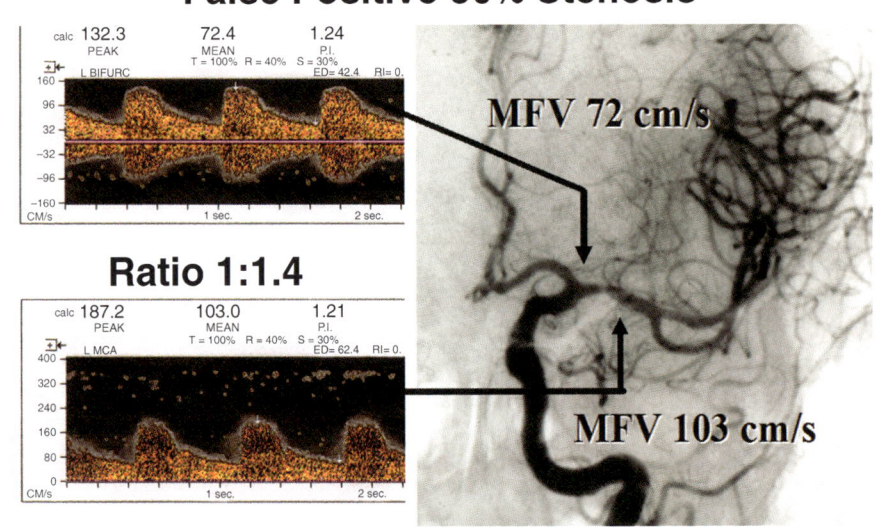

PART IV Ultrasound in Stroke Prevention and Treatment

Figure 14.3 An example of false-positive transcranial Doppler diagnosis of >50% stenosis in M1 MCA as estimated by WASID trial criteria. TCD mean flow velocity criteria are suggestive of a moderate (>50%) stenosis. However, WASID trial criteria measure only a 40% stenosis.

4 Microembolic signals found in the distal MCA (Figure 14.4).

A critical stenosis produces a focal flow velocity decrease or a "blunted" MCA waveform with slow or delayed systolic acceleration, slow systolic flow deceleration, low velocities and MCA MFV < ACA MFV or other intracranial arteries [41,42]. Decreased or minimal flow velocities with slow systolic acceleration can be found due to a tight elongated MCA stenosis or thrombus causing near occlusion or a proximal ICA obstruction [43,44]. The "blunted" waveform is

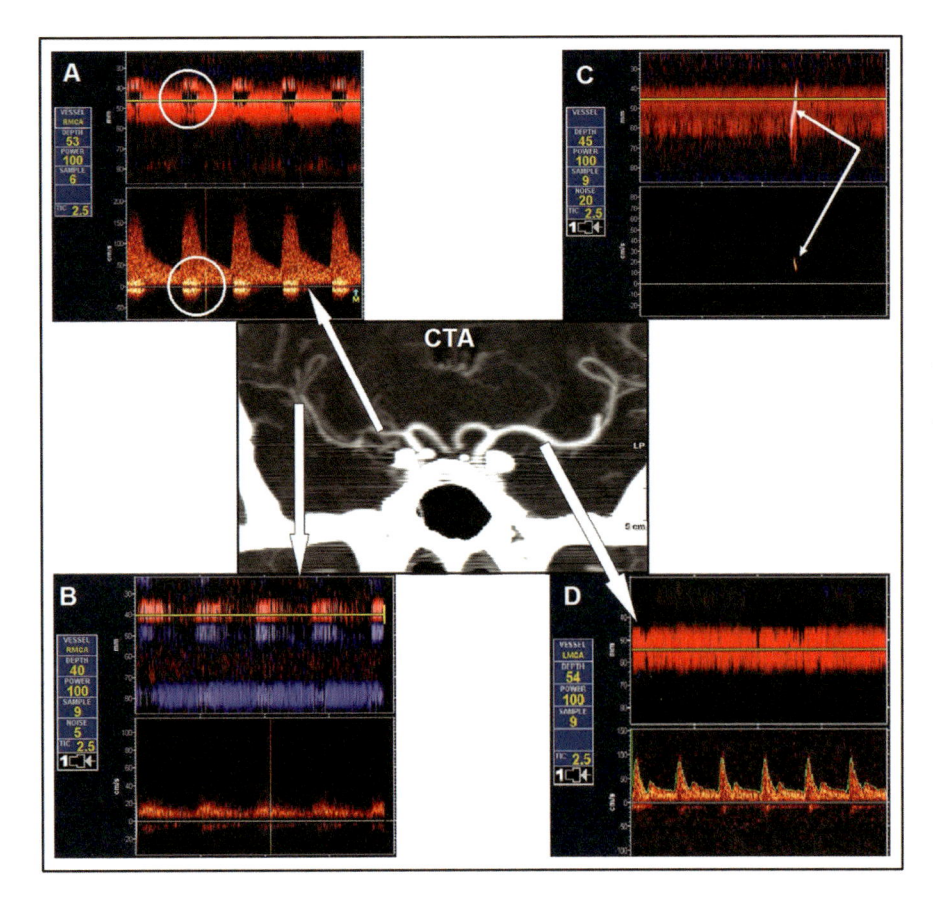

Figure 14.4 Salient TCD findings in a patient with severe stenosis of proximal MCA (confirmed by CT angiography in the central frame). Markedly elevated flow velocity is seen at proximal MCA (A) with a harsh systolic bruit represented by "black holes" on M-mode (within the circle in M-mode) and as higher intensity turbulent disturbance (within the circle on the spectral display). TCD signals obtained from the distal MCA show a "blunted" flow pattern (B). Continuous monitoring of distal left MCA detected a "spontaneous" embolus (C) seen as a bright, high-intensity "track" on M-mode (upper frame) and also on spectral display (lower frame with reduced gain). For comparison, normal flow pattern and velocity are seen from the TCD signals obtained from the contralateral and healthy MCA.

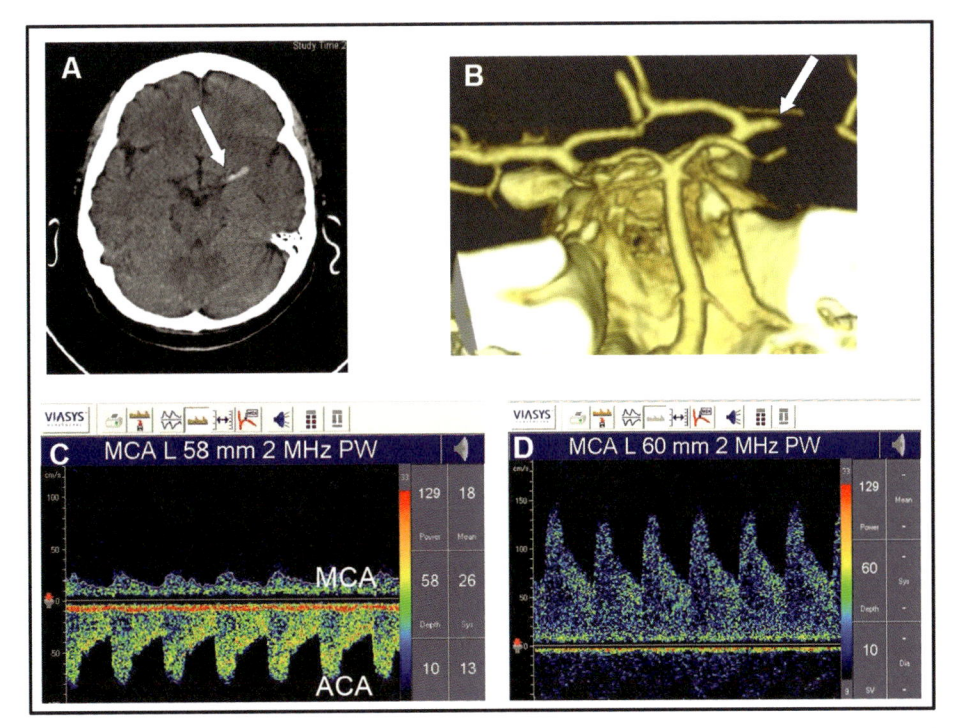

Figure 14.5 Imaging and TCD findings in a patient with acute left MCA infarction. Non-contrast CT scan of the brain performed 125 min after the symptom onset shows "hyperdense" left MCA sign (A). CT angiography performed immediately after the non-contrast CT scan shows MCA cut-off sign suggestive of an acute occlusion of left M1 MCA (B). Spectral TCD waveforms obtained from a depth of 58 mm, before intravenous tissue plasminogen activator (TPA) bolus shows blunted waveforms from left MCA along with "flow diversion" into the ipsilateral ACA (C). Continuous TCD monitoring was performed during the IV-TPA infusion and recanalization of left MCA was observed at 32 min from the TPA bolus, associated with significant clinical recovery. The resultant MCA waveforms after the recanalization show a stenotic pattern (D). Note that the spectral signals obtained from the left ACA become poor after the recanalization of the MCA.

common in patients with acute ischemic stroke, particularly in those presenting with a hyperdense MCA sign on non-contrast CT scan or a flow gap on MRA (Figure 14.5).

Anterior cerebral artery (ACA)

Primary findings in an ACA stenosis include a focal significant ACA MFV increase (ACA > MCA) and/or ACA MFV ≥ 80 cm s^{-1}, and/or a $\geq 30\%$ difference between the proximal and distal ACA segments, and/or a $\geq 30\%$ difference compared with the contralateral ACA [45]. Collateralization via the anterior communicating artery can be excluded by a normal contralateral ACA flow direction and the absence of stenotic signals at 75 mm. Usually, an A1 ACA stenosis can be detected at 60–75 mm. The differential diagnosis includes anterior cross-filling due to a proximal carotid artery disease on the contralateral side [46] (Figure 14.6). Additional findings may include turbulence and a flow diversion into the MCA and/or a compensatory flow increase in the contralateral ACA (Figure 14.5C) Decreased or minimal flow velocities at the A1 ACA origin may indicate a suboptimal angle of insonation from the unilateral temporal window, an atretic or tortuous A1 ACA segment and A1 ACA near occlusion. Since the A2 ACA segment cannot be assessed directly by TCD, its obstruction can be suspected only if a high-resistance flow is found in the distal dominant A1 ACA segment (70–75 mm).

Terminal ICA and ICA siphon

The paracellar and supraclinoid ICA segments are difficult to examine in their entirety. An orbital examination may reveal stenotic flow directed towards or away from the probe at 58–65 mm in adults. Deeper insonation is possible but vessel identification is less reliable since an ACA flow can be detected in the presence of a good orbital window. The terminal ICA bifurcation is located at 60–75 mm from the temporal window. A terminal ICA/siphon stenosis produces a focal significant MFV increase with ICA > MCA, and/or an ICA MFV ≥ 70 cm s^{-1}, and/or a $\geq 30\%$ difference between arterial segments [47]. The ICA siphon MFVs may decrease due to siphon near-occlusion (a blunted siphon signal) or distal obstruction (i.e. MCA occlusion or increased ICP).

The differential diagnosis includes a compensatory flow increase with contralateral ICA stenosis. Additional findings in the presence of an ICA stenosis may include turbulence, blunted unilateral MCA (post-stenotic flow), OA

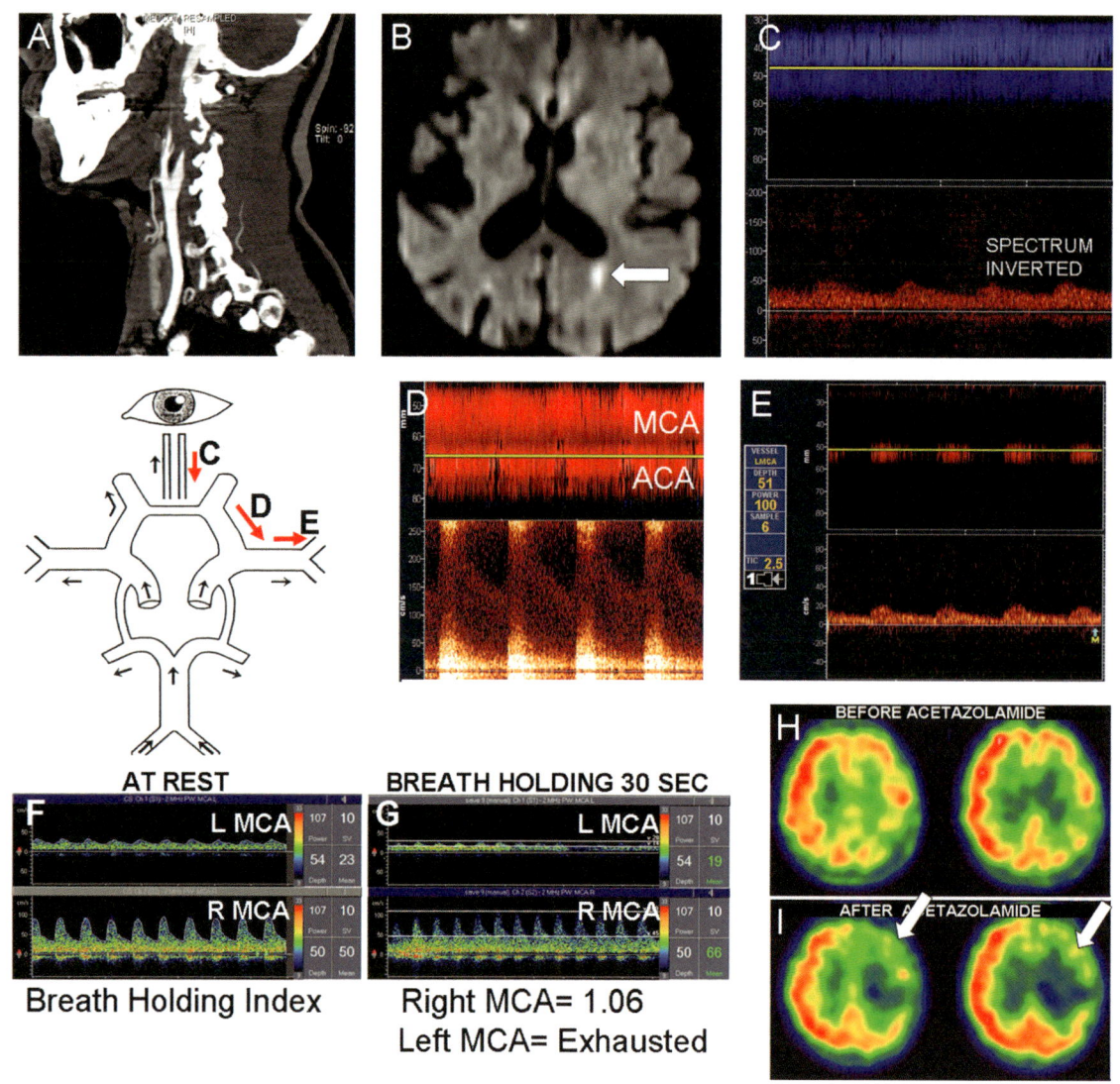

PART IV Ultrasound in Stroke Prevention and Treatment

Figure 14.6 Hemodynamic consequences of extracranial internal carotid artery (ICA) occlusive disease in a 56-year-old male. CT angiography of the neck shows a complete occlusion of left ICA just beyond the carotid bulb (A) with acute "water-shed" infarction on diffusion-weighted MRI (B). Transcranial Doppler examination revealed a reversed and lower resistance flow in the left ophthalmic artery (C) and a reversed flow (anterior cross-filling) in the left A1 ACA with an elevated flow velocity (D). Left MCA demonstrated a blunted flow. Vasomotor reactivity was assessed by breath-holding index (BHI) during simultaneous TCD monitoring of both MCAs. Right MCA demonstrated a normal response, with mean flow velocity increasing from 50 cm s^{-1} at rest (F) to 66 cm s^{-1} after 30 min of breath-holding (G). However, the mean flow velocity in the left MCA demonstrated a paradoxical reduction from 23 to 19 cm s^{-1}, suggesting an exhausted vasomotor reactivity. These findings were reliably replicated with HMPAO-SPECT with acetazolamide challenge (H and I). Significant reduction in the cerebral perfusion was noted in the MCA territory after acetazolamide injection, suggesting a "failed" vasodilatory reserve.

MFV increase and/or flow reversal with low pulsatility (Figure 14.6).

Common errors include vessel identification (MCA versus ICA), deep (>65 mm) transorbital insonation and collateralization of flow misinterpreted as an arterial stenosis.

Posterior cerebral artery (PCA)

A stenosis in the PCA produces a focal significant flow velocity increase: PCA MFV > ACA or ICA; and/or a PCA MFV ≥50 cm s^{-1} in adults [48]. The PCA flow is located at 58–65 mm; the P1 segment is directed towards the probe and the P2 segment is directed away from the probe. The top of the basilar and P1 PCA flow can be found originating at midline (75–65 mm). The differential diagnosis includes collateral flow via the posterior communicating artery (PcomA). Using transcranial color-coded duplex sonography (TCCD), it may be possible to differentiate PCA stenosis from collateralization of flow using color flow vessel identification and the peak systolic velocity [49]. Additional findings may include turbulence and a compensatory flow increase in the MCA.

Common sources of error include unreliable vessel identification (i.e. mixed PCA and MCA), the presence of an arterial occlusion and a top of the basilar stenosis.

Basilar artery (BA)

Primary findings in the presence of a BA stenosis include a focal significant velocity increase where a BA MFV > MCA or ACA or ICA, and/or MFV BA ≥60 cm s^{-1} in adults and/or ≥30% difference between arterial segment [50–53]. Although the depth range for basilar segments varied between previous studies [51,53], it is dependent on the size of the neck and skull and the technical skills allow insonation of the distal basilar artery with failure rates much less than 30% [52]. Our depth criteria are the following: the proximal basilar artery is located at 75–90 mm, the mid-BA segment is located at 90–100 mm and the distal BA is found at >100 mm in most adults [52,54]. The differential diagnosis includes terminal VA stenosis if elevated velocities are found proximally. If elevated velocities are found throughout the BA stem and VA, the differential diagnosis includes a compensatory flow increase due to anterior circulation abnormality.

Basilar artery sub-total stenosis or near-occlusion produces a focal FV decrease and/or BA < VA) with a blunted waveform [55]. The differential diagnosis includes a fusiform basilar artery with or without thrombus since an enlarged vessel diameter may reduce flow velocities. If end-diastolic flow is absent, the differential diagnosis includes BA occlusion. Additional findings may include:

1 signs of turbulence and disturbed signals distal to the stenosis;
2 high-resistance flow (PI > 1.2) proximal to the stenosis;
3 compensatory flow increase in VAs and PICAs indicating cerebellar collateralization;
4 collateral supply via PcomA to PCA and reversed distal basilar artery (Figure 14.7).

Common sources of error include tortuous basilar ("not found" does not always mean obstructed), elongated BA obstruction and distal BA lesions that were not reached by TCD insonation. Application of power Doppler, ultrasound contrast and duplex imaging may help detection of the tortuosity, distal basilar segment and distal branches [56,57].

Terminal vertebral artery (VA)

The terminal VA is found at 40–75 mm depending on the size of neck and skull (Figure 14.8). Primary findings of intracranial VA stenosis include a focal significant velocity

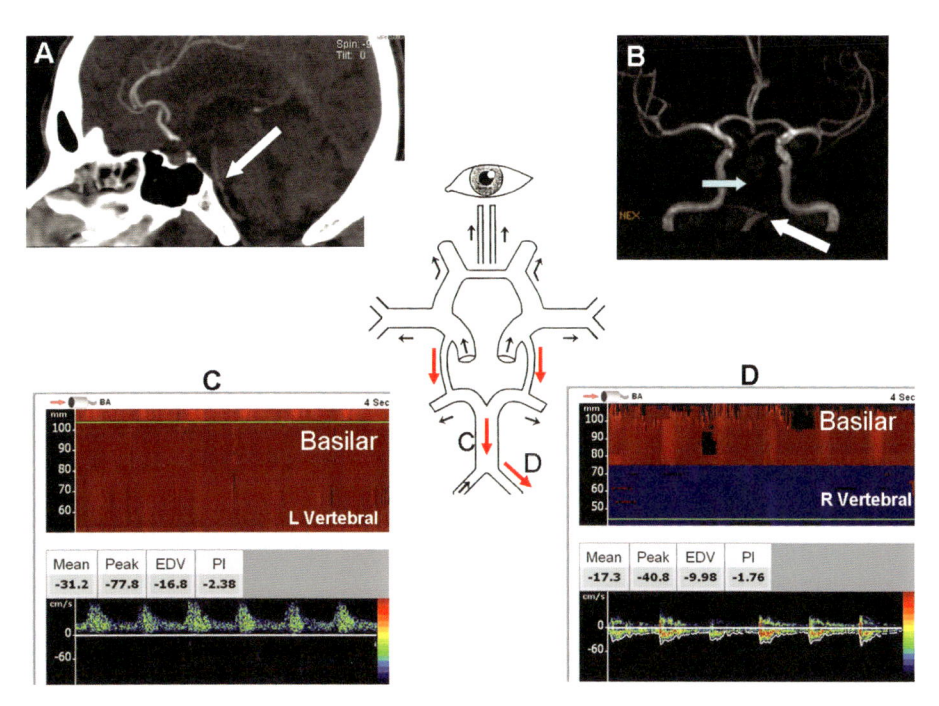

Figure 14.7 Hemodynamic consequences of a an vertebrobasilar occlusive disease in a 64-year-old man presenting with an acute brainstem stroke (NIHSS 13 points). An emergent non-contrast CT scan of the brain was unremarkable and a poor filling was noted in the vertebro-basilar arteries. A non-contrast time-of-flight MRA failed to detect any flow in the left vertebral and the entire basilar artery. TCD performed in the emergency room within 1 h of the CT angiography demonstrated a reversed flow in the entire basilar artery and also the left vertebral artery while a higher resistance flow was detected in the right vertebral artery. This patient made a good clinical recovery with a modified Rankin score of 0 at 3 months. However, the basilar artery maintained the reversed flow.

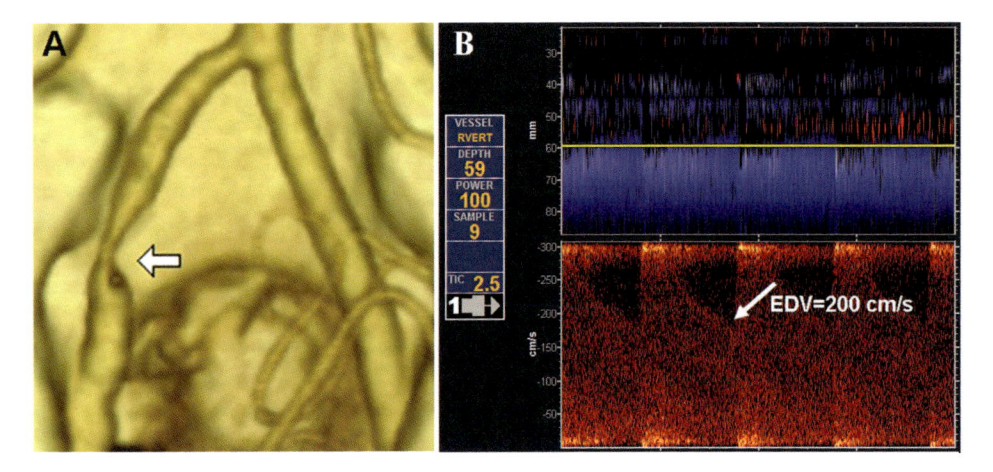

PART IV Ultrasound in Stroke Prevention and Treatment

Figure 14.8 Vertebral artery stenosis. A moderate stenosis is seen in the right intracranial vertebral artery on CT angiography (A) that presented with a markedly elevated flow velocity on TCD (B).

increase [48] where MFV VA > BA, and/or MFV VA ≥50 cm s^{-1} (adults), and/or ≥30% difference between VAs or their segments. [37,54]. A terminal VA stenosis may also cause a high-resistance (PI ≥ 1.2) flow in its proximal segment, and/or a blunted or minimal flow signal at or distal to the stenosis segment [55]. To detect ≥50% intracranial stenoses, the peak systolic velocity criteria were also developed for angle-corrected duplex ultrasound of the vertebral and other intracranial arteries [58].

The differential diagnosis includes proximal BA or contralateral terminal VA stenoses and a compensatory flow increase in the presence of a contralateral VA occlusion or carotid stenosis [59].

Additional findings may include:
1 signs of turbulence or disturbed flow signal distal to the stenosis;
2 a compensatory flow increase in the contralateral vertebral artery or its branches (cerebellar collaterals);
3 low BA flow velocities (hemodynamically significant lesion, hypoplastic contralateral VA) and low-resistance flow distal to stenoses (compensatory vasodilation);
4 high-resistance flow proximal to the stenoses.

Common sources of error include a compensatory flow increase due to hypoplastic contralateral VA, low velocities in both VAs due to suboptimal angle of insonation, extracranial VA stenosis or occlusion with well-developed muscular collaterals, elongated VA stenosis/hypoplasia and incorrect vessel identification, i.e. posterior inferior cerebellar artery.

Diffuse intracranial disease

A short segment of arterial stenosis produces focal velocity increases on the upslope of the so-called Spencer's curve of cerebral hemodynamics.(Figure 14.9). However, the relationship between flow velocity and diameter reduction is also affected by the length of the stenosis or the presence of multiple distal lesions [60,61]. TCD also provides information about impedance to flow by calculating the pulsatility index (PI), originally described by Gosling and King

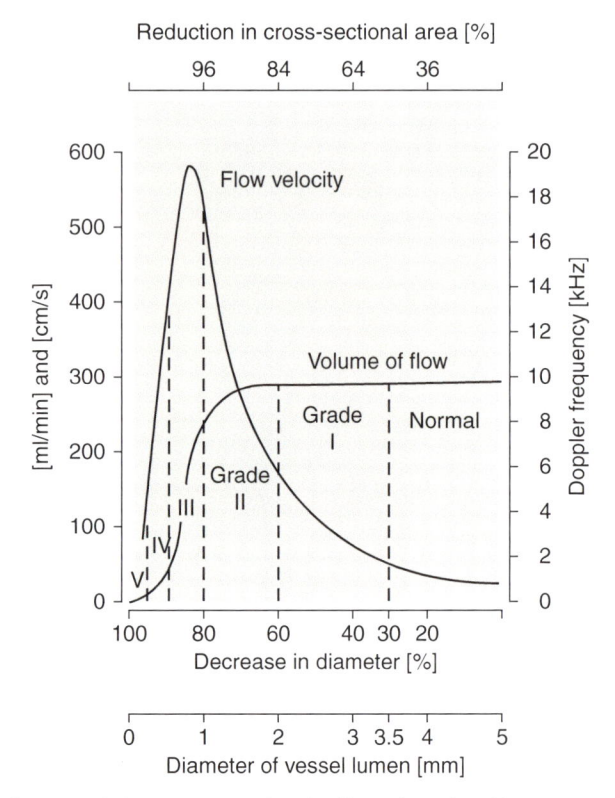

Figure 14.9 Spencer's curve of cerebral hemodynamics. This curve demonstrates the hemodynamic relationship among degree of an arterial stenosis, flow velocity and blood flow volume.

234

CHAPTER 14 Intracranial Stenosis

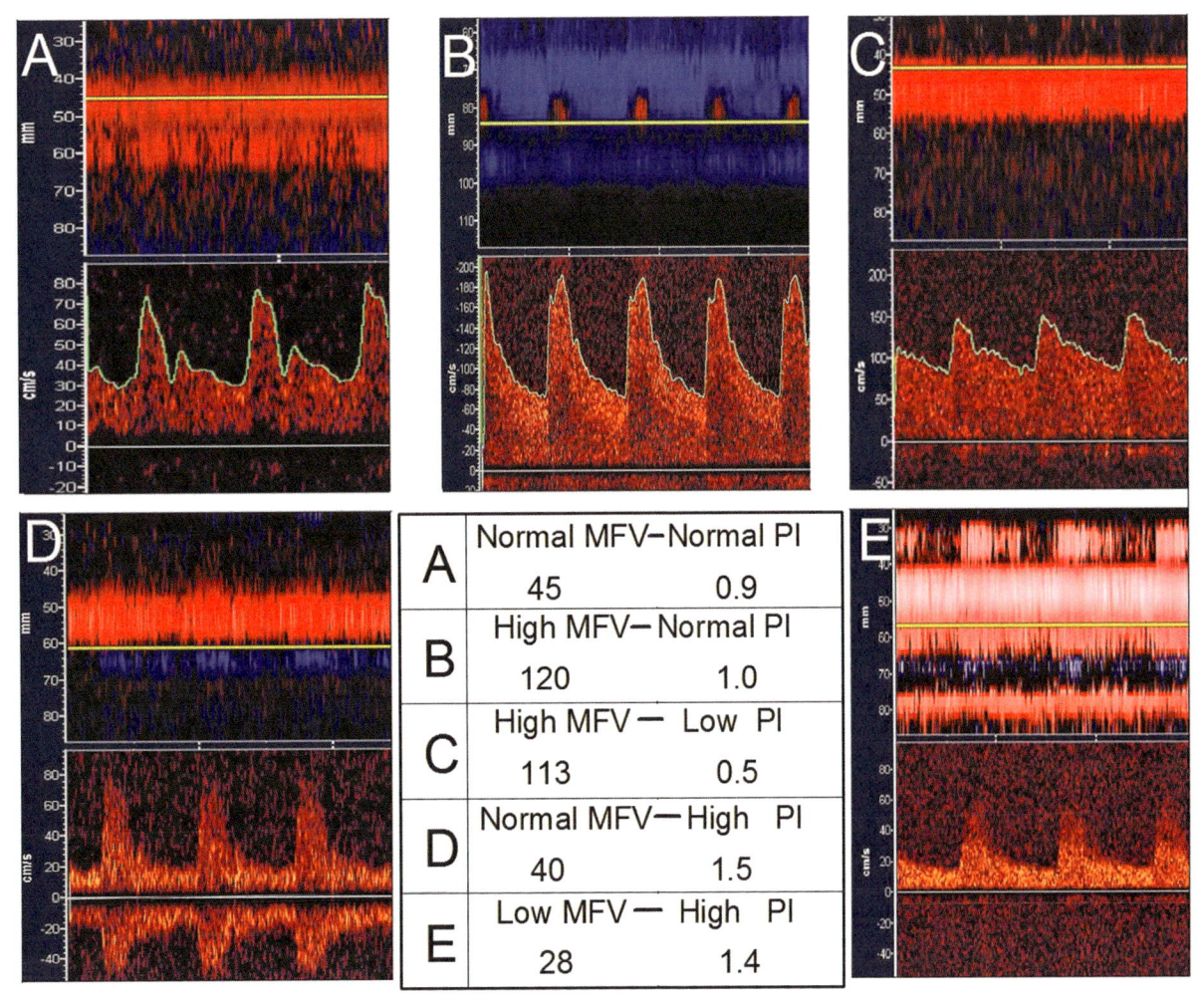

A	Normal MFV–Normal PI	
	45	0.9
B	High MFV–Normal PI	
	120	1.0
C	High MFV – Low PI	
	113	0.5
D	Normal MFV–High PI	
	40	1.5
E	Low MFV – High PI	
	28	1.4

Figure 14.10 M-mode and corresponding spectral TCD findings in patients with focal and diffuse intracranial disease. Various combinations of mean flow velocity and pulsatility index are seen which represent various physiological and disease states. Mean flow velocity (MFV) and pulsatility index (PI) values are shown in the table inset.

(PI calculated as PSV – EDV/MFV, where PSV is peak systolic velocity, EDV is end-diastolic velocity and MFV is mean flow velocity) [62,63]. The pulsatility of arterial blood flow can be affected by changes in cardiac output and also proximal and distal vascular resistance. Assuming stable central hemodynamics, an increase in the proximal resistance decreases pulsatility in the distal arterial segments (e.g. the middle cerebral artery acquires a low-resistance spectral pattern in the presence of a proximal internal carotid artery stenosis or occlusion) [64,65]. Similarly, an increase in resistance distal to the site of insonation results in an increased blood flow pulsatility [64,65].

With progression of the intracranial atherosclerotic process, the resulting long and severely narrowed vessels can reduce blood flow velocities on the down-slope of the Spencer's curve. The pulsatility index can differentiate a velocity reduction due to reduced cardiac output (low PI) from increased distal resistance (high PI) [66]. Many combinations of MFV and PI are possible and represent various distinct pathological states (Figure 14.10).

Current diagnostic criteria for intracranial disease such as those used in the WASID trial and prospective studies in a Chinese population, [8,21] take into account only increased flow velocities consistent with a ≥50% focal stenosis. Intracranial arterial stenosis increases flow velocities on the upslope of the Spencer's curve of cerebral hemodynamics. However, the velocity can decrease with long and severely narrowed vessels, multiple segments of focal stenosis along an artery or focal stenoses in multiple arteries. Therefore, a very severe or long stenosis and multiple stenoses in one artery can be missed (Figure 14.9). These patterns are associated with an elevated pulsatility index.

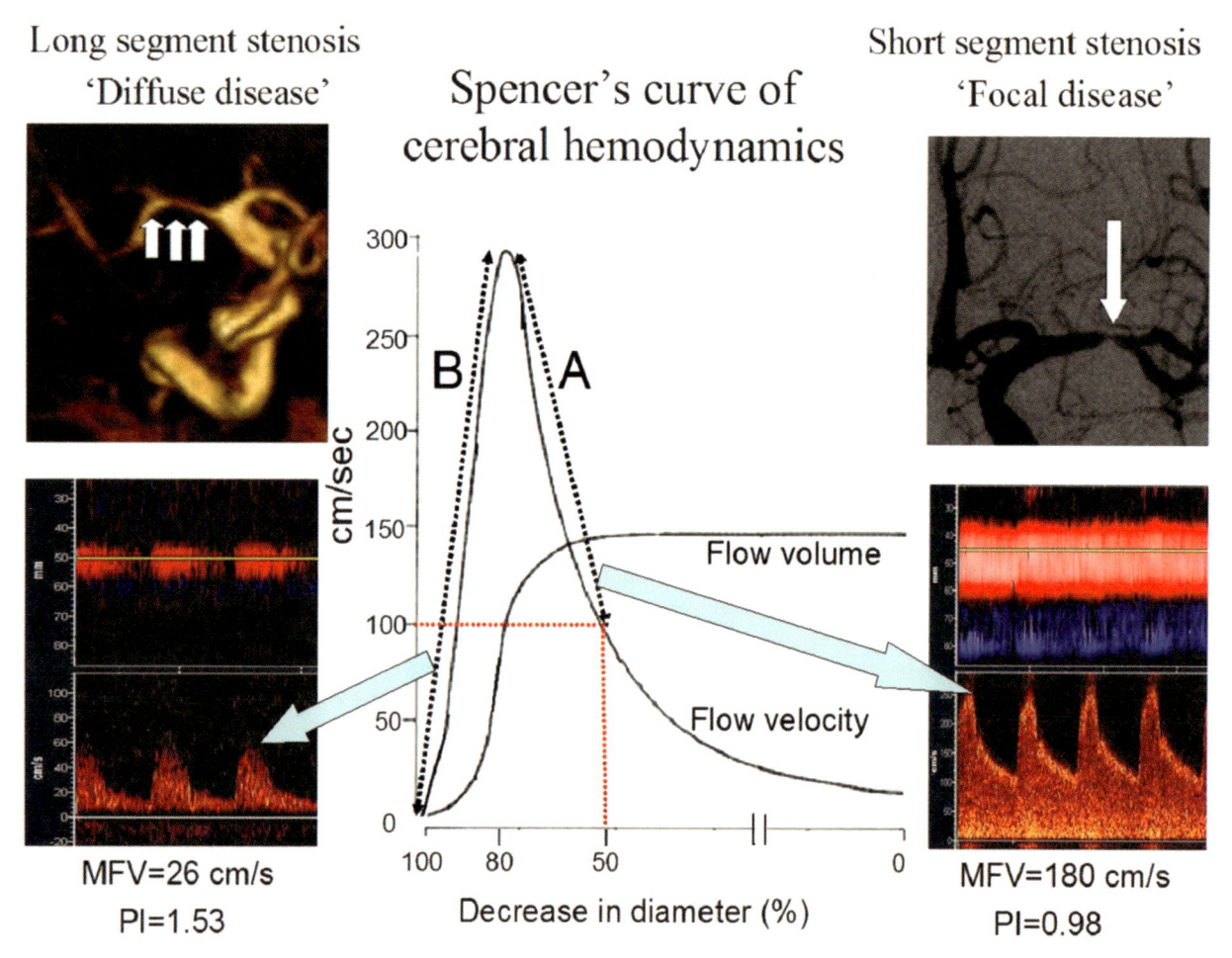

Figure 14.11 Blood flow patterns in the intracranial arteries due to the stenosis are determined by their position on the Spencer's curve of cerebral hemodynamics. Dotted line A corresponds to abnormally elevated flow velocities on the "up-slope" of the Spencer's curve caused by short and focal stenoses of ≥50% [20]. Upper right DSA image shows a focal >50% MCA stenosis with high mean flow velocities on TCD (bottom right image). Dotted line B shows the "down-slope" of the Spencer's curve when the velocities decrease due to increasing resistance with most severe or elongated lesions. The upper left CTA image shows a >1 cm long stenosis in the right MCA with low mean flow velocities and increased pulsatility index on TCD (bottom left image).

We have recently reported the abnormal TCD findings that low mean flow velocity in the presence of high pulsatility index is independently associated with the presence of diffuse intracranial disease after adjusting for demographic characteristics and stroke risk factors [67]. This pattern of diffuse intracranial disease was seen relatively commonly among the North American Stroke patients. The ability of TCD to detect diffuse intracranial disease increased with the number of arteries affected [67] (Figure 14.11). Low MFV/high PI were documented in multiple vessels by TCD in patients with diffuse intracranial disease on contrast angiography whereas the presence of low MFV/high PI in two or more intracranial arteries was highly specific for angiographically proven diffuse intracranial disease. Recent autopsy-based reports in patients with dementias also demonstrated correlation between a low-velocity/high-resistance flow pattern and degree of cumulative intracranial stenosis due to atheromatous disease [68,69].

Our study raises the possibility of increasing the yield of screening for intracranial disease and defining a broader spectrum of intracranial lesions for future clinical trials (Figure 14.12).

In conclusion, TCD has an established clinical value in the diagnostic workup of stroke patients and is suggested as an essential component of a comprehensive stroke center [70]. Well-established validated criteria exist for the diagnosis of focal intracranial stenosis; criteria were also recently developed for diffuse intracranial disease. Owing to the widespread availability of transcranial Doppler, this modality could be increasingly used in the evaluation of patients with cerebrovascular ischemia for diagnostic, therapeutic and prognostic indications.

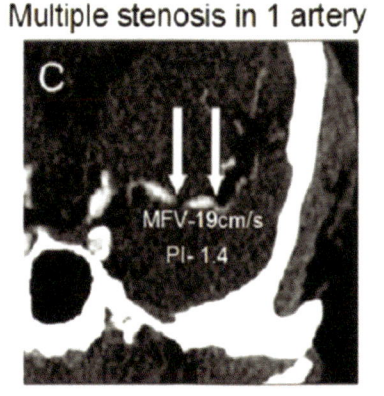

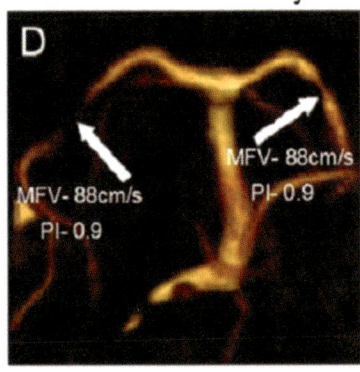

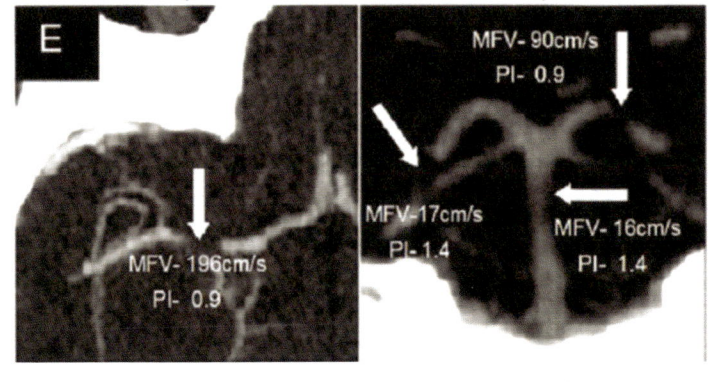

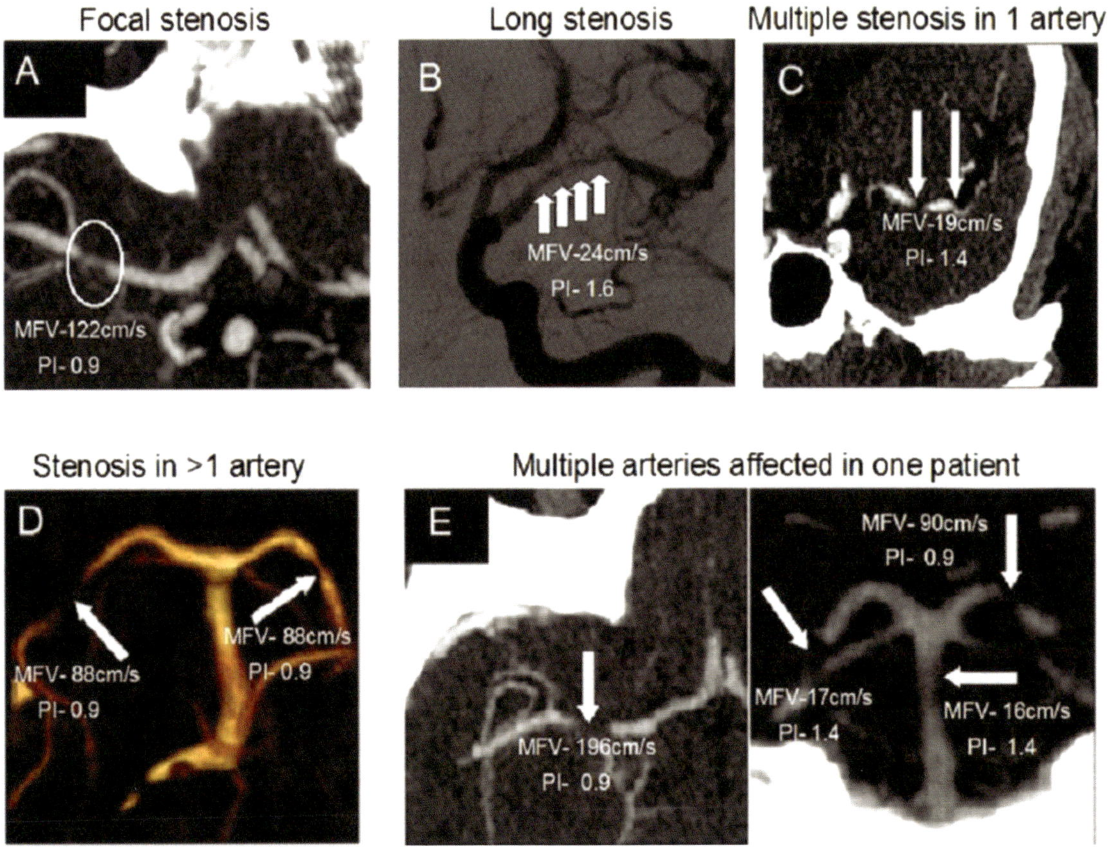

CHAPTER 14 Intracranial Stenosis

Figure 14.12 Spectrum of focal and diffuse intracranial lesions on contrast angiography with corresponding flow velocity and pulsatility values. (A) A focal stenosis in the M1 segment of the right MCA. (B) A long (>1 cm) stenosis in the left MCA. (C) Multiple segments with focal stenoses in the left MCA. (D) Stenoses in multiple segments of posterior circulation arteries. (E) Multiple stenoses in both anterior and posterior circulation vessels.

References

1 Sacco R, Kargman DE, Gu Q, et al. Race-ethnicity and determinants of intracranial atherosclerotic cerebral infarction: the Northern Manhattan Stroke Study. Stroke 1995;**26**: 14–20.
2 Wong KS, Huang YN, Gao S, et al. Intracranial stenosis in Chinese patients with acute stroke. Neurology 1998;**50**: 812–3.
3 Caplan LR, Gorelick PB, Hier DB. Race, sex and occlusive cerebrovascular disease: a review. Stroke 1986;**17**:648–55.
4 Gorelick PB, Caplan LR, Hier DB, et al. Racial differences in the distribution of anterior circulation occlusive disease. Neurology 1984;**34**:54–9.
5 Nishimaru K, McHenry LK, Toole JF. Cerebral angiographic and clinical differences in carotid system transient ischemic attacks between American Caucasian and Japanese patients. Stroke 1984;**15**:56–9.
6 Wityk RJ, Lehman D, Klag M, et al. Race and sex differences in the distribution of cerebral atherosclerosis. Stroke 1996;**27**: 1974–80.
7 The International Cooperative Study of Extracranial/Intracranial Arterial Anastomosis (EC/IC Bypass Study). Methodology and entry characteristics. The EC/IC Bypass Study Group. Stroke 1985;**16**:397–406.
8 Chimowitz MI, Lynn MJ, Howlett-Smith H, et al.; Warfarin-Aspirin Symptomatic Intracranial Disease Trial Investigators. Comparison of warfarin and aspirin for symptomatic intracranial arterial stenosis. N Engl J Med 2005;**352**:1305–16.
9 Bendszus M, Koltzenburg M, Burger R, et al. Silent embolism in diagnostic cerebral angiography and neurointerventional procedures: a prospective study. Lancet 1999;**354**:1594–7.
10 Skutta B, Furst G, Eilers J, et al. Intracranial stenoocclusive disease: double-detector helical CT angiography versus digital subtraction angiography. AJNR Am J Neuroradiol 1999;**20**:791–9.
11 Knauth M, von Kummer R, Jansen O, et al. Potential of CT angiography in acute ischemic stroke. AJNR Am J Neuroradiol 1997;**18**:1001–10.
12 Katz DA, Marks MP, Napel SA, et al. Circle of Willis: evaluation with spiral CT angiography, MR angiography and conventional angiography. Radiology 1995;**195**:445–9.
13 Nguyen-Huynh MN, Wintermark M, English J, et al. How accurate is CT angiography in evaluating intracranial atherosclerotic disease? Stroke 2008;**39**:1184–8.

14 Babikian VL, Feldmann E, Wechsler LR, et al. Transcranial Doppler ultrasonography: year 2000 update. *J Neuroimaging* 2000;**10**:101–15.
15 Markus H. Transcranial Doppler ultrasound. *J Neurol Neurosurg Psychiatry* 1999;**67**:135–7.
16 Tsivgoulis G, Sharma VK, Lao AY, et al. Validation of transcranial Doppler with computed tomography angiography in acute cerebral ischemia. *Stroke* 2007;**38**:1245–9.
17 Wong KS, Li H, Lam WW, et al. Progression of middle cerebral artery occlusive disease and its relationship with further vascular events after stroke. *Stroke* 2002;**33**:532–6.
18 Arenillas JF, Molina CA, Montaner J, et al. Progression and clinical recurrence of symptomatic middle cerebral artery stenosis: a long term follow up transcranial Doppler ultrasound study. *Stroke* 2001;**32**:2898–904.
19 Komotar RJ, Wilson DA, Mocco J, et al. Natural history of intracranial atherosclerosis: a critical review. *Neurosurgery* 2006;**58**:595–601.
20 Marinoni M, Ginanneschi A, Forleo P, et al. Technical limits in transcranial Doppler recording: inadequate acoustic windows. *Ultrasound Med Biol* 1997;**23**(8):1275–7.
21 Wong KS, Li H, Chan YL, et al. Use of transcranial Doppler ultrasound to predict outcome in patients with intracranial large-artery occlusive disease. *Stroke* 2000;**31**:2641–7.
22 Kasner SE, Chimowitz MI, Lynn MJ, et al.; Warfarin Aspirin Symptomatic Intracranial Disease Trial Investigators. Predictors of ischemic stroke in the territory of a symptomatic intracranial arterial stenosis. *Circulation* 2006;**113**:555–63.
23 Samuels OB, Joseph GJ, Lynn MJ, et al. A standardized method for measuring intracranial arterial stenosis. *AJNR Am J Neuroradiol* 2000;**21**:643–6.
24 Bragoni M, Feldmann E. Transcranial Doppler indicies of intracranial hemodynamics. In: Tegeler CH, Babikian VL, Gomez CR, eds. *Neurosonology*. St. Louis, MO: Mosby, 1996:129–39.
25 Lindegaard KF, Bakke SJ, Aaslid R, et al. Doppler diagnosis of intracranial artery occlusive disorders. *J Neurol Neurosurg Psychiatry* 1986;**49**:510–8.
26 de Bray JM, Joseph PA, Jeanvoine H, et al. Transcranial Doppler evaluation of middle cerebral artery stenosis. *J Ultrasound Med* 1988;**7**(11): 611–6.
27 Ley-Pozo J, Ringelstein EB. Noninvasive detection of occlusive disease of the carotid siphon and middle cerebral artery. *Ann Neurol* 1990;**28**:640–7.
28 Schwarze JJ, Babikian V, DeWitt LD, et al. Longitudinal monitoring of intracranial arterial stenoses with transcranial Doppler ultrasonography. *J Neuroimaging* 1994;**4**:182–7.
29 Rother J, Schwartz A, Rautenberg W, et al. Middle cerebral artery stenoses: assessment by magnetic resonance angiography and transcranial Doppler ultrasound. *Cerebrovasc Dis* 1994;**4**:273–9.
30 Alexandrov AV, Bladin CF, Norris JW. Intracranial blood flow velocities in acute ischemic stroke. *Stroke* 1994;**25**:1378–83.
31 Segura T, Serena J, Castellanos M, et al. Embolism in acute middle cerebral artery stenosis. *Neurology* 2001;**56**(4): 497–501.
32 Arenillas JF, Molina CA, Montaner J, et al. Progression and clinical recurrence of symptomatic middle cerebral artery stenosis: a long-term follow-up transcranial Doppler ultrasound study. *Stroke* 2001;**32**(12): 2898–904.

33 Felberg RA, Christou I, Demchuk AM, et al. Screening for intracranial stenosis with transcranial Doppler: the accuracy of mean flow velocity thresholds. *J Neuroimaging* 2002;**12**(1): 9–14.
34 Mattle H, Grolimund P, Huber P, et al. Transcranial Doppler sonographic findings in middle cerebral artery disease. *Arch Neurol* 1988;**45**(3):289–95.
35 Brass LM, Duterte DL, Mohr JP. Anterior cerebral artery velocity changes in disease of the middle cerebral artery stem. *Stroke* 1989;**20**(12):1737–40.
36 Navarro JC, Lao AY, Sharma VK, et al. The accuracy of transcranial Doppler in the diagnosis of middle cerebral artery stenosis. *Cerebrovasc Dis* 2007;**23**:325–30.
37 Babikian V, Sloan MA, Tegeler CH, et al. Transcranial Doppler validation pilot study. *J Neuroimaging* 1993;**3**:242–9.
38 Adams RJ, McKie V, Nichols F, et al. The use of transcranial ultrasonography to predict stroke in sickle cell disease. *N Engl J Med* 1992;**326**:605–10.
39 Mattle H, Grolimund P, Huber P, et al. Transcranial Doppler sonographic findings in middle cerebral artery disease. *Arch Neurol* 1988;**45**(3): 289–95.
40 Brass LM, Duterte DL, Mohr JP. Anterior cerebral artery velocity changes in disease of the middle cerebral artery stem. *Stroke* 1989;**20**(12):1737–40.
41 Alexandrov AV, Demchuk AM, Wein TH, et al. Yield of transcranial Doppler in acute cerebral ischemia. *Stroke* 1999;**30**:1604–9.
42 Alexandrov AV, Demchuk AM, Felberg RA, et al. Intracranial clot dissolution is associated with embolic signals on transcranial Doppler. *J Neuroimaging* 2000;**10**(1):27–32.
43 Lindegaard K, Bakke S, Grolimund P, et al. Assesment of intracranial hemodynamics in carotid artery disease by transcranial Doppler ultrasound. *J Nuerosurg* 1985;**63**:890–898.
44 Schneider P, Rossman M, Bernstein E, et al. Effect of internal carotid artery occlusion on intracranial hemodynamics: transcranial Doppler evaluation and clinical correlation. *Stroke* 1988;**19**:589–93.
45 Lindegaard KF, Bakke SJ, Aaslid R, et al. Doppler diagnosis of intracranial artery occlusive disorders. *J Neurol Neurosurg Psychiatr.* 1986;**49**:510–8.
46 Zanette EM, Fieschi C, Bozzao L, et al. Comparison of cerebral angiography and transcranial Doppler sonography in acute stroke. *Stroke* 1989;**20**:899–903.
47 Razumovsky AY, Gillard JH, Byran RN, et al. TCD, MRA and MRI in acute cerebral ischemia. *Acta Neurol Scand* 1999;**99**:65–76.
48 Steinke W, Mangold J, Schwartz A, et al. Mechanisms of infarction in the superficial posterior cerebral artery territory. *J Neurol* 1997;**244**(9):571–8.
49 Kimura K, Minematsu K, Yasaka M, et al. Evaluation of posterior cerebral artery flow velocity by transcranial color-coded real-time sonography. *Ultrasound Med Biol* 2000;**26**(2): 195–9.
50 de Bray JM, Missoum A, Dubas F, et al. Detection of vertebrobasilar intracranial stenoses: transcranial Doppler Sonography versus angiography. *J Ultrasound Med* 1997;**16**(3):213–8.
51 Ringelstein EB. Ultrasonic diagnosis of the vertebrobasilar system. II. Transnuchal diagnosis of intracranial vertebrobasilar stenoses using a novel pulsed Doppler system (in German). *Ultraschall Med* 1985;**6**(2):60–7.

52 Budingen HJ, Staudacher T. Identification of the basilar artery with transcranial Doppler sonography (in German). *Ultraschall Med* 1987;**8**(2):95–101.

53 Volc D, Possnigg G, Grisold W, et al. Transcranial Doppler sonography of the vertebro-basilar system. *Acta Neurochir (Wien)* 1988;**90**(3-4):136–8.

54 Alexandrov AV. Transcranial Doppler sonography: principles, examination technique and normal values. Vasc. *Ultrasound Today* 1998;**3**:141–60.

55 Demchuk AM, Christou I, Wein TH, et al. Accuracy and criteria for localizing arterial occlusion with transcranial Doppler. *J Neuroimaging* 2000;**10**:1–12.

56 Droste DW, Nabavi DG, Kemeny V, et al. Echocontrast enhanced transcranial colour-coded duplex offers improved visualization of the vertebrobasilar system. *Acta Neurol Scand* 1998;**98**(3):193–9.

57 Postert T, Federlein J, Przuntek H, et al. Power-based versus conventional transcranial color-coded duplex sonography in the assessment of the vertebrobasilar-posterior system. *J Stroke Cerebrovasc Dis* 1997;**6**:398–404.

58 Baumgartner RW, Mattle HP, Schroth G. Assessment of ≥50% and <50% intracranial stenoses by transcranial color-coded duplex sonography. *Stroke* 1999;**30**(1):87–92.

59 Otis SM, Ringelstein EB. The transcranial Doppler examination: principles and applications of transcranial Doppler sonography. In: Tegeler CH, Babikian VL, Gomez CR, eds. *Neurosonology*. St. Louis, MO: Mosby, 1996:140–55.

60 Schwarze JJ, Babikian V, DeWitt LD, et al. Longitudinal monitoring of intracranial arterial stenoses with transcranial Doppler ultrasonography. *J Neuroimaging* 1994;**4**:182–7.

61 Spencer MP, Reid JM. Quantitation of carotid stenosis with continuous-wave (C-W) Doppler ultrasound. *Stroke* 1979;**10**:326–30.

62 Gosling RG, King DH. Arterial assessment by Doppler-shift ultrasound. *Proc R Soc Med* 1974;**67**:447–9.

63 Kontos HA. Validity of cerebral arterial blood flow calculations from velocity measurements. *Stroke* 1989;**20**:1–3.

64 Evans DH, Barrie WW, Asher MJ, et al. The relationship between ultrasonic pulsatility index and proximal arterial stenosis in a canine model. *Circ Res* 1980;**46**:470–5.

65 Giller CA, Hodges K, Batjer HH. Transcranial Doppler pulsatility in vasodilation and stenosis. *J Neurosurg* 1990;**72**:901–6.

66 Bude RO, Rubin JM. Stenosis of the main artery supplying an organ: effect of end-organ vascular compliance on the poststenotic peak systolic velocity. *J Ultrasound Med* 1999;**18**:603–13.

67 Sharma VK, Tsivgoulis G, Lao AY, et al. Noninvasive detection of diffuse intracranial disease. *Stroke* 2007;**38**:3175–85.

68 Roher AE, Esh C, Rahman A, et al. Atherosclerosis of cerebral arteries in Alzheimer disease. *Stroke* 2004;**35**:2623–7.

69 Roher AE, Garami Z, Alexandrov AV, et al. Interaction of cardiovascular disease and neurodegeneration: *transcranial Doppler ultrasonography and Alzheimer's disease*. *Neurol Res* 2006;**28**:672–8.

70 Alberts MJ, Latchaw RE, Selman WR, et al.; Brain Attack Coalition. Recommendations for comprehensive stroke centers: a consensus statement from the Brain Attack Coalition. *Stroke* 2005;**36**:1597–616.

15 Ultrasound in Acute Stroke: Diagnosis, Reversed Robin Hood Syndrome and Sonothrombolysis

Andrei V. Alexandrov[1], Robert Mikulik[2] & Andrew Demchuk[3]
[1]University of Alabama Hospital, Birmingham, AL, USA
[2]Masaryk University, Brno, Czech Republic
[3]University of Calgary, Calgary, Alberta, Canada

Introduction

Until recently, stroke was viewed as an irreversible disaster with grim prognosis for which nothing could be done. The first success in stroke treatment through systemic reperfusion therapy changed this paradigm [1,2]. Brain recovery after intravenous tissue plasminogen activator (TPA) administration made clinicians look for ways in which the brain and vessels could be imaged better. This chapter reviews how critical changes in blood supply can be detected non-invasively, in real time, at bedside and used to tailor therapeutic options.

We use transcranial ultrasound and carotid duplex as an extension of the neurological examination to identify the presence of a lesion amenable to reperfusion treatment and also the pathogenic mechanism of an ischemic insult. Ultrasound further provides real-time bedside monitoring of thrombus dissolution or re-occlusion, collaterals, cerebral embolization, etc. In addition to providing useful diagnostic information, ultrasound augments residual flow and speeds up thrombolysis, allowing patients to recover from stroke more rapidly.

Diagnosis of lesions amenable to intervention

An acute arterial occlusion is different from chronic since it is often partial and incomplete. In fact, the term occlusion could be too simplistic as these acute lesions encompass dynamic processes of often partial obstruction to flow, thrombus propagation, re-occlusion and sometimes spontaneous recanalization. Thrombi can develop over a pre-existing atheroma or lodge as emboli in a normal vasculature. As "time is brain," so "time is clot," since it can age and damage the vessel wall to which it attaches during this process. Perhaps a better term to use to describe such an obstruction is a "lesion amenable to intervention" [3].

Ultrasound can rapidly identify patients with these lesions regardless of baseline stroke severity. After clinicians started to perform angiography to localize these lesions in acute stroke patients [4,5], traditional assumptions such as "lacunar-type syndrome" presentation, mild stroke severity or even spontaneously resolved deficits offered some surprises as to the underlying vessel patency. Ultrasound provides a tool to detect a flow-limiting lesion, the residual flow around a thrombus, collateralization, ongoing embolization and failure of the vasomotor reserve. On the opposite side of the spectrum, ultrasound can also demonstrate early recanalization and normal vessel patency that point to a good prognosis [6–13].

Ultrasound testing can be performed at bedside using a *fast-track insonation protocol* [12] simultaneously with many activities in the emergency room causing no delay in TPA administration. This protocol should be used only by experienced TCD users with knowledge of the clinical status of the patient.

The choice of fast-track insonation steps is determined by a presumed arterial territory affected by ischemia based on clinical information. For example, if middle cerebral artery (MCA) symptoms are present, insonation begins with locating the MCA on the non-affected side to establish the presence of a temporal window, normal MCA waveform and velocity range. If time permits, insonation of the circle of Willis on the non-affected side should also provide the depth and velocity range for the M1, M2 MCA segments and the internal carotid (ICA) bifurcation. Next, the MCA on the affected side is located with insonation starting at the mid- to-proximal M1 MCA depth range, usually 50–60 mm. The waveform and systolic flow acceleration are compared to

Cerebrovascular Ultrasound in Stroke Prevention and Treatment, 2nd edition.
Edited by Andrei V. Alexandrov. © 2011 Blackwell Publishing Ltd.

the non-affected side. If a normal MCA flow is found, the distal MCA segments are insonated (range 30–45 mm) followed by the proximal MCA and ICA bifurcation assessment (range 45–60 mm and 60–70 mm). If a "blunted" waveform or no signals are found at 50–60 mm, the proximal MCA and ICA bifurcations are insonated before the distal segments. The absence of MCA flow signals can be confirmed by insonation across the midline from the contralateral window (depths 80–100 mm) when feasible. The ophthalmic artery (OA) flow direction and pulsatility are determined next on the affected side at depths of 50–60 mm followed by the ICA siphon assessment via transorbital window at depths of 60–65 mm. The basilar artery (BA) is insonated next to determine if compensatory flow velocity increase or a stenosis is present. Insonation of the vertebral arteries (VA), OA and ICA on the non-affected side, and also PCAs, is performed whenever time permits. Most studies can be accomplished within minutes and often while other patient assessments are ongoing, resulting in no time delays to treatment.

The key ultrasound findings for the *diagnosis of a lesion amenable to intervention* include:

1 one of four abnormal Thrombolysis in Brain Ischemia (TIBI) waveforms [14] in the vessel supplying a territory affected by ischemia; and

2 evidence of flow diversion or collateralization [15] to compensate for this lesion.

In the absence of flow diversion or collateralization, other findings can point to thrombus presence and location, such as stenotic velocities, embolic signals and flow pulsatility changes in vessels proximal and distal to the suspected obstruction [15,16]. With these criteria, a non-image-guided Doppler ultrasound can identify thrombus location with accuracy exceeding 90% for the middle cerebral (MCA) and internal carotid (ICA) arteries [17]. When combined with carotid duplex sonography, TCD can achieve practically 100% agreement with urgent catheter angiography in hyperacute stroke patients [18].

After determining the yield of TCD examination in the emergency room and formulation of the fast track TCD protocol [12], we started to combine TCD with portable bedside carotid/vertebral duplex examination of the cervical vessels [18]. In this subsequent study [18] we described *combined neurovascular ultrasound examination* steps. As with the fast track TCD protocol, this combined assessment is done at bedside and is guided by clinical findings.

Use portable devices with bright display overcoming room light and stand behind the patient headrest (Figure 15.1). Start with TCD since acute occlusion responsible for the neurological deficit is likely located intracranially. Extracranial carotid/vertebral duplex may reveal an additional lesion often responsible for intracranial flow disturbance.

Fast-track insonation steps follow clinical localization of patient symptoms [18].

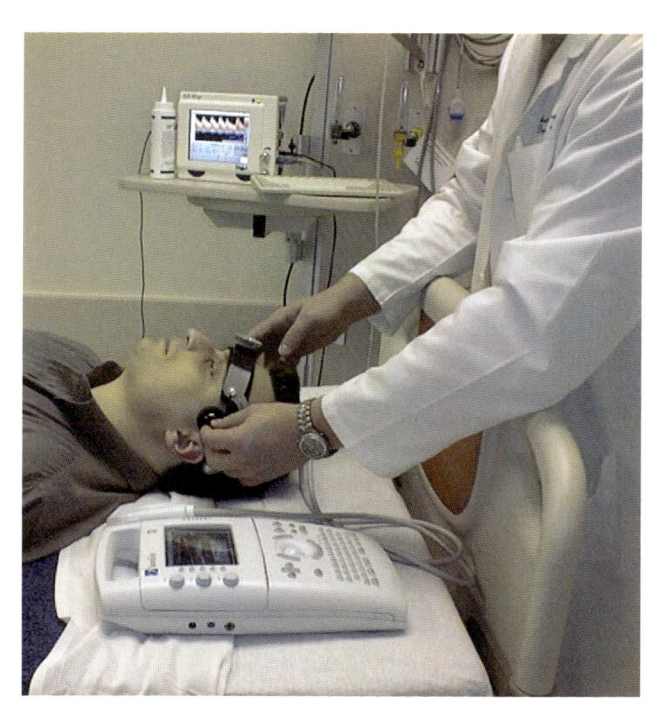

Figure 15.1 A neurovascular ultrasound examination with a portable TCD and carotid duplex system at bedside, ca 2000.

A. Clinical diagnosis of cerebral ischemia in the anterior circulation

STEP 1: Transcranial Doppler

1 If time permits, begin insonation on the *non-affected side* to establish the temporal window, normal MCA waveform (M1 depth 45–65 mm, M2 30–45 mm) and velocity for comparison to the affected side.

2 If short on time, start on *the affected side*: first assess MCA at 50 mm. If no signals are detected, increase the depth to 62 mm. If an antegrade flow signal is found, reduce the depth to trace the MCA stem or identify the worst residual flow signal. Search for possible flow diversion to the ACA, PCA or M2 MCA. Evaluate and compare waveform shapes and systolic flow acceleration.

3 Continue on the *affected side* (transorbital window). Check the flow direction and pulsatility in the ophthalmic artery (OA) at depths of 40–50 mm, followed by ICA siphon at depths of 55–65 mm.

4 If time permits or in patients with pure motor or sensory deficits, evaluate BA (depth 80–100+ mm) and terminal VA (40–80 mm).

STEP 2: Carotid/vertebral duplex

1 Start on the *affected side* in transverse B-mode planes followed by color or power-mode sweep from proximal to distal carotid segments. Identify CCA and its bifurcation on B-mode and flow-carrying lumens.

2 Document if ICA (or CCA) has a lesion on B-mode and corresponding disturbances on flow images. In patients with concomitant chest pain, evaluate CCA as close to the origin as possible.
3 Perform angle-corrected spectral velocity measurements in the mid-to-distal CCA, ICA and ECA.
4 If time permits or in patients with pure motor or sensory deficits, examine the cervical portion of the vertebral arteries (longitudinal B-mode, color or power mode, spectral Doppler) on the *affected side*.
5 If time permits, perform transverse and longitudinal scanning of the arteries on the *non-affected side*.

B. Clinical diagnosis of cerebral ischemia in the posterior circulation

STEP 1: Transcranial Doppler

1 Start suboccipital insonation at 75 mm (VA junction) and identify BA flow at 80–100+ mm.
2 If abnormal signals are present at 75–100 mm, find the terminal VA (40–80 mm) on the non-affected side for comparison and evaluate the terminal VA on the affected side at similar depths.
3 Continue with transtemporal examination to identify PCA (55–75 mm) and possible collateral flow through the posterior communicating artery (check both sides).
4 If time permits, evaluate both MCAs and ACAs (60–75 mm) for a possible compensatory velocity increase as an indirect sign of basilar artery obstruction.

STEP 2: Vertebral/carotid duplex ultrasound

1 Start on the affected side by locating CCA using longitudinal B-mode plane and turn the transducer downwards to visualize shadows from transverse processes of mid-cervical vertebrae.
2 Apply color or power modes and spectral Doppler to identify flow in intra-transverse VA segments.
3 Follow the VA course to its origin and obtain Doppler spectra. Perform a similar examination on the other side.
4 If time permits, perform bilateral duplex examination of the CCA, ICA and ECA as described above.

This combined neurovascular ultrasound examination can yield lesions amenable to intervention in over 90% of patients eligible for reperfusion therapies (Figure 15.2) and in over 40% of patients with transient ischemic attacks or spontaneously resolved symptoms [18]. With these ultrasound tests, one can quickly identify a lesion likely responsible for stroke symptoms, its severity, location and the likely pathogenic mechanism of stroke in the majority of patients, in minutes and at bedside.

To detect acute arterial obstructions and determine the residual flow at thrombus-blood interface, we developed the *Thrombolysis in Brain Ischemia (TIBI) flow grading system* [14]. In analogy with the Thrombolysis in Myocardial Infarction (TIMI) flow grades, TIBI waveforms were developed for TCD to predict intracranial vessel patency and this flow grading system was recently validated against invasive angiography with simultaneous TCD monitoring and intracranial catheter contrast injections [19]. The TIBI flow grading system with detailed definitions was shown in Chapter 6. In short, absent and minimal waveforms predict a complete TIMI 0–I occlusion, blunted and dampened waveforms correlate with persisting or partial occlusions with TIMI II flow and stenotic and normal waveforms indicate complete recanalization with TIMI III reperfusion with or without a residual stenosis.

TIBI flow grades can be used to detect and quantify the revascularization process as these waveforms reflect the beginning, speed, timing and completeness of recanalization [13] (Figure 15.3). Since TIBI waveforms also reflect an overall resistance to flow through changes in velocities during each cardiac cycle, they also are predictive of tissue reperfusion and TIMI flow grades. Recently, this important difference between a proximal recanalization and tissue reperfusion became a focus of scrutiny in acute interventional trials for stroke [20].

In addition to occlusion localization, understanding flow dynamics to and around it is also important since the majority of patients still arrive beyond the current window for reperfusion therapies or continue to have persisting occlusions despite treatment. Ultrasound can provide insights into how arterial blood flow is redistributed and how it responds to certain stimuli.

Reversed Robin Hood syndrome

Historically, the focus of ultrasound examination of intracranial occlusions has shifted from documentation of a simple velocity asymmetry between the homologous segments [7] to the analysis of waveform morphology in the areas of the residual flow–thrombus interface [14] and flow changes at bifurcations and even distal to an occlusion [21–23]. In fact, a combination of the antegrade residual flow, collaterals and potentially reversed filling of the vessels distal to an arterial obstruction [24] likely determine what is now being viewed as islets of penumbra and patches of severely insulted tissues. Ultrasound can provide direct sampling of and also some indirect clues about this arterial flow remodeling that attempts to compensate for an acute obstruction.

The natural way to compensate for an acute arterial occlusion is to steal blood flow, and this concept has been well known in cardiology since the 1960s [25]. Once a feeding vessel is blocked, arteries and arterioles distal to it dilate to decrease resistance and attract blood flow. This mechanism provides an incentive for the blood flow to travel a longer path across collaterals to reach areas distal to an occlusion. Therefore, tissues distal to occlusion steal blood from

CHAPTER 15 Ultrasound in Acute Stroke

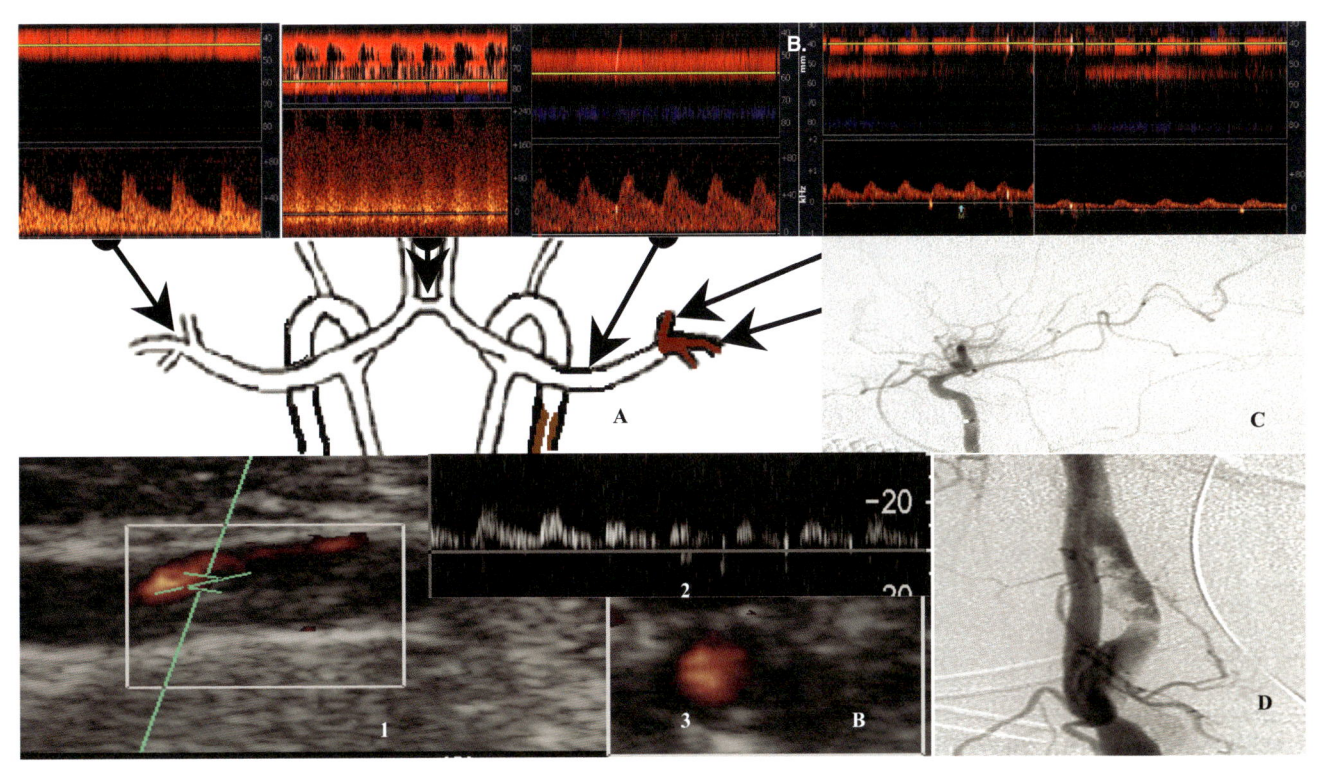

Figure 15.2 A lesion amenable for intervention: duplex scan on the neck and TCD waveforms showing tandem MCA–ICA thrombo-embolic occlusions.
A – Schematic drawing of a tandem acute lesion.
B – TCD waveforms from non-affected and affected sides.
C-D – Catheter angiograms of ICA and MCA lesions.
1,2,3 – Carotid duplex longitudinal image, spectral waveforms and transverse image.

normally perfused areas. Counterintuitively, the same collateral pathways that were recruited to compensate for a lesion can be reversed and steal from malperfused tissues if normal vessel dilate more. We detected this hemodynamic steal phenomenon with TCD in acute ischemic stroke patients and termed it the reversed Robin Hood syndrome in analogy with "rob the poor to feed the rich" [22].

If a stroke patient is challenged with a relative increase in carbon dioxide concentration in the blood stream (i.e. breath-holding), normal arterioles will dilate and the proximal intracranial vessels will show a velocity increase. The vessels distal to an occlusion cannot do it as efficiently and the result is either no change in velocity (exhausted vasomotor reactivity) or a paradoxical velocity decrease at the time when normal vessels start to dilate (Figure 15.4).

We performed a prospective study to establish how often this hemodynamic steal and associated clinical syndrome can be found in acute cerebral ischemia and what major risk factors are associated with these changes [23]. Approximately one in seven patients with acute ischemic stroke or TIA will have detectable and measurable steal on TCD in the proximal branches of the circle of Willis and half of them will have early neurological fluctuation attributable to the steal [22,23]. In the future, if we develop technologies that would allow us to look at bifurcations in real time with simultaneous assessment of flow in different arterial segments (i.e. multi-gate sampling, 3D perfusion imaging, etc.), we are likely to see this steal phenomenon more often [23,26,27] (see Chapter 6, section **Reversed Robin Hood syndrome**). This steal can occur at any level of the arterial tree, perhaps most commonly at the level of vessels distal to current insonation capabilities of TCD. Thus, we had the first glimpse into the real-time patho-physiology of a complex and dynamic process of brain perfusion changes in acute cerebral ischemia. Interestingly, the factors associated with the steal and clinical syndrome included younger age, large vessel atheromatous disease, persisting proximal arterial occlusion, recruitment of major collaterals and daytime sleepiness [23]. In the multivariate analysis, the key factors predictive of the steal were persisting arterial occlusion and daytime sleepiness [23].

Practical implications of this finding are as follows: most acute stroke patients have some level of persisting arterial occlusion and clinicians often see them lying sleepy in bed. This leads to hypoventilation and relative hypercapnia, triggering hemodynamic steal. If a patient has sleep apnea, further hypoxemia may contribute to continuing ischemic damage. The reversed Robin Hood syndrome may provide

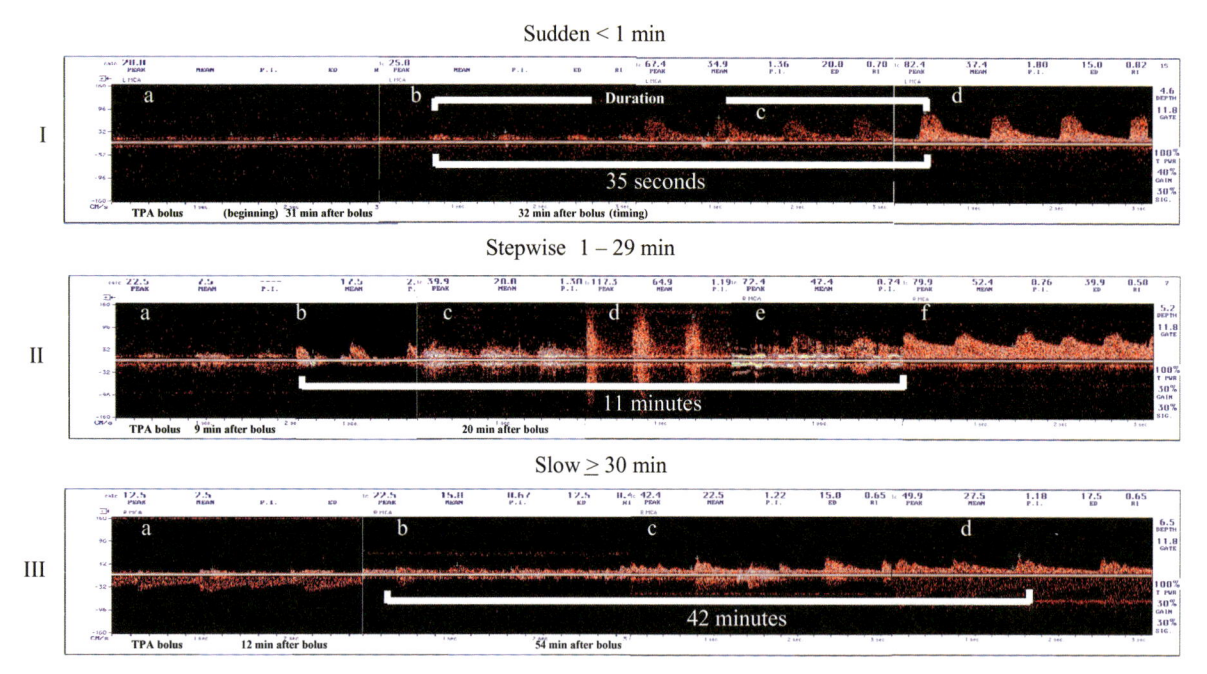

PART IV Ultrasound in Stroke Prevention and Treatment

Figure 15.3 Images I–III show types of recanalization with the beginning, speed, amount and timing of intracranial recanalization. **I: Sudden** (abrupt appearance of a normal or stenotic low resistance signal). (a) TCD shows a minimal signal in the middle cerebral artery (MCA) at the time of TPA bolus. (b) At 31 min after bolus the first improvement in signal intensity was noticed and marked as "beginning" of recanalization. (c) In less than 5 s, the first low-resistance signal was detected with normal waveform and 30 s later (d), a strong normal flow velocity signal was detected. Recanalization started at 31 min after TPA bolus; its duration was 35 s and timing of complete recanalization of the distal M1 MCA segment (TIMI grade III equivalent) was 32 min after TPA bolus. **II: Stepwise** (flow improvement over 1–29 min). (a) TCD shows a minimal signal in the mid-to-distal M1 MCA at the time of TPA bolus. (b) 9 min later TCD shows the first improvement in the amplitude of systolic velocities (beginning of recanalization); however, the absence of end-diastolic velocities still indicates minimal TIBI flow signal and persisting occlusion. (c) At 14 min, positive end-diastolic flow is detected with rounded systolic shape of the waveform (TIBI blunted signal) with flow improvement by 1 TIBI grade. Note high-intensity bruits during each cardiac cycle with possible embolic signals. (d) At 16 min, TCD shows high-resistance turbulent stenotic signals with elevated and variable systolic velocities which are replaced by normal waveforms at 18 min (e). At this point, TCD findings indicate that the M1 MCA patency at the site of insonation is restored. Further improvement in flow velocity, pulsatility and strength of the signal was detected between the 18th and 20th minutes after bolus (f), indicating continuous flow recovery, presumably due to distal clot migration beyond M2 MCA bifurcation. TCD shows the beginning of recanalization at 9 min, duration of 11 min and timing of complete (TIMI grade III equivalent) recanalization at 20 min after TPA bolus. **III: Slow** (30–60 min). (a) At the time of TPA bolus, TCD shows a minimal flow signal at the M1 MCA origin (above baseline) and a flow signal below baseline from the proximal A1 anterior cerebral artery (ACA) with mean flow velocity of 24 cm s^{-1}. (b) At 12 min after bolus, slow positive end-diastolic flow appears in the proximal M1 MCA, indicating the beginning of recanalization. A decrease in the ACA flow signal may indicate clot movement or break-up at its proximal part. Variable M1 MCA and A1 ACA flow velocities with dampened TIBI flow grade are seen during the next 40 min (c) with arrival of the dampened flow signal with the highest mean flow velocity of 28 cm s^{-1} and improved A1 ACA velocities of 54 cm s^{-1} at 54 min after TPA bolus (d). TCD findings indicate the beginning of recanalization at 12 min, duration of 42 min and timing of partial (TIMI grade II equivalent) recanalization with continuing flow diversion to ACA at 54 min after TPA bolus.

a missing link between acute thrombo-embolic occlusion, hypoventilation and sleep apnea and may identify patients for early non-invasive ventilatory correction and brain perfusion augmentation through blood pressure and flow volume manipulations [22,23]. The recurrent and common occurrence of the steal can provide a new target for the development of stroke therapies beyond conventional reperfusion windows.

Other pathogenic mechanisms

As an extension of the neurological examination, TCD provides diagnostic information that is helpful in identifying stroke pathogenic mechanisms in addition to occlusion localization and hemodynamic reserve. TCD is the gold standard to detect circulating emboli in real time. This information is useful for quantifying and localizing cerebral embolization [28,29], such as:

1 ongoing embolization despite anti-thrombotic therapy;
2 artery-to-artery embolization (from extra-and intracranial stenoses, dissections);
3 suspect cardiac sources of embolism;
4 detection of right-to left shunts (and refining findings by echocardiography) and ongoing paradoxical embolization (fat emboli, etc.);
5 peri-procedural or intra-operative emboli detection.

CHAPTER 15 Ultrasound in Acute Stroke

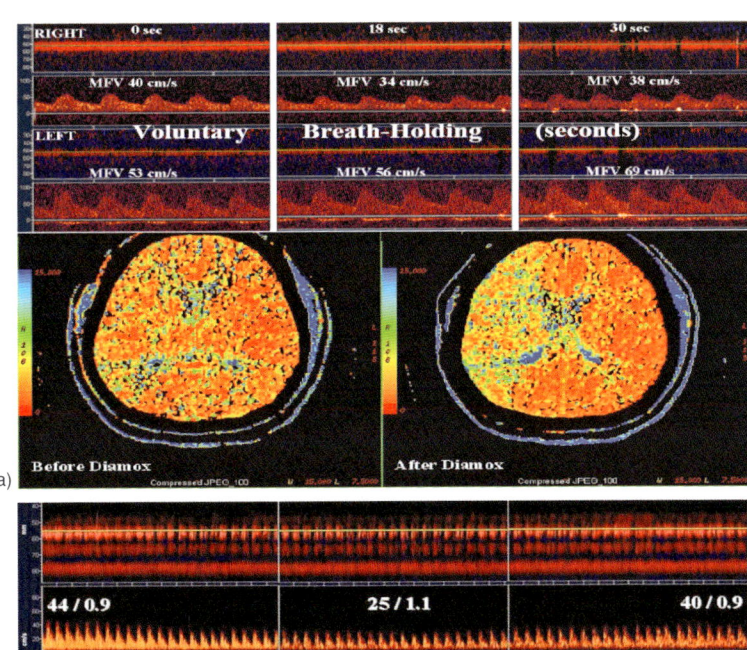

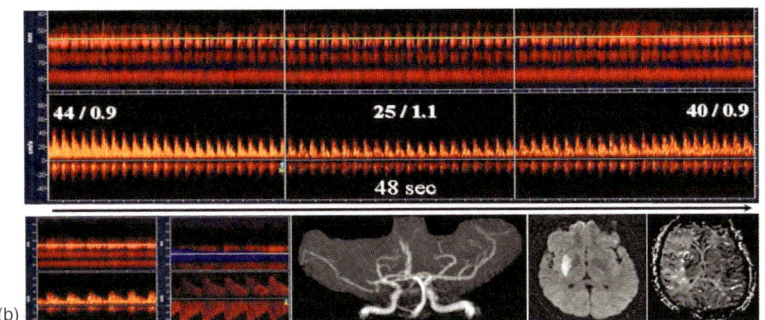

Figure 15.4 Examples of intracranial steal. (A) Voluntary breath-holding index induced paradoxical velocity decrease in the affected vessel at the time of a normal (contralateral) MCA vasodilatation with velocity increase. CT–perfusion images showing steal with administration of diamox. (B) Spontaneous velocity decrease in the affected MCA in a patient with distal M1 MCA occlusion and flow diversion to the ACA. See Chapter 6, section **Reversed Robin Hood syndrome**, for changes detectable by TCD in branching vessels.

TCD examination is complementary to CT- and MR-angiography studies as it compliments snap-shot images with real-time physiological information. TCD provides evidence of flow direction (that cannot be appreciated from static images), collateralization, emboli, short-term dynamic changes and reversed basilar artery [30,31]. The last item particularly underscores the value of TCD in the assessment of acute stroke patients including those with posterior circulation symptoms [31]. In one in 15 patients, TCD offered findings that could not have been appreciated from baseline CT-angiography and helped improve the interpretation of CTA, i.e. findings of M2 MCA branch occlusion and not flow-limiting thrombi manifesting only through distal micro-embolization or marginal velocity increases pointing to the presence of a non-occlusive thrombus [30].

Overall, learning diagnostic and monitoring skills of TCD performance and interpretation should be an integral part of training in vascular neurology. It broadens the clinician's ability to determine the mechanism of stroke, find lesions amenable to intervention and see in real time the results of treatment.

Monitoring thrombolytic therapy with ultrasound

Delaying TPA therapy within 4.5 h of symptom onset in favor of patient selection with imaging methods more time consuming than a non-contrast CT is unjustified since TPA efficacy decreases with time [32] and the first noticeable improvement of flow to the brain occurs at a median time of 17 min after TPA bolus [13]. The median time to completion of recanalization is 35 min after bolus [13] and those patients who complete recanalization before the end of 1 h of TPA infusion are 3.5 times more likely to achieve favorable outcome at 3 months [33].

Spontaneous complete recanalization of the MCA occlusion occurs at a rate of approximately 6% per hour during the first day after symptom onset [8–10,12]. Systemic TPA doubles the chance of complete MCA recanalization to almost 13% during the first hour of treatment [34]. The likelihood of early complete recanalization of the M2 MCA occlusion with systemic TPA is 44%, M1 MCA 30%, tandem MCA–ICA 27% and terminal ICA less than 6% [35] (Figure 15.5). Patients with persisting proximal occlusions have only about a 10% chance of recovering completely at 3 months [35,36] and this information can be used to discuss additional intra-arterial reperfusion procedures to lyse or remove thrombus with a catheter even after full-dose intravenous TPA.

Another unique piece if real-time information that TCD monitoring provides is detection of early arterial re-occlusion [36] (Figure 15.6). It can affect 15–25% of TPA-treated patients, more commonly those with partial or incomplete initial recanalization and large vessel atheromatous stroke mechanism [36,37]. Arterial re-occlusion

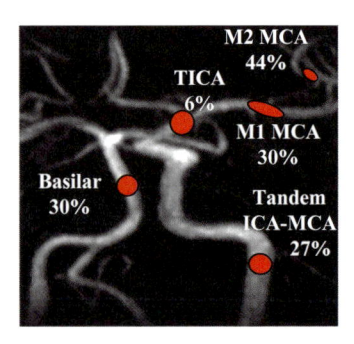

PART IV Ultrasound in Stroke Prevention and Treatment

Figure 15.5 Thrombus location and likelihood of its recanalization with systemic tPA.

accounts for two-thirds of patients who experience neurological deterioration following improvement with TPA therapy [36]. Intracranial arterial re-occlusion can even occur prior to or during TPA administration; however, the majority of these events happen after discontinuation of TPA infusion [36,37]. On average, re-occlusion occurs at 65 min after bolus [36]. After early re-occlusion there is a 33% chance of favorable outcome at 3 months compared with 50% in patients with stable early recanalization [36].

Early complete recanalization is closely associated with dramatic clinical recovery [38–40], and this is thought to be the mechanism by which a reperfusion therapy improves stroke outcomes [41]. Therefore, any effort to amplify the ability of systemic TPA to induce early recanalization should theoretically result in a faster and more complete recovery from stroke. This goal can be achieved through the phenomenon of ultrasound-enhanced thrombolysis.

Ultrasound-enhanced thrombolysis

In the past 30 years, numerous scientists have shown in experimental models that ultrasound facilitates the activity of fibrinolytic agents within minutes of its exposure to thrombus and blood containing drugs [42–51]. The mechanisms of ultrasound-enhanced thrombolysis include improved drug transport, reversible alteration of fibrin structure and increased TPA binding to fibrin for frequencies ranging from kilohertz to those used in diagnostic ultrasound [52–54]. Although kilohertz frequencies penetrate better with less heating, a combination of TPA with an experimental kilohertz delivery system resulted in excessive risk of intracerebral hemorrhage (ICH) in stroke patients [55].

We used diagnostic 2 MHz transcranial Doppler to evaluate acute stroke patients and reported an unexpectedly high rate of complete recanalization and dramatic clinical recovery when TPA infusion was continuously monitored with TCD for diagnostic purposes [38]. The analysis of phase I clinical data [56] allowed us to predetermine a sample size of a phase II clinical trial that, in addition to studying safety of TCD monitoring, was powered to demonstrate a 20% difference in the primary activity end-point of complete recanalization and dramatic clinical recovery within 2 h after TPA bolus [57].

The CLOTBUST trial (Combined Lysis of Thrombus in Brain ischemia using transcranial Ultrasound and Systemic TPA) was a phase II multi-center randomized clinical trial (Houston, Barcelona, Edmonton, Calgary) [34]. All patients with acute ischemic stroke were treated with 0.9 mg kg^{-1} intravenous TPA within 3 h of symptom onset. All patients had MCA occlusions on pretreatment TCD and were randomized to continuous monitoring with TCD (target group) or placebo monitoring (control). Safety end-point was symptomatic ICH. Primary combined activity end-point was complete recanalization on TCD or dramatic clinical recovery to a total National Institutes of Health Stroke Scale (NIHSS) score ≤3 or improvement by ≥10 NIHSS points within 2 h after TPA bolus. Secondary end-points included outcomes at 3 months by the modified Rankin score (mRS).

All projected 126 patients received TPA and were randomized 1:1 to continuous monitoring (median NIHSS 16) or control (median NIHSS 17) [34]. Age, occlusion location (M1 MCA or M2 MCA) on TCD and time to TPA bolus were similar. Symptomatic ICH occurred in three target patients (4.8% CI$_{95}$ 1.0–13.3) and three controls (4.8% CI$_{95}$ 1.0–13.3), $p =$ NS. Complete recanalization or dramatic clinical recovery within 2 h after TPA bolus (primary endpoint) was observed in 31 (49%, target) versus 19 (30%, control), $p = 0.03$. At 3 months, 22 (41.5% target) and 14 (28% control) patients achieved favorable outcomes (mRS 0–1), $p =$ NS.

In stroke patients treated with intravenous TPA, continuous TCD monitoring of intracranial occlusion safely augments TPA-induced arterial recanalization that is coupled with early dramatic clinical recovery (25% target versus 8% control, $p = 0.02$) at 2 h after treatment [34]. The CLOTBUST trial showed that TCD has a positive biological activity that aids systemic thrombolytic therapy and provided clinical evidence for the existence of ultrasound-enhanced thrombolysis in humans. Ultrasound can amplify the existing therapy for ischemic stroke with early brain perfusion augmentation, complete recanalization and dramatic clinical recovery being feasible goals for ultrasound-enhanced thrombolysis. Our international collaborative group focused on testing the ability of ultrasound-activated gaseous microspheres to amplify TPA activity further. More details of ultrasound and microspheres physics can be found in Chapter 16.

Gaseous microspheres and sonolysis

Molina *et al.* pioneered coupling of commercially available microspheres with TCD for the treatment of acute stroke

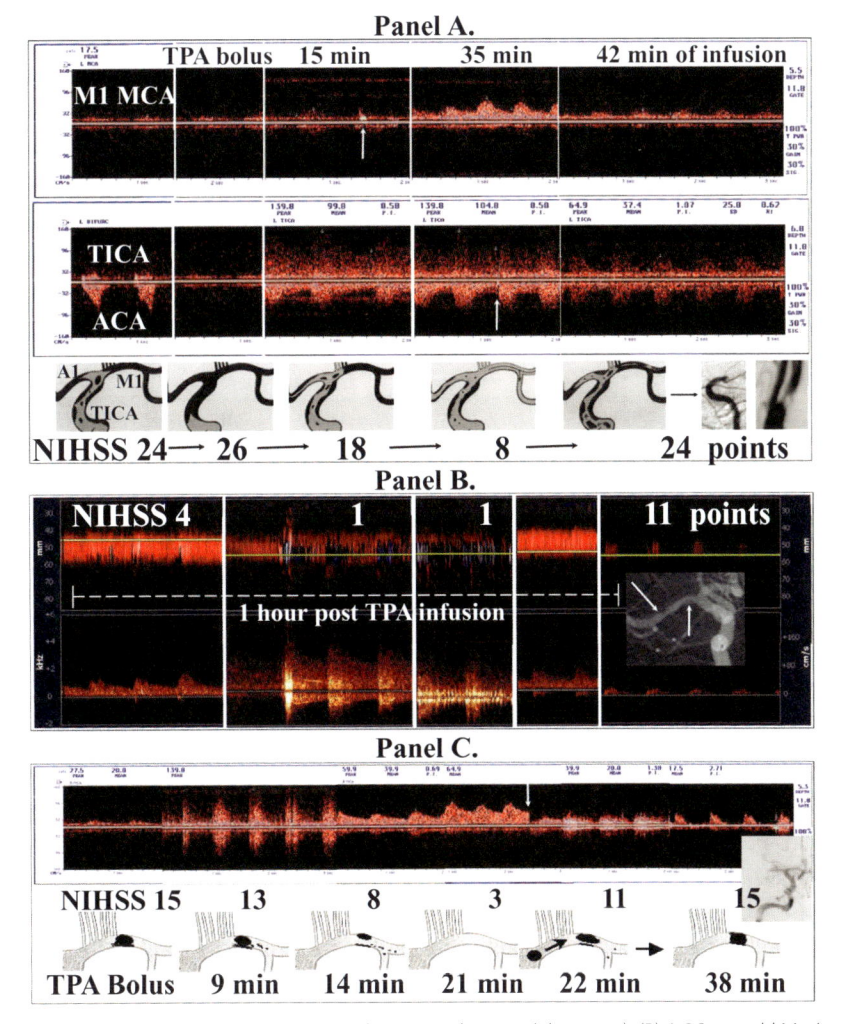

Figure 15.6 (A) A 42-year-old right-handed woman was seen 80 min after the acute onset of right hemiplegia, global aphasia, eye deviation to the left and a right homonymous hemianopsia (NIHSS score 24). TCD showed a proximal M1 MCA and A1 anterior cerebral artery (ACA) occlusion (top left Doppler spectra labeled M1 MCA, TICA and ACA beneath). Second set of Doppler spectra (left to right) shows rapid progression to the terminal internal carotid artery (TICA) occlusion at the time of TPA bolus. At this time, the patient became drowsy (NIHSS score 26). Intravenous tPA was started at 120 min from symptom onset using a standard dose of 0.9 mg kg^{-1}. At 10 min after TPA bolus, TCD showed terminal ICA recanalization with resumption of end-diastolic flow in the A1 ACA followed shortly by improvement in her level of consciousness. At 15 min of infusion, microembolic signals were heard in the M1 MCA accompanied by proximal M1 segment recanalization and resumption of low-resistance end-diastolic flow towards the lenticulostriate perforating arteries. Clinically, her right leg began to move followed by antigravity strength in the distal arm and improved facial weakness (NIHSS score 18). TCD showed a continuing recanalization of the A1 ACA at 20 min, followed by resolution of her gaze preference and continued improvement in her right-sided weakness by 30 min (NIHSS score 15). At 35 min, she had complete M1 MCA recanalization with multiple microembolic signals suggesting continuing proximal clot dissolution. By 37 min, the patient could lift her arm with a mild drift, verbalize simple words and follow axial and extra-axial commands (NIHSS score 8). At 42 min of infusion, TCD showed developing re-occlusion of the M1 MCA and dampening of the terminal ICA flow. At 44 min, the patient rapidly became drowsy and resumed her eye deviation, global aphasia and right hemiplegia (NIHSS score 24). Urgent DSA showed complete terminal ICA "T"-type occlusion and an 80% ulcerated proximal ICA stenosis (DSA images inserted in the bottom right corner). (B) A 26-year-old Mexican man was seen in the Emergency Department at 2 h after symptom onset. He had fluctuating left-sided weakness and episodes of neglect. Intravenous TPA was initiated at 2.5 h after symptom onset. His NIHSS scores were changing between 1 and 11 points during 1 h after TPA infusion. PMD–TCD images show continuing thrombus dissolution and re-occlusion. DSA image inset shows two parts of a thrombus in the right MCA. Continuing re-occlusion process was also seen during angiography at 4.5 h after symptom onset. A foreign body retrieval device was used to remove red thrombus from the MCA. (C) Upper image (left to right) represents sequential TCD monitoring spectra of the distal right M1 MCA. At the time of TPA bolus, the patient had an NIHSS score of 15 points and a blunted (TIBI grade II) residual flow signal, suggesting MCA near occlusion (cartoon). At 9 min after TPA bolus, TCD showed a stenotic (TIBI grade IV) flow signal with clusters of microemboli suggesting MCA clot dissolution (NIHSS score 13)]. At 14–21 min, TCD showed further MCA flow improvement to normal TIBI V flow grade indicating complete M1 MCA recanalization At this time his NIHSS score decreased to 3 points. At 22 min, a sudden drop in MCA flow was detected (white arrow), suggesting re-occlusion since the heart rate and blood pressure remained stable. This sudden M1 MCA obstruction was likely caused by a thrombus that lodged in the proximal MCA and then propagated to the site of insonation (next frame, NIHSS score 11). TCD shows a blunted (TIBI grade II) flow signal with clusters of emboli and bruits. At 38 min after bolus, TCD shows a minimal (TIBI grade I) flow signal that suggests a complete M1 MCA re-occlusion due to the absence of diastolic flow. Note the continuing appearance of emboli during the last cardiac cycle. The DSA image inset shows isolated MCA occlusion without evidence of ICA obstruction.

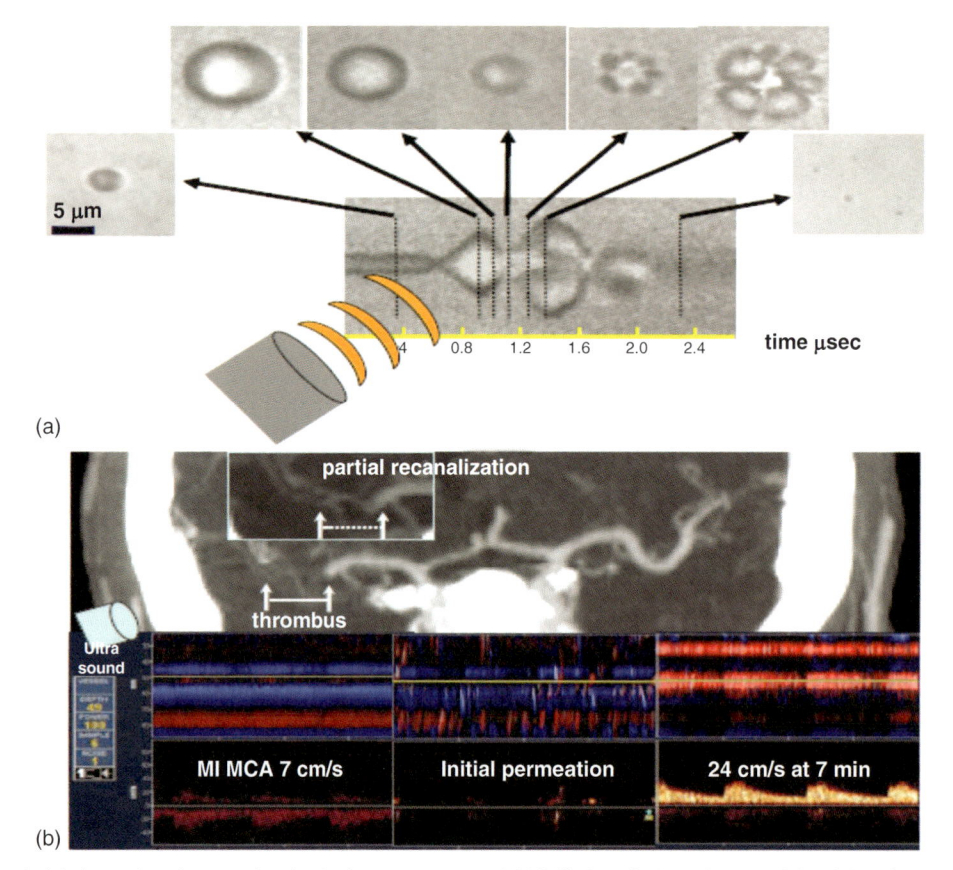

Figure 15.7 Images in (A) show microphotography of a single microsphere destruction by an ultrasound pulse. Time axis is in microseconds. Images in (B) show microsphere permeation around or through the MCA thrombo-embolic material to areas of no flow pretreatment (middle bottom image, "initial permeation"). It was possible to detect this phenomenon in our clinical feasibility study [62,63] due to initial dilution of microspheres and the ability of TCD to detect a single microsphere in the intracranial circulation. The bottom right image shows partial recanalization detected by TCD at 7 min of treatment with tPA + microspheres + TCD. This finding was confirmed by repeat CTA (image inset above "thrombus").

patients [58]. They compared the CLOTBUST target arm with a 2 MHz continuous TCD monitoring combined with Levovist air microspheres (Schering AG) [58]. They demonstrated that at 2 h after rt-PA bolus the rt-PA + TCD + Levovist group achieved a 55% sustained recanalization rate compared with 38% in the rt-PA + TCD group of the CLOTBUST trial.

Since then, several studies have been reported with different types of commercially available microspheres confirming higher recanalization rates with addition of microspheres [59–62]. The safety and feasibility of infusion of new and more stable C_3F_8 (perflutren-lipid) microspheres in patients treated with ultrasound-enhanced thrombolysis has recently been reported [62].

In a pilot clinical trial of perflutren-lipid microspheres with concurrent controls [62], microspheres permeated to areas with no pretreatment residual flow in 75% of patients, and in 83% the residual flow velocity improved at a median of 30 min from the start of microsphere infusion (range 30 s–120 min) by a median of 17 cm s^{-1} or 118% above pretreatment values (Figure 15.7) [63]. No sICH was found in both the target (rt-PA + 2 MHz TCD monitoring + microspheres) and in the control group (rt-PA + 2 MHz TCD monitoring) [62]. Moreover, microspheres were moving at velocities higher than the surrounding residual red blood cell flow in patients with middle cerebral artery occlusions (39.8 ± 11.3 versus 28.8 ± 13.8 cm s^{-1}, $p < 0.001$) [63]. As a signal-of-efficacy, perflutren-lipid microspheres, TCD and rt-PA completely lysed 50% of proximal MCA occlusions, which compares favorably with concurrent and historic controls receiving rt-PA alone [62].

Most recently, a multi-center microsphere dose escalation study called TUCSON (Transcranial Ultrasound in Clinical SONothrombolysis, NCT00504842) was completed [64]. Stroke patients with pretreatment proximal intracranial occlusions on TCD were randomized (2:1 ratio) to rt-PA with perflutren-lipid microspheres (MRX-801) infusion over 90 min (Cohort 1 1.4 ml, Cohort 2 2.8 ml) and continuous TCD insonation while controls received rt-PA and brief TCD assessments. Primary safety end-point was sICH within 36 h post-tPA. Among 35 patients (Cohort 1 = 12, Cohort 2 = 11, controls = 12), no sICH occurred in Cohort1 and controls whereas three (27%, with two fatal) sICHs occurred in Cohort 2 ($p = 0.028$). Sustained complete recanalization rates at the end of TCD monitoring were 67% Cohort 1, 46% Cohort 2 and 33% controls ($p = 0.255$). The median time to any recanalization tended to be shorter in Cohort 1 (30 min/IQR = 6) and Cohort 2 (30 min/IQR = 69) compared with controls (60 min, IQR 5; $p = 0.054$). Although patients with sICH had similar screening and pretreatment SBP levels in comparison with the rest, higher SBP levels were documented in sICH(+) patients at 30, 60 and 90 min and 24–36 h following rt-PA bolus [64].

Although the study was stopped half-way by the sponsor for administrative reasons, this trial showed that perflutren-lipid microspheres can be safely administered with rt-PA at the first dose tier, confirming the previous pilot study results [64].

The rates of recanalization and clinical recovery tended to be higher in both microsphere dose tiers compared with controls. However, it should be noted that sustained complete recanalization rates at the end of TCD monitoring were higher in Cohorts 1 and 2 without reaching statistical significance ($p = 0.255$). Similarly, the differences between groups in terms of functional outcomes were not significant ($p = 0.167$). In agreement with previous studies [58–62], addition of microspheres to rt-PA and ultrasound monitoring should reach at least 50% complete recanalization rate for proximal intracranial occlusions. In a recent meta-analysis, a combination of rt-PA, transcranial ultrasound in the low megahertz range with or without gaseous micro-spheres safely doubled the chance of rt-PA-induced recanalization [65].

Finally, Ribo et al. studied the safety and efficacy of local microsphere administration during intra-arterial thrombolysis and continuous TCD monitoring for the middle cerebral artery recanalization [66]. After no recanalization was achieved with rt-PA, nine patients underwent IA rescue procedures with addition of microspheres, suggesting that combination of ultrasound and intra-arterial microspheres and rt-PA may be a strategy to enhance the thrombolytic effect and increase recanalization rates [66].

Enhancing the only approved systemic therapy for stroke is desirable and microspheres together with ultrasound offer a promising way to reach this target. Microspheres combined with ultrasound may represent a more effective treatment initiation strategy that will help develop an intravenous–intra-arterial approach to recanalize thrombi most resistant to fibrinolysis alone.

To improve ultrasound and microsphere-assisted stroke therapies there is a need to replace an experienced sonographer in emergency situations with an operator-independent device that would reliably deliver ultrasound and activate microspheres at the thrombus–residual flow interface in often restless stroke patients. It would make this technology available to all emergency room and allow phase III clinical trials of ultrasound-enhanced thrombolysis.

References

1 The National Institutes of Neurological Disorders and Stroke rt-PA Stroke Study Group. Tissue plasminogen activator for acute ischemic stroke. *N Engl J Med* 1995;**333**:1581–7.

2 Hacke W, Kaste M, Bluhmki E, et al. Thrombolysis with alteplase 3 to 4.5 hours after acute ischemic stroke. *N Engl J Med* 2008;**359**:1317–29.

3 The IMS Study Investigators. Combined intravenous and intra-arterial recanalization for acute ischemic stroke: The Interventional Management of Stroke Study. *Stroke* 2004;**35**:904–12.

4 Fieschi C, Argentino C, Lenzi GL, et al. Clinical and instrumental evaluation of patients with ischemic stroke within six hours. *J Neurol Sci* 1989;**91**:311–22.

5 del Zoppo GJ, Poeck K, Pessin MS, et al. Recombinant tissue plasminogen activator in acute thrombotic and embolic stroke. *Ann Neurol* 1992;**32**:78–86.

6 Halsey JH Jr. Prognosis of acute hemiplegia estimated by transcranial Doppler ultrasonography. *Stroke* 1988:**19**:648–9.

7 Zanette EM, Fieschi C, Bozzao L, et al. Comparison of cerebral angiography and transcranial Doppler sonography in acute stroke. *Stroke* 1989;**20**:899–903.

8 Ringelstein EB, Biniek R, Weiller C, et al. Type and extent of hemispheric brain infarctions and clinical outcome in early and delayed middle cerebral artery recanalization. *Neurology* 1992;**42**:289–98.

9 Alexandrov AV, Bladin CF, Norris JW. Intracranial blood flow velocities in acute ischemic stroke. *Stroke* 1994;**25**:1378–83.

10 Toni D, Fiorelli M, Zanette EM, et al. Early spontaneous improvement and deterioration of ischemic stroke patients. A serial study with transcranial Doppler ultrasonography. *Stroke* 1998;**29**:1144–8.

11 Kaps M, Link A. Transcranial sonographic monitoring during thrombolytic therapy. *Am J Neuroradiol* 1998;**19**:758–60.

12 Alexandrov AV, Demchuk A, Wein T, et al. The yield of transcranial Doppler in acute cerebral ischemia. *Stroke* 1999;**30**:1605–9.

13 Alexandrov AV, Burgin WS, Demchuk AM, et al. Speed of intracranial clot lysis with intravenous TPA therapy: sonographic classification and short term improvement. *Circulation* 2001;**103**:2897–902.

14 Demchuk AM, Burgin WS, Christou I, et al. Thrombolysis in Brain Ischemia (TIBI) TCD flow grades predict clinical severity, early recovery and mortality in intravenous TPA treated patients. *Stroke* 2001;**32**:89–93.

15 Demchuk AM, Christou I, Wein TH, et al. Specific transcranial Doppler flow findings related to the presence and site of arterial occlusion with transcranial Doppler. *Stroke* 2000;**31**:140–6.

16 Alexandrov AV, Demchuk AM, Felberg RA, et al. Intracranial clot dissolution is associated with embolic signals on transcranial Doppler. *J Neuroimaging* 2000;**10**:27–32.

17 Burgin WS, Malkoff M, Felberg RA, et al. Transcranial Doppler ultrasound criteria for recanalization after thrombolysis for middle cerebral artery stroke. *Stroke* 2000;**31**:1128–32.

18 Chernyshev OY, Garami Z, Calleja S, *et al*. Yield and accuracy of urgent combined carotid/transcranial ultrasound testing in acute cerebral ischemia. *Stroke* 2005;**36**:32–7.

19 Tsivgoulis G, *et al*. TIBI validation. *Circulation* submitted.

20 Khatri P, Neff J, Broderick JP, *et al*.; IMS-I Investigators. Revascularization end points in stroke interventional trials: recanalization versus reperfusion in IMS-I. *Stroke* 2005;**36**(11):2400–3.

21 Kim YS, Meyer JS, Garami Z, *et al*. Arterial blood flow diversion on transcranial Doppler is associated with better improvement in patients with acute middle cerebral artery occlusion. *Cerebrovasc Dis* 2005;**28**:74–8.

22 Alexandrov AV, Sharma VK, Lao AY, *et al*. Reversed Robin Hood syndrome in acute ischemic stroke patients. *Stroke* 2007;**38**:3045–8.

23 Alexandrov AV, Ngyuen TH, Rubiera M, *et al*. Prevalence and risk factors associated with reversed Robin Hood syndrome in acute ischemic stroke. *Stroke* 2009;**40**:2738–42.

24 Liebskind DS. Understanding blood flow: the other side of an acute arterial occlusion. *Intl J Stroke* 2007;**2**:118–20.

25 Becker HM. Steal effect: natural principle of the collateralization of flow of arterial occlusions (in German). *Med Klin* 1969;**64**:882–6.

26 Tsivgoulis G, Sharma VK, Ardelt AA, *et al*. Reversed Robin Hood syndrome: correlation of neurological deterioration with intracerebral steal magnitude. *Stroke* 2008;**39**:725 (Abstract).

27 Alexandrov AV, Tsivgoulis G, Sharma VK, *et al*. Multigate Doppler ultrasound criteria for reversed Robin Hood syndrome in acute ischemic stroke patients. *Cerebrovasc Dis* 2007;**23**(Suppl 1): 25–6.

28 Sloan MA, Alexandrov AV, Tegeler CH, *et al*. Assessment: transcranial Doppler ultrasonography: report of the Therapeutics and Technology Assessment Subcommittee of the American Academy of Neurology. *Neurology* 2004;**62**:1468–81.

29 Alexandrov AV. *Cerebrovascular Ultrasound in Stroke Prevention and Treatment*. New York: Futura/Blackwell, 2004.

30 Tsivgoulis G, Sharma VK, Lao AY, *et al*. Validation of transcranial Doppler with computed tomography angiography in acute cerebral ischemia. *Stroke* 2007;**38**:1245–9.

31 Tsivgoulis G, Sharma VK, Hoover SL, *et al*. Applications and advantages of power motion-mode Doppler in acute posterior circulation cerebral ischemia. *Stroke* 2008;**39**:1197–204.

32 Hacke W, Donnan G, Fieschi C, *et al*.; ATLANTIS Trials Investigators; ECASS Trials Investigators; NINDS rt-PA Study Group Investigators. Association of outcome with early stroke treatment: pooled analysis of ATLANTIS, ECASS and NINDS rt-PA stroke trials. *Lancet* 2004;**363**(9411):768–74.

33 Labiche LA, Malkoff M, Alexandrov AV. Residual flow signals predict complete recanalization in stroke patients treated with TPA. *J Neuroimaging* 2003;**13**:28–33.

34 Alexandrov AV, Molina CA, Grotta JC, *et al*. Ultrasound-enhanced systemic thrombolysis for acute ischemic stroke. *N Engl J Med* 2004;**351**:2170–8.

35 Saqqur M, Uchino K, Demchuk AM, *et al*. Site of arterial occlusion identified by transcranial Doppler (TCD) predicts the response to intravenous thrombolysis for stroke. *Stroke* 2007;**38**:948–54.

36 Alexandrov AV, Grotta JC. Arterial re-occlusion in stroke patients treated with intravenous tissue plasminogen activator. *Neurology* 2002;**59**:862–7.

37 Molina CA, Ribo M, Rubiera M, *et al*. Predictors of early arterial reocclusion after tPA-induced recanalization. *Stroke* 2004;**35**:250 (Abstract).

38 Alexandrov AV, Demchuk AM, Felberg RA, *et al*. High rate of complete recanalization and dramatic clinical recovery during TPA infusion when continuously monitored by 2 MHz transcranial Doppler monitoring. *Stroke* 2000;**31**:610–4.

39 Christou I, Alexandrov AV, Burgin WS, *et al*. Timing of recnalization after TPA therapy determined by transcranial Doppler correlates with clinical recovery from ischemic stroke. *Stroke* 2000;**31**:1812–6.

40 Felberg RA, Okon NJ, El-Mitwalli A, *et al*. Early dramatic recovery during IV-TPA infusion: clinical pattern and outcome in acute MCA stroke. *Stroke* 2002;**33**:1301–7.

41 Rha JH, Saver JL. The impact of recanalization on ischemic stroke outcome: a meta-analysis. *Stroke* 2007;**38**:967–73.

42 Trubestein R, Bernard HR, Etzel F, *et al*. Thrombolysis by ultrasound. *Clin Sci Mol Med* 1976;**51**:697–8.

43 Tachibana K, Tachibana S. Ultrasonic vibration for boosting fibrinolytic effects of urokinase in vivo. *Thromb Haemost* 1981;**46**:211 (Abstract).

44 Lauer CG, Burge R, Tang DB, *et al*. Effect of ultrasound on tissue-type plasminogen activator-induced thrombolysis. *Circulation* 1992;**86**:1257–64.

45 Blinc A, Francis CW, Trudnowski JL, *et al*. Characterization of ultrasound-potentiated fibrinolysis in vitro. *Blood* 1993;**81**:2636–43.

46 Kimura M, Iijima S. Kobayashi K, *et al*. Evaluation of the thrombolytic effect of tissue-type plasminogen activator with ultrasound irradiation: *in vitro* experiment involving assay of the fibrin degradation products from the clot. *Biol Pharm Bull* 1994;**17**:126–30.

47 Akiyama M, Ishibashi T, Yamada T, *et al*. Low-frequency ultrasound penetrates the cranium and enhances thrombolysis in vitro. *Neurosurgery* 1998;**43**:828–32.

48 Suchkova V, Siddiqi FN, Carstensen EL, *et al*. Enhancement of fibrinolysis with 40-kHz ultrasound. *Circulation* 1998;**98**:1030–5.

49 Behrens S, Daffertshoffer M, Spiegel D, *et al*. Low-frequency, low-intensity ultrasound accelerates thrombolysis through the skull. *Ultrasound Med Biol* 1999;**25**:269–73.

50 Spengos K, Behrens S, Daffertshofer M, *et al*. Acceleration of thrombolysis with ultrasound through the cranium in a flow model. *Ultrasound Med Biol* 2000;**26**(5):889–95.

51 Behrens S, Spengos K, Daffertshofer M, *et al*. Transcranial ultrasound-improved thrombolysis: diagnostic vs. therapeutic ultrasound. *Ultrasound Med Biol* 2001;**27**(12):1683–9.

52 Daffertshoffer M, Hennerici M. Ultrasound in the treatment of ischaemic stroke. *Lancet Neurol* 2003;**2**:283–90.

53 Polak JF. Ultrasound energy and the dissolution of thrombus. *N Engl J Med* 2004;**351**:2154–5.

54 Alexandrov AV. Ultrasound enhanced thrombolysis for stroke. *Int J Stroke* 2006;**1**:26–9.

55 Daffertshofer M, Gass A, Ringleb P, *et al*. Transcranial low-frequency ultrasound-mediated thrombolysis in brain ischemia: increased risk of hemorrhage with combined ultrasound and

tissue plasminogen activator: results of a phase II clinical trial. *Stroke* 2005;**36**:1441–6.

56 Alexandrov AV, Demchuk AM, Burgin WS, *et al*. Ultrasound enhanced thrombolysis for acute ischemic stroke: phase I findings of the CLOTBUST trial. *J Neuroimaging* 2004;**14**:113–7.

57 Alexandrov AV, Wojner AW, Grotta JC. CLOTBUST: design of a randomized trial of ultrasound enhanced thrombolysis for acute ischemic stroke. *J Neuroimaging* 2004;**14**:108–12.

58 Molina CA, Ribo M, Rubiera M, *et al*. Microbubble administration accelerates clot lysis during continuous 2-MHz ultrasound monitoring in stroke patients treated with intravenous tissue plasminogen activator. *Stroke* 2006;**37**(2):425–9.

59 Larrue V, Viguier A, Arnaud C, *et al*. Transcranial ultrasound combined with intravenous microbubbles and tissue plasminogen activator for acute ischemic stroke: a randomized controlled study. *Stroke* 2007;**38**:472 (Abstract).

60 Perren F, Loulidi J, Poglia D, *et al*. Microbubble potentiated transcranial duplex ultrasound enhances IV thrombolysis in acute stroke. *J Thromb Thrombolysis* 2008;**25**:219–23.

61 Rubiera M, Ribo M, Delgado-Mederos R, *et al*. Do bubble characteristics affect recanalization in stroke patients treated with microbubble-enhanced sonothrombolysis? *Ultrasound Med Biol* 2008;**34**:1573–7.

62 Alexandrov AV, Mikulik R, Sharma VK, *et al*. A pilot randomized clinical safety study of sonothrombolysis augmentation with ultrasound-activated perflutren-lipid microspheres (μS) for acute ischemic stroke. *Stroke* 2008;**39**:1464–9.

63 Sharma VK, Tsivgoulis G, Lao AY, *et al*. Quantification of microspheres (μS) appearance in brain vessels: implications for residual flow velocity measurements, dose calculations and potential drug delivery. *Stroke* 2008;**39**:1476–81.

64 Molina CA, Barreto AD, Tsivgoulis G, *et al*. Transcranial ultrasound in clinical sonothrombolysis (TUCSON) trial. *Ann Neurol* 2009;**66**:28–38.

65 Tsivgoulis G, Saqqur M, Molina CA, *et al*. Safety and efficacy of ultrasound-enhanced thrombolysis: a meta-analysis of randomized and non-randomized studies. *Stroke* 2010;**41**:280–7.

66 Ribo M, Molina CA, Alvarez B, *et al*. Intra-arterial administration of microbubbles and continuous 2-MHz ultrasound insonation to enhance intra-arterial thrombolysis. *J Neuroimaging* 2009;Epub ahead of print).

16 Ultrasound and Gaseous Microspheres

Flemming Forsberg[1] & Andrei V. Alexandrov[2]
[1]Thomas Jefferson University, Philadelphia, PA, USA
[2]University of Alabama Hospital, Birmingham, AL, USA

Introduction

Gaseous microspheres (μS) have been used for over 20 years as ultrasound contrast agents [1–4], since conventional ultrasound has limited ability to detect blood flow in small vessels or in deep tissues owing to poor reflectivity of blood and strong echoes from surrounding soft tissues. Moreover, it is not always possible to achieve sufficient resolution in gray-scale imaging to differentiate between normal and diseased tissues [1–4].

Contrast agents are a routine part of diagnostic imaging modalities for stroke, including computed tomography (CT) and magnetic resonance imaging (MRI). Ultrasound contrast agents are used in Europe for neurovascular studies (Levovist®, Schering AG; SonoVue™, Bracco), particularly with transcranial Doppler (TCD) if poor temporal windows are encountered, and in the United States (Definity™, Lanteus Medical) for cardiac imaging. Overall, the sensitivity and specificity of diagnostic ultrasound imaging can be improved by intravenous injection of gaseous μS as intravascular contrast agents [1–4]. Microspheres significantly enhance the acoustic backscattering from blood in both Doppler and gray-scale modes, due to the large impedance difference between the gas and the surrounding blood. In this chapter, we describe the physics of gaseous μS interaction with ultrasound including *in vivo* artifacts with reference to emerging therapeutic applications of μS in the neurovascular field.

Ultrasound scattering from gaseous μS

The Rayleigh theory of scattering describes what happens when an ultrasound wave encounters a small spherical object comparable in size to its wavelength. It states that the backscattered wave from a single small scatterer can be considered spherical in the far field (this assumption is governed by the Born approximation). Therefore, the scattered ultrasound intensity I_s is a function of the incident intensity I_0 and the scattering cross-section of the scatterer σ to [5]

$$I_s = \frac{I_0 \sigma}{4\pi z^2} \quad (16.1)$$

where z is the distance between the receiving transducer and the scatterer. The scattering cross-section σ on differences between the adiabatic compressibility κ and the density ρ of the scatterer (index s) and the surrounding medium:

$$\sigma = \frac{4\pi}{9} k^4 r^6 \left\{ \left(\frac{\kappa_s - \kappa}{\kappa} \right)^2 + \frac{1}{3} \left[\frac{3(\rho_s - \rho)}{2\rho_s + \rho} \right]^2 \right\} \quad (16.2)$$

For multiple scatterers within a volume V, the combination of equations (16.1) and (16.2) yields [5]

$$\frac{I_s}{I_0} = \frac{1}{9} nV \frac{k^4 r^6}{z^2} \left\{ \left(\frac{\kappa_s - \kappa}{\kappa} \right)^2 + \frac{1}{3} \left[\frac{3(\rho_s - \rho)}{2\rho_s + \rho} \right]^2 \right\} \quad (16.3)$$

where n is the number density of the uniform scatterers. Of note, the scattering cross-section increases with frequency to the fourth power and scatterer size to the sixth power. This is true for all types of contrast media and the bracketed expression, therefore, holds the key to comparing different agents. Moreover, these equations provide a clue as to whether a "shielding" effect can be achieved if enough μS are "packed" on the way of an ultrasound beam. "Shielding" produces reflection and destruction of the ultrasound beam with no further propagation suitable for imaging. It is a phenomenon similar to shadowing discussed in previous chapters when an ultrasound beam encounters a bright reflector (such as calcium in a carotid plaque). If one imagines μS as small shields, the analogy would be 300 Spartans fighting in unison and successfully deflecting attacks of an enormous Persian army.

Different types of contrast agent materials were compared with interpretation of equation (16.3) by Ophir and Parker [1]. The most significant enhancement of the backscattered signal intensity occurs with gaseous contrast agents (Table 16.1). Maximum enhancement with gaseous reflectors ranges from 8.5 to 28 dB depending on the particular agent [6–9].

Cerebrovascular Ultrasound in Stroke Prevention and Treatment, 2nd edition.
Edited by Andrei V. Alexandrov. © 2011 Blackwell Publishing Ltd.

Table 16.1 Scattering cross-sections for different materials (assuming $r = 5$ μm and $f = 5$ MHz)[a]

Scatterer based on	Compressibility relationship	Density relationship	$\frac{4\pi}{9}k^4 r^6$	$\sigma(m^2)$
Gas	$\kappa_s \gg \kappa$	$\rho_s \ll \rho$	3.8×10^{-15}	~0.38
Solid	$\kappa_s \ll \kappa$	$\rho_s \gg \rho$	3.8×10^{-15}	~6.65×10^{-15}
Liquid	$\kappa_s \approx \kappa$	$\rho_s \approx \rho$	3.8×10^{-15}	~0

[a] κ = adiabatic compressibility; ρ = density of the scatterer; s = index; σ = scattering cross-section; r = radius of the scatterer; f = emitted frequency.

Backscattering and attenuation are interrelated and both depend on the concentration of the contrast agent. However, this dependence in not linear [10,11]. Scattering increases with low concentrations, whereas attenuation caused by multiple scattering dominates when the concentration is high enough (remember the Spartans analogy: surely one or 10 or 50 Spartans could not do the job but just 300 will in a narrow path!). This poses a concentration limit beyond which the agent cannot be used [11] (shielding effect). Furthermore, knowledge of the attenuation coefficient is required to calculate the absolute backscattering coefficient [12]. It has been shown that the frequency-dependent attenuation, $\alpha(f)$, represents a measure of μS concentration and size distribution [13]:

$$\alpha(f) = \int_{R_{min}}^{R_{max}} n(r)\sigma(r)dr \quad (16.4)$$

where the minimum and maximum μS radius are represented by R_{min} and R_{max}, respectively, and $n(r)$ represents μS concentration. This relationship has been used to calculate the μS size distribution of Levovist assuming that the attenuation measured at a given frequency is a relative indication of the number of μS having corresponding diameters. Of note, Levovist, the first commercially available ultrasound contrast agent, had room air bubbles surrounded by a galactose–palmitic shell, and this composition produced less stable spheres of variable diameter relative to later-generation agents such as SonoVue™ and Definity™. Nevertheless, equation (16.4) predicts gaseous contrast behavior and the resulting μS diameters were found to be in reasonable agreement with values measured using optical methods [14].

Contrast microspheres in the circulation

To deploy gaseous μS as ultrasound contrast agents, their diameter has to be less than 8 μm since larger spheres are removed by the lungs or adhesion [15]. However, μS smaller than 8 μm persist for a only few seconds without a protective shell in a fluid with normal values of surface tension [16]. This is much less than the duration required for a contrast agent to pass from a peripheral vein (i.e. the site of injection) to the end-organ target for insonation (see Table 16.2). Consequently, gaseous μS have to be stabilized somehow in order for the agent to achieve sufficiently long persistence and also to survive the pressure changes in the heart and surface tension and adhesion through the lung circulation acting as a filter. Interestingly, artificial heart valves produce a substantial number of nitrogen cavitational microbubbles that probably become coated with lipids and protein from surrounding blood at their creation. It is speculative, but the frequency of these bubbles detection by TCD decreases by 40% after patients with artificial valves have undergone hyperbaric oxygenation [17].

Most contrast agents are stabilized against dissolution and against coalescence by the presence of additional materials at the gas–liquid interface [18,19]. This material could be an elastic solid shell, which enhances stability by supporting a strain to counter the effect of surface tension. Otherwise, the material could be one or a combination of two or more surfactants, which promote stability by greatly reducing the surface tension at the interface. Although sulfur hexafluoride, nitrogen and air are used as μS filling gases [4], the majority of newer agents utilize perfluorochemicals due to their low solubility in blood and high vapor pressure.

Table 16.2 Persistence requirements for an ultrasound contrast agent injected intravenously as a bolus

Route	Time (s)
Peripheral vein to right side of heart	2
Right side of heart to left atrium	4–10
Left atrium to end-organ	8–15
Total duration	12–27

The amount of filling gas imparts sufficient pressure to counter the sum of the Laplace pressure (surface tension) and blood pressure [20,21]. In theory and experiments, despite initial stabilization, contrast μS will undergo significant change in size over time [18–22]. Activation of μS through a 45 s mechanical agitation of gas with future shell components produces initial and fairly consistent μS size adjustment that for Definity™ translates into most of the μS population being 1–2 μm in size. However, body temperature and arterial and venous blood pressure exert forces on μS leading to either swelling or shrinkage depending on the partial pressure of gas in the μS. This is followed by a period of slow diffusion of gas into the blood stream. These changes were originally modeled by van Liew and Burkard assuming a single μS containing a mixture of a filling gas and air of concentrations C_F and C_A, respectively [20,21]. The model equations were presented by Kabalnov et al. [18,19] as

$$(C_F + C_A)RT = \frac{2\sigma_{ST}}{r} + p_B + p_{atm} \quad (16.5)$$

$$-\frac{d}{dt}\left(C_F r^3\right) = 3r D_F L_F C_F \quad (16.6)$$

$$-\frac{d}{dt}\left(C_A r^3\right) = 3r D_A L_A \left(C_A - \frac{p_{atm}}{RT}\right) \quad (16.7)$$

where R is the gas constant, T the absolute temperature and D_F, L_F, D_A and L_A are the diffusion and Ostwald coefficients for the filling gas and for air, respectively. The condition that the vapor pressure of the gas mixture equals the sum of the Laplace pressure, the systemic blood pressure p_B (which here includes the partial pressures of the gases dissolved in the blood) and the atmospheric pressure p_{atm} (101 kPa) is described by equation (16.5). According to Kabalnov et al., the fluctuations in p_B are large with a mean value of 4.3 ± 10 kPa [18]. The gas concentrations and also the μS radius are functions of time and the following boundary conditions apply:

$$r(0) = r_0 \quad (16.8)$$

$$[C_F(0) + C_A(0)]RT = \frac{2\sigma_{ST}}{r_0} + p_B + p_{atm} \quad (16.9)$$

$$(1 - X_F)C_F(0) = X_F C_A(0) \quad (16.10)$$

where r_0 is the bubble size and X_F the mole fraction of the filling gas at the time of injection (i.e. $t = 0$). These equations hold the key to diffusivity of gaseous component and overall longevity of μS in circulation.

Resonance of contrast microspheres

Free air μS can act as harmonic oscillators (i.e. resonate) within a liquid. In fact, their appearance (single, multi-ple, shower or curtain) and clinical value are described in Chapter 10. The Rayleigh–Plesset equation describes the μS behavior within a large volume of incompressible fluid [23]:

$$\rho r \ddot{r} + \frac{3}{2}\rho \dot{r}^2 = p_g - p_B - \frac{2\sigma_{ST}}{r} - \frac{4\mu}{r}\dot{r} \quad (16.11)$$

where p_g is the internal gas pressure of the μS:

$$p_g = (C_A + C_F)RT \quad (16.12)$$

in accordance with equation (16.5) and μ is the viscosity of the liquid. The resonance frequency f_0 of a μS acting as a harmonic oscillator was given by Houghton [24] as

$$f_0 = \frac{1}{2\pi r}\sqrt{\frac{3\lambda}{\rho}\left[P_0 + \left(1 - \frac{1}{3\gamma}\right)\frac{2\sigma_{ST}}{r}\right] - \left(\frac{2\mu}{r\rho}\right)^2} \quad (16.13)$$

One approximation to the resonance frequency commonly applied is [25]

$$f_0 \approx \frac{1}{2\pi r}\sqrt{\frac{3\gamma P_0}{\rho}} \quad (16.14)$$

where γ denotes the adiabatic ideal gas constant and P_0 is the ambient fluid pressure. The assumptions made to derive equation (16.14) are that the damping caused by the surrounding medium is negligible and that there are no effects due to μS surface tension or thermal conductivity. Parameters used for theoretical calculations are given in Table 16.3. The resonance frequency of different sized air μS is given in Table 16.4.

Table 16.3 Parameters used in the theoretical calculations; the values of nitrogen are used as the diffusion and Ostwald coefficients for air

Compound	κ (m²/N)	ρ (kg m⁻³)	$D \times 10^{-9}$ (m² s⁻¹)	$L \times 10^{-6}$
Air	7.05×10^{-6}	1.29	19	14480
C_4F_{10}	7.05×10^{-6}	10.62	6.9	202
SF_6	7.05×10^{-6}	6.52	6.7	2300

Table 16.4 Resonance frequencies of different microsphere sizes

Bubble diameter (μm)	Resonance frequency (MHz)
1	9.5
3	2.4
5	1.3
8	0.8
10	0.6

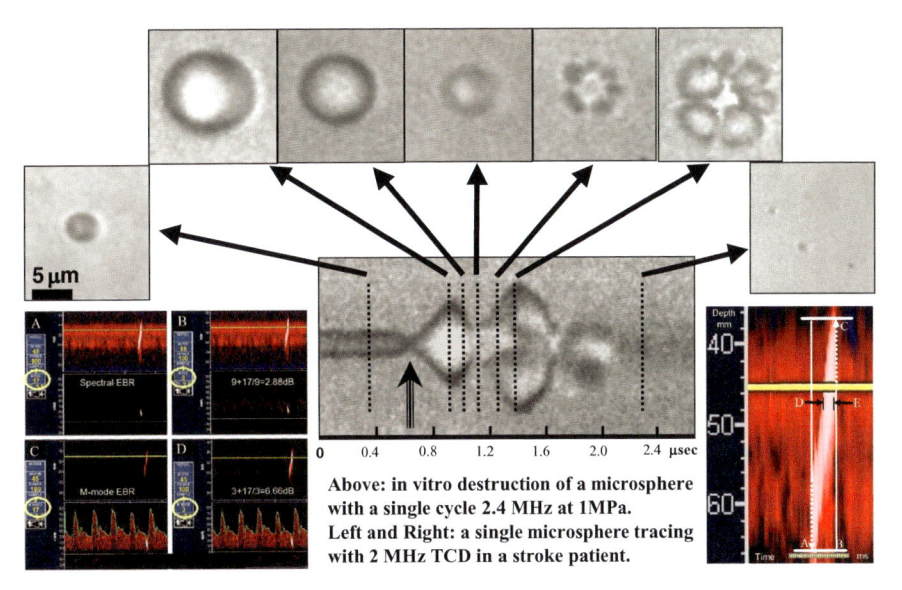

CHAPTER 16 Ultrasound and Gaseous Microspheres

Figure 16.1 Fast *in vitro* destruction and longer reflection times in stroke patients from a single microsphere. High-resolution photographs (courtesy of Kathy Ferrara, UC-Davis) demonstrate "balloon angioplasty"-like inflation and break-up of a microsphere activated and destroyed by ultrasound over just 2 μs. In stroke patients, a standard TCD beam detects microspheres over several milliseconds and over 2–3 cm of intra-beam propagation, This is possible likely due to oscillation rather than rapid destruction. In any case, both destruction and oscillation transmit mechanical energy momentum to surrounding residual flow that could be useful for therapeutic applications. On spectral and power motion TCD, microspheres appear as transient high-intensity signals. EBR is embolus-to-blood ratio measured in decibels (dB).

There is an important effect resulting from resonance of a gaseous μS. The resonance can produce scattering cross-sections 2–3 orders of magnitude larger than their geometric cross-sections. This may have detrimental effects on the accuracy of structural or functional imaging but may have a very useful impact on stagnant residual flow agitation or mechanical energy momentum transmission to the clot. The latter could be useful in therapeutic applications whereby μS act as microscopic balloons inflated transiently by an ultrasound wave to produce microscopic "balloon angioplasty" to the thrombus (Figure 16.1).

The scattering cross-section varies dramatically with the emitted frequency of ultrasound. A second-order expression for the scattering cross-section of a single air-filled μS in water, including losses, was presented by Anderson and Hampton [26]:

$$\sigma = \frac{4\pi r^2}{\left[\left(\frac{f_0}{f}\right)^2 - 1\right]^2 + \left(\frac{f_0}{f}\right)^4 \delta^2} \quad (16.15)$$

where the damping constant, δ, can be written as the sum of the thermal, the viscous and the re-radiation damping constants that can be calculated via Eller's expressions [27].

Thermal damping is the most important parameter below the resonance frequency, whereas re-radiation dominates at frequencies above resonance. As an example, see Figure 16.1, where the scattering cross-section (or physical expansion of reflective surfaces) follows the numeric solution of equation (2.11). At resonance, the scattering cross-section reaches its maximum, which could be 100 times greater than its geometric cross-section. This process is reflected in echoes that are of higher intensity than those registered by ultrasound scanner from surrounding blood. This is measured in decibels (dB). It is unlikely that resonance occurs with 2 MHz TCD, particularly when the beam is further attenuated by the temporal bone. Furthermore, the average size perflutren-lipid microspheres would require resonance frequencies above 2.4 MHz (Table 16.4). We recently evaluated perflutren-lipid microsphere propagation in normal and occluded vessels of acute stroke patients undergoing experimental thrombolysis [28]. For comparison, we used large air-filled microspheres that are detected by TCD in patients with the right-to-left shunts such as patent foramen ovale.

Ultrasound can detect backscatter from a single microsphere (μS) [29], and we recorded single μS traces within a few seconds from the beginning of continuous μS infusion when dilution is maximum. Subsequent traces documented the arrival of multiple clusters of μS and continuous "curtain"-like flow enhancement. Perflutren-lipid μS traces were termed "small" μS since their mean size is 1–2 μm, with 99% of these μS being <7 μm [30]. and almost 100% of <8 μm in size given their stable passage through the lung circulation [31].

The comparison group consisted of air μS (Figure 16.2A) that lack engineered protective shells and are normally filtered out by lung circulation in patients without right-to-left shunts. Therefore, the size of most air μS is likely to be

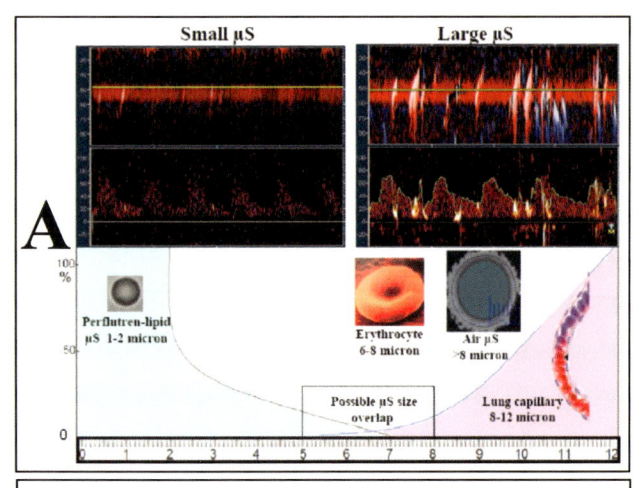

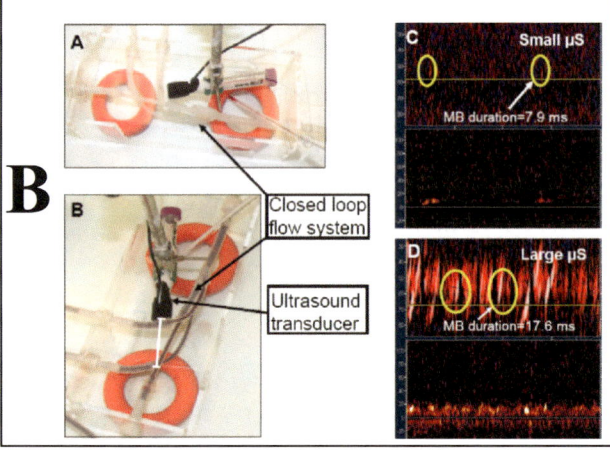

Figure 16.2 Power M-mode and spectral appearance of small and large microspheres in stroke patients (A) and *in vitro* (B). Section A shows sizes of microspheres relative to erythrocytes and lung capillaries. Section B shows calibrated dilution to produce a single microsphere trace in a flow loop model. Modified from Eller [27].

greater than 8 μm, making them larger than erythrocytes (6–8 μm) or the smallest lung capillaries (8 μm) [31]. Even if smaller air μS could exist, they are likely to be unstable and collapse early after injection. These characteristics make TCD testing with agitated saline at least equivalent to echocardiography for the detection of right-to-left shunts such as patent foramen ovale [32–37]. Experimental data suggest that perflutren-lipid μS larger than 5 μm are eliminated from the circulation by adhesion in capillaries [38], while air μS cannot be detected without a shunt (these are filtered out by lung capillaries of 8–12 μm diameter). Therefore, a theoretical overlap for the 5–8 μm range in both size groups becomes negligible (Figure 16.2A). Air μS were termed "large" and these traces were obtained in chronic stroke patients with patent middle cerebral arteries (MCA) who were diagnosed positive for right-to-left shunts (RLS) with routine diagnostic TCD testing. We used normal saline agitated with air according to standard diagnostic protocol (9 cm³ saline + 1 cm³ air) as recommended by the International Consensus Group [32].

We obtained single and multiple μS traces of both estimated sizes in the M1 segment of MCA on the multi-gate power-motion Doppler (PMD 100, Spencer Technologies). A single-crystal pulsed wave 2 MHz TCD beam intercepted the M1 MCA at 40–60 mm depths from the trans-temporal acoustic window [39] with at least 1.5 cm long MCA segment displayed at an assumed 0° angle of insonation. All traces were obtained with a PMD sweep speed of 4 s per frame.

Signal intensities (decibels) were calculated for the μS traces and background cerebral blood flow, both on the motion-mode and spectral display (Figure 16.1B). The embolus-to-blood ratio (EBR), originally proposed for grading emboli size [40], was calculated in decibels using the equation

$$\mathrm{EBR} = \frac{\sigma_\mathrm{B} + \sigma_\mathrm{E}}{\sigma_\mathrm{B}} \quad (16.16)$$

where σ_B is backscatter cross-section of blood flowing within the sample volume and σ_E represents the backscatter cross-section of the embolus.

We also measured (Figure 16.1, left and right PMD–TCD insets):

1 Maximum time width of a high-intensity, horizontal, single μS trace in a small (3 mm) motion-mode gate. This was termed maximum "μS duration" for brevity and displayed in milliseconds.
2 Total duration of μS trajectory through multiple adjacent motion-mode gates (multi-gate travel time-MGTT), in milliseconds.
3 Total distance (millimeters) that μS traveled on the motion-mode display in the M1 MCA (depth range 60–40 mm).
4 μS propagation velocity (distance divided by MGTT), in centimeters per second.

In order to validate our findings from human subjects, we conducted an *in vitro* experiment in a closed-loop flow system mimicking the size of the arteries of the circle of Willis (Figure 16.2B). Plastic tubes resembling the MCA were immersed in a water tank at 37 °C. Normal saline and bovine blood were perfused through the closed loop by a motorized pump that induced pulsatile and unidirectional flow. A 2 MHz transcranial Doppler ultrasound transducer (PMD 100, Spencer Technologies) was aimed to intercept the tube at a 5 cm distance from the transducer surface at a 30° angle of incidence.

The same perflutren-lipid μS were used to obtain small μS traces. Since 1.0 ml of activated agent solution contains 1.2×10^{10} small μS, we performed serial dilutions with normal saline to achieve a total of less than 100 small μS per milliliter of saline. This solution was slowly injected into the

65 ml of circulating bovine blood in the closed loop to obtain single µS traces *in vitro*.

We analyzed 101 single and multiple µS traces from 50 RLS-positive and 10 TPA + µS-treated patients [28]. The median maximum µS duration in a single motion-mode gate and multi-gate travel time (MGTT) of a single large µS (*n* = 62) was 30.8 ms [interquartile range (IQR) 22.0 ms] and 58.6 ± 19.3 ms compared with small µS (*n* = 3 9): duration 8.3 ms (IQR 4.3 ms), MGTT 43.2 ± 13.9 ms, $p < 0.001$.

Small µS had higher intensity ratios (EBR 17.5, IQR 9.3) than large µS (7.5, IQR 4.0), $p < 0.001$, due to reduced cerebral blood flow intensity with acute MCA occlusions (median 1.0 dB, interquartile range 0.2) compared with flow intensities with normal patency in the RLS-positive patients (median 4.0 dB, IQR 3.0, $p < 0.001$).

The receiver-operating characteristic (ROC) curve areas were: duration 0.989 [95% confidence interval (CI) 0.968 to 1.000], MGTT 0.766 (95% CI 0.672 to 0.859) and EBR 0.927 (95% CI 0.871 to 0.982), all $p < 0.001$. After adjustment for all motion-mode and Doppler parameters, including blood flow and µS velocities, a multivariate logistic regression model showed that maximum µS duration [odds ratio (OR) per 1 ms increase: 2.00, 95% CI 1.34 to 2.98; $p = 0.001$] and motion-mode EBR (OR per 1-point decrease: 2.43, 95% CI 1.32 to 4.52; $p = 0.005$) were independently associated with large-sized µS. A longer than 15.1 ms single µS trace duration discriminated large from small µS with sensitivity 98.4%, specificity 100%, PPV 100%, NPV 97.5% and 99% accuracy.

Since the median maximum µS duration was 30.8 ms for large and 8.3 ms for small µS, the median µS number needed to arrive sequentially to produce a continuous or curtain-like appearance of flow enhancement on a 4 s sweep was calculated as 130 (range 51–260) for large µS and 500 (range 265–588) for small µS.

Monitoring of the cerebral blood flow velocities and µS propagation speed showed that despite cerebral blood flow intensity and velocity reductions with acute MCA occlusions, small µS velocities in obstructed vessels (39.8 ± 11.8 cm s^{-1}) were similar to large µS velocities in patent vessels (40.8 ± 11.5 cm s^{-1}; $p = 0.719$). Furthermore, small µS were moving on average 11 cm s^{-1} faster than the residual red blood cell flow at the time of µS appearance (28.8 ± 13.8 cm s^{-1}, $p < 0.001$) while large µS were moving at velocities similar to the surrounding cerebral blood flow. Therefore, we further examined the propagation of small µS in the unobstructed anterior cerebral arteries (ACA) in patients with persisting MCA occlusions. ACA flow signals were detected by motion-mode gates at 60–70 mm simultaneously with µS propagation in the obstructed MCAs. Small µS in the unobstructed vessels moved with a single-gate duration of 8.2 ms (*n* = 10, IQR 1.5), which was similar to the duration in obstructed MCA vessels (8.3 ms, IQR 4.3, $p > 0.9$). Additionally, small µS propagation velocities in patent ACAs were similar to small µS velocities in the obstructed MCAs and large µS velocities in patent vessels (small µS/patent ACA 38.9 ± 13.7 versus small µS/obstructed MCA 39.8 ± 11.3 versus large µS/patent MCA 40.8 ± 11.5 cm s^{-1}, $p > 0.9$).

Single traces for both small and large µS in a controlled closed-loop flow system (Figure 16.1D) showed a median maximum duration for small µS (*n* = 20) of 7.9 ms (IQR 1.6 ms) compared with large µS traces (*n* = 20): median 29.2 ms, IQR 19.9, $p < 0.001$. Mean propagation velocities of small µS (45.5 ± 12.4 cm s^{-1}) were similar to those of large µS (37.6 ± 18.1 cm s^{-1}, $p = 0.129$). EBR could not be obtained since neither motion-mode nor spectral display detected any background signals from circulating bovine blood. A longer than 15.1 ms single µS trace duration discriminated large from small µS in the *in vitro* experiment with sensitivity 95.0%, specificity 100%, PPV 100%, NPV 95.2% and 97.5% accuracy.

This study showed that in patients with normal or reduced flow conditions, the duration of activated µS passage through a small power motion Doppler gate correlates with µS size range and can provide preliminary estimates of µS numbers delivered to an intracranial vessel. While activating µS as potential therapeutic or drug-delivery agents, real-time ultrasound monitoring can determine the minimum number of µS needed to achieve constant flow enhancement, a potentially useful finding for targeted drug delivery.

One unexpected finding in this study is how small µS propagate in patent and obstructed vessels. Although small µS traveled in areas of slower blood flow velocities with acute arterial occlusions, their propagation velocity was comparable to the velocity of small and large µS that traveled through unobstructed vessels with higher blood flow velocities. In other words, µS propagation velocity is comparable to the surrounding blood flow velocity in patent vessels, whereas small µS move faster than the residual blood flow around acute obstructions. This finding may indicate that perflutren-lipid µS smaller than erythrocytes may actually travel with either (a) a velocity that is dependent on the size of µS, the size of the residual lumen and pressure gradients across acute but incomplete obstructions, or (b) the velocity of residual flow around thrombus that is so reduced that it could not be detected without the presence of µS. Of note, these velocity measurements were derived from µS traces on power motion-mode and not from spectral displays. The advantage of power motion-mode is its ability to track the front edge of the returned signal intensity over time. This makes µS velocity measurements independent of artifacts that occur with fast Fourier transformation on spectral analysis.

Since µS can change the signal-to-noise ratio and artificially increase velocities detected by spectral Doppler, an artifact such as "blooming" [41] could affect spectral measurements. However, µS traces were obtained from first-arriving microspheres at concentrations far less lower those

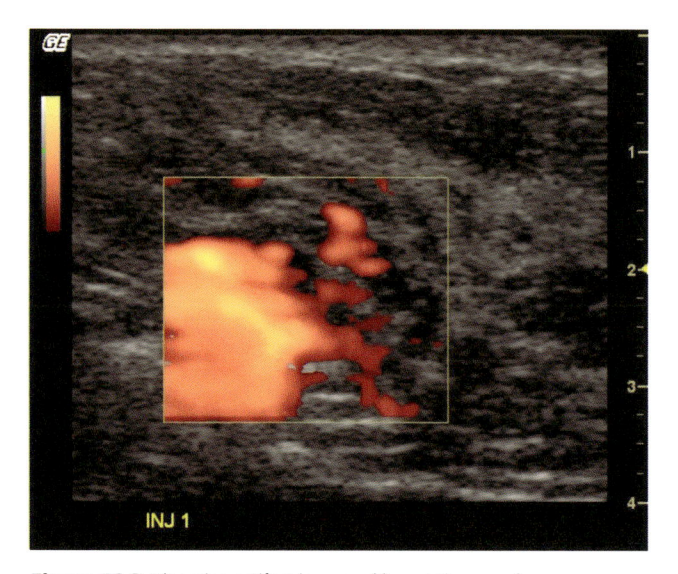

PART IV Ultrasound in Stroke Prevention and Treatment

Figure 16.3 Blooming artifact in normal breast tissue and a fibroadenoma following injection of Optison.

used for imaging (i.e. 1.4 cm³ given as a bolus). Therefore, blooming at the very beginning of continuous infusion of diluted µS should be minimal, if any. If our findings are confirmed in subsequent clinical trials, µS may provide a tool for residual flow assessment around and beyond acute arterial occlusions.

Artifacts and contrast microbubbles

The specific artifacts associated with ultrasonic contrast agent studies are color blooming, spectral bubble noise and increased maximum Doppler shifts [41]. Color blooming occurs immediately after the bolus injection and is seen as pixels changing to color in regions where blood flow is not possible. In Figure 16.3, the post-contrast injection images show large regions of normal breast tissue filling with power mode signal (uni-color scale) caused by the contrast-induced increase in Doppler signal intensity, which effectively lowers the threshold below which weak flow signals are excluded from display (the so-called color reject threshold). Color blooming can be eliminated either by reducing the overall color gain, by waiting for the peak enhancement to pass or by employing a continuous infusion of contrast instead of a bolus injection [41,42]. Spectral bubble noise is seen as very large excursions in the spectral display (Figure 16.4) associated with microsphere rupture within the Doppler sample volume. Both microsphere noise and color blooming are easy to identify and, thus, of limited clinical significance.

The increase in maximum Doppler shifts is a more controversial artifact. Increases in peak Doppler frequency shifts ranging from 15 to 45% have been observed *in vitro* and *in vivo* [41,43–46]. In Figure 16.5, a 33% relative increase in Doppler shifts occurred (from 3.0 to 4.0 kHz) in a rabbit contrast study. Such changes are believed by some researchers to be an artifact arising from the limited dynamic range of the spectral display [41]. When the Doppler signal power increases, the highest frequency shown also increases to accommodate the increased signal-to-noise-ratio (SNR) within the limited dynamic range of the scanner, as explained in a simulation model [47]. However, another simulation study reported a downward shift in mean and maximum Doppler frequencies after contrast administration [48], while other groups have reported no contrast-induced velocity changes in a series of *in vitro* and *in vivo* experiments

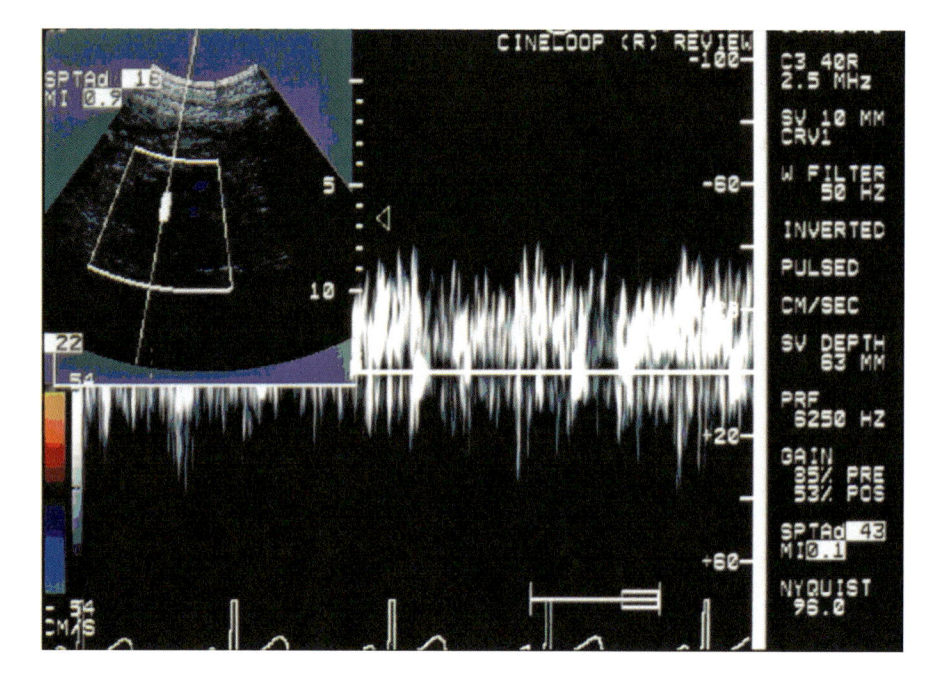

Figure 16.4 Noise artifact seen in the spectral display due to microsphere rupture.

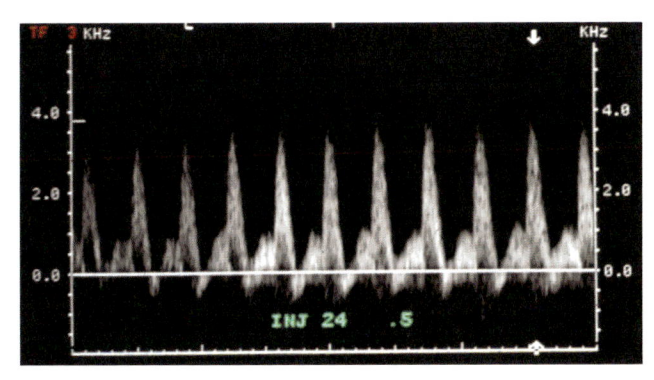

Figure 16.5 Example of the increase in peak Doppler shift (from 3.0 to 4.0 kHz or 33%) observed after contrast administration in a rabbit model.

[49–51]. These contradictions undoubtedly stem from the different experimental conditions employed – Doppler angles >60° in one study and changes in gain settings from pre- to post-assessments in another – or even from different definitions of what constitutes a velocity measurement. Moreover, many other parameters will influence the measured (or simulated) Doppler shift such as the transmitted and received spectral bandwidth, the concentration of microspheres, bubble resonance phenomena and attenuation from intervening tissues [47,48]. Finally, marked spectral broadening has been observed at high acoustic powers due to the destruction of microspheres, which would also impact the velocity measurements [52].

It is clearly not trivial to account correctly for the influence of all these parameters on the final Doppler spectral display. If no signal can be obtained pre-injection (i.e. under poor SNR conditions), this impact is clearly beneficial. Conversely, if an adequate Doppler signal exists pre-injection (i.e. a moderate to good SNR), the impact on peak velocity can be more ambiguous. At least some studies indicate that whether significant peak velocity changes occur or not, the spectral indices appear unaffected [45,50,53]. However, resolving this issue completely will require further studies.

One such study was recently published using a multi-gate power-motion Doppler system to study 60 stroke patients (10 before and after injection of contrast microspheres) [28]. This system bypasses many of the potential artifacts associated with a single-gate pulsed Doppler system. The authors found that microspheres in patent vessels moved with the same velocities as the red blood cells, whereas in obstructed vessels the microspheres flowed 11 cm s^{-1} faster, similar to the plasma flow. It is important to note that in acute stroke patients bolus injections of Levovist likely resulted in an artificial increase in spectral velocity (in the presence of a good temporal window), since occlusions with minimal TIBI residual flow signals often persisted after the initial bolus of bubbles cleared from circulation (Figure 16.6 > [54]. Perhaps continuously infused and diluted microspheres cause less artificial spectral velocity increase [28,55], but better modeling and understanding of these phenomena is required to derive reliable criteria for grading recanalization during mesosphere infusion.

Summary

Gaseous microspheres are by far the most effective scatterers for an ultrasound contrast agent, due to their large

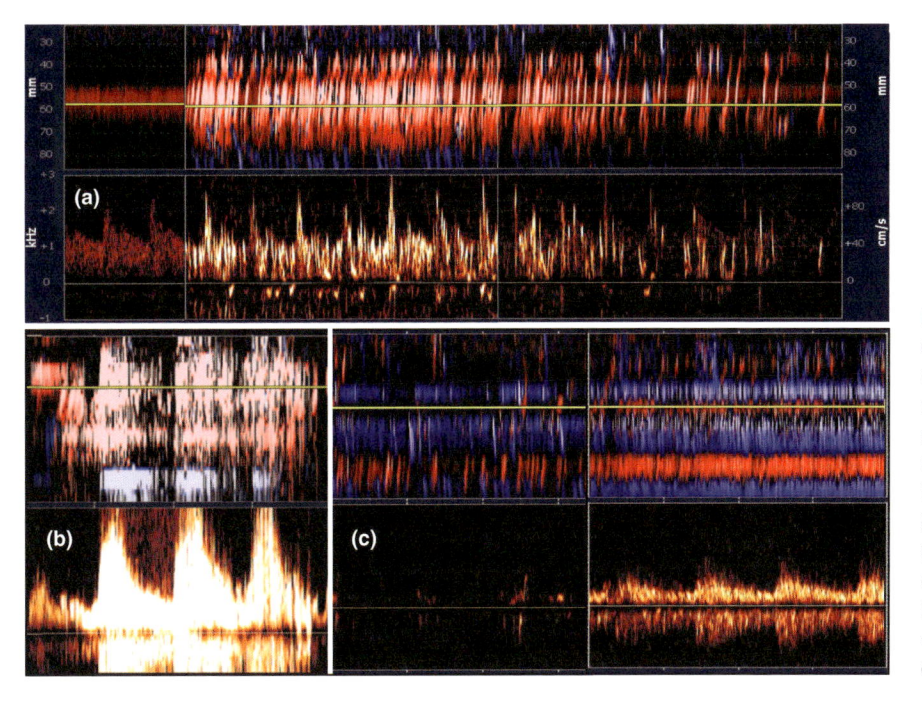

Figure 16.6 Spectral overload due to arrival of too many large air microspheres. (A) Curtain-type appearance of large air-filled microbubbles in a patient with functional patent foramen ovale (bolus injection of normal saline agitated with room air); (B) bolus injection of Levovist in an acute stroke patient; (C) continuous infusion of 2 cm^3 perflutren-lipid microspheres (Definity™) diluted in 100 cm^3 normal saline over 60 min in an acute stroke patient. Diluted small microspheres enhance the spectrum without overloading it.

differences in compressibility compared with the surrounding blood. Microspheres can resonate at a fundamental frequency producing up to three orders of magnitude increases in backscattering. To increase persistence and reduce susceptibility to pressure effects, most contrast agents are stabilized by either an elastic solid shell or a combination of two or more surfactants at the gas–liquid interface. Moreover, the majority of newer agents use higher molecular weight gases in the microbubbles due to their low solubility in blood. Microspheres are being tested in randomized clinical trials [54,55,57,58] and the results are discussed in Chapter 15.

Finally, the latest advances in microsphere technology include targeted or immuno-bubbles, which can recognize receptors (such as GPIIb/IIIa of activated platelets in a thrombus) [56]. These microspheres first can be injected to find the thrombus using delayed ultrasound imaging, i.e. when free circulating microspheres are excreted from circulation. Once thrombus has been located, another injection of targeted microspheres can deliver micro-doses of clot-busting medications to facilitate fibrinolysis at the occlusion site, sparing the rest of the brain from over-exposure to potentially harmful downstream effects of these drugs on ischemic tissues. In conclusion, microspheres appear to be a promising technology for both diagnosis and targeted therapy delivery.

References

1 Ophir J, Parker KJ. Contrast agents in diagnostic ultrasound. *Ultrasound Med Biol* 1989;**15**:319–33.

2 Goldberg BB, Liu JB, Forsberg F. Ultrasound contrast agents: a review. *Ultrasound Med Biol* 1994;**20**:319–33.

3 Needleman L, Forsberg F. Contrast agents in ultrasound. *Ultrasound Q*, 1996;**13**:121–38.

4 Goldberg BB. *Ultrasound Contrast Agents*. London: Martin Dunitz, 1997.

5 Morse PM, Ingard KV. *Theoretical Acoustics*. New York: McGraw-Hill, 1968.

6 Burns PN, Hilpert P, Goldberg BB. Intravenous contrast agent for ultrasound Doppler: in vivo measurement of small tumor vessel dose-response. *Proc. IEEE Eng Med Biol Soc* 1990;**12**:322–4.

7 Forsberg F, Liu JB, Merton DA, *et al.* Parenchymal enhancement and tumor visualization using a new sonographic contrast agent. *J. Ultrasound Med* 1995;**14**:949–57.

8 Frush DP, Babcock DS, White KS, *et al.* Quantification of intravenous contrast-enhanced Doppler power spectrum in the rabbit carotid artery. *Ultrasound Med Biol* 1995;**21**:41–7.

9 Forsberg F, Wu Y, Makin IRS, *et al.* Quantitative acoustic characterization of a new surfactant based ultrasound contrast agent. *Ultrasound Med Biol* 1997;**23**:1201–8.

10 Fan P, Czuwale PJ, Nanda NC, *et al.* Comparison of various agents in contrast enhancement of color Doppler flow images: an *in vitro* study. *Ultrasound Med Biol* 1993;**19**:45–57.

11 Uhlendorf V. Physics of ultrasound contrast imaging: scattering in the linear range. *IEEE Trans Ultrason Ferroelec Freq Control* 1994;**41**:70–9.

12 Shung KK, Sigelman RA, Reid JM. Scattering of ultrasound by blood. *IEEE Trans. Biomed. Eng* 1976;**BME-23**:460–7.

13 de Jong N, ten Cate FJ, Lancee CT, *et al.* Principles and recent developments in ultrasound contrast agents. *Ultrasonics* 1991;**29**:324–30.

14 Schlief R, Schurmann R, Balzer T, *et al.* Saccharide-based contrast agents and their application in vascular Doppler ultrasound. *Adv Echocontrast* 1994;**3**:60–76.

15 Hoff L, Christiansen C, Skotland T. Consideration about the contribution to acoustic backscatter from Albunex microspheres with different sizes. *J Ultrasound Med* 1994;**13**:181–2.

16 Epstein PS, Plesset MS. On the stability of bubbles in liquid–gas solutions. *J Chem Phys* 1950;**18**:1505–9.

17 Kaps M, Hansen J, Weiher M, *et al.* Clinically silent microemboli in patients with artificial prosthetic aortic valves are predominantly gaseous and not solid. *Stroke* 1997;**28**:322–5.

18 Kabalnov A, Klein D, Pelura T, *et al.* Dissolution of multicomponent microbubbles in the bloodstream: 1. Theory. *Ultrasound Med Biol* 1998;**24**:739–49.

19 Kabalnov A, Bradley JA, Flam S, *et al.* Dissolution of multicomponent microbubbles in the bloodstream: 2. Experiment. *Ultrasound Med Biol* 1998;**24**:751–60.

20 van Liew HD, Burkard ME. Bubbles in circulating blood: stabilization and simulations of cyclic changes of size and content. *J Appl Physiol* 1995;**79**:1379–85.

21 van Liew HD, Burkard ME. Behavior of bubbles of slowly permeating gas used for ultrasonic imaging contrast. *Invest Radiol* 1995;**30**:315–21.

22 Forsberg F, Basude R, Liu JB, *et al.* Effect of filling gasses on the backscatter from contrast microbubbles: theory and in vivo measurements. *Ultrasound Med Biol* 1999;**25**:1203–11.

23 Plesset MS, Prosperetti A. Bubble dynamics and cavitation. *Annu Rev Fluid Mech* 1977;**9**:145–85.

24 Houghton G. Theory of bubble pulsation and cavitation. *J Acoust Soc Am* 1963;**35**:1387–93.

25 Minnaert M. On musical air bubbles and the sound of running water. *Philos Mag* 1933;**16**:235–48.

26 Anderson AL, Hampton LD. Acoustics of gas-bearing sediments: I. Background. *J Acoust Soc Am* 1980;**67**:1865–89.

27 Eller AI. Damping constants of pulsating bubbles.. *J Acoust Soc Am* 1970;**47**:1469–70.

28 Sharma VK, Tsivgoulis G, Lao AY, *et al.* Quantification of microspheres (µS) appearance in brain vessels: implications for residual flow velocity measurements, dose calculations and potential drug delivery. *Stroke* 2008;**39**:1476–81.

29 Sboros V, Moran CM, Pye SD, *et al.* The behaviour of individual contrast agent microbubbles. *Ultrasound Med Biol* 2003;**29**:687–94.

30 Unger EC, Porter T, Culp W, *et al.* Therapeutic applications of lipid-coated microbubbles. *Adv Drug Deliv Rev* 2004;**56**:1291–314.

31 Lewis WH, ed.. *Henry Gray's Anatomy of the Human Body*, 20th edn. Philadelphia, PA: Lea & Febiger, 1918.

32 Jauss M, Zanette E. Detection of right-to-left shunt with ultrasound contrast agent and transcranial Doppler sonography. *Cerebrovasc Dis* 2003;**10**:490–6.

33. Belvis R, Leta RG, Marti-Fabregas J, et al. Almost perfect concordance between simultaneous transcranial Doppler and transesophageal echocardiography in the quantification of right-to-left shunts. *J Neuroimaging* 2006;**16**:133–8.

34. Devuyst G, Despland PA, Bogousslavsky J, et al. Complementarity of contrast transcranial Doppler and contrast transesophageal echocardiography for the detection of patent foramen ovale in stroke patients. *Eur Neurol* 1997;**38**:21–5.

35. Droste DW, Schmidt-Rimpler C, Wichter T, et al. Right-to-left-shunts detected by transesophageal echocardiography and transcranial Doppler sonography. *Cerebrovasc Dis* 2004;**17**:191–6.

36. Uzuner N, Horner S, Pichler G, et al. Right-to-left shunt assessed by contrast transcranial Doppler sonography: new insights. *J Ultrasound Med* 2004;**23**:1475–82.

37. Souteyrand G, Motreff P, Lusson JR, et al. Comparison of transthoracic echocardiography using second harmonic imaging, transcranial Doppler and transesophageal echocardiography for the detection of patent foramen ovale in stroke patients. *Eur J Echocardiogr* 2006;**7**:147–54.

38. Lindner JR, Song J, Jayaweera AR, et al. Microvascular rheology of Definity microbubbles after intra-arterial and intravenous administration. *J Am Soc Echocardiogr* 2002;**15**:396–403.

39. Monsein LH, Razumovsky AY, Ackerman SJ, et al. Validation of transcranial Doppler ultrasound with a stereotactic neurosurgical technique. *J Neurosurg* 1995;**82**:972–5.

40. Moehring MA, Klepper JR. Pulse Doppler ultrasound detection, characterization and size estimation of emboli in flowing blood. *IEEE Trans Biomed Eng* 1994;**41**:35–44.

41. Forsberg F, Liu JB, Burns PN, et al. Artifacts in ultrasonic contrast agent studies. *J Ultrasound Med* 1994;**13**:357–65.

42. Albrecht T, Urbank A, Mahler M, et al. Prolongation and optimization of Doppler enhancement with a microbubble US contrast agent by using continuous infusion: preliminary experiences. *Radiology* 1998;**207**:339–47.

43. Wang SH, Chang PP, Shung KK, et al. Some considerations on the measurements of mean frequency shifts and integrated backscatter following administration of Albunex®. *Ultrasound Med Biol* 1996;**22**:441–51.

44. Strauss AL, Veller KD. Arterial parameters under echo contrast enhancement. *Eur J Ultrasound* 1997;**5**:31–8.

45. Needleman L, Forsberg F, Malguria NO, et al. US contrast does not change canine renal Doppler pulsatility indices. *Radiology* 1998;**209**(P): 461 (Abstract).

46. Khan HG, Gailloud P, Bude RO, et al. The effect of contrast material on transcranial Doppler evaluation of normal middle cerebral artery peak systolic velocity. *AJNR Am J Neuroradiol* 2000;**21**:386–90.

47. Sponheim N, Myhrum M. An in vitro study on the influence of the limited frequency resolution on contrast agent-enhanced Doppler signals. *Ultrasonics* 1996;**34**:599–601.

48. Lo MT, Tsao J, Su D. Volume scattering of distributed microbubbles and its influence on blood flow estimation. *IEEE Trans Ultrason Ferroelectr Freq Control* 2003;**50**:1699–710.

49. Petrick J, Zomack M, Schlief R. An investigation of the relationship between ultrasound echo-enhancement and Doppler frequency shift using a pulsatile arterial flow phantom. *Invest Radiol* 1997;**32**:225–35.

50. Gutberlet M, Venz S, Zendel W, et al. Do ultrasonic contrast agents artificially increase maximum Doppler shift? In vivo study of human common carotid arteries. *J Ultrasound Med* 1998;**17**:97–102.

51. Kröger K, Massalha K, Rudofsky G. The use of the echo-enhancing agent Levovist does not influence the estimation of the degree of vascular stenosis calculated form peak systolic ratio, diameter reduction and cross-section area reduction. *Eur J Ultrasound* 1998, **8**:17–24.

52. Shi WT, Forsberg F, Oung H. Spectral broadening in conventional and harmonic Doppler measurements with gaseous contrast agents. *Proc IEEE Ultrasonics Symp* 1997; 1575–8.

53. Forsberg F, Needleman L, Goldberg BB, et al. Contrast enhancement of breast masses. *Ultrasonic Imaging* 1998;**20**:52–3 (Abstract).

54. Molina CA, Ribo M, Rubiera M, et al. Microbubble administration accelerates clot lysis during continuous 2-MHz ultrasound monitoring in stroke patients treated with intravenous tissue plasminogen activator. *Stroke* 2006;**37**(2):425–9.

55. Alexandrov AV, Mikulik R, Sharma VK, et al. A pilot randomized clinical safety study of sonothrombolysis augmentation with ultrasound-activated perflutren-lipid microspheres (μS) for acute ischemic stroke. *Stroke* 2008;**39**:1464–9.

56. Alonso A, Della Martina A, Stroick M, et al. Molecular imaging of human thrombus with novel abciximab immunobubbles and ultrasound. *Stroke* 2007;**38**(5):1508–14.

57. Molina CA, Barreto AD, Tsivgoulis G, et al. Transcranial ultrasound in clinical sonothrombolysis (TUCSON) trial. *Ann Neurol* 2009;**66**:28–38.

58. Tsivgoulis G, Saqqur M, Molina CA, et al. Safety and efficacy of ultrasound-enhanced thrombolysis: a meta-analysis of randomized and non-randomized studies. *Stroke* 2010;**41**:280–7.

17 Neurosonology Pearls

Georgios Tsivgoulis[1], Clotilde Balucani[2] & Vijay K Sharma[3]

[1]University of Alabama Hospital, Birmingham, AL, USA and Democritus University of Thrace, Alexandroupolis, Greece
[2]University of Alabama Hospital, Birmingham, AL, USA and University of Perugia, Perugia, Italy
[3]National University Hospital, Singapore, Singapore

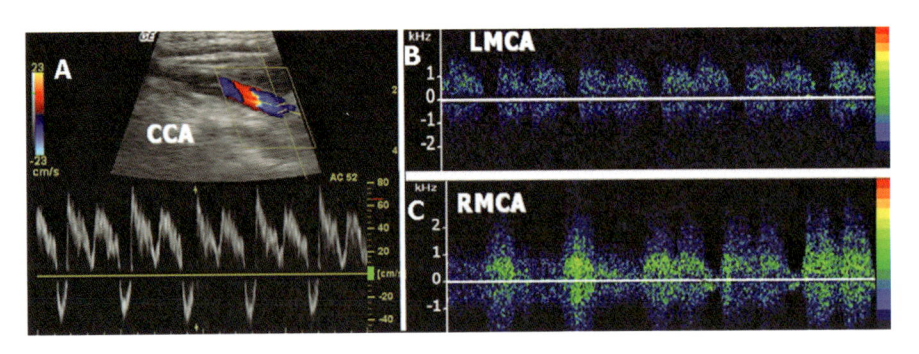

Figure 17.1 Spectral waveform in the CCA and MCA in a patient with intra-aortic balloon pump (IABP). Note that the timing of IABP causes reversal of end-diastolic flow in CCA and flow gaps in the MCA. This can be corrected with proper IABP timing.

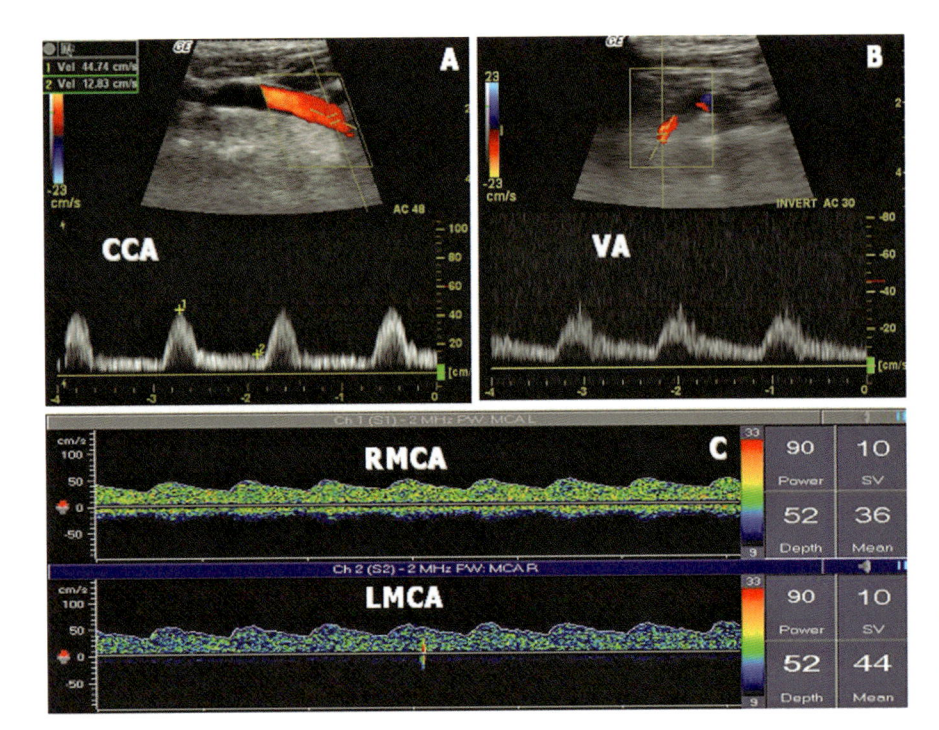

Figure 17.2 Delayed systolic flow acceleration in pre-cerebral vessels and bilaterally blunted MCA waveforms in a patient with severe aortic stenosis.

Cerebrovascular Ultrasound in Stroke Prevention and Treatment, 2nd edition.
Edited by Andrei V. Alexandrov. © 2011 Blackwell Publishing Ltd.

CHAPTER 17 Neurosonology Pearls

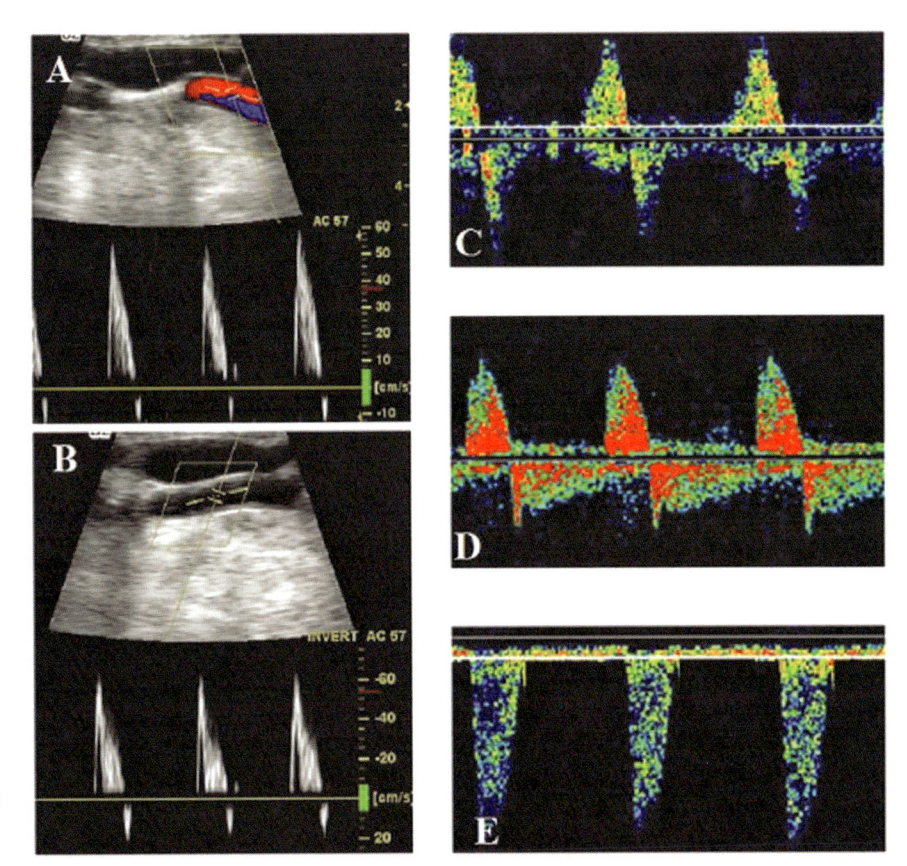

Figure 17.3 Reverberating flow signals in the CCA, MCA and vertebral arteries in a patient with severe aortic valve insufficiency. At the time of examination the patient was arousable and followed commands.

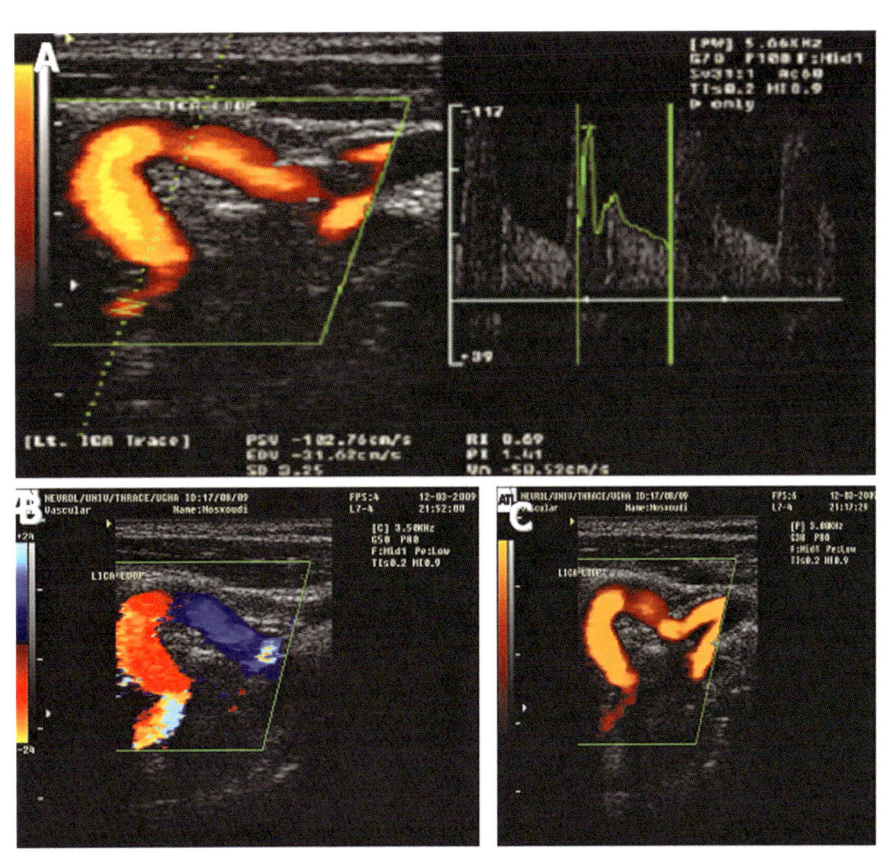

Figure 17.4 Examples of carotid artery loops that cause no significant stenosis (power mode and color flow mode). The presence of aliasing does not indicate stenosis but is caused by low flow-velocity scale setting.

263

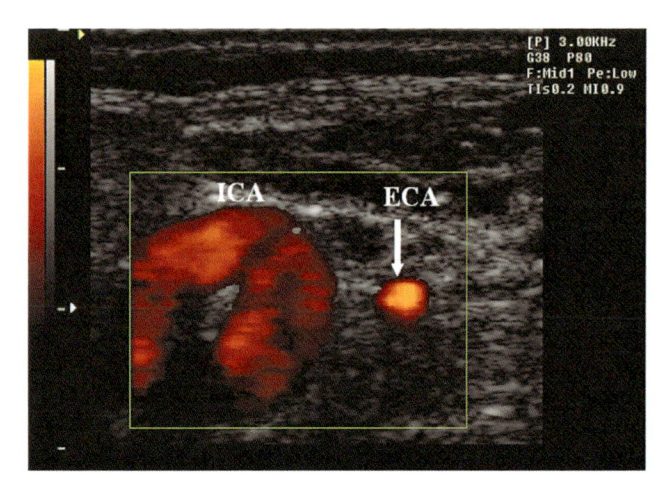

PART IV Ultrasound in Stroke Prevention and Treatment

Figure 17.5 Transverse view demonstrating a loop in the ICA.

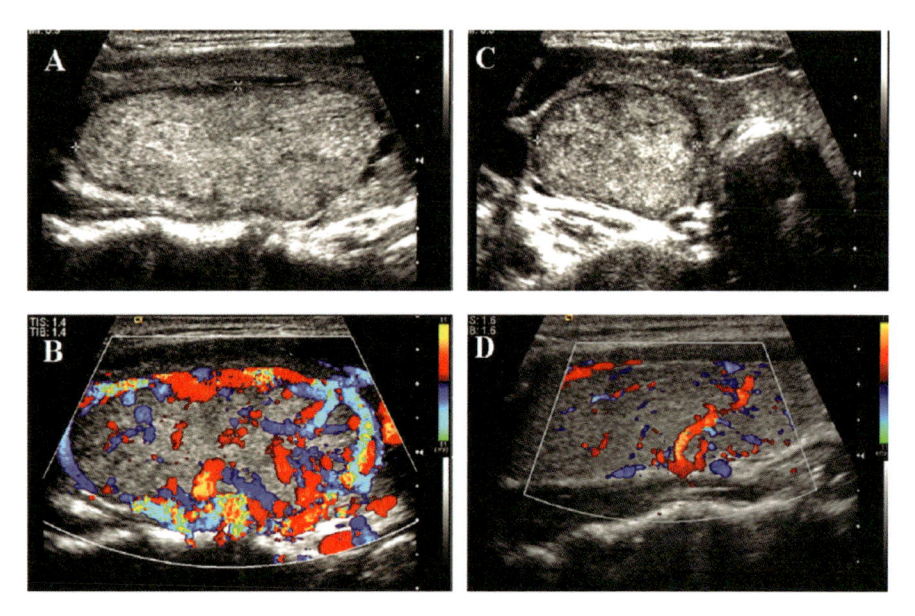

Figure 17.6 Pregnancy-induced vascularity in thyroid mass. Cervical duplex ultrasound in a pregnant woman with transverse view on right side (A) demonstrating a large homogeneous mass in the region of right lobe of the thyroid gland. Color Doppler shows the highly vascularized nature of the mass (B). A repeat ultrasound examination performed 3 months after the delivery shows a considerable reduction in both the size (C) and the vascularity (D) of the thyroid mass.

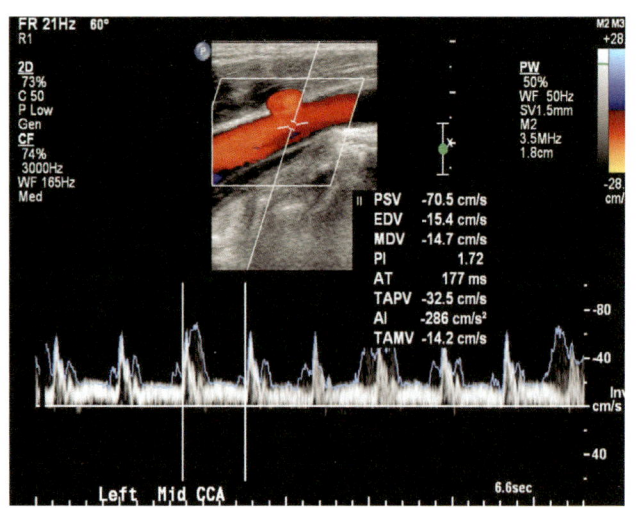

Figure 17.7 Pseudoaneurysm in the CCA caused by internal jugular vein (IJV) line placement.

264

CHAPTER 17 Neurosonology Pearls

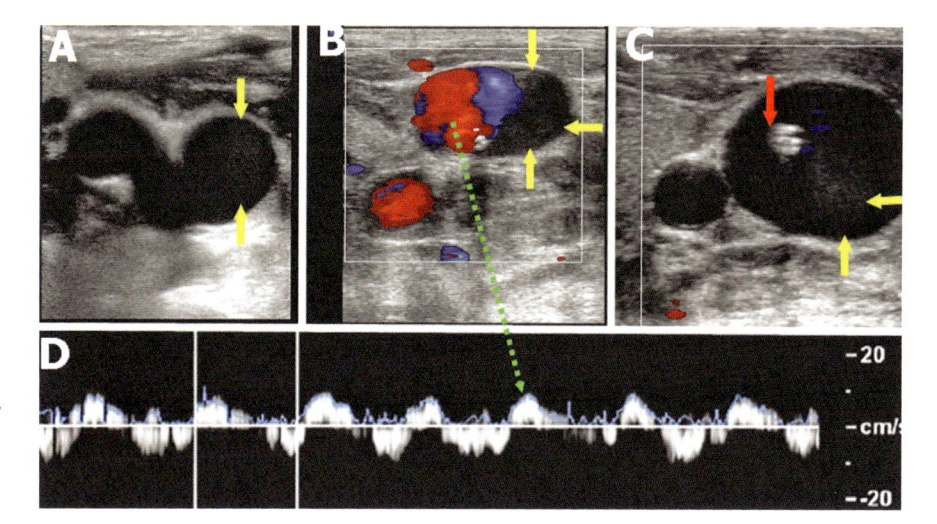

Figure 17.8 Yellow lines indicate thrombus in the internal jugular vein (IJV) adjacent to IJV line placement (red arrow). Note the high-resistance alternating flow in the IJV (waveform) consistent with thrombosis.

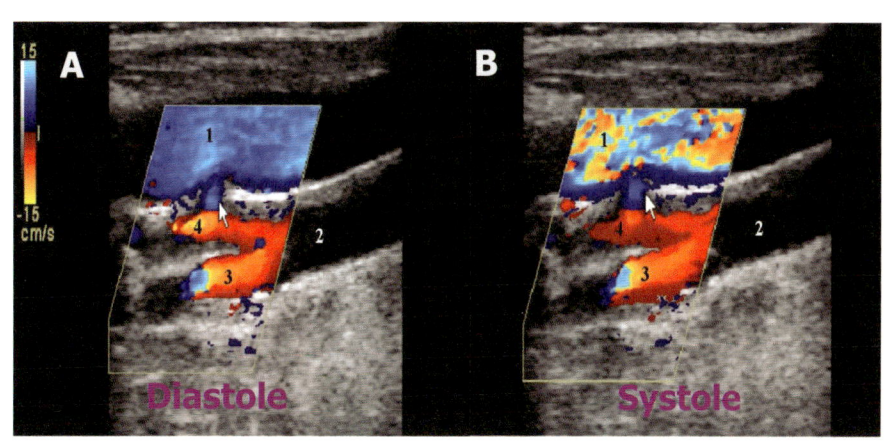

Figure 17.9 Cervical duplex findings in a patient presenting with bruit on the right side of her neck. She had history of repeated episodes of high-output cardiac failure in the past and needed mechanical ventilation during one of the episodes. A central line into the internal jugular vein was inserted during the admissions. She gave a history of a pulsatile swelling on her right side of neck that persisted for many months. (A) Longitudinal view of the right carotid bifurcation during diastole. Although a flow signal is present in the fistula (arrow), normal venous flow is observed in the internal jugular vein. (B) Longitudinal view of the right carotid bifurcation during systole. Note the presence of a color flow signal through a fistula (arrow) between the external carotid artery and the internal jugular vein, causing turbulence in the internal jugular vein. 1, Internal jugular vein; 2, common carotid artery; 3, internal carotid artery, 4: external carotid artery.

Figure 17.10 Systolic flow gaps due to turbulence and bruit that are subtracted by power motion-mode Doppler (PMD). These areas indicate a disturbed flow signal and can lead to better identification of intracranial stenosis.

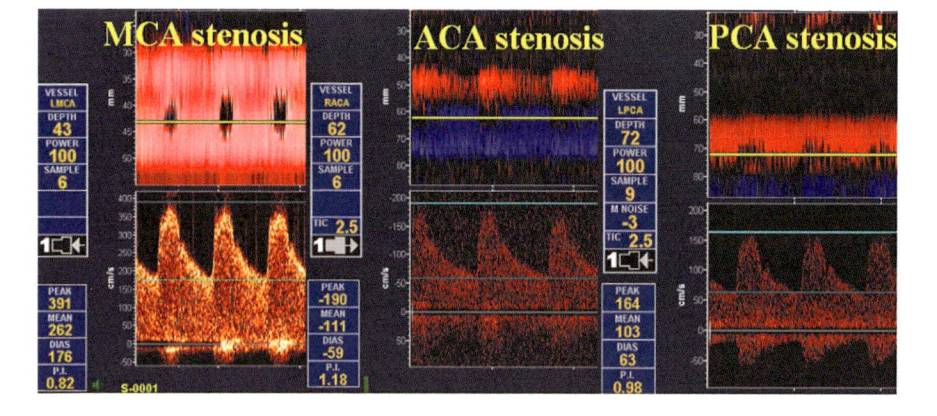

265

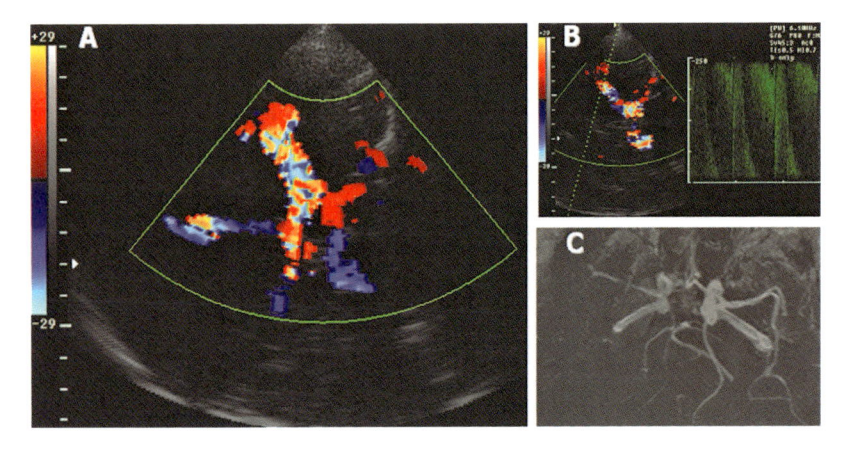

PART IV Ultrasound in Stroke Prevention and Treatment

Figure 17.11 Aliasing and blooming during contrast enhanced duplex sonography (A) in a patient with a severe right M1 MCA stenosis (C). Note the double aliasing in a unidirectional spectral insert (B) during non contrast-enhanced velocity measurements (PSV exceeds 500 cm s^{-1}, maximum scale setting 250 cm s^{-1}). The only measurement not affected by aliasing is the EDV that is approximately 230 cm s^{-1}.

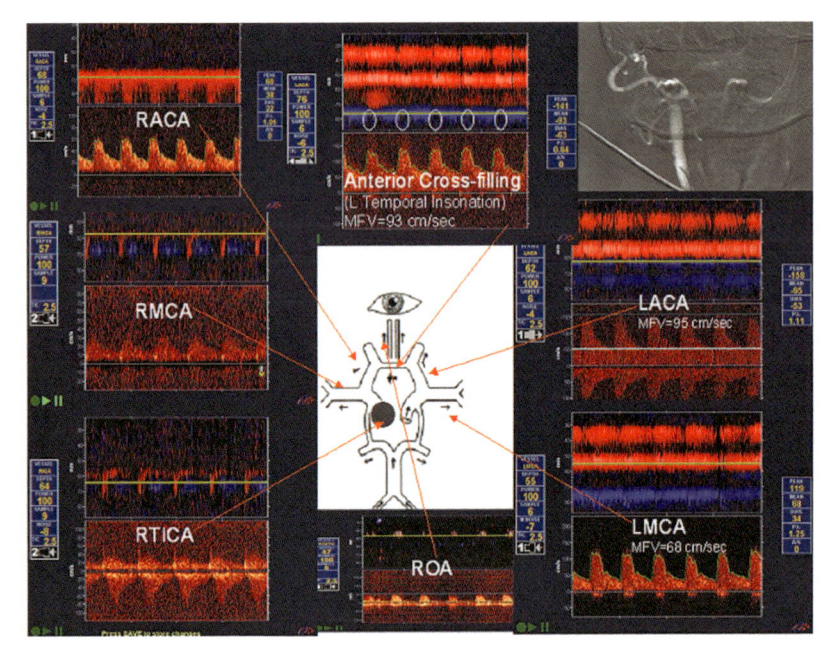

Figure 17.12 Patient with right proximal ICA (internal carotid artery) occlusion, left-to-right anterior cross-filling and retrograde filling of the right ICA siphon. Note the high-resistance flow reversal in the terminal ICA and antegrade flow in the right OA (ophthalmic artery).

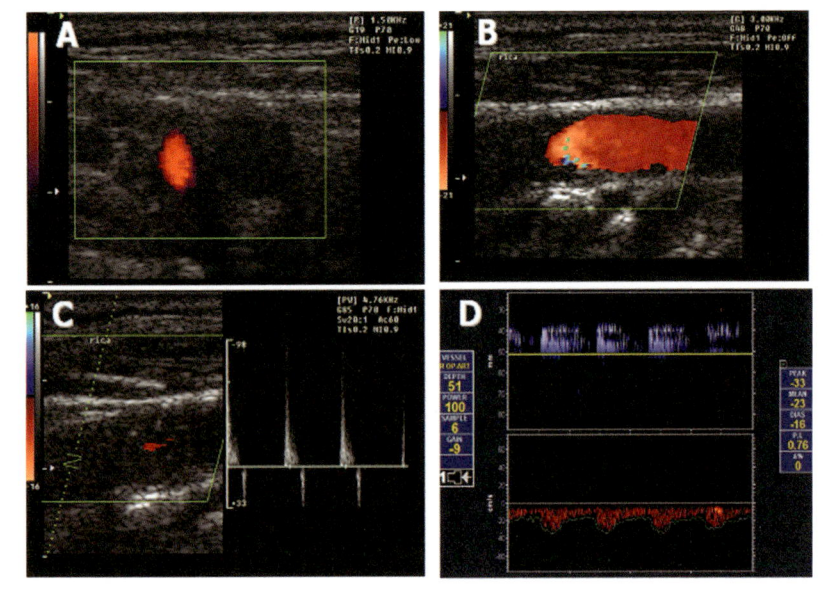

Figure 17.13 Proximal ICA (internal carotid artery) thrombosis with OA (ophthalmic artery) flow reversal. Only ECA has detectable flow in transverse scanning (A). Distal CCA (common carotid artery) flow just proximal to ICA thrombosis (B). Reverberating drum-like waveform in the ICA indicating complete occlusion (C). Low-resistance reversed flow in OA (D).

CHAPTER 17 Neurosonology Pearls

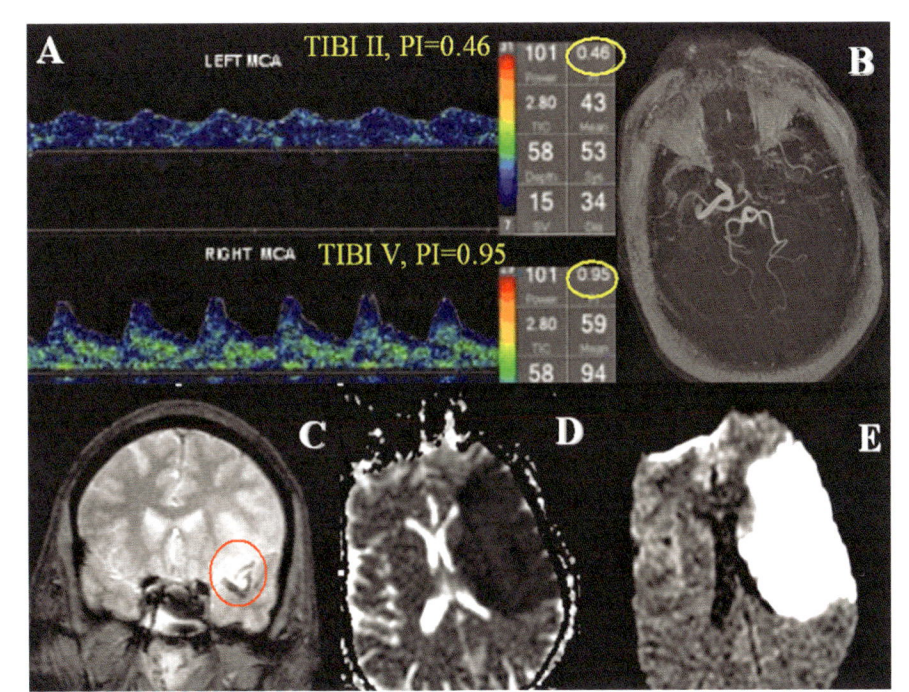

Figure 17.14 Acute left L-type TICA (terminal internal carotid artery) thrombosis with thrombus extending in left M1MCA. MRA overestimates the degree of obstruction by showing complete flow void. TCD shows blunted left M1 MCA (middle cerebral artery) signal representing residual flow around the thrombus in the proximal left MCA. [(C) MR gradient echo image showing thrombus in left M1MCA, red circle.] MR DWI and ADC images indicating large hemispheric acute stroke with restricted diffusion.

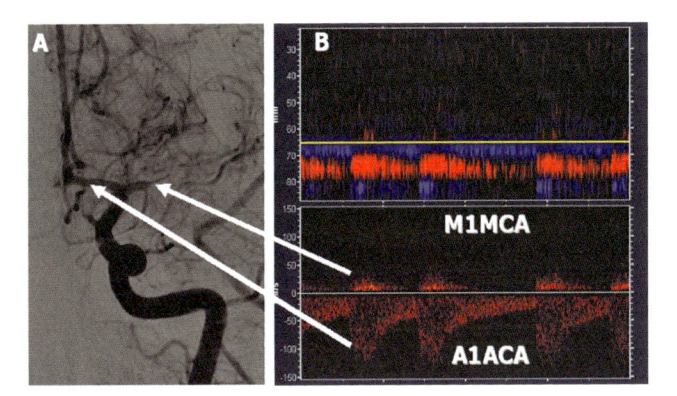

Figure 17.15 Typical appearance of a M1 MCA occlusion with flow diversion to ACA. Note also irregular heart rhythm (the patient has a history of atrial fibrillation).

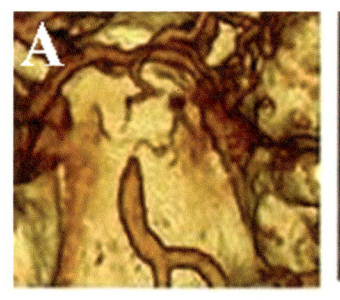

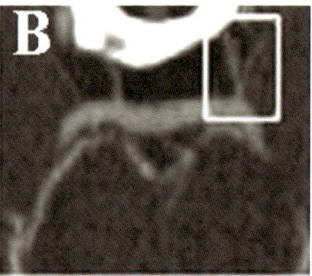

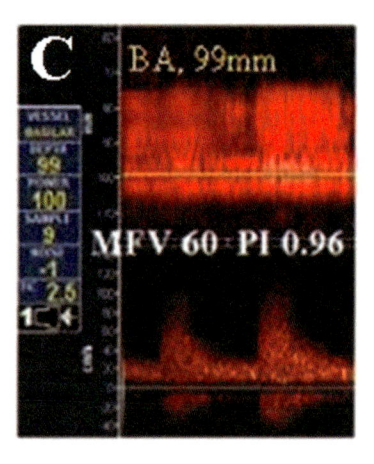

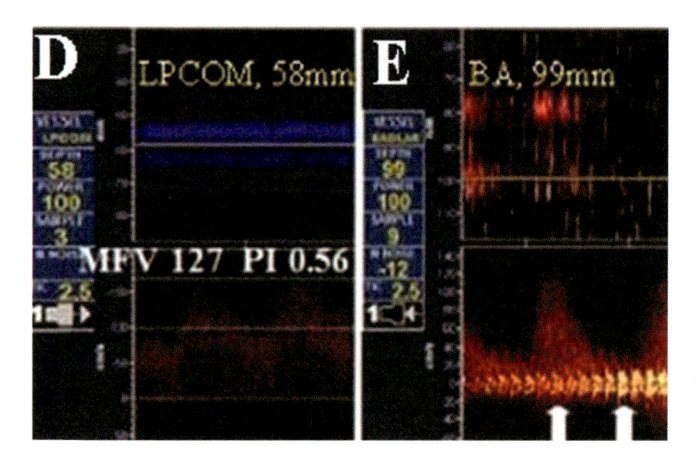

PART IV Ultrasound in Stroke Prevention and Treatment

Figure 17.16 Reversed mid and distal BA flow signatures on PMD (C) in a patient with a proximal BA occlusion on CTA (A). Both PMD and spectrogram showed a response to the left carotid tapping (white arrows, E) indicating that the reversed BA flow is supplied from the anterior circulation vessels. Transtemporal insonation showed the stenotic-like, low-resistance flow directed away from the probe in the left PCom (D) also seen on axial CTA sequences (B; white square).

CHAPTER 17 Neurosonology Pearls

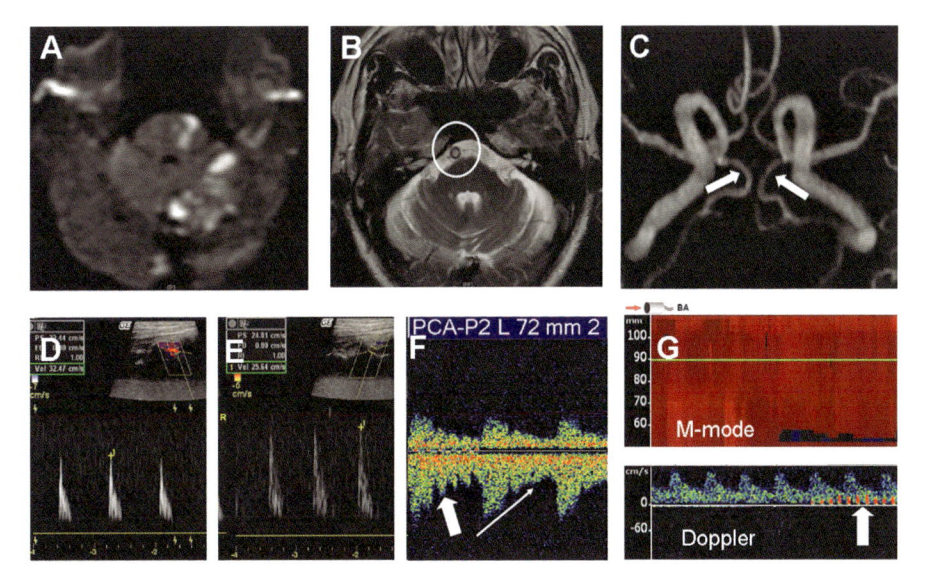

Figure 17.17 Reversed flow in the basilar artery in a patient with acute thrombosis of distal vertebral and proximal basilar arteries. Brain MRI shows acute brainstem infarction (A), occluded proximal basilar artery (B) and prominent posterior-communicating (PCOM) arteries (C). High-resistance flow in cervical segments of the vertebral arteries (D, E) is consistent with distal severe steno-occlusive disease. Transcranial Doppler (TCD) shows flow spectra obtained from the PCOM artery with transmitted tapping (thick arrow during the first cardiac cycle) of left carotid in neck (F). Reversed flow is observed in the entire basilar artery and the distal left vertebral artery (note that the expected normal flow in the vertebrobasilar system is away from the probe and represented on power-motion Doppler TCD as blue in color) with transmitted signals during the tapping of carotid arteries in the neck, performed to assess the parent source of blood supply to the vertebrobasilar system (G). The vertebrobasilar system was assessed through a transforaminal acoustic window.

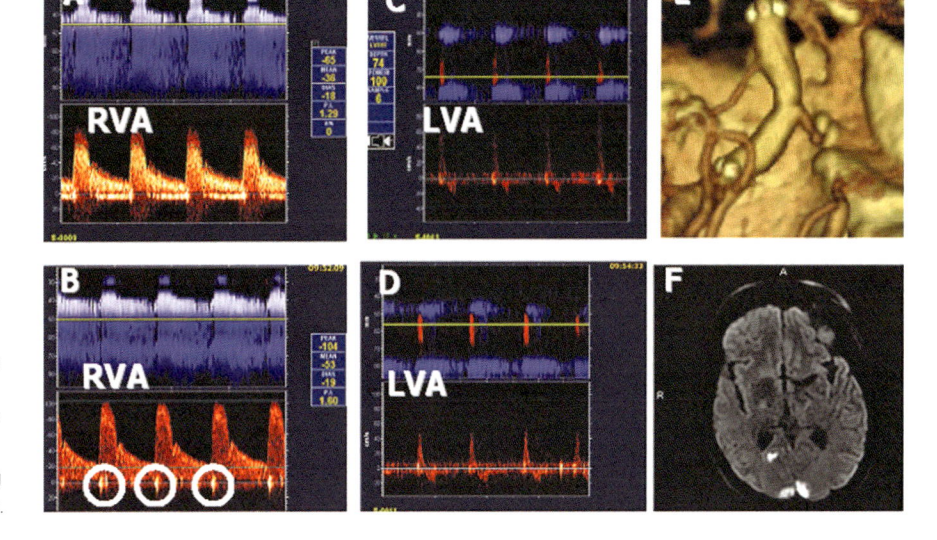

Figure 17.18 Acute terminal left VA occlusion (E; arrow) beyond the origin of the PICA with reversed reverberating flow from right to left VA (vertebral artery; C, D). Patent right vertebral artery with knock-type signals (B) that likely represent an artifact induced by reverberation of flow in the neighboring occluded vessel (left VA). DWI image showing acute infarctions in bilateral occipital lobes (F).

269

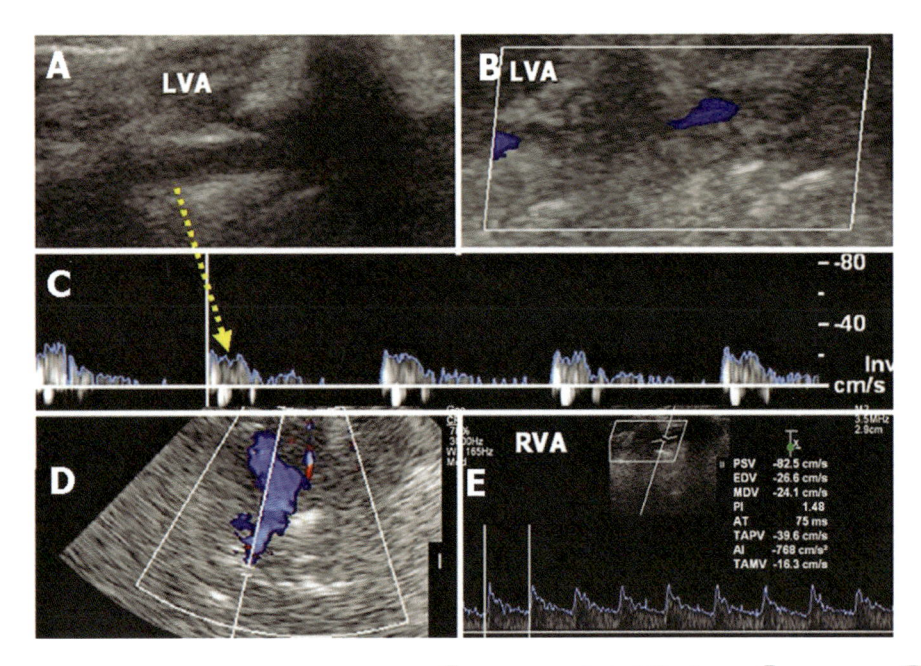

PART IV Ultrasound in Stroke Prevention and Treatment

Figure 17.19 Minimal flow signal in occluded left VA and reversal flow at the terminal portion of left VA (vertebral artery) in TCCD (transcranial color-coded duplex; D). Antegrade flow is shown in right VA(E).

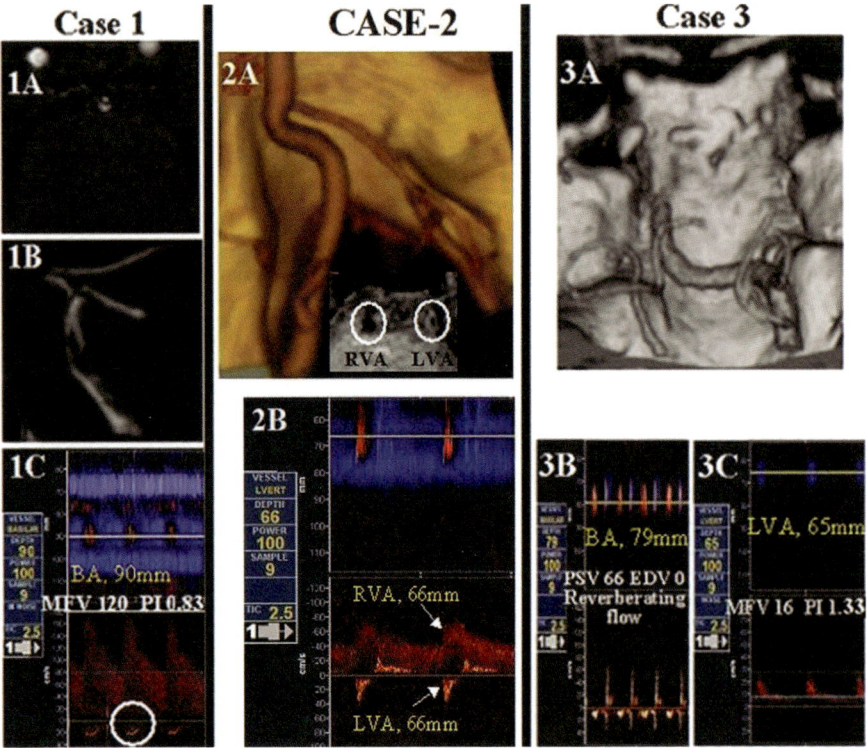

Figure 17.20 Case 1: PMD signatures in a patient with BA dissection depicted on brain MRI (A; axial T1 sequence showing intimal flap in the BA lumen, "double lumen sign") and MRA (B; dynamic contrast-enhanced sequence showing smooth tapering of the mid-BA portion, a characteristic feature of dissection resulting from poor contrast enhancement in the false lumen). Insonation of the mid-BA portion with PMD–TCD (90 mm) shows antegrade flow on PM display (depicted as a continuous blue band) with elevated MFV (120 cm s^{-1}) on spectral display corresponding to the true lumen as well as high-resistance retrograde flow on PMD display (depicted as intermittent narrow red bands) with systolic spikes (white circles) and absent diastolic flow in the spectral display corresponding to the false lumen. Case 2: alternating flow signals in the left VA in a patient with intracranial LVA dissection on CTA (1) and MRA (1, inset; fat-saturation axial T1 sequence depicting the intramural hematoma). PMD–TCD showed alternating flow signatures with high-resistance flow reversal during systole (narrow red bands on PMD display) in the left VA (C) and normal low-resistance antegrade flow in the right VA at a depth of 66 mm. No flow reversal augmentation was found during the hyperemia cuff test and the left subclavian artery stenosis was also excluded by neck CTA. Case 3: Reverberating PMD flow signatures with oscillating flow on spectral display (B) in a patient with a proximal BA occlusion on CTA (A). PMD and spectrogram showed high-resistance flows (PI = 1.3) in the left VA (C). PI indicates Gosling–King pulsatility index.

CHAPTER 17 Neurosonology Pearls

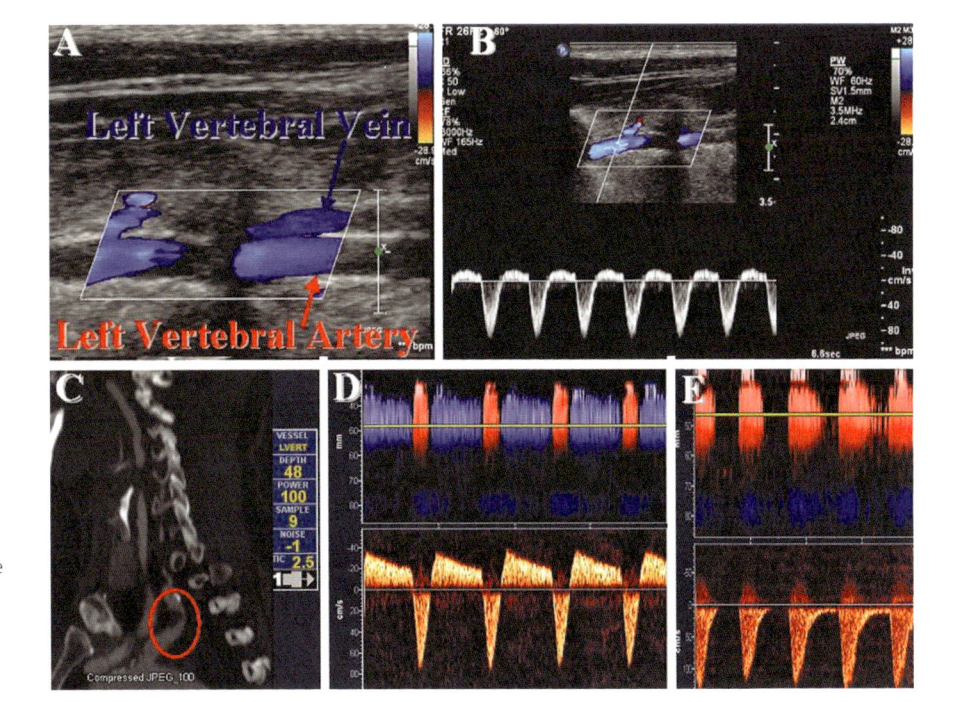

Figure 17.21 Examples of subclavian steal waveforms with alternating flow signals in extracranial and intracranial vessels. (B), (D) Waveforms at rest; (E) during hyperemia ischemia cuff-test with the third cardiac cycle from the left showing the appearance of reversed diastolic flow towards the arm; (C) shows the lesion in the subclavian artery causing the steal.

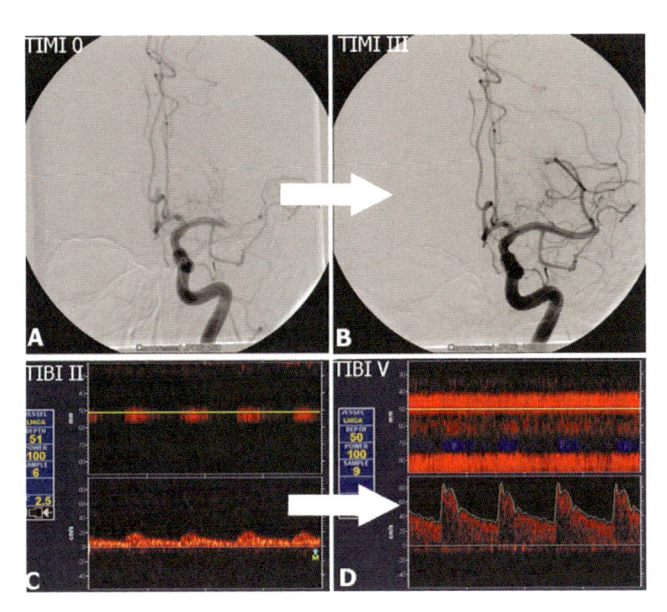

Figure 17.22 Corresponding TIBI and TIMI grades during complete recanalization (TIBI II ⇒ TIBI V and TIMI 0 ⇒ TIMI III).

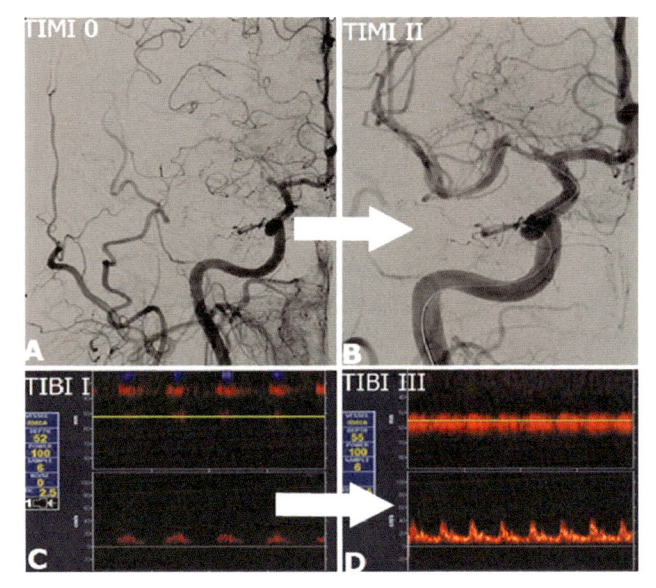

Figure 17.23 Corresponding TIBI and TIMI grades during partial recanalization (TIBI I ⇒ TIBI III and TIMI 0 ⇒ TIMI II).

271

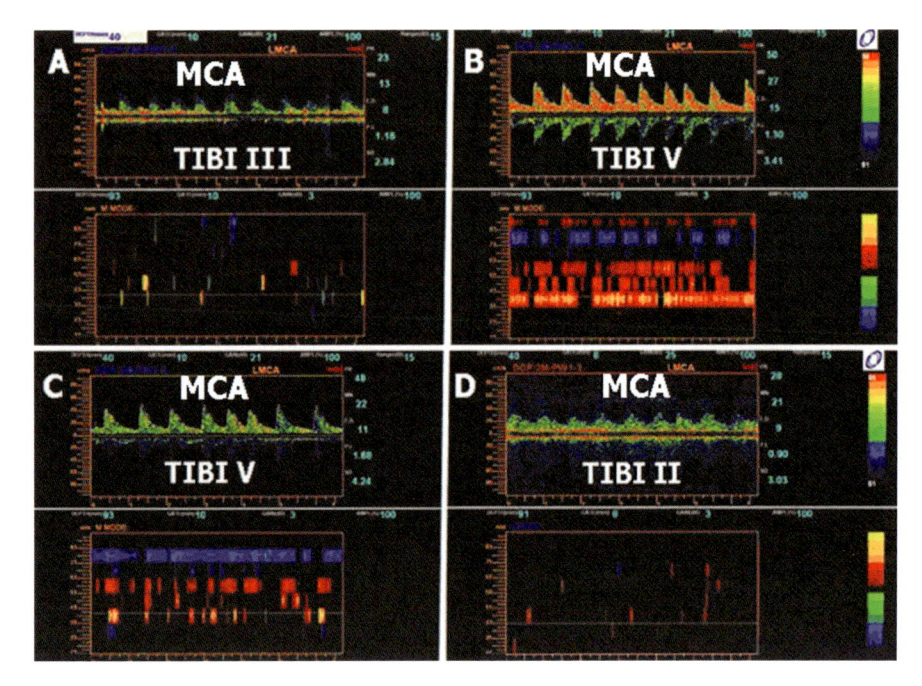

PART IV Ultrasound in Stroke Prevention and Treatment

Figure 17.24 Documentation of reocclusion on TCD followed tPA-induced recanalization. (A) Left M2 MCA (middle cerebral artery) occlusion (TIBI II) before the onset of intravenous thrombolysis (MFV = 13 cm s^{-1}, high-resistance flow on M-mode spectrum). (B) Complete recanalization was achieved 28 min after tPA bolus (TIBI V; MFV = 27 cm s^{-1}, low-resistance flow on M-mode spectrum). (C) Complete recanalization is sustained at 42 min following tPA bolus (TIBI V) but high-resistance flow signatures appear on M-mode spectrum, while spectral interrogation reveals an increase in pulsatility index [from 1.3 in (B) to 1.7]. (D) Re-occlusion occurred at 56 min following tPA bolus (TIBI II)

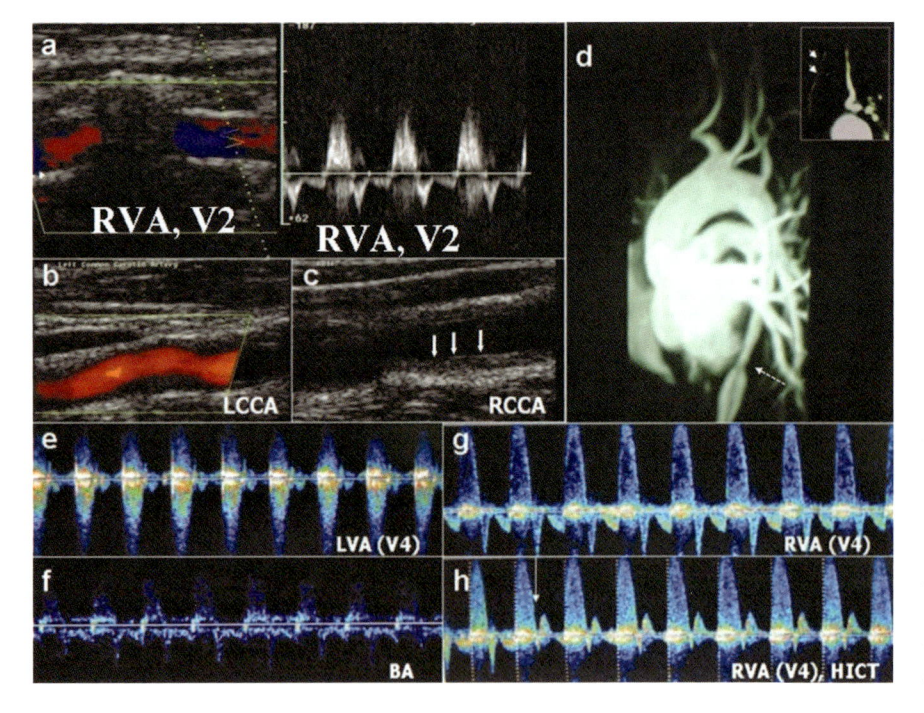

Figure 17.25 Carotid duplex and TCD findings in a patient with Takayashu Arteritis (A)–(C) (Carotid duplex): alternating-flow in transverse-segment of right-vertebral artery. Homogeneous, mildly hyper-echogenic eccentric wall thickening in left (B) and right (C) common carotid artery. (D) (Aortic arch MRA): right subclavian-artery occlusion and subdiaphragmatic descending aorta stenosis (dotted-arrow). Note the delayed retrograde filling of right vertebral artery following contrast injection (inset/arrowheads). (E)–(G) (Transcranial Doppler): antegrade flow in intracranial-segment of left vertebral artery and alternating flow in right intracranial vertebral (F) and basilar artery (G). H (Transcranial Doppler/hyperemia–ischemia cuff test): complete flow-reversal in right vertebral artery after cuff deflation (arrow).

CHAPTER 17 Neurosonology Pearls

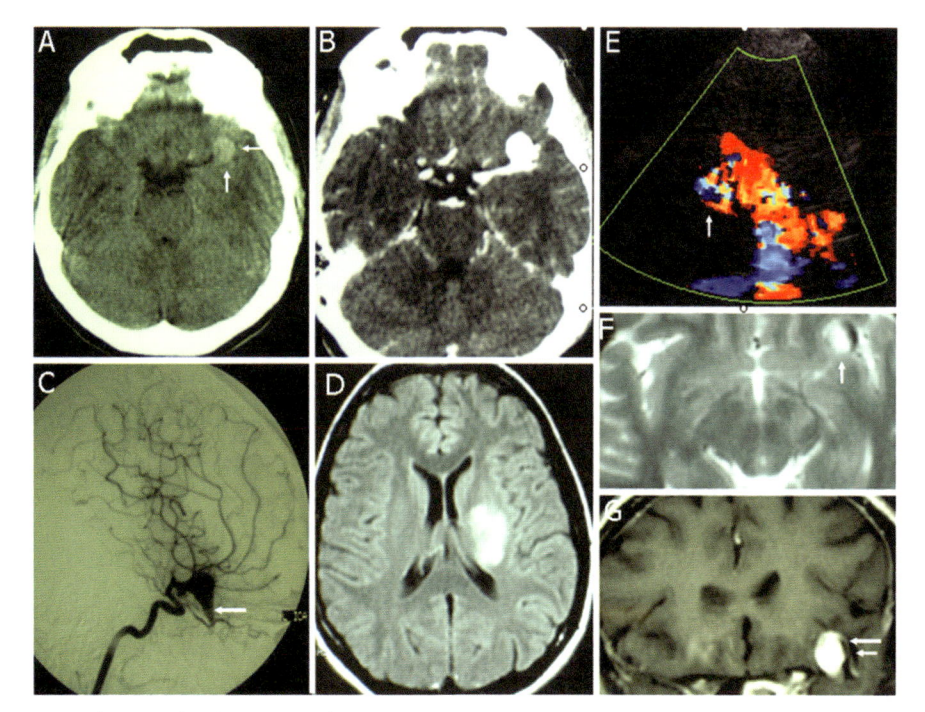

Figure 17.26 (A) Non-contrast brain CT showing segmental hyperattenuation of left middle cerebral artery (MCA; arrow). (B) Contrast brain CT showing an aneurysmal dilatation in proximal left MCA. (C) DSA (left anterior oblique projection) confirming a giant (maximum diameter 33 mm) dissecting LMCA aneurysm. Note multiple distal MCA branches originating from the dome of the aneurysm including external lenticulostriate arteries. (D) Brain MRI showing a hyperintense ischemic lesion affecting the left basal ganglia. (E) TCCD (left transtemporal insonation, axial midbrain plane) depicting an aneurysmal dilatation (arrow) in left distal M1MCA (depicted as red band; left anterior cerebral artery is depicted as blue band). Note the intrasacullar turbulent flow (alternating blue and red colors inside the aneurysm lumen). (F) Brain MRI (axial T2 sequence) showing a crescent-like hyperintense area inside the intrasacullar flow void of the aneurysm (suggestive of partial thrombosis). (G) Gadolinium-enhanced brain MRI (coronal T1 sequence) depicting the tail of the aneurysm (arrow).

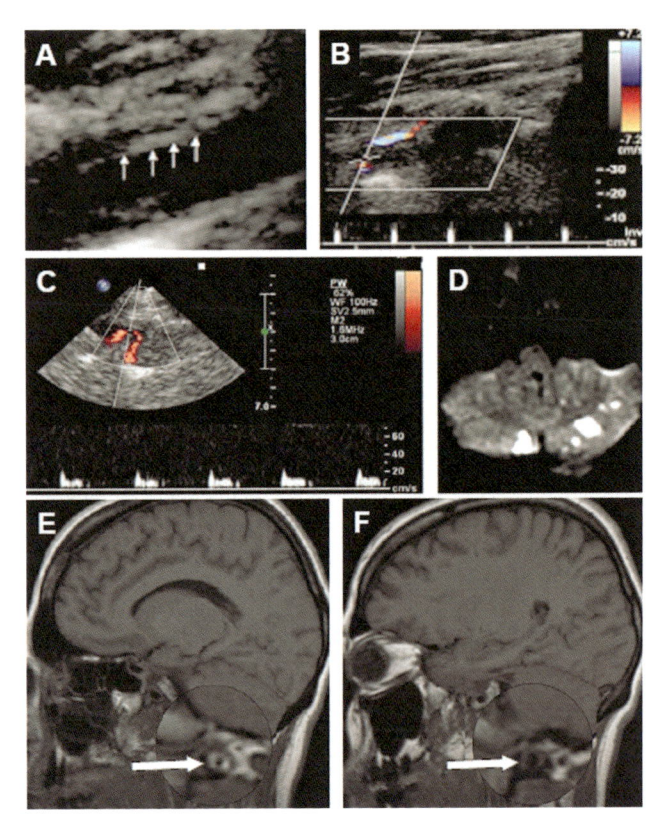

PART IV Ultrasound in Stroke Prevention and Treatment

Figure 17.27 Extracranial duplex B-mode image showing an intimal flap with vessel wall irregularities at the exit of the left VA from the C2 vertebra transverse foramen (transition zone from V2 to V3 segment of vertebral artery). Minimal systolic flow, with absent diastolic flow, is detected inside the true lumen of the artery (B). Insonation of the V3 segment with TCCD shows a high-resistance flow pattern, i.e. minimal flow during systole and absent diastolic flow (C). MRI revealed bilateral multiple acute cerebellar infarcts on diffusion-weighted series (D). T1 sagittal images demonstrate a "fried egg" appearance of the left VA at the C1–2 level, extending intracranially, consistent with dissection [arrows in (E), the affected artery, and (F), the normal artery for comparison].

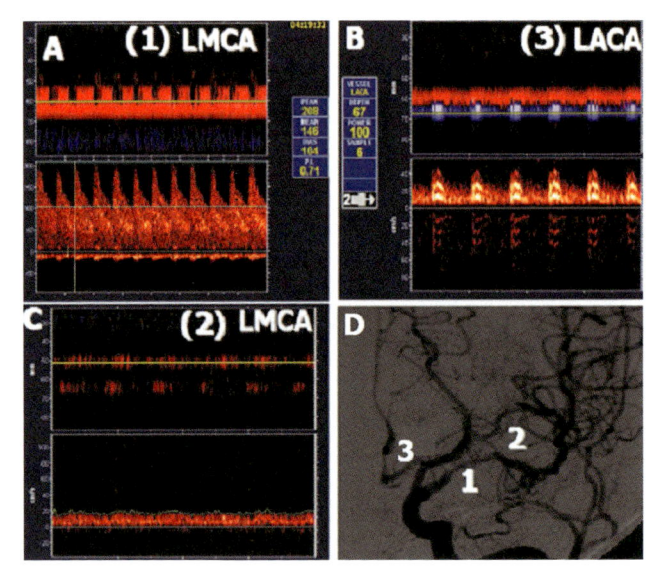

Figure 17.28 Proximal M1 MCA (middle cerebral artery) severe stenosis (D) with stenotic flow signals at proximal MCA (A) and harmonic bruit at the origin of A1 ACA (anterior cerebral artery) (B). Note the severely blunted flow in the distal M1 MCA (C)

Index

Page numbers in *italics* represent figures, those in **bold** represent tables.

Aaslid, Rune 14
ACE inhibitors 169
afterload 52
age, and cerebral blood flow 150
aliasing 7, 78–81, *79–81*, 97, 266
alpha-adrenoreceptors 53
American Society of Neuroimaging 13
aneurysms 30–1, 33, *33*, *38*, 207
   anterior communicating artery *34*
   atrial septal 188
   middle cerebral artery *273*
   posterior cerebral artery *43*
   superior cerebellar artery *33*
   see also subarachnoid hemorrhage
angiography 3
   carotid stenosis 92–4, *92*
   CT 228
   digital subtraction 228
   magnetic resonance 93, 228
angioplasty 209, 211
   balloon *210*, 211, 221
   hyperperfusion syndrome after 117
   patient selection 116
   vasospasm 211
angle-corrected Doppler velocimetry 98–9, *98*, *99*
angle of Louis 54
anterior cerebral artery (ACA) 33–5, *34*, *35*
   stenosis 109, 231, *232*
anterior choroidal artery *32*, 33
anterior circulation 27–30, *28–30*
anterior communicating artery (ACA) 13, 34, *36*
   aneurysm *34*
   collateral flow patterns 119–20
anterior inferior cerebellar arteries 39, *39*
antidiuretic hormone (ADH) 53
aortic arch 3, 26
   anomalies 26–7, *27*, *28*
aortic stenosis *262*
aortic valve insufficiency *263*
aphasia 74, 183, 194, 247
arterial bifurcations 71–2
arterial blood pressure (ABP) 53, 68, 151
   hemodynamic assessment 59–66
   mean arterial pressure 50, **55**
   raised *see* hypertension
arterial supply 26–44
   anterior circulation 27–30, *28–30*
   aortic arch 3, 26–7, *28*

great vessel origins 26–7, *28*
   posterior circulation 37–9, *37–9*
   see also individual arteries
arterial vasospasm *see* vasospasm
arterial wall pulsation 88, *89*
arteries
   anatomical variation 151
   bifurcation and blood flow *4*, *5*, *10*
   cerebral *see* anterior cerebral artery; middle cerebral artery; posterior cerebral artery
   compliance 88
   hyperdense 109, *110*, *128*, 231, *231*
   occlusion *see* occlusion, arterial
   perfusion 51
   stenosis 69–70, 79, 81–3, *81–3*, 151
   see also hemodynamics; and individual arteries
arteriovenous malformations (AVMs) 151
artifacts
   aliasing 7, 78–81, *79–81*, 97, 266
   mirror images 7, *8*, *21*, 26, 80, 152–3
   reflection 7, *9*
   shadowing 7, 94, 96, *96*, 97, 102, 167, 252
Asymptomatic Carotid Artery Surgery (ACAS) Trial 161–2
Asymptomatic Carotid Stenosis and Risk of Stroke (ACSRS) study 159
Asymptomatic Carotid Surgery Trial (ACST) 159
Asymptomatic Cervical Bruit Study 159
Atherosclerosis Risk in Communities (ARIC) study 160
atherosclerotic plaque *see* plaque
atrial contraction 50
atrial fibrillation 77
atrial natriuretic factor (ANF) 53
atrial septal aneurysm 188
auditory perception 181
automaticity 52, 53
autoregulation 47, 71
axial resolution 7

Bainbridge reflex **54**
balloon angioplasty *210*, 211, 221
baroreceptor reflex **54**
basilar artery 13
   dissection *270*
   occlusion 126, *128*, *268*
   reversed flow 120, *269*
   stenosis 111–12, *112*, 233, *233*

basilar-vertebral-subclavian steal syndrome *see* subclavian steal syndrome
Bayliss effect 71
Bernoulli equation 70
beta-adrenoreceptors 53
beta-blockers 169
B-flow imaging 9, *9*
bleeding artifact 8, *8*
blood flow *see* cerebral blood flow
blooming 266
blunted flow signal 77
B-mode imaging 7
   atherosclerotic plaque 164–8
   carotid stenosis 94–7, *94–7*
   color duplex 21, *22*
bovine aortic arch 26, *27*
brachiocephalic artery 26
brain death 203–4, *204*
brain retroperfusion *see* retrograde cerebral perfusion
breath-holding index (BHI) 71
brightness-mode imaging *see* B-mode imaging
bruits 79, *81*
   right-sided 265
   systolic flow gaps 265

calcified plaque 168
calcium channel blockers 169
   vasospasm 210–11
callosomarginal artery 35, *35*
capillary pressure 51
capnography 56
carbon dioxide, effects of 150–1
carbon monoxide, non-invasive monitoring 59
cardiac arrhythmias 76–7, *76*, *77*
cardiac cycle 48–51, *49*, *50*
cardiac index (CI) 51, **55**
cardiac output (CO) 51, **55**, 151
   blood flow velocities and 150–3, **150**
   neuroendocrine mediation 53–4, **54**
cardiac surgery monitoring 222–5
   retrograde cerebral perfusion 222–3
   ultrasound findings 223–5, *223*, *224*
Cardiovascular Health Study (CHS) 160
cardiovascular risk factors 165
   carotid plaque 160–1, *161*
   intimal-medial thickening 94

275

Index

carotid arteries
  common *see* common carotid artery
  dissection 105, 106
  external *see* external carotid artery
  internal *see* internal carotid artery
  loops 263
  occlusion 105–6, *105*, *106*
  plaque *see* carotid plaque
  stenosis *see* carotid stenosis
  tandem lesions 103–5, *103–5*
  see also carotid endarterectomy
carotid-basilar anastomosis 42
carotid bifurcation *4*, *5*
  transverse scanning *10*
carotid bulb 3, 89
carotid clamping 215–16
carotid Doppler 161–2
carotid endarterectomy (CEA) 91, **91**, 214–20
  diagnostic considerations 214
  findings with carotid clamping 215–16
  findings pre-clamp 214–15, *215*
  intraluminal thrombosis *104*
  NASCET trial *see* North American Symptomatic Carotid Endarterectomy Trial (NASCET)
  post-operative ultrasound 101–2, *102*
  shunt and cross-clamp removal 218–20, *219*, *220*
  shunt placement 216–18, *217*
carotid intima-media thickness 158, 165, 168–71, *169*
  clinical trials 169
  image analysis 170–1, *170*
  measurement 169–70, *170*
  measurement protocol 170
  prediction of vascular events 169
carotid plaque *161*
  area 160–1, *161*
  non-stenotic 160
  planimetry 92
  size/burden 160
Carotid Revascularization Endarterectomy versus Stent Trial (CREST) 163
carotid siphon 5, 24, 31
carotid space 27
carotid stenosis
  asymptomatic 158–9, 165
    risk factors 159
    stroke risk 159–62, **159**, *160*
  diagnosis 91–2, **91**, *92*
    angiography 92–4, *92*
    angle-corrected Doppler velocimetry 98–9, *98*, *99*
    bilateral, grading of 102–3
    color Doppler imaging 97, *97*
    Society of Radiologists in Ultrasound criteria **98**, *99*
    ultrasound 94–7, *94–7*, 99–100
  multi-center clinical trials 163–4
  screening for 158–9
  ultrasound detection 162–4, *163*, **163**
carotid stents 101–2, *102*, 220–2, *222*
carotid ultrasound 158–76
  asymptomatic disease 158–9
  carotid stenosis 162–4, *163*, **163**

epidemiological studies 164
  quality assurance 164
carotid/vertebral duplex 241–2
central venous pressure (CVP) 51, **55**
  measurement 56–7, *56–7*
cerebral arteries *see* anterior cerebral artery; middle cerebral artery; posterior cerebral artery
cerebral autoregulation 200
cerebral blood flow (CBF) 47–8, 59, 68
  cardiac determinants of 51–3, *52*
  collateralization 78
  turbulent 48, *81*
  vasomotor reactivity 71
  vasospasm 209–10, **209**, *210*
  see also hemodynamics
cerebral embolization 120–2, *121*, *122*
cerebral hemodynamics 68–84
cerebral ischemia
  anterior circulation 241–2
  posterior circulation 242
cerebral oxygenation *see* oxygenation
cerebral perfusion, retrograde 222–3
cerebral perfusion pressure (CPP) 59, 68
  neurocritical care 198–9
cerebral salt-wasting syndrome 208
cerebral vasospasm *see* vasospasm
cerebrovascular anatomy
  arterial system *3*, *4*, *5*, *6*, *29*
  circle of Willis *see* circle of Willis
  see also individual vessels
cerebrovascular resistance 69
cervical aortic arch 27, *28*
cervical carotid arteries *28*
chemoreceptors **54**
children
  sickle cell disease 147–57
  transcranial Doppler 148–50, *149*
choroid plexus *21*, *33*, *38*, *39*, *40*
circle of Willis 5, 13, *14*, *33*, 41, *41*
  in children 149
circulatory arrest 83–4, *83*, 123–5, *124*
clinical outcome prediction 200–1
  intracerebral hemorrhage 201
  traumatic brain injury 200–1
CLOTBUST trial 246
cognitive tasks 178–9, *178*, *179*, **182**
collateral flow 118–19, *118*
  anterior communicating artery 119–20
  distribution of 71–2
  posterior communicating artery 120
color bar, zero baseline (PRF) 11, *12*
color box 8, *10*, *12*, *21*, *23*
color desaturation *12*
color Doppler flow imaging *see* color-flow Doppler imaging
color-flow Doppler imaging (CDFI)
  carotid stenosis 97, *97*
  flow dynamics 10
  image 8, *8*, 21–2, *22*
  optimization of 11–12
color gain 8, 12, 22, 258
color velocity imaging 8
color velocity scale 22

common carotid artery (CCA) 26, *27*
  anatomy 3, *4*
  normal flow 88–9, *89*
  pseudoaneurysm *264*
  transverse scanning *10*
Common Carotid (C) method, carotid stenosis measurement 93
compliance flow 88
compound imaging 9, *9*
computed tomography (CT)
  angiography 228
  cranial 201
  single-photon emission *see* SPECT
  stroke 252
  xenon 210
continuity principle 70
continuous-wave (CW) Doppler imaging 5, 7–9, *7*
  B-flow and compound imaging 9, *9*
  B-mode image *7*
  color-flow Doppler image 8, *8*
  color velocity image *8*
  Doppler velocity spectral display *9*
  harmonic imaging *9*
  power Doppler image 8, *8*
contractility 52
contrast agents 252
  gaseous microspheres *see* gaseous microspheres
corpus callosum *33*, *34*, *34*, *35*
CREST trial, percutaneous carotid stenting 163–4
critical closing pressure 69
CT *see* computed tomography

decompression sickness, and patent foramen ovale 189–90
delayed ischemic neurological deficits (DIND) 207
  clinical and diagnostic features 208–9, *209*
diabetes 159
diagnostic criteria 87–143
  arterial occlusion, recanalization and re-occlusion 125–30
  arterial vasospasm and hyperemia 114–20
  carotid artery occlusion/dissection 105–14
  carotid stenosis 91–2, **91**, *92*
    angiography 92–4, *92*
    angle-corrected Doppler velocimetry 98–9, *98*, *99*
    bilateral, grading of 102–3
    color Doppler imaging 97, *97*
    Society of Radiologists in Ultrasound criteria **98**, *99*
    ultrasound 94–7, *94–7*, 99–101, *101*
  carotid stents 101–2, *102*
  cerebral circulatory arrest 123–5, *124*
  cerebral embolization and right to left shunts 120–2, *121*, *122*
  increased intracranial pressure 122–3, *123*
  normal findings 87–91
    arterial wall pulsation 88, *89*
    common carotid artery 88–9, *89*
    external carotid artery 89–90
    internal carotid artery 88, *89*
    intracranial flow 90–1, **91**

276

laminar flow 87–8, *88*
vertebral arteries 90, *90*
post-carotid endarterectomy 101–2, *102*
reversed Robin Hood syndrome 131–3, *132, 133*
subclavian steal syndrome 130–1, *130, 131*
tandem carotid lesions 103–5, *103–5*
see also specific arteries/conditions
diffuse intracranial disease 234–7, *235–7*
diffusion coefficient 254, **254**
digital subtraction angiography (DSA) 228
distensibility, vascular 50
Doppler shift 9
Doppler ultrasound
cardiac surgery monitoring 223–5, *223, 224*
carotid endarterectomy 101–2, *102*
carotid stenosis 94–7, *94–7*, 99–100
extracranial duplex *see* extracranial duplex ultrasound
spectral analysis
flow dynamics 10–11, *11*
transcranial color Doppler imaging 21–2, *21, 22*
transcranial *see* transcranial Doppler
velocity spectral display 9
see also specific techniques
double aortic arch 26
double lumen sign *270*
duplex imaging *see* color duplex imaging
duplex ultrasound, extracranial *see* extracranial duplex ultrasound

echodense plaque 166–7, *166, 167*, 168
echolucent plaque 168
embolization 120–2, *121, 122*
end-expiration measurement 56, *56, 60*
ensemble length 12
European Carotid Surgery Trial (ECST) 93
European (E) method, measurement of carotid stenosis 93
examination technique *see specific techniques*
executive functions 181–2
external carotid artery (ECA)
anatomy 5, *6*, 29
normal flow 89–90
transverse scanning *10*
extracranial duplex ultrasound 9–10, *10*
longitudinal plane 9
transverse plane 9
extracranial ultrasound examination 3–12
extrasystole 76

fast Fourier transform 121
fast-track insonation 240
fever 151
Fisher classification 96
flashing artifact 8
flow dynamics
color flow ultrasound evaluation 10
Doppler spectral evaluation 10–11, *11*
flow resistance 68–9, *69*
focal intracranial disease 228–34, *229*
anterior cerebral artery 231, *232*
basilar artery 233, *233*

middle cerebral artery stenosis 229–31, *230, 231*
posterior cerebral artery 232–3
terminal internal carotid artery and siphon 231–2, *232*
terminal vertebral artery 233–4, *234*
frame rate 12, 21
Framingham Study 158, 161, **164**, 165
Frank-Starling law 52, *52*
functional transcranial Doppler 177–86
applications 181–3, **182**
auditory perception 181
executive functions 181–2
language and motor activation 181
neurological disorders 182–3
vision and visual perception 181
cognitive tasks 178–9, *178, 179*, **182**
devices, hardware and software 178
limitations 180–1
physiological background 177–8
undershooting reaction 179, *179*
validation studies 179–80, **180**

gaseous microspheres 252–61
artifacts and contrast microbubbles 258–9, *258, 259*
in circulation 253–4, **253**
diffusion coefficient 254, **254**
Ostwald coefficient 254, **254**
resonance frequency **254**
resonance of 254–8, **254**, *255, 256, 258*
in stroke treatment 246, 248–9, *248*
ultrasound scattering 252–3, **253**
Glasgow Coma Scale 207
glitazones 169
global vascular risk assessment 165
Gosling-King pulsatility index 74, 199, 234
gray-scale imaging *see* B-mode imaging
gray-scale median index 167–8, *167*

Hagen-Poiseuille law 68
harmonic imaging 9
head injury *see* traumatic brain injury
hematocrit 150
hemodynamics 47–67
arterial perfusion and venous return 51
autoregulation 47
bedside assessment 54–9
blood flow 47–8
blood flow velocity 150–3, **150**
anatomic variables 151
angle of insonation 152
Doppler signal 152
instrument settings 152–3
physiologic factors 150–1, **151**
technique and equipment variables 151–2
visual display 152
waveform follower 152
cardiac cycle 48–51, *49, 50*
case studies 62–4
systemic vs intracranial 59–66
turbulent flow 48, *81*
vasomotor reactivity 71
venous return 51

waveforms *see* waveforms
see also cardiac cycle; cardiac output; and specific parameters
hemodynamic steal phenomenon 131
hemoglobin SS *see* sickle cell disease
hemorrhagic transformation 202
hepatojugular reflex 54–5
hollow-skull phenomenon *204*
holoprosencephaly 34
Huebner's recurrent artery 34, *34*
Hunt-Hess grading system 207, **208**
hypercapnia 20, **54**, 71, 131, 177, 243
hyperdense artery sign 109, *110, 128*, 231, *231*
hyperechoic plaque 166–7, *166, 167*, 168
hyperemia 114–15, *115, 116*
hyperemic reperfusion 117, *118*
hyperperfusion syndrome 117
hypertension 20, 159
and blood flow 50–1, 74
and carotid artery disease 159, *160*
diagnosis 199
and left ventricular afterload 52
hypoechoic plaque 168
hypoglycemia, and blood flow velocity 151
hypoxia, and blood flow velocity 151

Imaging in Carotid Angioplasty and Risk of Stroke (ICAROS) study 168
innominate artery 3
inotropic agents 52, 53
internal carotid artery (ICA) 13, 30–1, *30, 31*
anatomy 3–5, *4, 5*
intracranial branches 31–3, *32, 33*
loop in *264*
normal flow *88*, 89
occlusion *128, 129, 266*
terminal 110–11
stenosis 231–2, *232*
thrombosis *266, 267*
transverse scanning *10*
internal carotid siphon 110–11
retrograde filling *266*
stenosis 231–2, *232*
internal jugular vein, thrombosis *265*
intimal-medial thickness (IMT) 94
intra-aortic balloon pump waveform (IABPW) 66, *66*
intracerebral hemorrhage, outcome prediction 201
intracranial flow, normal 90–1, **91**
intracranial parenchymal assessment 201–2
intracranial pressure (ICP) 68
increased, diagnosis 122–3, *123*
management *61*
neurocritical care 199, *199*
waveform 60, *60*
intracranial steal *245*
intracranial stenosis *108*, 228–9
diffuse intracranial disease 234–7, *235–7*
focal intracranial disease 228–34, *229*
anterior cerebral artery 231, *232*
basilar artery 233, *233*
middle cerebral artery stenosis 229–31, *230, 231*

277

Index

intracranial stenosis (*Cont.*)
    posterior cerebral artery 232–3
        terminal internal carotid artery and siphon 231–2, *232*
        terminal vertebral artery 233–4, *234*
intracranial ultrasound 13–25
    see also transcranial color duplex imaging; transcranial Doppler
intra-operative monitoring 214–27
    cardiac surgery 222–5
    carotid artery stenosis 220–2
    carotid endarterectomy 214–20
invasive procedures, localization during 202–3, *203*
ischemic penumbra 12
isovolumetric contraction 49
isovolumetric relaxation 50

jugular venous oxygen saturation ($S_{jv}O_2$) 60
jugular venous pressure (JVP) 54

Kuopio heart study 169
Kussmaul's sign 54

lacunar-type syndrome 240
laminar flow 48, 87–8, *88*
language 181
Laplace pressure 254
Laplace's law 48, *49*
length-tension relationship 52
lenticulostriate arteries 36
Lindegaard ratio 81
Louis, angle of 54

magnetic resonance angiography (MRA) 93, 228
Marey's law of the heart **54**
mass effect after stroke 202, *202*
mean arterial pressure (MAP) 50, **55**
meningohypophyseal artery 32
metabolic coupling 177
metabolic syndrome 159
middle cerebral artery (MCA) 5, 35–7, *36*, *37*
    aneurysm *273*
    occlusion *128*, *129*, *267*
    reocclusion *272*
    segmental hyperattenuation *273*
    stenosis 108–9, *109*, 229–31, *230*, *231*, *266*, *274*
        sub-total 109, *110*
    trifurcation 36
    vasospasm *209*
    see also vasospasm
middle communicating artery 13
migraine, and patent foramen ovale 188–9, **188**
mirror artifacts 7, *8*, *21*, *26*, 80, 152–3
M-mode imaging *see* power mode Doppler
Moehring, Mark 19
Monro-Kellie hypothesis 59
motor activation 181
moya-moya phenomenon 147

neurocritical care 198–206
    brain death 203–4, *204*
    cerebral autoregulation 200
    cerebral perfusion pressure 198–9
    clinical outcome prediction 200–1
        intracerebral hemorrhage 201
        traumatic brain injury 200–1
    duplex ultrasound imaging 201
    hemorrhagic transformation 202
    intracranial parenchymal assessment 201–2
    intracranial pressure 199, *199*
    localization during procedures 202–3, *203*
    mass effect after stroke 202, *202*
    pulsatility index 199–200, *200*
    vasospasm assessment 198
neurological disorders 182–3
neurovascular coupling 177
nimodipine 114
nitric oxide (NO) 54, 177
nitrogen 253
North American (N) method, measurement of carotid stenosis 92
North American Symptomatic Carotid Endarterectomy Trial (NASCET) 161–2
Northern Manhattan Study (NOMAS) 160
Nyquist limit 79

occlusion, arterial 125–30
    basilar artery 126, *128*, *268*
    carotid arteries 105–6, *105*, *106*
    middle cerebral artery *128*, *129*, *267*
    signal pattern 79, 81–3, *81–3*
    vertebral artery 130, *132*, *269*, *270*
    see also reocclusion; and specific vessels
Ohm's law 48, 58
oligemia 60, *61*
oncotic pressure 51
ophthalmic artery 5, 13, *30*, 32, 241
    reversed 119, *119*
optic nerve 17, 22, 24, 31, 32, 33
optimization of Doppler signal 11–12, 78–81, *79–81*
orbitofrontal artery 35
Ostwald coefficient 254, **254**
oxygenation 47, 58–9, 60
    calculations 60, **61**
    fall in 71
    hyperbaric 253

papaverine 211
patent foramen ovale 187–97
    closure devices 188
    and decompression sickness 189–90
    detection methods 190–1, **190**, **191**
    and ischemic stroke 287–8, **288**
    and migraine 188–9, **188**
    prevalence 187, *188*
    see also right-to-left shunts
peak systolic velocity 98
pencil probe 5
percussion wave 59
perfluorochemicals 253
pericallosal arteries 34, *34*, 35
phantom image 7
phlebostatic axis 55–6
pial to pial anastomotic flow 41, *42*

plaque
    calcifications *96*
    calcified 168
    carotid *see* carotid plaque
    characterization 165–6, *166*
    composition 94, *95*, **95**
    echogenicity/echodensity 166–7, *166*, *167*
    echolucent (hypoechoic) 168
    formation 91–2
    gray-scale imaging 164–8
    gray-scale median index 167–8, *167*
    homogeneous 94, *95*
    length 94
    location 94
    pathological changes 96
    surface 95, *96*, **96**, *97*
    see also stenosis
plasma colloid pressure 51
Poiseuille's law 48, 70
positive inotropic agents 52
posterior cerebral artery (PCA) 39–41, *40*, *41*
    aneurysm *43*
    stenosis 111, *111*, 232–3
posterior circulation 37–9, *37–9*
    branches 37–9, *38*, *39*
posterior communicating artery (PComA) 13, 32–3, *33*
    collateral flow 120
posterior inferior cerebellar arteries 38, *38*
power mode Doppler (PMD) 19–21, *21*
    image 8, *8*
    patent foramen ovale 190–1, *191*
preload 52, *52*
pressure 47
pressure gradient 68
primitive anastomoses 41–3, *43*
pseudoaneurysm *264*
pulmonary artery end-diastolic pressure (PAEDP) 57–8, *58*
pulmonary artery pressure (PAP) **55**
pulmonary artery wedge pressure (PAWP) **55**, 57, *58*
pulmonary vascular resistance (PVR) **55**
pulsatility index 74–6, *74–6*, 91
    neurocritical care 199–200, *200*
pulse pressure 50–1
pulse repetition frequency (PRF) 79

rapid ventricular ejection 49, 59
Rayleigh-Plesset equation 254
recanalization, arterial 125–30
reflection artifacts 7, *9*
reocclusion 245
    middle cerebral artery *272*
resistance, blood flow 47, 48
resistance flow 88
resistance index 91
restenosis criteria 102
retrograde cerebral perfusion (RCP) 222–3
reverberation 7, 83, *269*
reversed Robin Hood syndrome 242–4, *244*
Reynolds number 70
right aortic arch 26

Index

right-to-left shunts 120–2, *121, 122*
    grading/quantitation 191–2, **192**
    patent foramen ovale *see* patent foramen ovale
    TCD detection 191
        clinical applications 192–3, *193,* 194
Robin Hood syndrome, reversed 131–3, *132, 133*

salt-wasting syndrome 208
shadowing artifacts 7, 94, 96, *96,* 97, 102, 167, 252
shunt placement 216–18, *217*
sickle cell disease 147–57
    arterial lesions *148*
    moya-moya phenomenon 147
    STOP TCD protocol 148
    stroke risk 147, 154–5
signal optimization 78–81, *79–81*
single-photon emission computed tomography *see* SPECT
Society of Radiologists in Ultrasound, criteria for carotid stenosis measurements **98**, 99
sonolysis 246, 248–9, *248*
Soustiel's ratio 115, *116*
SPECT 177, 210
spectral analysis 22
    flow dynamics 10–11, *11*
spectral broadening 87, *89*
Spencer, Merrill 5
Spencer's curve *98,* 114, *236*
Spencer's logarithmic scale 191
square-wave test *56*
Starling equilibrium 51
statins 169
steal phenomenon *see* subclavian steal
stenosis, arterial 151
    carotid 91–2, **91**, *92*
    flow velocity 70–1
    pressure-flow relationship 69–70
    signal pattern 79, 81–3, *81–3*
    see also individual arteries
stents, carotid 101–2, *102,* 220–2, *222*
Strandness, Eugene 5
stroke 240–51
    ischemic penumbra 12
    lesions amenable to intervention 240–2, *241, 243*
    mass effect after 202, *202*
    reversed Robin Hood syndrome 242–4, *244*
    risk factors
        carotid stenosis 159–62
        echodense (hyperechoic) plaque 168
        echolucent (hypoechoic) plaque 168
        patent foramen ovale 287–8, **288**
        sickle cell disease 147–57
    treatment
        gaseous microspheres and sonolysis 246, 248–9, *248*
        thrombolytic therapy 245–6, *246*
        ultrasound-enhanced thrombolysis 246, *247*
    see also subarachnoid hemorrhage
Stroke Outcomes and Neuroimaging of Intracranial Atherosclerosis (SONIA) trial 112, 113

Stroke Prevention in Sickle Cell Disease (STOP) trial 147–57
    questions on 156
    reading of 153–4, *154, 155*
    scanning protocol 153
stroke volume 51, **55**
subarachnoid hemorrhage
    delayed ischemic neurological deficits 207
        clinical and diagnostic features 208–9, *209*
    Fisher grading **208**
    Hunt-Hess grading 207, **208**
    vasospasm after 114–15, *115,* 117, 207–13
        biologic and physiological aspects 207, *208,* **208**
        clinical and diagnostic features 208–9, *209*
        TCD and cerebral blood flow studies 209–10, *209, 210*
        treatment 210–11
    see also aneurysms
subclavian arteries 26, *27*
subclavian steal *37,* 130–1, *130, 131,* 271
sulfur hexafluoride 253
superficial temporal artery 27, *29*
superior cerebellar artery 39
    aneurysm *33*
systemic immune response syndrome 58
systemic vascular resistance (SVR) 50, **55**, 58
systolic flow acceleration 77–8, *77, 78*
systolic flow gaps *265*

Takayasu's arteritis *272*
TAMM velocity 147, 150
    factors affecting 150–3, **151**, **152**
    measurements 153–4, *154*
TCD *see* transcranial Doppler
TCDI *see* transcranial color duplex imaging
thoracic electrical bioimpedance 6
thrombolysis 235–6, *246*
    ultrasound-enhanced 246, *247*
Thrombolysis in Brain Infarction (TIBI) flow grading system 125, *126, 127,* 241, 242, 271
Thrombolysis in Myocardial Infarction (TIMI) flow grading system 125, *126, 127,* 271
thrombosis detection 79, 81–3, *81–3*
thyroid mass *264*
tidal wave 59, *60*
time-averaged mean of maximum velocity *see* TAMM velocity
time-gain compensation (TGC) 9
Tower of Hanoi puzzle 179
transcranial color duplex imaging (TCDI) 21–5, *21, 22*
    advantages 24
    anatomical variations 151
    B-mode imaging 21, *22*
    color Doppler imaging 21–2, *22*
    Doppler spectral analysis 22
    examination technique 22–3
    foramenal window 23–4
    limitations 24–5
    neurocritical care 201
    orbital window 24
    submandibular window 24
    transtemporal window 22–3

transcranial Doppler (TCD) 13–25
    acoustic windows *14*
    cerebral ischemia 241, 242
    children 148–50, *149*
    examination technique 13–14, *14*
    M-mode technique 19–21, *21*
    power-motion mode 19–21, *21*
    procedure 14–19, *14–18*
    protocols
        fast-track 240
        instrument settings 152–3
    proximal intracranial segments 15
    sickle cell disease 147–57
    submandibular insonation 18, *18*
    transforaminal insonation 15–18, *17, 18*
    transorbital insonation 15, *17*
    transtemporal insonation 15, *16*
    waveform follower 152
    see also individual applications
transesophageal echocardiography, with contrast injection 190
transient ischemic attacks *160*
transthoracic echocardiography 190
traumatic brain injury
    outcome prediction 200–1
    vasospasm 209–10, *209, 210*
Treppe phenomenon 52
triple-H therapy 81, 114
    vasospasm 210–11
TUCSON study 248
turbulent blood flow 48, *81*

ultrasound *see* Doppler ultrasound

vagus nerve 53
vascular distensibility 50
vasoconstriction 53
vasodilation 53
vasomotor reactivity (VMR) 71
    see also vasospasm
vasospasm 114–15, *115*
    arterial 114–15, *115*
    assessment of 198
    distal 114
    grading of 115–20, *116*
    post-traumatic 209
    proximal 114
    subarachnoid hemorrhage 114–15, *115,* 117, 207–13
        biologic and physiological aspects 207, *208,* **208**
        clinical and diagnostic features 208–9, *209*
        TCD and cerebral blood flow studies 209–10, *209, 210*
        treatment 210–11
venous oxygen saturation **55**, 58
venous pressure 68
venous return 51
ventricular diastole 50
ventricular systole 49
vertebral artery 13, *37,* 37
    anatomy 5, *6*
    intimal flap *274*
    normal flow 90, *90*

Index

vertebral artery (*Cont.*)
  occlusion 130, *132, 269, 270*
  reversed flow *270*
  stenosis 106–8, *107*
  terminal, stenosis 112–13, *113*, 233–4, *234*
vertebrobasilar arterial system 37
viscosity 48
visual perception 181
von Reutern, Michael 5

Wada test 179–80
Warfarin Aspirin Stroke in Intracranial Disease (WASID) trial 108, 229, *229*, 235

waveform follower 152
waveform recognition
  atrial fibrillation *77*
  blunted flow signal 77
  branch occlusion *82*
  cardiac arrhythmias 76–7, *76, 77*
  cardiac cycle 48–51, *49, 50*
  extrasystole 76
  increased flow pulsatility 74–6, *74–6*
  normal findings 73–4, *73, 74*
  percussion wave 59
  pulsatility 74–6, *74–6, 91*
  reading of 72–3, *73*

  signal optimization 78–81, *79–81*
  'stump' 105
  systolic flow acceleration 77–8, *77, 78*
  visual display 152
Willis, Thomas 13
Windkessel effect 50
Wisconsin Card Sorting Tesst 179, 181

xenon CT 210

zero baseline 11, 12

CPSIA information can be obtained
at www.ICGtesting.com
Printed in the USA
BVIC01n0515060117
472721BV00002B/5